Cartilage Tympanoplasty

Mirko Tos, MD D. Sc.

Professor Emeritus
ENT Dep. Gentofte Hospital
University of Copenhagen; Denmark
Professor of Otorhinolaryngology at the
University of Maribor; Slovenia

1155 illustrations

Thieme
Stuttgart · New York

Library of Congress Cataloging-in-Publication Data
Tos, Mirko.
　Cartilage tympanoplasty / Mirko Tos.
　　p. ; cm.
　Includes bibliographical references.
　ISBN 978-3-13-145091-3 (alk. paper)
　1. Tympanoplasty. 2. Articular cartilage I. Title.
　[DNLM: 1. Tympanoplasty–methods. 2. Ear Cartilage–surgery.
WV 225 T713c 2009]
　RF126.T67 2009
　617.8′059–dc22
　　　　　　　　　　　　　　2009012403

Illustrator: Regitze Steinbruch, Denmark

Important note: Medicine is an ever-changing science undergoing continual development. Research and clinical experience are continually expanding our knowledge, in particular our knowledge of proper treatment and drug therapy. Insofar as this book mentions any dosage or application, readers may rest assured that the authors, editors, and publishers have made every effort to ensure that such references are in accordance with **the state of knowledge at the time of production of the book.**

Nevertheless, this does not involve, imply, or express any guarantee or responsibility on the part of the publishers in respect to any dosage instructions and forms of applications stated in the book. **Every user is requested to examine carefully** the manufacturers' leaflets accompanying each drug and to check, if necessary in consultation with a physician or specialist, whether the dosage schedules mentioned therein or the contraindications stated by the manufacturers differ from the statements made in the present book. Such examination is particularly important with drugs that are either rarely used or have been newly released on the market. Every dosage schedule or every form of application used is entirely at the user's own risk and responsibility. The authors and publishers request every user to report to the publishers any discrepancies or inaccuracies noticed. If errors in this work are found after publication, errata will be posted at www.thieme.com on the product description page.

© 2009 Georg Thieme Verlag,
Rüdigerstrasse 14, 70469 Stuttgart, Germany
http://www.thieme.de
Thieme New York, 333 Seventh Avenue,
New York, NY 10001, USA
http://www.thieme.com
Cover design: Thieme Publishing Group
Typesetting by Primustype Hurler, Notzingen, Germany
Printed in India by Replika Press PVT LTD.
ISBN　　978-3-13-145091-3　　　　　　1 2 3 4 5 6

Some of the product names, patents, and registered designs referred to in this book are in fact registered trademarks or proprietary names even though specific reference to this fact is not always made in the text. Therefore, the appearance of a name without designation as proprietary is not to be construed as a representation by the publisher that it is in the public domain.

This book, including all parts thereof, is legally protected by copyright. Any use, exploitation, or commercialization outside the narrow limits set by copyright legislation, without the publisher's consent, is illegal and liable to prosecution. This applies in particular to photostat reproduction, copying, mimeographing, preparation of microfilms, and electronic data processing and storage.

Preface

The first and main goal of this book is to teach otologists who are in training cartilage tympanoplasty methods, using step-by-step demonstration of the surgery.

This is the first book on cartilage tympanoplasty and represents the very first collection of all known cartilage tympanoplasty methods. I hope, therefore, that experienced otosurgeons may also profit from this book.

In recent years cartilage tympanoplasties have been used more and more often in otosurgical practice and several new methods have been published, allowing me in this book to classify 23 original cartilage tympanoplasty methods. In the individual chapters each method is thoroughly defined, illustrated, and described, which is the second goal of this book.

The third goal is to analyze the anatomical and functional results of surgery, to illustrate functional differences between the various methods, and to promote clinical and basic research in cartilage tympanoplasty.

I have used cartilage for reconstruction of the ear canal wall and obliteration of the attic, antrum, and mastoid cavity since the early 1960s. Inspired by Heermann, who also was a frequent teacher on the Bochum tympanoplasty courses, I started sporadically with cartilage palisades in the 1990s. In Volume 1 of the Manual of Middle Ear Surgery (1993) I included a chapter on cartilage tympanoplasty, with illustration of the annular graft method, posterior cartilage–perichondrium composite island graft method, micro sliced cartilage methods, and the cartilage palisade techniques of Heermann. In Volume 2 (1995) the methods of reconstruction of the ear canal wall with cartilage and the methods of obliteration of the mastoid cavity were described and illustrated. During 1995–2000 I reconstructed the eardrum in half of the children with cholesteatoma at the Gentofte Hospital with cartilage palisades and in the other half with fascia. Three years and again ten years after surgery, the anatomical and functional results were significantly better in the palisade group than in the fascia group. These results convinced me that cartilage tympanoplasty is a good method, especially for difficult cases. From 1995 to my retirement from the Gentofte Hospital in 2001 and during the following 3 years of surgery outside my hospital, I used most often the cartilage methods. In 2004 I started to write this book.

Writing such book from the age of 73 to 77 years, at home, without a secretary and with my two-finger typing, is not easy and demands enormous discipline and a strong will to finish it. At the start I did not dream that the book would end with 28 chapters, but several new methods have been published and included, resulting in 23 original methods.

With only one exception, all the illustrations were made especially for this book in the same manner as in my previous books: I sketched each illustration in pencil on parchment paper, then the artist, Regitze Steinbruch, copied it and redrew it in ink on another parchment. Regitze also made the figures for Volumes 1 and 2 and partly for Volume of 4 of Manual of Middle Ear Surgery in the same way.

I would like to thank Dr. SV Fernandes, from Newcastle, Australia, the author of the "Triple C" Technique (Chapter 26), for great help in reading and correcting the text of most of the chapters, and Dr. MW Yung for correcting the text of Chapter 14.

The staff of the Gentofte Hospital Library were very helpful in finding the literature I needed.

I also wish to thank many friends and authors for discussion about and help with explanation of their cartilage methods: M Bernal-Sprekelsen, AE Ferekidis, SV Fernandes, F Hitari, J Heermann, K-B Hüttenbrink, K Jahnke, J. Klacansky, H Martin, C Milewski, B Morra, and D Portmann.

Finally I would like to thank my beloved wife Nives for her help and patience during the retirement and the cartilage tympanoplasty years. I was never able to answer her constant question: Do you really need this book?

Mirko Tos

Foreword

While cartilage has been used to a limited extent in otosurgical procedures for many years, its utility in major reconstruction of the tympanic membrane has become increasingly recognized. While routine acceptance of cartilage tympanoplasty has been hampered by anticipated worsening of hearing results with the use of a thick graft, many studies comparing cartilage to more traditional grafting materials have shown no difference in hearing post-operatively. Likewise, the rigidity and stability of cartilage, especially in the hostile middle ear environment often found in the surgical ear, have made it invaluable in cases of cholesteatoma, atelectasis, and recurrent perforations.

The techniques involved in cartilage tympanoplasty do present a few nuances that must be appreciated, such as graft harvest, cartilage shaping, and placement. Likewise, the creation of an opaque ear drum must be anticipated in the post-operative period. Intubation of the tympanic membrane, if deemed necessary, can be difficult. As a result of this, several techniques have evolved with modifications in graft thickness, placement, and degree of drum reconstruction based on the clinical situation or surgeon's preference. Some represent minor variations of existing techniques while others are quite novel and intuitive.

Mirko Tos has written a remarkable book, the only comprehensive text to my knowledge, on cartilage tympanoplasty. Since reading his manuals of middle ear surgery over 15 years ago, I have appreciated Professor Tos' ability to classify, organize, and explain middle ear surgery in a clear but detailed way. This book continues in that tradition and clearly reflects his 40 years of experience in otosurgery. The book is well illustrated and is unique in the fact that the initial drawings were produced by Professor Tos. As a result, they are straightforward and easy to follow from a surgeon's perspective.

There is no question that this book will not only be valuable to the otologist in training, but also to more advanced surgeons. As a surgeon experienced and published in cartilage tympanoplasty, I was astounded by Mirko Tos' ability to provide such a comprehensive treatise of techniques, from so many different surgeons, and explain them in a way that only an experienced ear surgeon could. I read this book from cover to cover and learned a great deal. The entire community of otologic surgeons will benefit from this contribution.

John Dornhoffer M.D., F.A.C.S
Professor of Otolaryngology
Director of Otology and Neurotology
Samuel McGill Chair in Otolaryngology Research
University of Arkansas for Medical Sciences
Little Rock, Arkansas, USA

Table of Contents

1 History of Cartilage Tympanoplasty 1
　Introduction 1
　Cartilage in Ossiculoplasty in Tympanoplasty Type 2
　with Intact Stapes 1
　Cartilage Slices in Tympanoplasty
　Type 2 with Intact Stapes 1
　Cartilage in Ossiculoplasty in Tympanoplasty Type 3
　with Missing Stapedial Arch 1
　Myringoplasty Using Autogenous Septal Cartilage
　by Salen—the First Cartilage Tympanoplasty.... 3
　The Heermann Cartilage Bridge from the Stapes
　Columella to the Inferior Annulus............. 4
　The Broad Heermann Stapes–Annulus Cartilage
　Bridges................................... 6
　The Tunnelplasty 7
　Cartilage Palisade Tympanoplasty............. 7
　The Goodhill Annular Graft—the First Cartilage-
　Perichondrium Composite Graft 8

2 Classifications and Definitions 10
　Classification of Cartilage Tympanoplasty
　Methods 10
　Cartilage Grafts............................ 10
　　Cartilage Palisades....................... 11
　　Cartilage Strips.......................... 12
　　Cartilage Foils, Thin Plates, and Thick Plates.. 13
　　Cartilage–Perichondrium Composite Island
　　Grafts................................. 15
　　Special Cartilage–Perichondrium Composite
　　Island Grafts 16
　　Composite Islands Grafts for Minor,
　　Medium-sized, and Subtotal Perforations 18
　　Special Cartilage Methods in Small and
　　Medium-Sized Perforations 20
　Classification of Tympanoplasty 20
　　Cartilage Tympanoplasty 20
　　Classification of Tympanoplasty in Relation
　　to Ossiculoplasty 20
　Pictorial Key to the Drawings in this Book...... 23
　　Pieces of Cartilage and Cartilage Palisades.... 23
　　Cartilage Strips, Foils, and Plates............ 24
　　Composite Cartilage–Perichondrium Grafts .. 25
　　Soft Tissues............................. 26
　　Bony Tissues............................ 27
　　Other Elements 28

3 Approaches and Harvesting of Cartilage 30
　Approaches................................ 30
　　Transmeatal Approach through Fixed Ear
　　Speculum 30
　　Endaural Approach with Intercartilaginous
　　Incision 33
　　Retroauricular Approach.................. 35
　Harvesting of Cartilage 40
　　Harvesting of Tragal Cartilage 40
　　Harvesting of Cartilage from the Auricle 42
　　Harvesting of Cartilage in Endaural
　　Approaches............................. 45
　　Thinning the Cartilage.................... 46
　　The Hüttenbrink Cartilage Guide 49
　　The Groningen Cartilage Cutting Device 50

**4 Cartilage Palisades in Underlay Tympanoplasty
　Techniques** 52
　Definition 52
　Indications for Surgery 52
　Harvesting and Shaping of Palisades 52
　Surgical Techniques......................... 53
　　Posterior Perforation..................... 53
　　Inferior Perforation 53
　　Total Perforation 58
　　Underlay Cartilage Palisade Technique and
　　Ossiculoplasty.......................... 64
　Modifications of Cartilage Palisade Technique .. 74
　　Ferekidis Chondrotympanoplasty.......... 74
　　Covering Palisades with the Perichondrium .. 78
　　Cartilage Palisades and Fascia 79
　Results of Surgery with Palisades in Underlay
　Tympanoplasty Techniques 82
　　Results in Pars Tensa Cholesteatoma in
　　Children................................ 82
　　Comparing Results of Cartilage Palisades
　　with Fascia 83
　　Comparing Functional Results and
　　Tympanometry.......................... 83
　　Comparison of Underlay Cartilage Palisades
　　with Fascia—Recent Results 83
　　Late Results in Underlay Palisade Technique.. 83
　　Ten-year Results of Cartilage Palisades versus
　　Fascia in Eardrum Reconstruction after Surgery
　　for Sinus or Tensa Retraction Cholesteatoma in
　　Children................................ 84
　Author's Comments and Proposals 84

Clinical Research on Cartilage Tympanoplasty
Is Needed 84
Placement of the Palisades 84
Gelfoam in the Tympanic Cavity or Not? 85
Small On-lay Perichondrium Grafts 85
Why Not Perichondrium Covering on Both
Sides of the Palisade? 85

**5 Cartilage Palisades in On-lay Tympanoplasty
Techniques** 87
Definitions 87
Full-Thickness Palisades..................... 87
Half-Thickness Palisades and Perichondrium
Flaps 87
Harvesting and Shaping of the Palisades....... 88
Harvesting of the Palisades 88
Shaping of the Palisades.................... 88
Curling of the Cartilage Grafts.............. 89
Indications for On-lay Palisade Technique 89
Surgical Techniques with On-lay Placement
of Palisades.................................. 89
Anterior Perforation 90
Inferior Perforation........................ 92
Total Perforation 95
Results of On-lay Cartilage Tympanoplasty
Techniques................................... 101
Author's Comments on On-lay Palisade
Techniques................................... 101
Clinical Research in On-lay Cartilage
Technique is Needed....................... 101

6 Tympanoplasty with Broad Cartilage Palisades .. 103
Definition 103
Harvesting and Shaping of Broad Palisades 103
Indications for Tympanoplasty with Broad
Cartilage Palisades 104
The Bernal-Sprekelsen Broad Palisade
Techniques................................... 104
Total Perforation with Intact Ossicular Chain .. 104
Total Perforation with Missing Ossicles....... 104
Total Perforation with Missing Long Process
of Incus 104
Retracted and Adherent Malleus Handle in a
Total Perforation with Defective Incus........ 106
Broad Palisades and Various
Tympanomastoidectomies..................... 110
Closure of an Atticotomy with Broad Cartilage
Palisades.................................. 110
Results in Tympanoplasty with Broad Cartilage
Palisades..................................... 110
Anatomical Results 110
Functional Results......................... 110
Author's Comments and Recommendations..... 112
The Longest Follow-up Period............... 112
Evaluation of Hearing Results in
Tympanoplasty Type 1 with Broad Cartilage
Palisades Is Needed........................ 112
Support of Broad Palisades by Small Pieces
of Cartilage................................ 112

**7 Cartilage Strips in Underlay Tympanoplasty
Techniques** 114
Definition................................... 114
Harvesting and Shaping of the Cartilage Strips .. 115
Cutting and Shaping of the Cartilage Strips ... 115
Indications for Cartilage Strips in Underlay
Techniques................................... 117
Surgical Techniques 117
Posterior Perforation 117
Inferior Perforation........................ 118
Total Perforation 118
Tunnelplasty 122
Reconstruction of the Eardrum and the Attic
Wall with Cartilage Strips 123
Covering the Cartilage Strips with
Perichondrium............................. 124
Results of Surgery 124
Comparison of Results of Underlay Cartilage
Strip Technique with Fascia Grafting 125
Conclusion on Results of the Underlay
Cartilage Strip Technique................... 125
Author's Comments and Recommendations..... 125

**8 Cartilage Strips in On-lay Tympanoplasty
Techniques** 127
Definition................................... 127
Harvesting and Shaping of the
Cartilage Strips 127
Indications for Surgery....................... 128
The On-lay Cartilage Strip Techniques.......... 128
Anterior Perforation 128
Inferior Perforation........................ 130
Total Perforation 132
On-lay Cartilage Strips in ossiculoplasty 132
Results of Surgery 137
Author's Comments and Recommendations..... 137
Need for Clinical Research 137

9 The Dornhoffer Cartilage Mosaic Tympanoplasty 138
Definition................................... 138
Harvesting and Trimming of the Cartilage 138
Indications for Cartilage Mosaic Tympanoplasty . 139
Surgical Techniques of Cartilage Mosaic
Tympanoplasty 139
Posterior Perforation 139
Inferior Perforation........................ 141
Subtotal Perforation 141
Total Perforation 143
Results of Surgery 144
Author's Comments and Recommendations..... 146

10 Underlay Tympanoplasty with Cartilage Foils and Thin Plates ... 147
Definition ... 147
Harvesting and Elaboration of Cartilage Foils and Thin Plates ... 148
   Portmann's Tangential Cutting of Conchal Thin Plates and Lamellae ... 148
Indications for Surgery ... 149
Underlay Techniques with Foils and Thin Plates. 149
   Posterior Perforation ... 149
   Inferior Perforation ... 149
   Total Perforation ... 149
   The Portmann Mosaic Underlay Cartilage Tympanoplasty with Foils or Thin Plates ... 152
Results after Surgery with Cartilage Foils or Thin Plates Covered with Perichondrium ... 152
Author's Comments and Recommendations ... 153

11 On-lay Tympanoplasty with Cartilage Foils and Thin Plates ... 155
Definition ... 155
Harvesting and Elaboration of Cartilage Foils and Thin Plates ... 155
Indications for On-lay Tympanoplasty with Cartilage Foils and Thin Plates ... 155
On-lay Techniques with Foils and Thin Plates ... 155
   Anterior Perforation ... 156
   Inferior Perforation ... 156
   Total Perforation ... 157
Results after On-lay Tympanoplasty with Cartilage Foils ... 160
Author's Comments and Recommendations ... 160

12 On-lay Tympanoplasty with Thick Cartilage Plates ... 162
Definitions ... 162
Harvesting and Elaboration of the Cartilage Plates ... 162
On-lay Techniques with Thick Cartilage Plates ... 162
   The Jansen Cartilage Plate On-lay Tympanoplasty ... 163
   Tympanoplasty Type 2 or Type 3 and Cartilage Plates ... 163
   "Cartilage Boards" On-lay Technique ... 163
   Cartilage Plates in Stabilization of the Columella ... 163
   Full-Thickness Cartilage Plate ... 163
Results of Surgery with Cartilage Plates ... 165
   Results of the Early On-lay Techniques ... 165
Author's Comments and Recommendations ... 165
Effect of the Thickness of The Cartilage Disk on Hearing ... 167
Experimental Investigation of the Use of Cartilage in Tympanic Membrane Reconstruction ... 168
   Methods ... 168
   Sound Pressure Response ... 168
Clinical Research on the Thickness of Cartilage Grafts ... 169
   Problems with Curling ... 169
   Optimal Graft Thickness for Different Sizes of the Perforation ... 170

13 Underlay Tympanoplasty with Thick Cartilage Plates ... 172
Definitions ... 172
Harvesting and Elaboration of the Autogenous Cartilage Plates ... 172
The Underlay Tympanoplasty Techniques with Thick Cartilage Plates ... 172
   Cartilage Plate Covered with Fascia ... 172
   Cartilage Plate Covered with Areolar Tissue— a Cartilage Shield Tympanoplasty? ... 173
   Cartilage Shield Tympanoplasty of Moore ... 173
   Tympanoplasty with Cartilage Plates Only ... 173
   Tympanoplasty with Crushed Autogenous Cartilage Plate ... 173
   Tympanoplasty with Irradiated Homogenous Rib Cartilage Plates ... 175
   Reinforcement of the Tympanic Membrane with Cartilage Plates after Removal of Congenital Cholesteatoma ... 176
Results of Surgery with Cartilage Plates ... 176
   Results of Recent Underlay Techniques ... 176
Author's Comments and Proposals ... 177
   Classification of Cartilage Shield Tympanoplasty ... 177

14 Superior (or Attic) Cartilage–Perichondrium Composite Island Graft Tympanoplasty ... 179
Definition ... 179
Indications for Surgery ... 179
Surgical Methods for Closure of Bony Defects of the Scutum ... 181
   McCleve Technique ... 181
   Fleury Technique ... 181
   Adkins Technique ... 183
   Black Technique ... 183
   Honda Scutumplasty ... 185
   Quinn Technique ... 185
Results of Surgery ... 187
   Lateral Attic Reconstruction (LAR) Technique: Preventive Surgery for Epitympanic Retraction Pockets ... 188
Author's Comments and Proposals ... 189
   Difficulties in Comparison of the Various Series ... 189

15 Posterior Cartilage–Perichondrium Composite Island Graft Tympanoplasty ... 194
Definition ... 194
Harvesting and Shaping of the Graft ... 195
   Shaping of the Posterior Cartilage–Perichondrium Island Graft ... 196
Indications for Surgery ... 196
Surgical Techniques with Posterior Cartilage–Perichondrium Composite Island Graft ... 197

Transmeatal Technique with Posterosuperior Island Graft... 197
Transmeatal Removal of a Posterior Retraction... 198
Transmeatal Removal of the Sinus Cholesteatoma... 201
Removal of a Large Sinus Cholesteatoma... 203
Retrograde Atticoantrotomy in a Large Sinus Cholesteatoma... 205
Posterior Ear Canal Wall Reconstruction with a Composite Cartilage Titanium Mesh Graft... 206
Cartilage Ossiculoplasty and Myringoplasty by Lever Method... 207
Results of Surgery with the Posterior Island Graft... 207
Author's Comments and Recommendations... 208
When to Operate a Posterior Retraction?... 209
Pathogenesis of Sinus Cholesteatoma... 211
When to Operate a Posterior Perforation?... 212

16 Superior and Posterior Cartilage–Perichondrium Composite Island Graft Tympanoplasty... 215
Definition... 215
Harvesting and Shaping of the Graft... 215
Indications... 215
Surgical Methods... 217
Technique of Levinson... 217
Technique of Poe and Gadre... 220
Two Separate Grafts of Couloigner... 223
Results of Surgery... 223
Levinson Series... 223
Series of Poe and Gadre... 224
Pediatric Series with Two Separate Cartilage–Perichondrium Composite Island Grafts... 224
Author's Comments and Recommendations... 224
Vibratile and Non-vibratile Island Grafts... 224
Prevalence and Classification of Attic Retractions... 225
Attic Precholesteatoma... 226
Pathogenesis of Attic Cholesteatoma... 226
The Incidence of Cholesteatoma... 227

17 Total Pars Tensa Cartilage–Perichondrium Composite Island Graft Tympanoplasty... 228
Definitions... 228
The Tolsdorff and the Nitsche Grafts... 228
Harvesting and Shaping of the Cartilage Graft... 228
Shaping of the Tolsdorff Graft... 228
Shaping of the Dornhoffer Graft... 229
Klacansky Small Total Pars Tensa Composite Island Graft... 230
Other Pars Tensa Composite Grafts... 232
Indications for Surgery... 232
Surgical Techniques... 232
The Nitsche On-lay Technique... 232
The Tolsdorff Technique... 235
The Würzburg Clinic Techniques... 235
The Dornhoffer Technique... 239

Results of Surgery with the Total Tensa Composite Graft... 239
The First Würzburg Series (1982–1987)... 239
The Second Würzburg Series (1989–1994)... 239
The Dornhoffer Series... 241
Outcomes by Surgical Indication... 241
Pediatric Series... 242
Comparison of the Cartilage–Perichondrium Graft with the Fascia Graft... 242
Series with Posterior and Total Pars Tensa Grafts... 243
Author's Comments and Recommendations... 243

18 Annular Cartilage–Perichondrium Composite Graft Tympanoplasty... 245
Definition... 245
Previous Applications of the Annular Graft... 246
Harvesting and Shaping of the Annular Graft... 246
The Klacansky Chondrotome... 246
Circular Graft and U-Graft... 246
Indications for Application of Annular Grafts... 248
Surgical Techniques with Annular Grafts... 249
Goodhill's On-lay Annular Graft Technique... 249
Annular Graft in Tympanoplasty Type 2 with Interposition Techniques... 249
Annular Graft in Tympanoplasty Type 3 with a Columella... 257
The Klacansky Annular Graft Technique with Removal of Fibrous Annulus and Eardrum Remnant... 261
Further Development of the Klacansky Annular Graft... 261
The Borkowski Underlay Annular Graft Technique... 261
Retracted Malleus Handle and Annular Graft... 261
Missing Malleus Handle and Annular Graft... 270
Circular Annular Graft in Case of Missing Entire Malleus... 271
U-shaped Annular Graft in Large Inferior Perforation... 274
Annular Graft in the Reconstruction of the Tympanic Cavity after a Canal Wall Down Mastoidectomy... 274
Results of Surgery with the Annular Graft... 280
Author's Comments and Proposals... 280
Need for Future Research on Clinical Series with Annular Graft... 280

19 "Crown Cork" Cartilage–Perichondrium Composite Graft Tympanoplasty... 282
Definition... 282
Harvesting and Construction of the "Crown Cork" Graft... 282
Harvesting of Tragal Cartilage... 282
Harvesting of Conchal Cartilage... 282
Indications for "Crown Cork" Tympanoplasty... 287
Congenital Malformations... 287
Acquired Ear Canal Lesions... 287

Surgical Techniques of "Crown Cork"
Tympanoplasty.......................... 288
   Schematic Illustration of Surgical Principle in
   Congenital Type 2a Atresia Reconstructed
   with Crown Cork Tympanoplasty 288
   Surgery of Congenital Type 2b Atresia
   Applying Crown Cork Graft 290
   Removal of Fibrous Tissue in Blunting
   Phenomena When Applying Crown Cork
   Tympanoplasty......................... 290
Results of the "Crown Cork" Tympanoplasty.... 290
Author's Comments and Recommendations 295

20 Cartilage Shield T-Tube Tympanoplasty 296
Definition 296
Harvesting and Construction of the Cartilage
Shield T-Tube Grafts 297
   Construction of the Hall Cartilage Shield
   T-Tube Graft in Intact Eardrum 297
   Construction of the Duckert Cartilage Shield
   T-Tube Graft 297
   Construction of the Dornhoffer Cartilage
   Shield T-Tube Graft 298
   The Elsheikh U-shaped Cartilage–
   Perichondrium T-Tube Graft 298
Indication for Cartilage Shield T-Tube
Tympanoplasty............................ 299
Surgical Techniques........................ 300
   The Hall Technique 300
   The Duckert Technique................... 302
   The Dornhoffer Technique 316
   Application of the Elsheikh Graft 318
Postoperative Care and Problems 322
   Accidental or Intentional Removal of the Tube 322
   Reinsertion of the T-Tube in a Cartilage Shield
   Graft.................................. 323
   Malfunction of the T-Tube due to Plugged
   Cerumen 323
   Formation of Granulation Tissue at the
   Tube–Perichondrium Interface 323
   Infection and Otorrhea 324
   Medialization of the Cartilage Graft 324
Results of Cartilage Shield T-Tube
Tympanoplasty............................ 324
   Hall's Series of Children 324
   The First Series of Duckert and Co-workers .. 324
   The Later Series of Duckert and Co-workers.. 325
   The Series of Danner and Dornhoffer 325
   The Randomized Prospective Study of Elsheikh
   and Co-workers 325
Author's Comments and Recommendations 326
   Proposal of an Inferior Cartilage Shield T-Tube
   Graft.................................. 326
   Comments on Tubal Function 326
   Need for Testing of Tubal Function 328
   Cartilage Shield T-Tube Tympanoplasty
   Provides Ideal Opportunities for Long-Term
   Research on Tubal Function 328

21 Underlay Tympanoplasty Techniques with
Cartilage–Perichondrium Composite Island Graft 331
Definition 331
Harvesting and Shaping of the Island Graft..... 331
Indication for Application of the Underlay Island
Graft.................................... 331
Surgical Techniques........................ 331
   Anterior Perforation 331
   Inferior Perforation 337
   Subtotal Perforation 337
   Cartilage Graft in Type 1 Tympanoplasty—
   A Modification without Perichondrium Flaps . 338
Results of Surgery with the Island Graft 341
   Comparison with Fascia 342
Author's Comments and Recommendations 343
   Drilling a Hole or a Groove into the Bony
   Annulus............................... 343
   Modifications of the Techniques 344

22 In-lay Underlay Tympanoplasty Techniques with
Cartilage–Perichondrium Composite Island Graft 345
Definition 345
Harvesting and Shaping of the Graft........... 345
Indications for In-lay Underlay Technique...... 346
The In-lay Underlay Techniques 346
   Anterior Perforation 346
   Inferior Perforation 346
   Posterior Perforation..................... 351
   Subtotal Perforation 351
Results of Surgery 352
Author's Comments and Recommendations 352

23 On-lay Tympanoplasty Techniques with
Cartilage–Perichondrium Composite Island Graft 353
Definition 353
Harvesting and Elaboration of the On-lay Island
Graft.................................... 354
   Thinning, Trimming, and Shaping of On-lay
   Island Grafts 354
Indications for Surgery 354
Surgical Techniques of On-lay Tympanoplasty
with Island Grafts 355
   Anterior Perforation 355
   Inferior Perforation 357
   Total and Subtotal Perforations 358
Results of Surgery with On-lay Techniques..... 362
Author's Comments and Recommendations 363
   Research on Epithelialization of the Cartilage
   Grafts is Needed........................ 364

24 In-lay On-lay Tympanoplasty Techniques with
Cartilage–Perichondrium Composite Island Graft 365
Definition 365
Harvesting and Elaboration of the Graft 365
Indications for Application of the In-lay On-lay
Graft.................................... 366

The In-lay On-lay Technique 366
    Anterior Perforation 366
    Posterior Perforation 368
    Inferior Perforation. 368
    Subtotal Perforation 368
    Total Perforation 371
    Pediatric Interleave Tympanoplasty. 371
Results of Surgery. 373
    Results of Pediatric Cartilage Interleave
    Tympanoplasty 374
Author's Comments and Recommendations. 375
    Minimally Invasive Surgery. 375
    Composite Island Grafts for Small and
    Medium-sized Perforations. 375

25 In-lay Butterfly Cartilage Tympanoplasty 376
Definition 376
Indications 376
Harvesting and Shaping of the Butterfly Cartilage
Graft 376
The In-lay Butterfly Cartilage Technique. 378
    Grafting of a Small Anterior Perforation 378
    Grafting of a Medium-Sized Inferior
    Perforation. 378
    Butterfly Technique in Large Perforations. 378
    Butterfly Prosthesis Placed onto the Bony
    Annulus. 378
Results of the In-lay Butterfly Technique 381
Author's Comments and Recommendations. 381
    Problems with Epithelialization of the Graft . . 384
    Elevation of the Epithelium Instead of
    Removal 385
    Closure of Large Perforations and
    Postoperative Hearing 385
    Future Research Needed 385

26 Composite Chondroperichondrial Clip
Tympanoplasty: The Triple "C" Technique. 387
Definition 387
Indications for the Triple "C" Techniques 387
Harvesting and Preparation of the Graft. 388
Surgical Techniques 389
    Anterior Perforation 389
    Inferior Perforation. 391
    Posterior Perforation 396
Results of Triple "C" Technique. 402
Author's Comments and Proposals. 402

27 The Fate of Implanted Cartilage Grafts 403
The Nourishment of the Cartilage 403
Experiments on the Fate of Transplanted
Cartilage 403
    Living Cartilage Implanted into Animals. 403
    Living Cartilage Implanted into Humans. 403
    Otological Research on Cartilage Grafts. 404
    The Fate of Cartilage Columellae and Struts . . . 404
    The Fate of Cartilage Grafts after
    Myringoplasty 405
Author's Comments and Recommendations. 406
The Fate of the Implanted Cartilage and Clinical
Consequences 407

28 Clinical Research in Cartilage Tympanoplasties . . 410
Postoperative Results without Comparison with
Other Series 410
    Comparison of Functional Results within the
    Same Cartilage Tympanoplasty in Relation
    to the Preoperative Tubal Function 410
    Comparison of Functional Results within the
    Same Cartilage Tympanoplasty in Relation
    to the Postoperative Tubal Function 410
Comparison of the Results in Cartilage
Tympanoplasty Methods with the Results in
Tympanoplasty Methods Using Fascia or
Perichondrium Graft. 411
    Tympanoplasty with Total Pars Tensa
    Cartilage–Perichondrium Composite Island Graft
    Compared with Tympanoplasty with
    Perichondrium Graft. 411
    Underlay Tympanoplasty with Cartilage
    Palisades Compared with Underlay
    Tympanoplasty with Fascia Graft 411
    Tympanoplasty with Total Pars Tensa Cartilage-
    Perichondrium Composite Island Graft
    Compared with Tympanoplasty with Fascia
    Graft 411
    Underlay Tympanoplasty with Cartilage Strips
    Compared with Underlay Tympanoplasty with
    Fascia. 411
Comparison of Results between Various Cartilage
Tympanoplasty Methods 411
Proposals for the Methods of Clinical Research
in Cartilage Tympanoplasty. 411
    Comparison of Results within Group A 411

Index 414

Cross references occasionally appear in the text of this book labeled MMES_1, MMES_2, MMES_3, and MMES_4. These refer to figures contained in the four-volume series *Manual of Middle Ear Surgery*, written by Professor Mirko Tos, published by Thieme Publishers between 1993 and 2000.

MMES_1: Vol. 1. Approaches, Myringoplasty, Ossiculoplasty, Tympanoplasty (1993)
MMES_2: Vol. 2. Mastoid Surgery and Reconstructive Procedures (1995)
MMES_3: Vol. 3. Surgery of the External Auditory Canal (1997)
MMES_4: Vol. 4. Surgical Solutions for Conductive Hearing Loss (2000)

1 History of Cartilage Tympanoplasty

Introduction

- In this chapter, the very first cartilage ossicular prostheses will be briefly mentioned.
- The first series of cartilage myringoplasty techniques published in 1963 by Salen will be described and illustrated by redrawing his diagrams.
- The beginning and evolution of Heermann's palisade techniques will be described in detail and illustrated by redrawing his illustrations.
- The very first cartilage–perichondrium composite graft—the annular graft of Goodhill (1967)—will be illustrated.
- The historical aspects of other cartilage methods, such as cartilage strips, cartilage foils or plates, various cartilage–perichondrium composite grafts, and some specific, recently published new methods will be described at the beginning of the respective chapters involving these methods.

Cartilage in Ossiculoplasty in Tympanoplasty Type 2 with Intact Stapes

The classification of tympanoplasty used in this book is described in Chapter 2 and in Tos (2008), and also in Volume 1 of *Manual of Middle Ear Surgery* (Tos 1993).

The first ear surgeon to apply cartilage in middle ear surgery was Utech (1959, 1960, 1961). In the latter 1950s, Utech placed a rectangular piece of tragal cartilage without perichondrium onto the stapes tendon and brought the cartilage prosthesis into contact with the eardrum (**Fig. 1.1a**). Utech was also responsible for placing the cartilage prosthesis onto the head of the stapes and under the eardrum (**Fig. 1.1b**). Other cartilage prostheses placed on the stapes head have been inspired by Utech (**Fig. 1.1c–f**).

In the late 1950s, Jansen used an allogenous septal cartilage plate as a short T-prosthesis in cases of missing incus and intact stapes (**Fig. 1.2a, b**) (Jansen 1963). In the early 1960s, Glasscock and Shea (1967) applied a solid "horse-rider" prosthesis shaped from septal cartilage in situations where an intact stapes was present (**Fig. 1.3**).

During the last 40 years, various cartilage partial ossicular replacement prostheses (PORPs) have been developed and are illustrated in Tos (1993). Subsequently all PORPs made of allogenous cartilage were abandoned. PORPs made of autogenous cartilage are still in use.

Cartilage Slices in Tympanoplasty Type 2 with Intact Stapes

Waltner (1966) published a curious ossiculoplasty technique using thin and long cartilage slices placed onto the head of the stapes (**Fig. 1.4a–c**). The tragal cartilage is cut 3 mm wide and 10–12 mm long. The pieces are then split to one-half or one-third of their thickness. The slices do not touch the promontory and are supposed to grow together with the fascial graft that will cover the eardrum perforation. The slice is either placed under the remnant of the long process of the incus (**Fig. 1.4a**) or replaces the incus (**Fig. 1.4b**), or two slices replace both the incus and the malleus (**Fig. 1.4c**). The use of the thin slices was inspired by Heermann's stapes–annulus bridges (see **Fig. 1.7a, b**).

Cartilage in Ossiculoplasty in Tympanoplasty Type 3 with Missing Stapedial Arch

Utech (1959, 1960, 1961) was also the first surgeon to use a cartilage stapes columella in cases with a missing stapes (**Fig. 1.5a**). Jansen (1963) applied a T-shaped allogenous septal cartilage graft in the early 1960s in similar situations (**Fig. 1.5b**). Pfatz used tragal and conchal cartilage in 1962, mainly as a columella after stapedectomy but also in chronic otitis media cases with a missing stapedial arch (Pfatz and Piffko 1968). In the early 1960s, Goodhill used a tragal cartilage strut as a columella (**Fig. 1.5c**) and also a tragal cartilage–perichondrial composite T-columella (**Fig. 1.5 d**) (Goodhill 1967). Glasscock and Shea (1967) applied a tragal cartilage strut columella (**Fig. 1.5e**).

All columellae made of allogenous cartilage have been abandoned. Practically all columellae made of autogenous cartilage have also been abandoned, because the grafts became soft over a period of years (Steinbach and Pusalkar 1981).

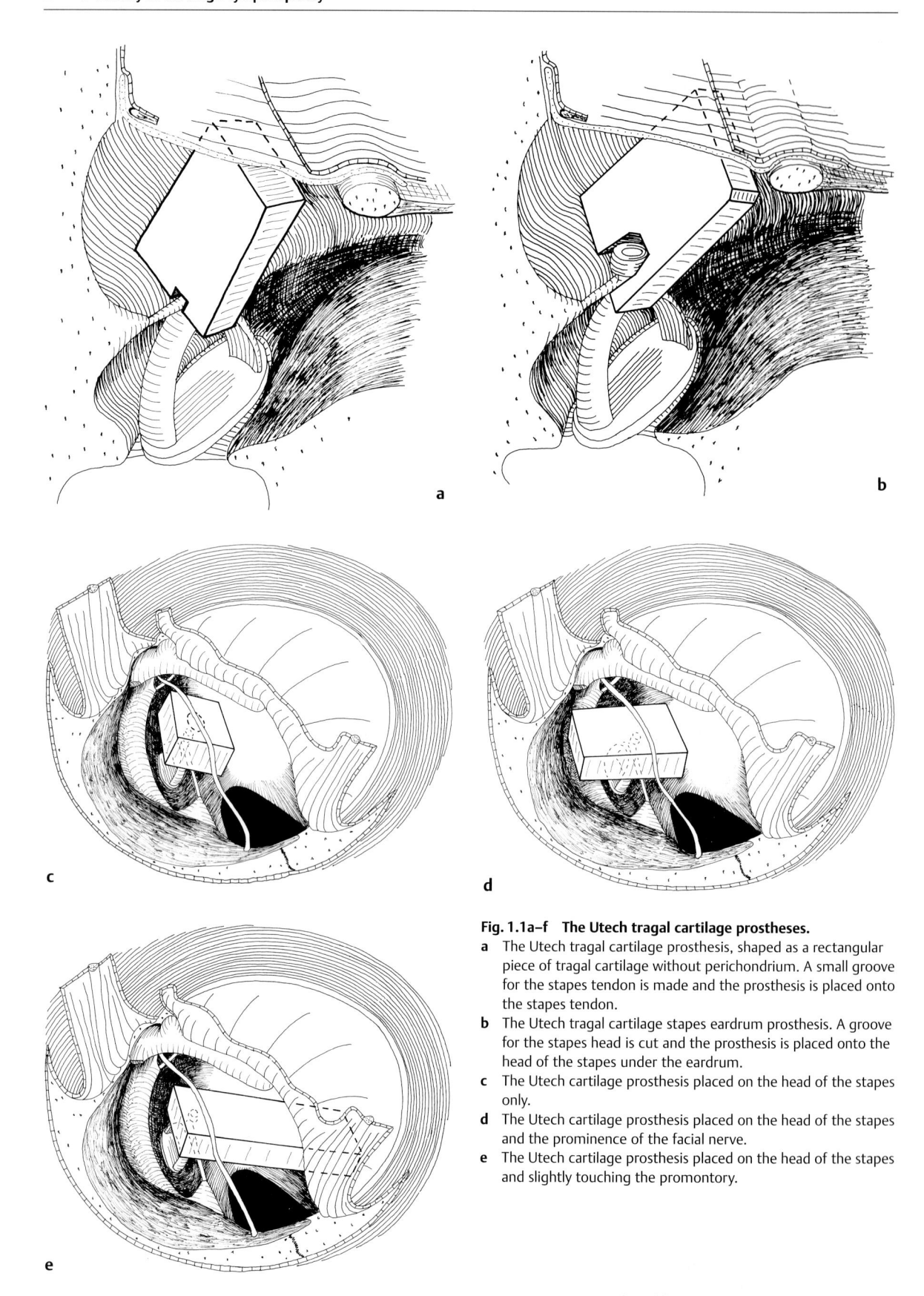

1 History of Cartilage Tympanoplasty

Fig. 1.1a–f The Utech tragal cartilage prostheses.
a The Utech tragal cartilage prosthesis, shaped as a rectangular piece of tragal cartilage without perichondrium. A small groove for the stapes tendon is made and the prosthesis is placed onto the stapes tendon.
b The Utech tragal cartilage stapes eardrum prosthesis. A groove for the stapes head is cut and the prosthesis is placed onto the head of the stapes under the eardrum.
c The Utech cartilage prosthesis placed on the head of the stapes only.
d The Utech cartilage prosthesis placed on the head of the stapes and the prominence of the facial nerve.
e The Utech cartilage prosthesis placed on the head of the stapes and slightly touching the promontory.

Fig. 1.1f

f The Utech cartilage prosthesis placed on the head of the stapes and on the posterosuperior bony annulus.

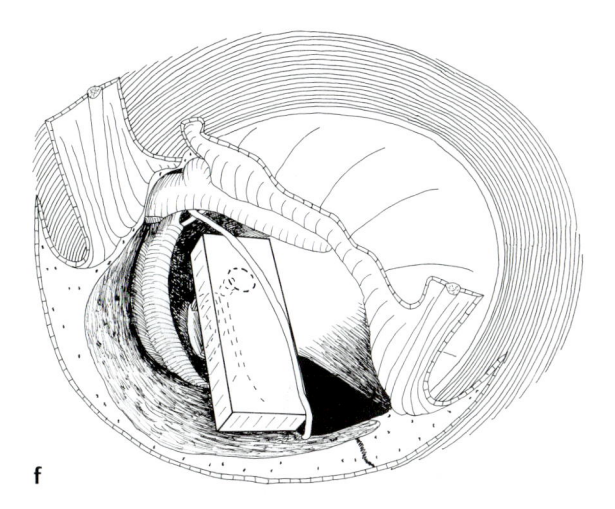

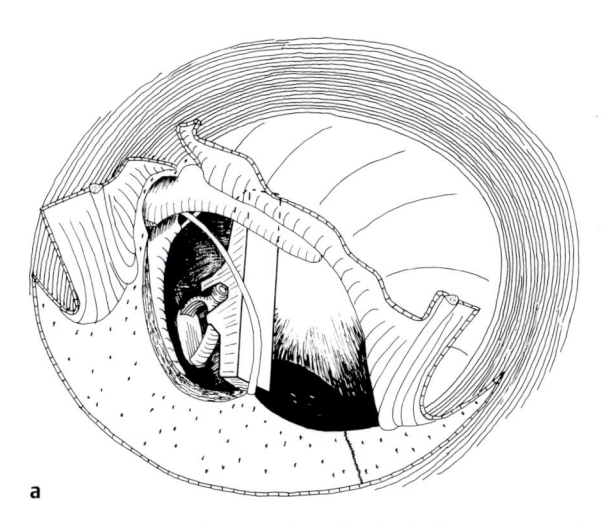

Fig. 1.2a, b Jansen's short T-prosthesis of allogenous septal cartilage.
a A groove is made for the head of the stapes and the cartilage prosthesis is placed onto the head of the stapes. Posteriolateral view.
b Inferior view of Jansen's septal cartilage prosthesis.

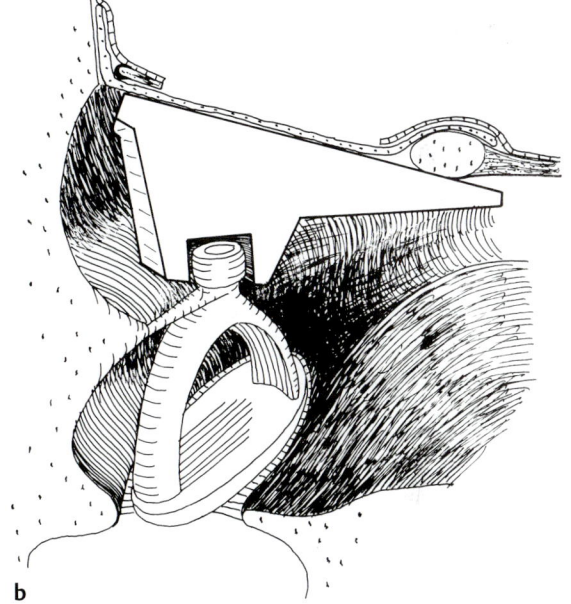

Myringoplasty Using Autogenous Septal Cartilage by Salen—the First Cartilage Tympanoplasty

In 1964, Salen from Sweden published good hearing results following myringoplasty on 25 patients with total and subtotal perforation using autogenous septal cartilage with nasal mucosa on one side.

The septal graft is harvested by an anteroinferior incision through the nasal mucosa and perichondrium on one side. The mucosa and perichondrium are elevated and preserved on this side. A circular excision 12 mm in diameter of cartilage, contralateral perichondrium, and mucosa is made (**Fig. 1.6a**). This relatively thick "composite" graft is trimmed by substantial thinning of the cartilage. The thinning is more pronounced at the periphery of the graft (**Fig. 1.6b**).

The edges of the tympanic membrane perforation are cleared of epithelium. The epithelium from the eardrum is elevated together with the ear canal skin (**Fig. 1.6c**). The trimmed round septal cartilage–perichondrium–mucosa graft is placed onto the annulus and the epithelium and the ear canal skin are replaced (**Fig. 1.6d**).

The graft healed in 23 ears. The average improvement of hearing was 16 dB in tympanoplasty type 1, and 20 dB in type 2 with intact stapes.

This seems to be the first report on an outcome of a cartilage tympanoplasty.

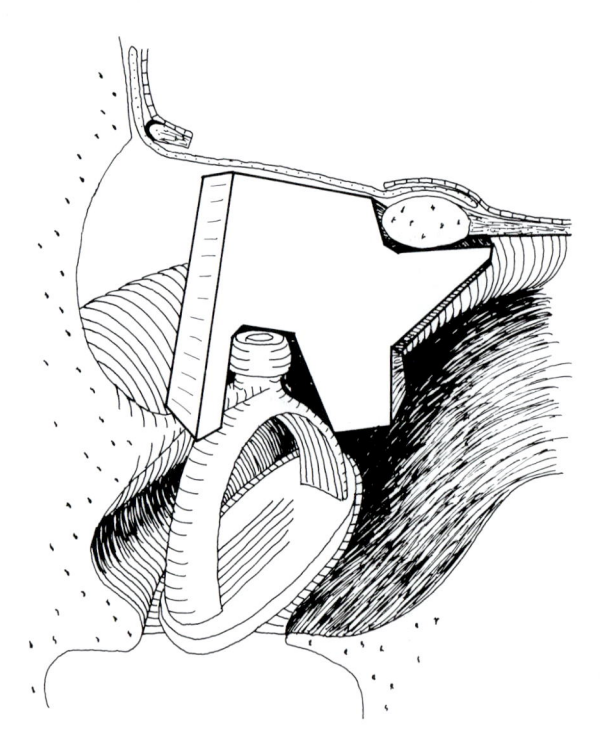

Fig. 1.3 **Glasscock tragal cartilage prostheses** with a groove for the stapes head, contacting the tendon of the stapes head as well as the anterior crus.

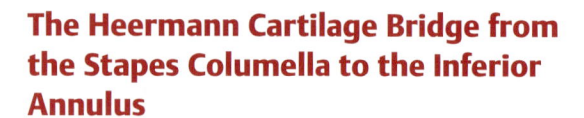

The Heermann Cartilage Bridge from the Stapes Columella to the Inferior Annulus

The beginning of the cartilage palisade techniques is presumably the Heermann cartilage plate between the cartilage columella (or the stapes) and the inferior annulus (Heermann 1962a, 1962b). In cases of missing stapedial arch, Heermann constructed a cartilage columella with a groove (**Fig. 1.7a**). Onto this columella (or stapes head) a long and relatively thin cartilage plate is placed. The plate continues in the direction of the long process of the incus down to the inferior fibrous annulus. The lower end of the plate is placed either under the eardrum remnant and fibrous annulus or onto the eardrum remnant and fibrous annulus.

Later Heermann (1962c, 1963) applied a cartilage plate with two legs (**Fig. 1.7b**). The purpose of the cartilage bridge was an ossiculoplasty with expected hearing improvement and which also provided a support for the fascial grafting. At that time use of fascia dominated the reconstruction of the eardrum and Heermann used it in myringoplasty as an on-lay technique and as an underlay technique (Heermann and Heermann 1967; Heermann et al. 1970).

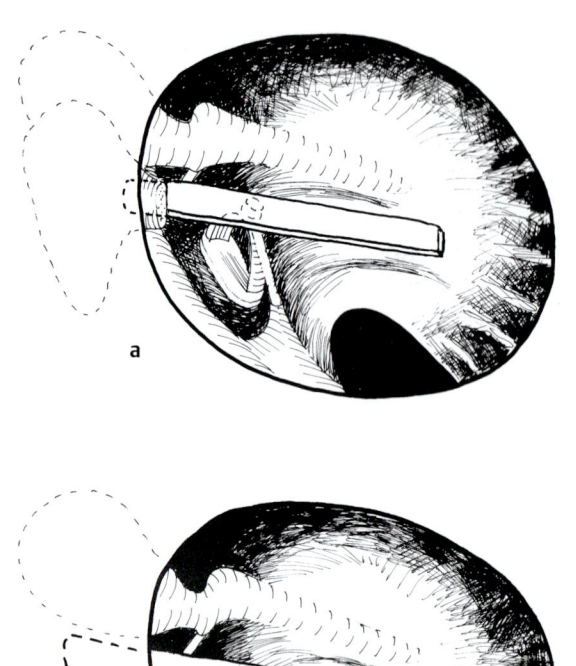

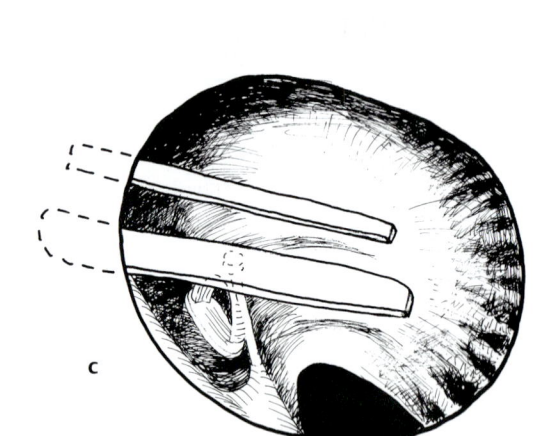

Fig. 1.4a–c Waltner's type 2 ossiculoplasty with 3 mm wide and 10–12 mm long cartilage slices placed onto the head of the stapes.
a The superior end of the slice is placed medial to the missing long process of the incus.
b The slice replaces the entire incus.
c Two slices are placed, replacing both the malleus and incus. The slices do not touch the promontory and will be included in the fascial graft.

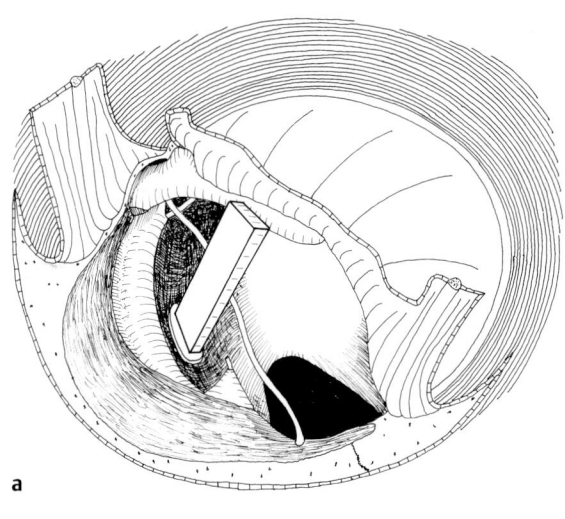

Fig. 1.5a–e Cartilage columellae.
a Utech cartilage columella. A thin cartilage columella is placed onto the footplate and under the eardrum, close to the malleus handle.
b Jansen's T-shaped allogenous septal cartilage columella.
c Goodhill's tragal cartilage strut as columella.
d Goodhill's tragal cartilage–perichondrium composite T-columella.
e Glasscock's tragal cartilage strut.

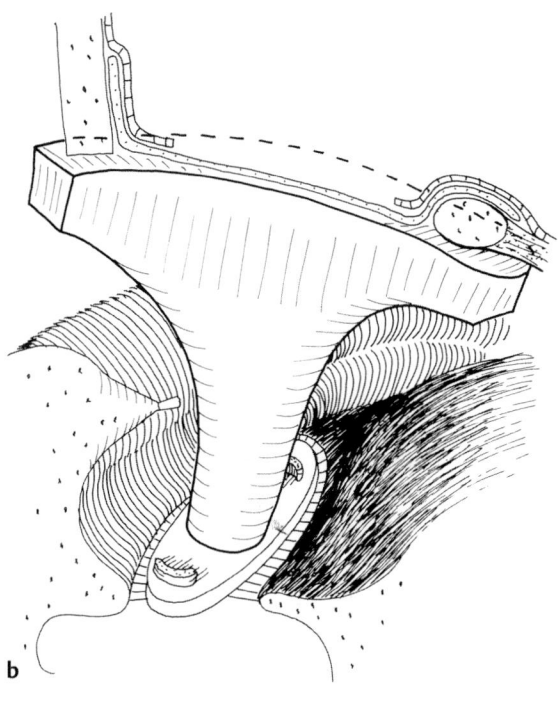

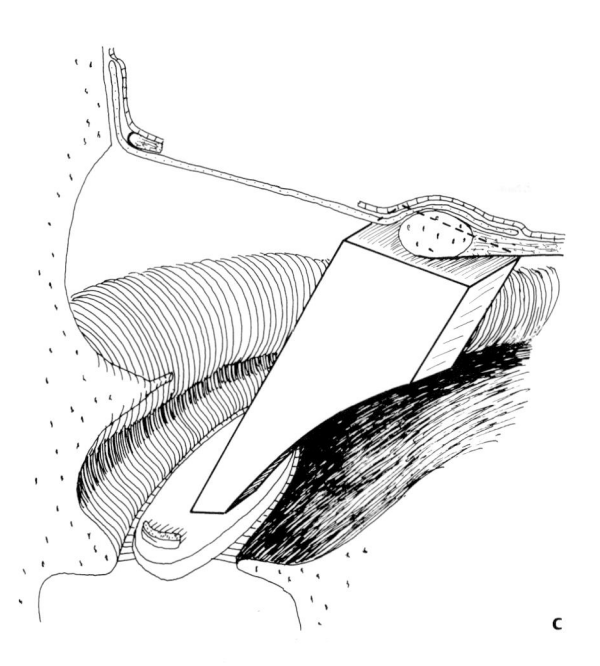

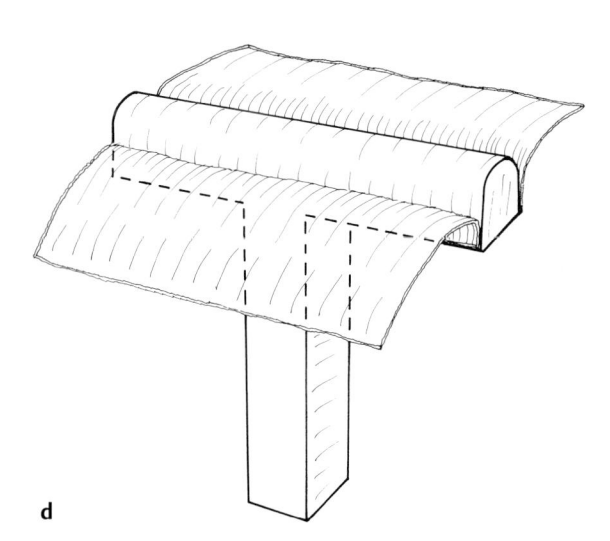

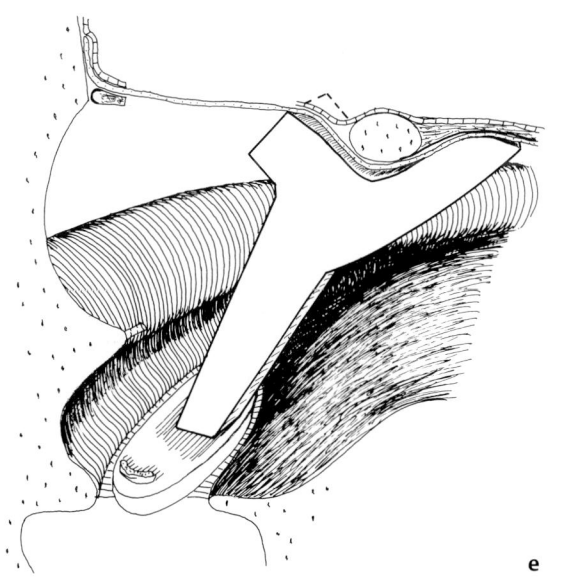

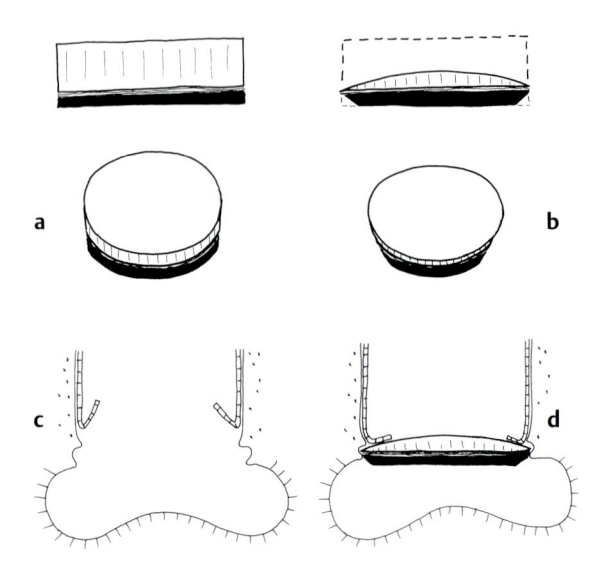

The Broad Heermann Stapes–Annulus Cartilage Bridges

With time, the cartilage plates became broader. They are used to protect the promontory and the hypotympanum and additionally they serve as a solid ossiculoplasty (**Fig. 1.8a**). In a canal wall down mastoidectomy situation, without ossicles and eardrum, the cartilage plate is placed onto the cartilage columella and onto the inferior bony annulus. The tympanic cavity will subsequently be covered with fascia (Heermann et al. 1970).

In a similar situation, without ossicles and eardrum, a very large cartilage plate is placed onto the cartilage columella and onto the tunnelplasty (**Fig. 1.8b**).

With an intact malleus handle and intact stapes, the posterior perforation is covered with a broad cartilage plate, placed onto the stapes head and onto deepithelialized eardrum remnant and the fibrous annulus (**Fig. 1.8c**). Thus this is again an example of on-lay tympanoplasty (Heermann et al. 1970).

Fig. 1.6a–d **The Salen cartilage tympanoplasty using autologous septum cartilage.** (Redrawn from Salen [1964].)
a A round and thick cartilage–perichondrium–nasal mucosa composite graft is harvested from the nasal septum.
b The graft is trimmed and the cartilage is thinned, especially at the edges.
c The epithelium from the eardrum remnant is elevated, together with the ear canal skin.
d The round trimmed composite graft is placed onto the annulus and the epithelial flaps are replaced.

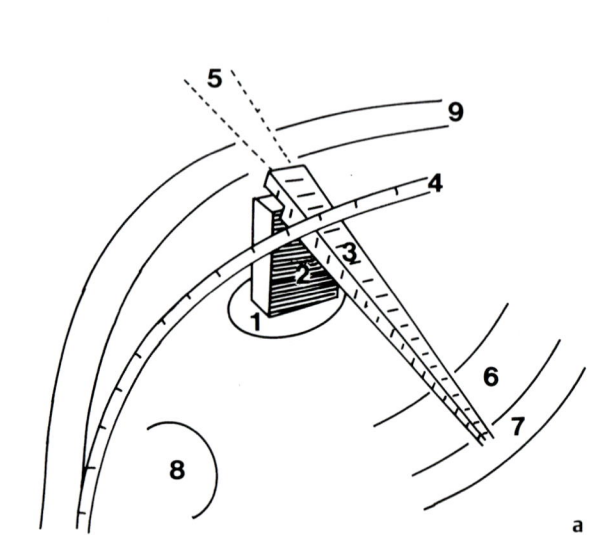

Fig. 1.7a, b **The Heermann stapes–annulus cartilage plate in the right ear.** (Redrawn from the original schematic drawing of Heermann [1962a].)
a A piece of tragal cartilage, with the perichondrium, is shaped as a stapes columella and a groove for the cartilage plate is created. The columella (2) is placed onto the footplate (1). The cartilage plate (3) is placed onto the groove of the cartilage columella in the direction of the long process of the incus (5) and under the eardrum remnant (6) and under the fibrous annulus (7). The chorda tympani (4) supports and stabilizes the cartilage plate. The round window (8) and the facial nerve (9) are indicated.
b A two-leg stapes–annulus cartilage plate (3) is placed onto the groove of the cartilage columella (2) and onto the inferior eardrum remnant (6) and the inferior annulus (7). The plate has the same direction as the long process of the incus (5). The footplate (1) and oval window (4) are also shown.

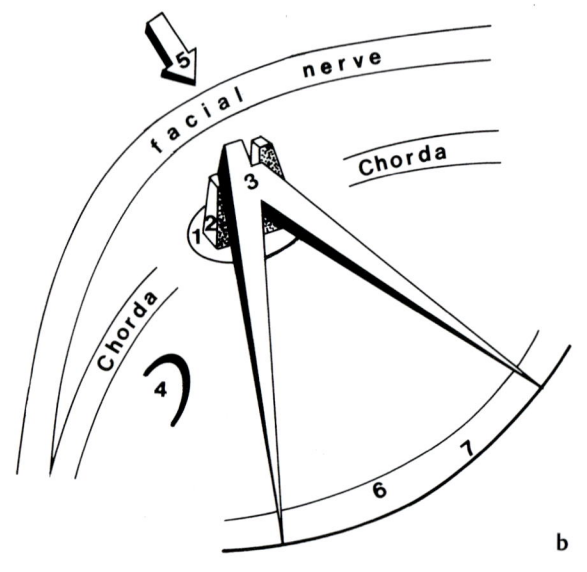

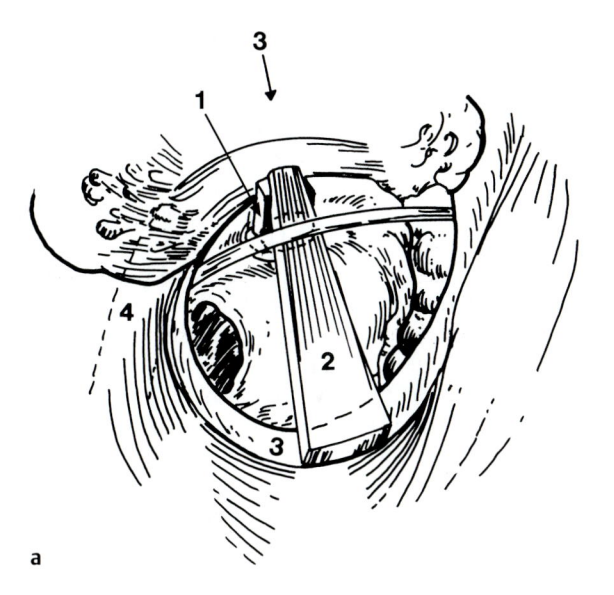

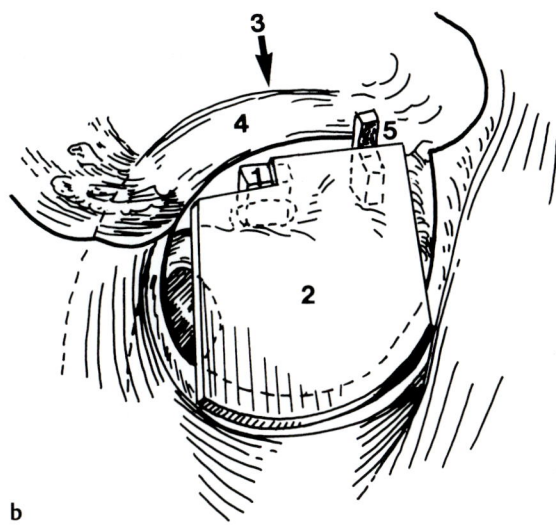

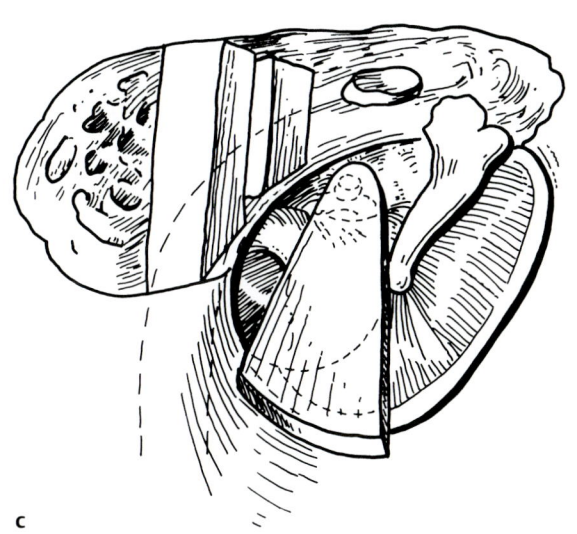

Fig. 1.8a–c Heermann broad cartilage stapes–annulus bridge.

a In a situation without ossicles and without eardrum, a broad cartilage plate (2) is placed onto a stapes columella (1) and onto the inferior bony annulus (3). The chorda tympani stabilizes the cartilage plate and a fascia graft will cover the tympanic cavity. The position of the facial nerve (4) is indicated. (Redrawn from Heermann et al. [1970].)

b In a tympanic cavity with absent ossicles and eardrum, a very large plate (2) is placed onto the stapes columella (1) and onto a piece of cartilage involved in the tunnelplasty (5). Inferiorly, the cartilage plate is placed onto the bony annulus and will be covered with fascia. The axis of the long process of the incus (3) and the position of the facial nerve (4) are indicated. (Redrawn from Heermann et al. [1970].)

c In a situation subsequent to an attico-antrostomy and a posterior eardrum perforation with an intact stapes and malleus handle, a broad cartilage plate is placed onto the intact stapes head and onto the inferior eardrum remnant and fibrous annulus. The eardrum remnant is deepithelialized. The cartilage plates reconstruct the posterior meatal wall. (Redrawn from Heermann et al. [1970].)

The Tunnelplasty

To stabilize the first palisade, which was placed under the bony annulus, and to maintain open the orifice of the eustachian tube, Heermann placed a rectangular piece of tragal cartilage onto the eminence of the tensor tympani muscle (**Figs. 1.9, 1.10**). He called this procedure a **tunnelplasty** (Heermann et al. 1970; Heermann 1978).

Cartilage Palisade Tympanoplasty

After 1962, Heermann used cartilage fragments for the reconstruction of the tympanic membrane. Initially cartilage was used to stabilize the fascial graft, first with small cartilage plates and later with broad plates of cartilage. It has been shown that large pieces of cartilage may twist after some years, so again the cycle shifted to small palisades (Heermann et al. 1970; Heermann 1992).

The palisades were usually placed parallel to the malleus handle. In a total perforation the first palisade is placed under the anterior bony annulus at the entrance of the eustachian tube. The palisade is closely connected to the bone. Heermann calls this palisade the "*simmering*" (**Fig. 1.11**). At the upper part of the tubal orifice this

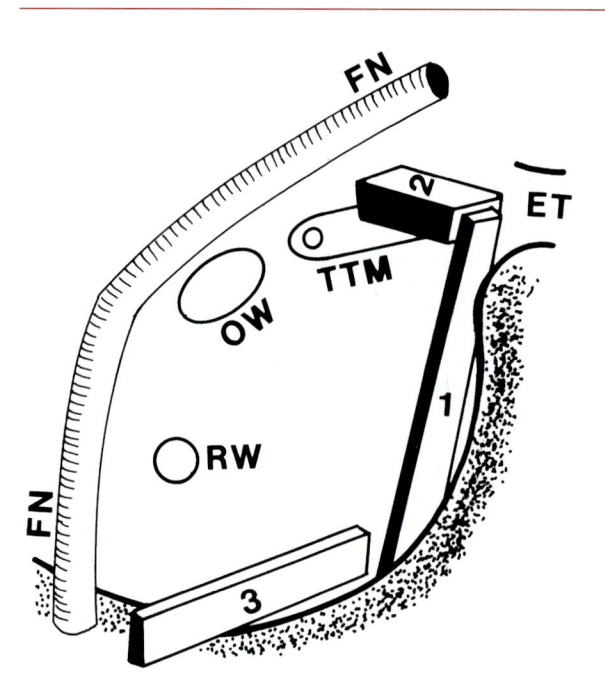

Fig. 1.9 Tunnelplasty. A rectangular piece of cartilage (2) is placed onto the eminence of the tensor tympani muscle (TTM) close to the entrance of the eustachian tube (ET). The first palisade (1) is placed under the bony annulus and onto the rectangular piece of cartilage (2). The third cartilage plate (3) is placed over the bony annulus in the posterior hypotympanum, and under the bony annulus in the anterior hypotympanum. The oval window (OW), round window (RW), facial nerve (FN), and tensor tympani tendon (TTM) are indicated. The diagram is adapted to the right ear and is redrawn from Heermann and Heermann (1967).

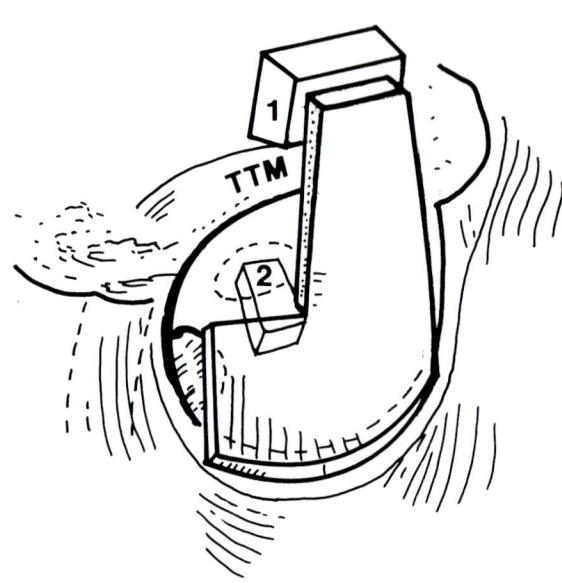

Fig. 1.10 Tunnelplasty with a large cartilage plate in a canal wall down situation without ossicles and eardrum (Heermann 1977). A rectangular piece of tragal cartilage (1), termed the "architrave", is placed onto the eminence of the tensor tympani muscle (TTM). A large cartilage plate is positioned onto a cartilage stapes columella (2) and onto the "architrave" (1). (Redrawn from Heermann [1978].)

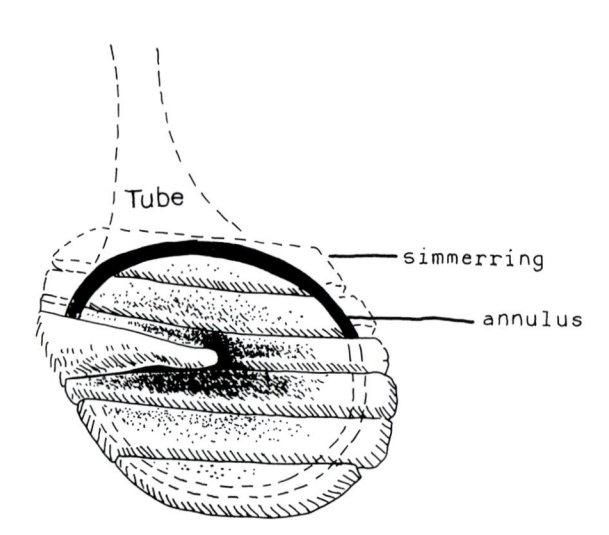

Fig. 1.11 The cartilage palisade tympanoplasty in the presence of the malleus. The most anterior cartilage plate, termed by Heermann the *simmering*, is placed medial to the bony annulus and on the "architrave" and the second palisade is placed under the bony annulus. The two following palisades at the malleus handle are cut funnel-shaped, and are placed onto the bony annulus. The posterior palisades are placed onto the bony annulus but under the fibrous annulus. (Redrawn from Heermann [1992].)

palisade rests on the "architrave," which is a rectangular piece of cartilage placed onto the eminence of the tensor tympani muscle (see **Fig. 1.10**). The architrave is the main cartilage in tunnelplasty. The other palisades at the promontory level and at the malleus handle are placed onto the bony annulus and under the fibrous annulus (**Fig. 1.11**).

The Goodhill Annular Graft—the First Cartilage–Perichondrium Composite Graft

Goodhill (1962) introduced perichondrium harvested from the tragal dome to cover the oval window niche after stapedectomy and later to reconstruct the eardrum in tympanoplasty (Goodhill et al 1964). In 1967 Goodhill published his "circumferential cartilage batten still attached to one surface of a total perichondrial autograft" (**Fig. 1.12**) (Goodhill 1967). This cartilage aids in maintaining a lateral position of the central perichondrium graft, which covers only the stapedial capitulum and does not contact any other surface (**Fig. 1.13**).

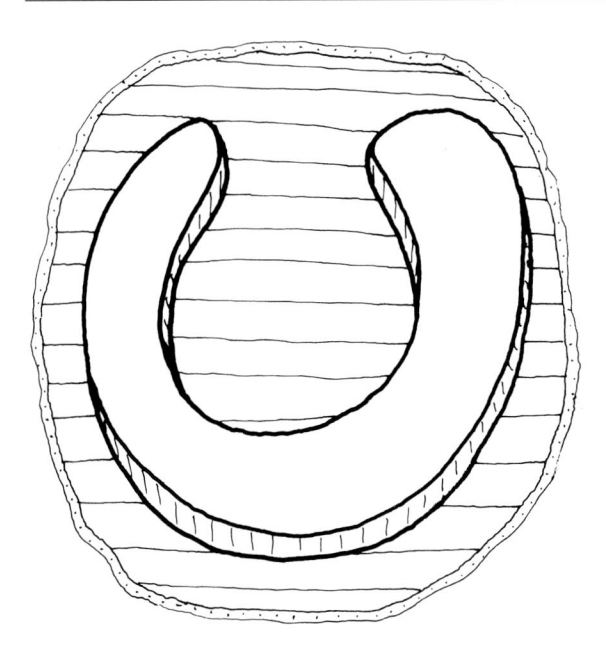

Fig. 1.12 The Goodhill annular graft: the composite cartilage–perichondrium graft. In a total perforation, Goodhill placed the cartilage ring onto the denuded remnant of the eardrum. The central perichondrium acts as the new eardrum. The peripheral perichondrium is placed onto the bone of the ear canal and suspends the annular graft.

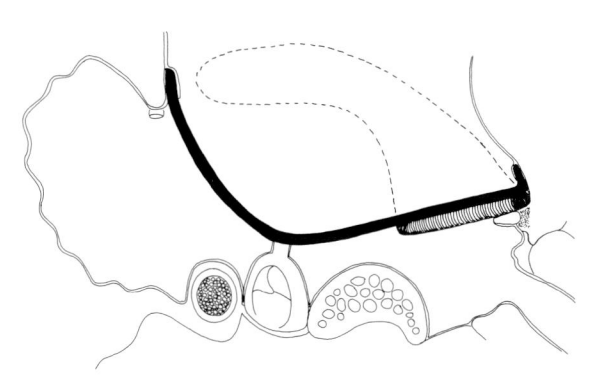

Fig. 1.13 Sagittal cross-section of the tympanic cavity, attic, and antrum with the implanted Goodhill annular composite cartilage–perichondrium graft in a situation with total perforation and an intact stapes as the only ossicle. The ear canal skin and the epithelium from the eardrum were elevated and the annular graft was placed onto the fibrous annulus and covered with the epithelium. The perichondrium is in contact with the head of the stapes as a myringostapediopexy. Superiorly, at the pars flaccida region there is no cartilage.

References

Glasscock ME, Shea MC. Tragal cartilage as an ossicular substitute. Arch Otolaryngol 1967;86:308–317.

Goodhill V. Surgical correction of deafness. Annu Rev Med 1962;13:447–470.

Goodhill V. Tragal perichondrium and cartilage in tympanoplasty. Arch Otolaryngol 1967;85:480–491.

Goodhill V, Harris I, Brockman SJ. Tympanoplasty with perichondral graft. Arch Otolaryngol 1964;79:131–137.

Heermann J. [Experiences with free transplantation of facia-connective tissue of the temporalis muscle in tympanoplasty and reduction of the size of the radical cavity. Cartilage bridge from the stapes to the lower border of the tympanic membrane.] Z Laryngol Rhinol Otol 1962a;41:141–155.

Heermann J. [Tympanoplasty with enlargement of the tympanum into the auditory canal for the prevention of adhesions in poor mucosal relations or moderate tubal function.] Z Laryngol Rhinol Otol 1962b;41:235–241.

Heermann J. Trichterförmige Faszienplastik des Trommelfells aus mehreren Stücken mit Knorpelbrücke zum Stapes nach Radikaloperation des Ohres und das Gehör bei dickeren Trommelfell. Arch Ohren Nasen Kehlkopfheilkd 1962c;180:556–562.

Heermann J. [Syndesmosis in tympanic sclerosis. Lining atrophic scars and small perforations with inclusion of a cartilage bridge without scalping the ear drum. Leveling of the radical cavity.] Acta Otolaryngol 1963;56:1–10.

Heermann J. [Development from skin- to fascia- and to cartilage tympanoplasty (epitympanon-antrum-mastoidplasty) (author's transl.)] Laryngol Rhinol Otol (Stuttg) 1977;56:267–270.

Heermann J. Auricular cartilage palisade tympano-, epitympano-, antrum- and mastoid- plasties. Clin Otolaryngol Allied Sci 1978;3:443–446.

Heermann J. Autograft tragal and conchal palisade cartilage and Perichondrium in tympanomastoid reconstruction. Ear Nose Throat J 1992;71:344–349.

Heermann J, Heermann H. [Seven years of fascia-cartilage-tegmen tympanoplasty and antrum-mastoidoplasty] Z Laryngol Rhinol Otol 1967;46:370–382.

Heermann J, Heermann H, Kopfstein E. Fascia and cartilage palisade tympanoplasty. Nine years' experience. Arch Otolaryngol 1970;91:228–241.

Jansen C. Cartilage tympanoplasty. Laryngoscope 1963;73:1288–1302.

Pfatz CR, Piffko P. Substitution of the stapedial arch by free cartilage grafts. Arch Otolaryngol 1968;87:29–33.

Steinbach E, Pusalkar A. Long- term histological fate in ossicular reconstruction. J Laryngol Otol 1981;95:1031–1039.

Salen B. Myringoplasty using septum cartilage. Acta Otolaryngol 1964;(Suppl 188):82–93.

Tos M. Manual of Middle Ear Surgery. Vol. 1. Approaches, Myringoplasty, Ossiculoplasty, Tympanoplasty. New York: Thieme; 1993:245–382.

Tos M. Cartilage tympanoplasty methods: proposal of a classification. Otolaryngol Head Neck Surg 2008;139:747–58.

Utech H. [Tympanotomy in disorders of sound conduction; its diagnostic & therapeutic possibilities.] Z Laryngol Rhinol Otol 1959;38:212–221.

Utech H. [Improved final hearing results in tympanoplasty by changes in the operation technic.] Z Laryngol Rhinol Otol 1960;39:367–371.

Utech H. Über die Verwendung von Knorpelgewebe bei der Tympanoplastik und Stapeschirurgie. [Abstract] HNO 1961;9:232–233.

Waltner JG. Cartilage tympanoplasty. A new technique in ossicular problems. Ann Otol Rhinol Laryngol 1966;75:1117–1123.

2 Classifications and Definitions

Classification of Cartilage Tympanoplasty Methods

An exact classification of cartilage tympanoplasty methods is very important when presenting and elaborating new techniques. Furthermore, the methods should be widely known, discussed, and used in daily surgical practice. To initiate a discussion, I have made a classification of all the known cartilage tympanoplasty methods (Tos 2008). The various methods are divided into several main groups:

Group A: Cartilage tympanoplasty with palisades, strips, and slices
1. Cartilage palisades in underlay tympanoplasty techniques (Chapter 4).
2. Cartilage palisades in on-lay tympanoplasty techniques (Chapter 5).
3. Tympanoplasty with broad cartilage palisades (Chapter 6).
4. Cartilage strips in underlay tympanoplasty techniques (Chapter 7).
5. Cartilage strips in on-lay tympanoplasty techniques (Chapter 8).
6. The Dornhoffer underlay cartilage slice mosaic tympanoplasty (Chapter 9).

Group B: Cartilage tympanoplasty with foils, thin plates, and thick plates
7. Underlay tympanoplasty with cartilage foils and thin plates (Chapter 10).
8. On-lay tympanoplasty with cartilage foils and thin plates (Chapter 11).
9. On-lay tympanoplasty with thick cartilage plates (Chapter 12).
10. Underlay tympanoplasty with thick cartilage plates (Chapter 13).

Group C: Tympanoplasty with cartilage–perichondrium composite island grafts
11. Superior (attic) cartilage–perichondrium island graft tympanoplasty (Chapter 14).
12. Posterior cartilage–perichondrium composite island graft tympanoplasty (Chapter 15).
13. Superior and posterior cartilage–perichondrium composite island graft tympanoplasty (Chapter 16).
14. Total pars tensa cartilage–perichondrium composite island graft tympanoplasty (Chapter 17).

Group D: Tympanoplasty with special total pars tensa cartilage–perichondrium composite grafts
15. Annular cartilage–perichondrium composite graft tympanoplasty (Chapter 18).
16. "Crown cork" cartilage–perichondrium composite graft tympanoplasty (Chapter 19).
17. Cartilage shield T-tube tympanoplasty (Chapter 20).

Group E: Cartilage–perichondrium composite island graft tympanoplasty for anterior, inferior, and subtotal perforations
18. Underlay tympanoplasty techniques with cartilage–perichondrium composite island graft (Chapter 21).
19. In-lay underlay tympanoplasty techniques with cartilage–perichondrium composite island graft (Chapter 22).
20. On-lay tympanoplasty techniques with cartilage–perichondrium composite island graft (Chapter 23).
21. In-lay on-lay tympanoplasty techniques with cartilage–perichondrium composite island graft (Chapter 24).

Group F: Special cartilage tympanoplasty methods
22. In-lay butterfly cartilage tympanoplasty (Chapter 25).
23. Composite chondroperichondrial clip tympanoplasty: The triple "C" technique (Chapter 26).

For the oldest method, the cartilage palisade underlay tympanoplasty, some important modifications are described in Chapter 4, such as Ferekidis chondroplasty (Ferekidis et al. 2003), where the palisades are always placed under the bony annulus. In a further modification in which the palisades are covered by fascia or by perichondrium. Wiegand (1978) used palisades covered by perichondrium on both sides.

Cartilage Grafts

In contrast to the fascia and perichondrium grafts, cartilage grafts have many variations in their construction, thickness, and shape. Placement of the graft in relation to the eardrum remnant, fibrous annulus, and bony annulus may also vary. Here only a short overview of variations and definitions will be presented; the details will be pre-

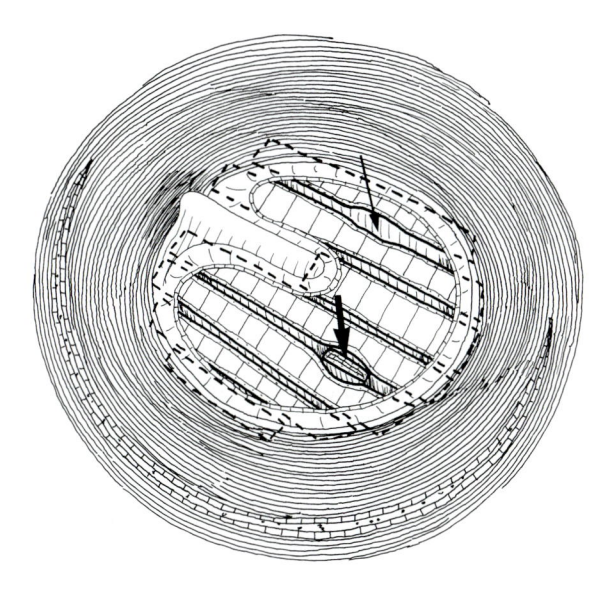

Fig. 2.1 Underlay palisade grafting of a total perforation with a relatively large distance between two palisades at two sites. The anterior site is closed spontaneously by the epithelium but represents a weak spot for later retraction (thin arrow). The posterior place has been closed immediately with a very small palisade (thick arrow).

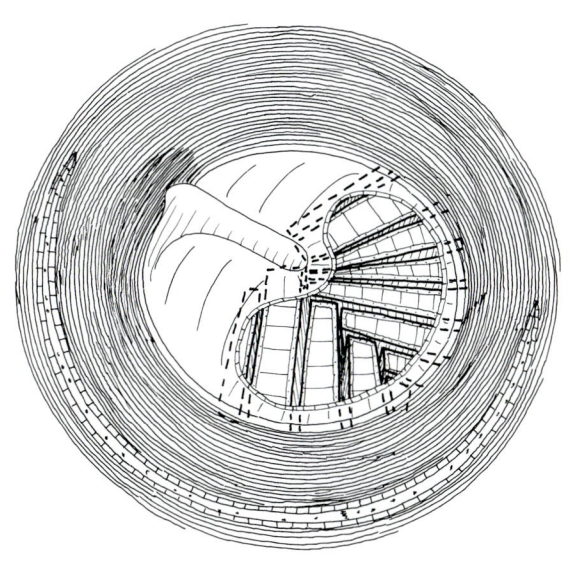

Fig. 2.2 Underlay palisade grafting of a large inferior perforation with oblique placement of the palisades centered on the umbo. Gelfoam balls support the palisades, especially around the umbo.

sented in the respective chapters as noted above. It is very important that all methods of cartilage tympanoplasty are clearly defined and classified so that they can be collated in the appropriate groups.

Cartilage Palisades

The 0.5–3 mm broad palisades of Heermann are placed close to each other, but there will always be a small distance between neighboring palisades. They are cut from a piece of tragal or conchal cartilage, covered on the concave side with the perichondrium. When placed into the tympanic cavity, the perichondrium is on the ear canal side only, promoting fibrous connection between the two parallel palisades and faster epithelialization. Such fibrous connections between the palisades are mostly very stable, but when the distance is 1 mm (**Fig. 2.1**) the fibrous connection may be only a thin membrane, with the attendant risk of a later retraction. Immediate closure of the defect between two palisades with a small palisade prevents retraction.

The length of the palisades depends on the size of the perforation.

Usually the palisades are placed in superoinferior direction but they can be placed in posteroanterior direction or oblique direction as well and can be connected to the umbo (**Fig. 2.2**). Some surgeons use Gelfoam balls placed in the tympanic cavity to support the palisades, others do not use Gelfoam. Some palisades will need support to stay in the proper position.

Small palisades of 0.5–3 mm can be applied to cover small bony defects around the tympanic cavity, such as a posterosuperior bony defect caused by drilling, or spontaneous defects of the scutum. Additionally, small palisades can bridge the defects from the annulus to the interposed ossicle in tympanoplasty type 2 or to the columella in tympanoplasty type 3 (see Chapters 4 and 5). Small defects between palisades or along their borders to the bone can be additionally covered with small palisades at any place.

Broad palisades of full cartilage thickness covered on the ear canal side with the perichondrium measure 3.5–5 mm in width (Bernal-Sprekelsen and Barberan 1997; Bernal-Sprekelsen et al. 1997, 2003). For reconstruction of the eardrum in a total perforation, only two or three palisades are used as underlay grafts (see Chapter 6).

Underlay Palisade Technique

Most surgeons used underlay grafting of the eardrum (Heermann and Heermann 1967; Heermann et al. 1970; Heermann 1977, 1978; Wiegand 1978; Amedee et al. 1989; Pere 1989; Heermann 1992; Milewski 1993; Helms 1995; Hildmann et al. 1996; Andersen et al. 2002, 2004; Uzun et al 2003; Neumann and Jahnke 2005; Tos et al. 2005). The anterior palisades are placed under the bony annulus (**Fig. 2.1**) and are supported by architrave (see Chapter 4) or Gelfoam. The posterior palisades are placed onto the bony annulus, but under the fibrous annulus and do not need a support. It is my own experience that the palisades in posterior perforation do not need to be placed onto the inferior bony annulus. Support with Gelfoam was suffi-

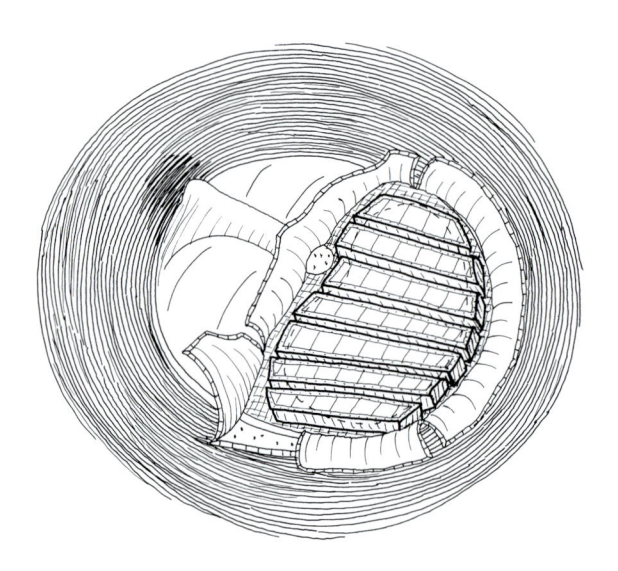

Fig. 2.3 On-lay palisade technique in a large inferior perforation. The epithelium is mostly elevated around the perforation and partly removed. A very small belt of the denuded eardrum is needed for placement of the palisades as on-lay grafts.

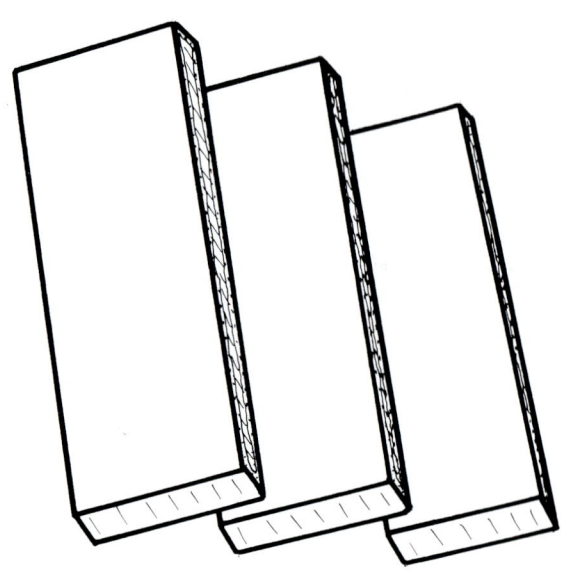

Fig. 2.4 Cartilage strips cut in an oblique manner. Using oblique cutting it is possible to cut thin and wide strips.

cient, and all palisades adhered to the under surface of the eardrum (Tos et al. 2005).

On-lay Palisade Technique

The on-lay technique seems to be a reliable technique (see Chapter 5) without risk of dislocation of the palisades into the tympanic cavity because, after elevation of the epithelium, the palisades are placed onto the denuded eardrum remnant or fibrous annulus (**Fig. 2.3**). The palisades can be thinned at the ends or even along the entire length depending on the size of the perforation. Some curling may be expected after thinning of the palisades. There is no need for support of the palisades in the tympanic cavity. My experience with on-lay cartilage palisade technique has been positive.

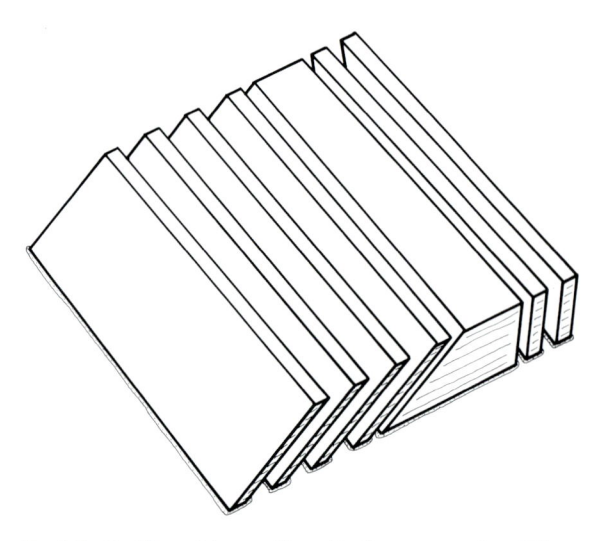

Fig. 2.5 Cartilage strips positioned in the manner of roof tiles.

Cartilage Strips

Cartilage strips (or slices) differ from the cartilage palisades in several ways:
a) The grafts, harvested from the tragus, concha, or cymba, are cut in an oblique manner, resulting in cartilage strips that are wider than the thickness of the original graft (**Fig. 2.4**).
b) The strips are thinner than the palisades and can be wide.
c) Successive strips are positioned on the edge of the previous strip, slightly overlapping like roof tiles (**Fig. 2.5**) (Neumann 1999).
d) The belt of perichondrium covering each cartilage strip on the ear canal side is considerably smaller than the perichondrium of the palisades, but the perichondrium is important for the epithelialization and nutrition of the cartilage.

Because of these differences, in particular the difference in positioning the strips by the "roof tiles method" and of the palisades according to the "close to each other method," these methods are dealt with in separate chapters. Even today there are very few papers on cartilage strips, but they will hopefully appear in the future and allow comparison of the results of these two distinct methods. The palisade technique is blamed for causing the thin mem-

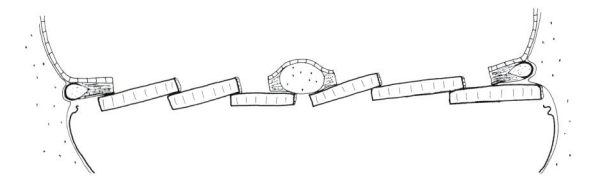

Fig. 2.6 Side view of the underlay cartilage strip method. The most anterior strip is placed under the bony annulus. The most posterior strip is placed under the eardrum remnant. The strips around the malleus can be placed under or at the level of the malleus handle.

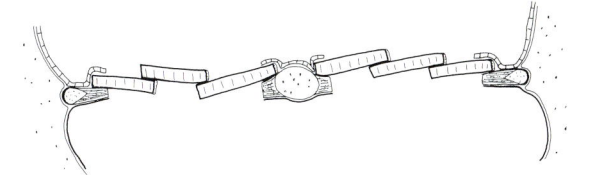

Fig. 2.7 The on-lay cartilage strip method. The posterior and anterior palisades are placed onto the lamina propria of the cleaned eardrum remnant. The epithelium of the eardrum remnant can be either elevated or removed.

branes between the palisades to retract and may lead to cholesteatoma, but such a membrane should not exist in the cartilage strips method.

Cartilage Strips in Underlay Technique

The positioning of the most anterior strip is under the bony annulus; the following strips are placed onto the bony annulus but under the fibrous annulus (**Fig. 2.6**) (see Chapter 7). Cartilage strips as underlay grafts were first used by Neumann (1999) and only a few reports on results have been published in recent years (Neumann et al. 2002, 2003; Kazikdas et al. 2007).

Cartilage Strips in On-lay Technique

Similarly to palisades, cartilage strips can also be applied in on-lay technique. The cartilage strips are placed onto the denuded lamina propria of the eardrum remnant (**Fig. 2.7**). The epithelium of the eardrum remnant is either removed or elevated. There are no publications on the on-lay cartilage strip method, but I have used the on-lay technique with cartilage strips relatively often during the last 4 years. The method used in various pathologies will be described and illustrated in Chapter 8.

Underlay Cartilage Slice Mosaic Tympanoplasty Techniques

The full-thickness slices (or pieces) of cartilage, covered on the ear canal side with the perichondrium, are pieced together, like the pieces of a jigsaw puzzle (Chapter 9), to reconstruct a total perforation. In contrast to the strict Heermann technique, the Dornhoffer mosaic technique is more "liberal," allowing slices of various shapes and sizes (Dornhoffer 1997, 2000, Danner and Dornhoffer 2001).

The Dornhoffer mosaic cartilage tympanoplasty can be applied as an on-lay method as well, by placing the cartilage slices onto the denuded lamina propria of the eardrum remnant, but apparently no-one has yet tried this method.

Cartilage Foils, Thin Plates, and Thick Plates

Cartilage foils are thin plates of cartilage without perichondrium of thickness 0.2–0.3 mm. They may be of various shapes and various sizes. Some are elongated, like lamellae; some have a size of a quarter of the eardrum; the largest may measure 1 cm × 1 cm. The thickness of the normal eardrum is 0.1 mm; thus the eardrum reconstructed with foils of the indicated thickness will still be thicker than a normal eardrum but it will have the acoustic quality of a normal eardrum. Thin cartilage plates may have a thickness of 0.4 mm and may be applied in similar way to the method for strips, i.e. overlapping (**Figs. 2.8a, b, 2.9**).

The foils and thin plates are usually cut with the Kurz Precise Cartilage Knife (Kurz Medical, Dusslingen, Germany). The placement of the foils is similar to placement of a dried fascia graft. They can be placed as underlay or as on-lay grafts (see Chapters 10 and 11). One may expect papers giving methods and results to appear in the literature in the future. The foils were introduced and used by K. B. Hüttenbrink (personal communication, 2001) in Dresden and by his co-workers (Mürbe et al. 2002). Experimentally, the Dresden group has shown that in poor tubal function an overlapping placement of thin cartilage foils, like the leaves of a tulip, can provide good stabilization of the reconstructed eardrum (Mürbe et al. 2002).

Half-thickness plates of 0.5 mm, three-quarter-thickness plates of 0.6–0.8 mm, and full-thickness plates are not covered with the perichondrium. They are applied in a similar way as composite grafts. The methods using thick cartilage plates are illustrated in Chapter 22.

Underlay Technique with Cartilage Foils and Thin Plates

As in underlay techniques with fascia or perichondrium, the tympanomeatal flap with the eardrum remnant has to be elevated and the foils adapted to the undersurface of the eardrum remnant, which with large foils may be more difficult than with large fascia. Accordingly, several small foils may be placed to cover a total perforation (**Fig. 2.8**). Using three foils, for example, the second foil is partly placed under the first foil and the third foil is partly placed

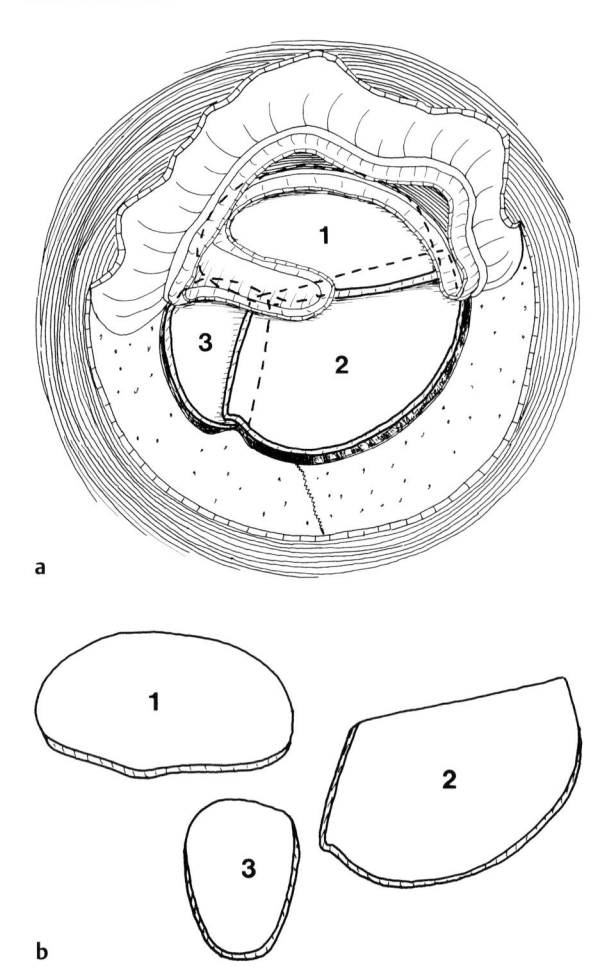

Fig. 2.8a, b Underlay technique with cartilage foils in a total perforation and intact ossicular chain. Removal of the edges of the perforation and scarification of the mucosa of the medial surface of the eardrum remnant provides a better attachment of the naked cartilage (without perichondrium) foils as expected, but Gelfoam balls can be placed into the tympanic cavity for support. The anterosuperior foil (1) is placed first and is supported by Gelfoam. The posteroinferior foil (2) is placed partly under the first and partly over the third foil (3). The posterior foil partly overlaps the posteroinferior foil.

under the second foil so that the foils are "underlapping" each other (Chapter 10).

On-lay Technique with Cartilage Foils and Thin Plates

The cartilage foils are placed onto the denuded eardrum remnant (**Fig. 2.9**). The foils can be cut exactly in relation to the size of the perforation and the overlapping of the foils can easily be performed. No support of the foils is needed. In fascia tympanoplasty of anterior, inferior, subtotal, and total perforations, I prefer transcanal on-lay techniques, mainly because such methods are minimally invasive and need no support. Cartilage foils seem to be a good material

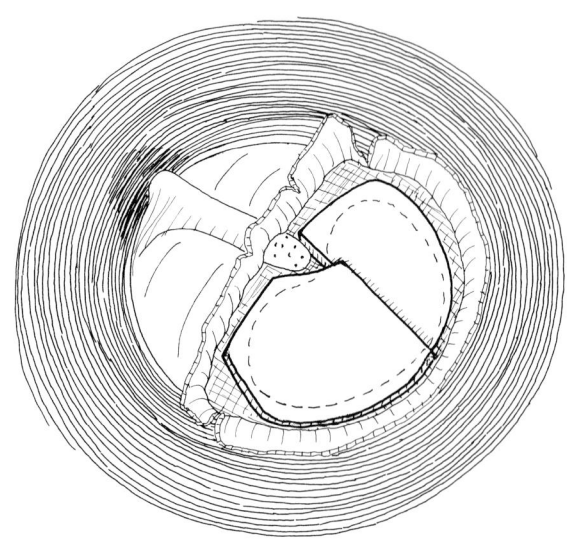

Fig. 2.9 On-lay technique with cartilage foils in an inferior perforation. The epithelium is elevated as flaps all the way around the perforation. The anterior foil covers the anterior half of the perforation. The posterior foil partly overlaps the anterior foil. The epithelial flaps are replaced.

for on-lay closure of any perforation, regardless of size (Chapter 11)

On-lay Tympanoplasty with Thick Cartilage Plates

"Cartilage plate" denotes a cartilage disk of a thickness between 0.4 and 1.1 mm (**Fig. 2.10**), but without attached perichondrium. The thickness of a plate may vary at different locations on the plate, depending on the cuts made with the scalpel. The on-lay tympanoplasty with cartilage plates had already been used since the early 1960s (Jansen 1963, 1968; Kleinsasser and Glanschneider 1969; Kleinfeldt et al. 1975). The cartilage plates are placed onto the denuded edge of the lamina propria.

Cartilage plates differ considerably from the cartilage composite island grafts suspended by perichondrium flaps. Also, at the end of the tympanoplasty the cartilage plates are covered with fascia or with free perichondrium (Chapter 12).

Underlay Technique with Thick Plates

In the underlay technique, the cartilage plates are of the same thickness as in the on-lay technique. Martin (1979) applied cartilage plates in the reinforcement of the eardrum. Puls (2003), in 161 patients, presented good results with reconstruction of the eardrum with cartilage plates without perichondrium (see Chapter 13). The cartilage plates are placed as an underlay graft and covered with perichondrium or fascia.

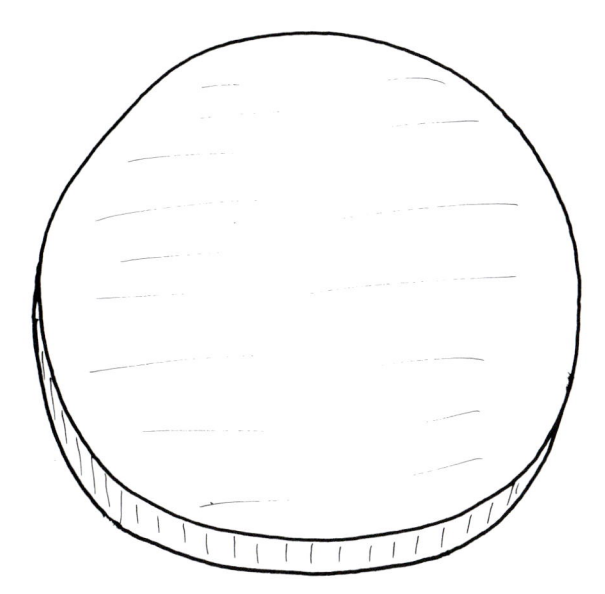

Fig. 2.10 Cartilage plate of half to full thickness, most often without perichondrium, cut usually with a scalpel or with the Kurz Precise Cartilage Knife (Kurz Medical, Dusslingen, Germany).

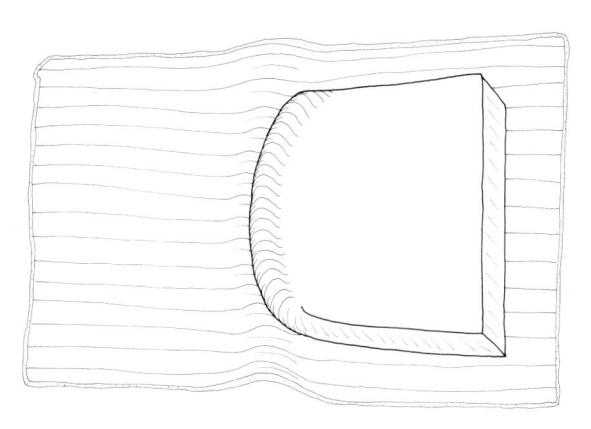

Fig. 2.12 Very large superior composite cartilage–perichondrium island graft. The graft includes the dome of the tragus and the perichondrium from both sides of the cartilage as a large perichondrium flap.

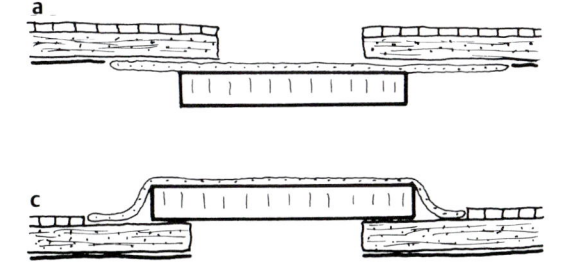

Fig. 2.11a–d The four methods of application of the various composite cartilage–perichondrium flaps.
a Underlay island graft with relatively large perichondrium flaps.
b In-lay underlay graft. The cartilage disk is positioned in the perforation and is covered with perichondrium on both sides. The perichondrium flaps are under the eardrum.
c On-lay island graft placed onto the edges of the perforation. The perichondrium flap is placed onto the denuded eardrum remnant.
d In-lay on-lay graft with the cartilage disk placed into the perforation and the perichondrium flap onto the denuded eardrum. The perichondrium flap may be partly covered by the epithelial flaps of the eardrum.

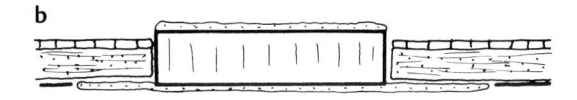

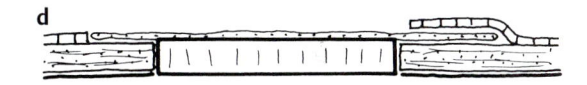

Cartilage–Perichondrium Composite Island Grafts

A cartilage–perichondrium composite (or compound) island graft is defined as a piece of cartilage covered on one side with perichondrium, which surrounds the cartilage disk as a flap and fixates or suspends the cartilage disk (**Fig. 2.11a–d**). There are large differences between the various grafts in the shape and size of the cartilage as well as of the surrounding perichondrium. The differences depend on location and function of the graft. All island grafts should prevent retraction and all—except the attic island graft—should also optimally vibrate and transmit the sound. All pars tensa grafts are supposed to vibrate.

Superior or Attic Composite Island Graft

The function of the superior or attic island graft is primarily to prevent a postoperative attic retraction but also to maintain a smooth superior ear canal wall, facilitating proper epithelial migration and self-cleaning of the ear canal. Attic grafts are of various shapes and sizes to fit into the superior bony defect (see Chapter 14). The perichondrium flaps are as large as possible (McCleve 1969), especially the superior flap (**Fig. 2.12**). Some surgeons make double flaps by using perichondrium from both sides of the cartilage (Fleury et al.1974), others cover the attic island graft with fascia (Adkins and Osguthorpe 1984).

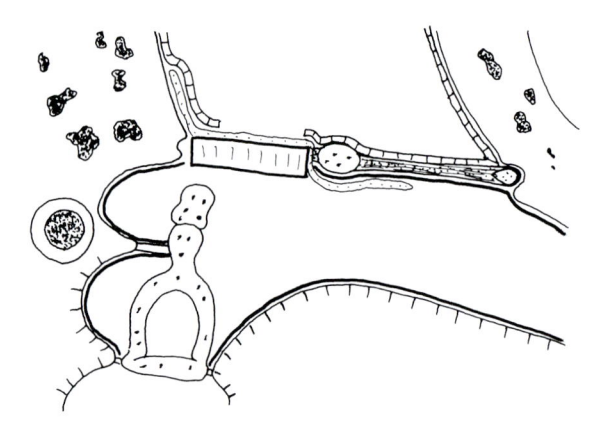

Fig. 2.13 Posterosuperior composite cartilage–perichondrium island graft. The graft consists of an oval cartilage disk and is placed between the malleus handle and the posterior bony annulus. On the ear canal side, the cartilage is covered with perichondrium, which continues in an anterior flap placed under the eardrum and in a posterior flap placed on the posterior ear canal wall.

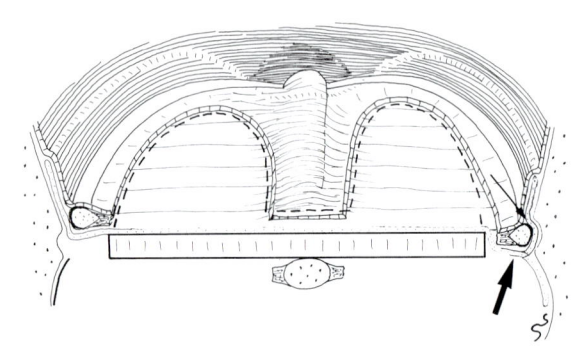

Fig. 2.14 Side view with some perspective at the level of the umbo of a total pars tensa cartilage–perichondrium island graft, positioned as an underlay graft. Posteriorly the perichondrium is placed under the fibrous annulus and onto the bony annulus and ear canal bone. Anteriorly, the perichondrium is also placed under the fibrous annulus and either onto the bony annulus and the anterior ear canal bone (thin arrow) or under the bony annulus and the anterior wall of the tympanic cavity (thick arrow).

Posterior Composite Island Graft

A posterior cartilage–perichondrium composite island graft (Linde 1973; Martin 1979; Glasscock et al. 1982) is employed relatively often and prevents the common posterosuperior retraction. The composite island graft consists of an oval cartilage disk, covered and surrounded by a perichondrium flap (see Chapter 15). The small inferior and superior perichondrium flaps cover the inferior and superior edges of the perforation. The anterior flap covers the undersurface of the malleus handle and the longest posterior flap covers the posterior ear canal wall (**Fig. 2.13**).

Posterior and Superior or Attic Composite Island Graft

In case of attic retraction or attic cholesteatoma and posterosuperior retraction in the same ear operated at the same time (see Chapter 16), one graft has been fashioned to cover both retractions or both bony defects with one graft only. Two such grafts are described (Levinson 1987; Poe and Gadre 1993) (see **Figs. 16.1, 16.2**), but they are apparently not often used. Most surgeons prefer a separate attic island graft and a separate posterosuperior island graft.

Total Pars Tensa Composite Island Graft

The total pars tensa composite cartilage–perichondrium island graft covers the entire tympanic cavity and is suspended by the perichondrium flap. At the beginning, the perichondrium flap is placed as an on-lay graft onto the anterior and posterior fibrous annulus (Tolsdorff 1983; Nitsche 1985). Most often, the graft is positioned as an underlay graft, i.e., the perichondrium flap is placed anteriorly under the fibrous annulus, but either onto or under the bony annulus (**Fig. 2.14**).

Principally, the cartilage disks of a total pars tensa composite graft are round, measuring 7–9 mm in diameter (Tolsdorff 1983), but to accommodate the graft to the malleus handle, wedges of cartilage of various sizes or shapes are excised (Nitsche 1985). Dornhoffer (1997, 2000, 2006) excises a 1–2 mm wide belt of cartilage. Jahnke excises three very small belts of cartilage, resulting in four cartilage belts (Neumann and Jahnke 2005) (**Fig. 2.15a–d**). The Dornhoffer graft and the Jahnke graft are far more flexible during insertion than the Tolsdorff and Nitsche grafts.

Special Cartilage–Perichondrium Composite Island Grafts

Special composite grafts are used in special situations and have special constructions. An **annular graft** has the shape of a ring; it is placed onto or instead of the fibrous annulus in total and subtotal perforations. A **crown cork graft** is a total pars tensa graft with very long perichondrium flaps applied in acquired and congenital atresias and blunting of the external auditory canal. In a **cartilage shield T-tube graft**, a T-tube is incorporated for permanent ventilation of the middle ear cavity.

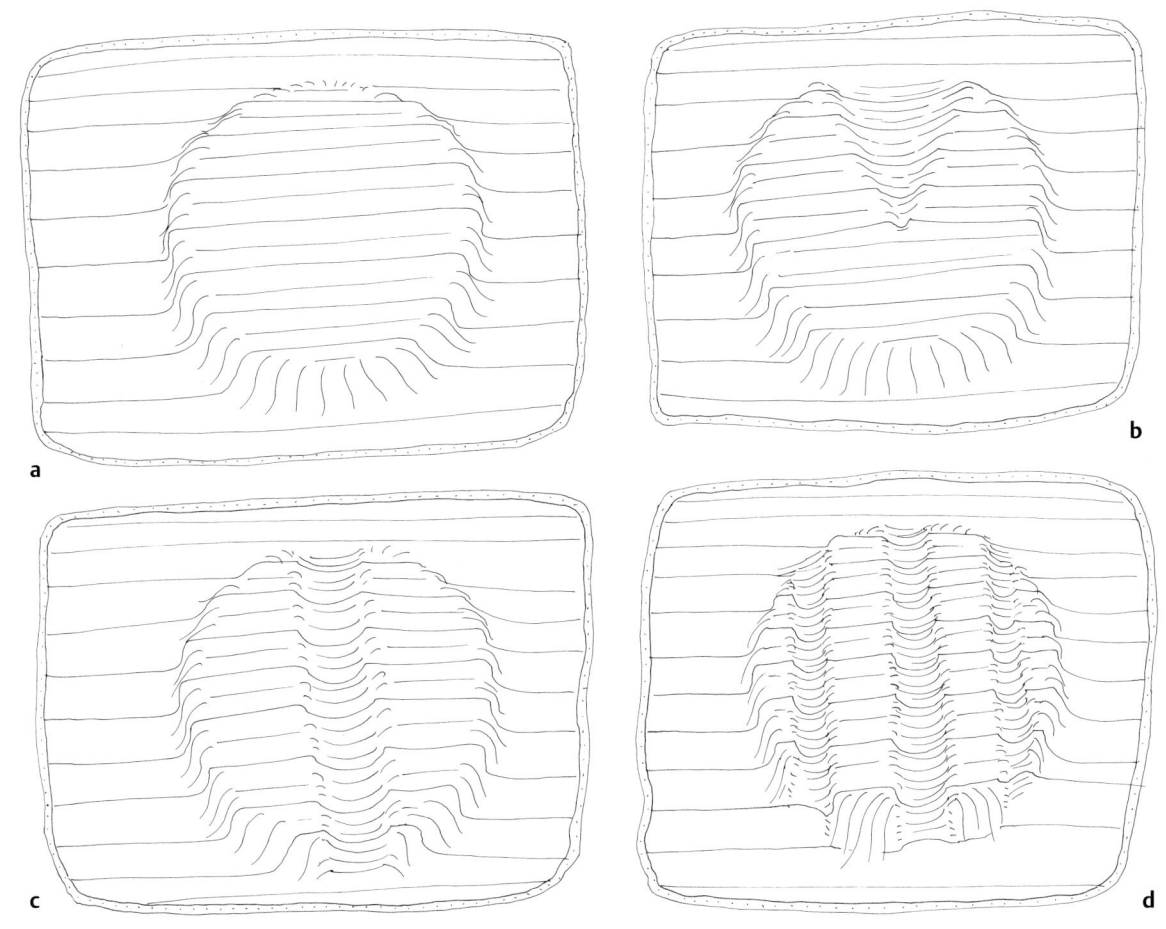

Fig. 2.15a–d The four types of a total pars tensa cartilage–perichondrium island graft.
a The round cartilage disk without a wedge.
b Nitsche graft with a wedge.
c Dornhoffer graft.
d Jahnke graft.

Annular Graft

The annular cartilage–perichondrium composite graft was the very first composite cartilage–perichondrium graft (Goodhill 1967). It is a 1.5–3 mm wide, horseshoe-shaped, circular, or U-shaped cartilage ring attached to perichondrium which continues beyond the cartilage as a circumferential peripheral extension. The cartilage ring of the annular graft is placed either onto the fibrous or the bony annulus or into the tympanic cavity at the level of the bony annulus (**Fig. 2.16**). The central perichondrium serves as the eardrum and is placed either under or onto the malleus handle. The peripheral perichondrium is placed onto the bone of the ear canal, suspending and stabilizing the cartilage ring (see Chapter 18).

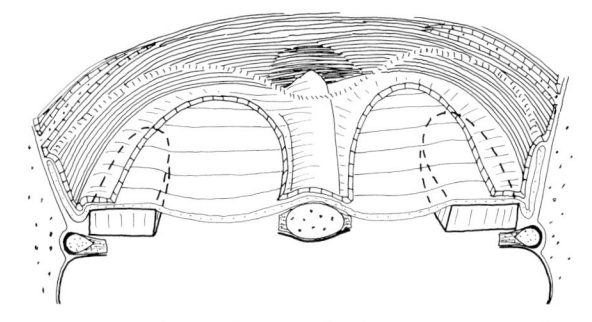

Fig. 2.16 Annular cartilage–perichondrium composite graft in total perforation. Side view with some perspective. The on-lay cartilage graft is placed onto the fibrous annulus and eardrum remnant. The central perichondrium is placed onto the denuded malleus handle; the peripheral flap is placed onto the bone of the ear canal.

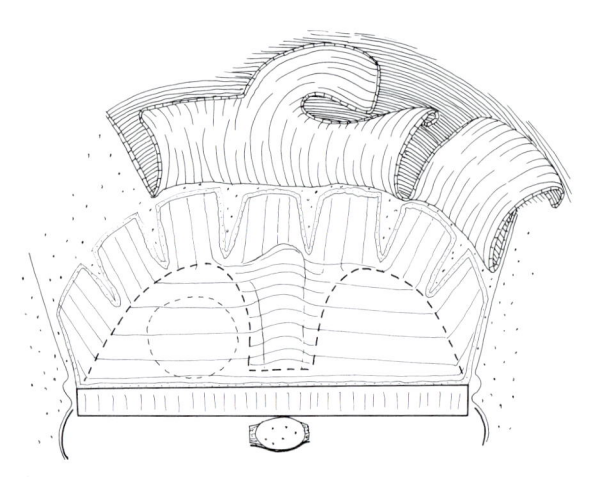

Fig. 2.17 Crown cork cartilage–perichondrium tympanoplasty in total perforation with missing stapes arch and incus and with severe blunting of the anterior ear canal. A rectangular wedge in the cartilage disk is made to accommodate the malleus handle. The cartilage–perichondrium graft is placed into the tympanic cavity at the level of the bony annulus and the large perichondrium flaps are folded out to cover the denuded ear canal bone all the way around.

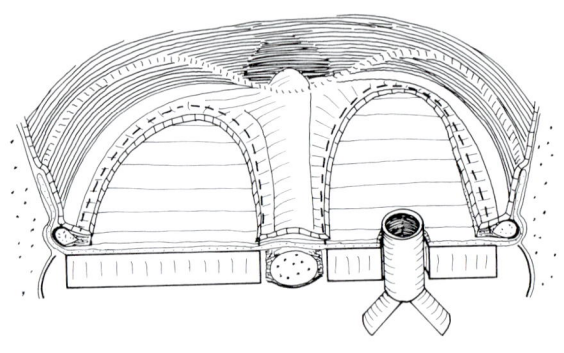

Fig. 2.18 Side view with some perspective in total perforation and poor tubal function closed with a Dornhoffer cartilage shield T- tube composite island graft. The tube is placed in the anterior part of the cartilage graft. The graft is suspended by the perichondrium.

Crown Cork Graft

The graft consists of a round piece of cartilage, covered on the ear canal side with perichondrium, which continues in large peripheral, radial perichondrium flaps, resembling a crown cork (**Fig. 2.17**) (Hartwein et al. 1992). The diameter of the cartilage is 9 mm, slightly smaller than the diameter of the ear canal at the level of the bony annulus. Indications for crown cork tympanoplasty are conditions with involvement of the ear canal and the eardrum. These conditions include congenital and acquired atresia and severe blunting (see Chapter 19).

Cartilage Shield T-Tube Graft

A T-tube is incorporated in this total pars tensa cartilage–perichondrium island graft,. Such a graft is placed into the tympanic cavity at the level of the bony annulus. The cartilage disk with the T-tube is suspended by the surrounding perichondrium flap, placed onto the ear canal bone (**Fig. 2.18**). The goal of placement of the permanent tube is the prevention of repeated insertions of ventilating tubes, especially in children with severe chronic secretory otitis media (Hall 1990). In adults, Duckert, Müller, Makielski, and Helms (1995) used a cartilage–T-tube device for the long-term ventilation of the tympanic cavity in cases with total perforation of the eardrum and chronically severe poor tubal function. Danner and Dornhoffer (2001) used the cartilage shield T-tube in selected cases, such as craniofacial abnormalities, Down syndrome, nasopharyngeal adenoid cystic carcinoma, and previous head and neck cancer involving the nasopharynx, and in patients with recurrences of chronic otitis media and a history of multiple surgery (see Chapter 20).

Composite Island Grafts for Minor, Medium-sized, and Subtotal Perforations

Very little has been published on the four techniques described in the following, which are mainly applied in anterior, inferior, and subtotal perforations. There may be several reasons, for example, posterior retraction or perforation is well treated with a posterior composite cartilage–perichondrium island graft as an underlay technique, or subtotal and total perforations are treated with a composite island graft, mainly as an underlay technique.

Two of the four techniques that need to be mentioned here are mainly underlay techniques: the **pure underlay technique** (see **Fig. 2.11a**) for all types of perforation of various sizes (see Chapter 21) and the **in-lay underlay technique** (see **Fig. 2.11b**) for posterior, anterior, inferior, and subtotal perforations, which is also sometimes used for total perforation (see Chapter 22).

The two other techniques are mainly on-lay techniques: The **on-lay technique** (see **Fig. 2.11c** and Chapter 23) and the **in-lay on-lay technique** (see **Fig. 2.11d** and Chapter 24) are used in anterior and inferior perforations as well as occasionally in subtotal and total perforations. Both methods are, in my opinion, able to compete in the future with the underlay total pars tensa island graft method (see Chapter 17).

Underlay Technique

The underlay cartilage–perichondrium composite island graft technique is similar to tympanoplasty with underlay placement of fascia or perichondrium. After cleansing of the edges of the perforation, the tympanomeatal flap is elevated, the mucosa around the perforation is scarified or removed, and a cartilage–perichondrium composite island graft is placed under the perforation (**Fig. 2.19**). In my practice I support the graft with Gelfoam (see Chapter 21). The thickness of the cartilage disk may be half or one-third of the thickness of the tragus.

In-lay Underlay Technique

In the in-lay underlay technique with a composite cartilage-perichondrium island graft, the perichondrium flaps lie under the eardrum remnant, while the cartilage disk is positioned into the perforation (**Fig. 2.20**). The surgical principles and methods are the same as for the underlay technique, but instead of placement of the cartilage disk under the edges of the perforation, it can be pushed though the perforation. The cartilage disk may even be suspended from the edges of the perforation and support of the graft with Gelfoam may not be necessary (see Chapter 22).

On-lay Technique

The on-lay technique with a composite cartilage–perichondrium island graft is similar to fascia or perichondrium grafting: Epithelium has to be elevated or removed from a 1–3 mm belt around the perforation and the edges of the perforation have to be cleaned as well (**Fig. 2.21**). A full-thickness graft or a half- or one-third-thickness graft can be placed onto the edges of the perforation surrounded by the perichondrium flap (see Chapter 23). The most appropriate thickness will be a half- or one-third-thickness graft because a small or medium-sized perforation does not need a thick cartilage slice.

In-lay On-lay Technique

The cartilage disk of the in-lay on-lay graft is placed into the perforation; the surrounding perichondrium is placed onto the denuded eardrum remnant (**Fig. 2.22**). This technique is a transcanal, minimal invasive on-lay technique, without a larger skin incision and without entering the tympanic cavity. The epithelium surrounding the perforation is usually elevated and replaced onto the perichondrium with fast and safe reepithelialization (see Chapter 24).

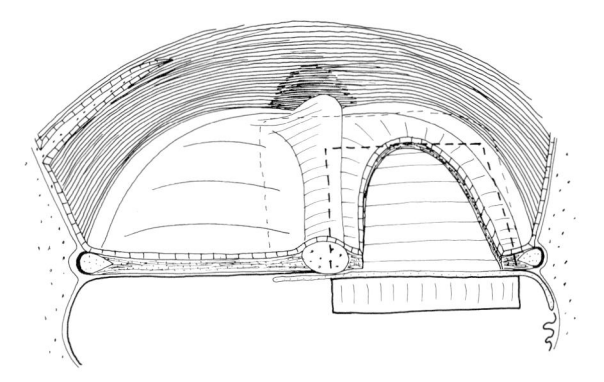

Fig. 2.19 Underlay technique for closure of an anterior perforation with a cartilage–perichondrium composite island graft; side view with some perspective. The graft is placed under the malleus handle and under the anterior eardrum remnant and onto the mucosa.

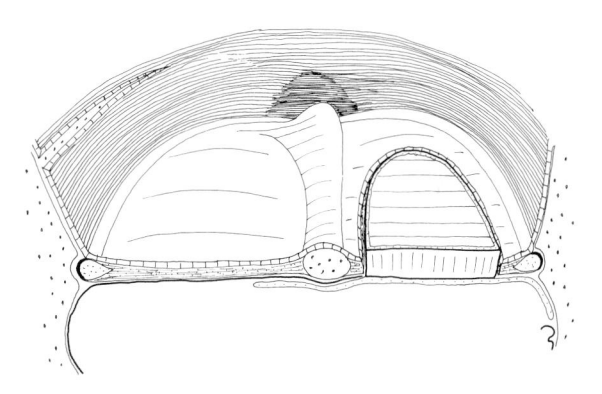

Fig. 2.20 In-lay underlay technique in closure of an anterior perforation. The cartilage disk is placed into the perforation and protrudes slightly into the ear canal. The perichondrium flap is placed under the eardrum remnant.

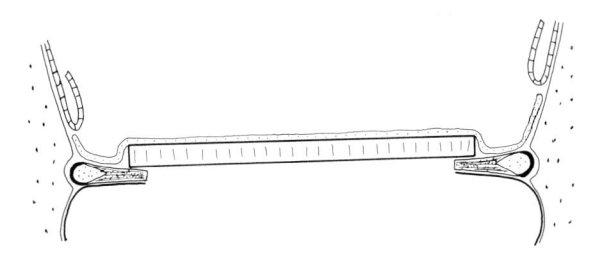

Fig. 2.21 On-lay technique with a thinned cartilage–perichondrium composite island graft in closure of an inferior perforation. The epithelium around the perforation is elevated. A composite island graft with a thinned cartilage disk is placed onto the edge of the perforation. The perichondrium flap is folded out over the denuded eardrum. The elevated epithelial flaps will be replaced.

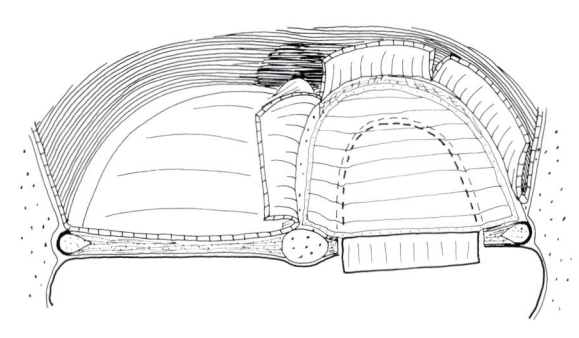

Fig. 2.22 In-lay on-lay cartilage–perichondrium island graft in an anterior perforation; side view with some perspective. The epithelium around the perforation is elevated, the cartilage disk is placed into the perforation, the perichondrium is placed onto the denuded eardrum, and the epithelial flaps are replaced.

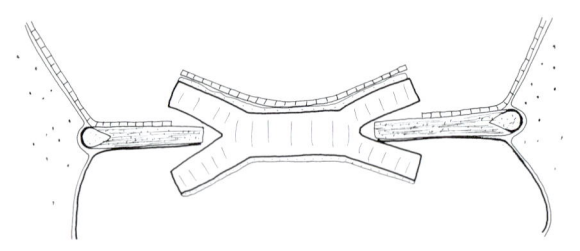

Fig. 2.23 Side view of the Eavey butterfly graft placed in a relatively large inferior perforation. The diameter of the graft is 2 mm larger than the diameter of the perforation. A split-skin graft is placed onto the graft.

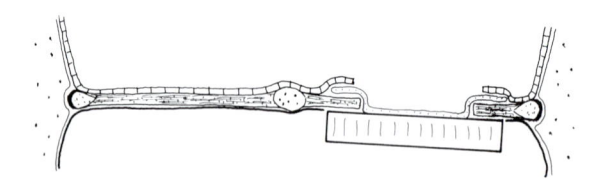

Fig. 2.24 Composite chondroepithelial clip tympanoplasty (triple "C" technique) of an anterior perforation, side view. The cartilage disk is larger than the extent of the perforation. It is positioned as an underlay graft under the eardrum and is suspended by the perichondrium positioned as an on-lay graft on the denuded remnant of the eardrum.

Special Cartilage Methods in Small and Medium-Sized Perforations

In recent years some new cartilage tympanoplasty methods have been presented as minimally invasive transcanal procedures without incision or tympanotomy. The indications were closure of small or medium-sized dry perforations with intact ossicular chain.

Butterfly Technique

This technique is partly an on-lay technique, partly an underlay technique, but most of the graft lies on the level of the eardrum as an in-lay graft (**Fig. 2.23**). The graft resembles a grommet without a hole. A round piece of cartilage covered on both sides with perichondrium is cut in the middle, parallel to the perichondrium on either side (see Chapter 25). The circumferentially incised edges of the cartilage curl apart, like the wings of a butterfly, hence the name "in-lay butterfly technique" (Eavey 1998). The graft is larger then the perforation and is rotated into the perforation.

Methods of closure of large perforations with the butterfly graft have been published recently (Ghanem et al. 2006).

Even if the cartilage disk is covered on both sides with perichondrium, the graft is not a composite graft because it does not have a perichondrium flap and is not suspended by one.

Triple "C" technique

The triple "C" technique of Fernandes (2003) is an on-lay and an underlay technique (**Fig. 2.24**). The three "C"s derive from "composite chondroperichondrial clip tympanoplasty." The 2 mm larger cartilage disk is positioned under the eardrum, the perichondrium covers the lateral side of the cartilage, but a 1 mm belt of the perichondrium has been elevated from the cartilage, resulting in a perichondrium flap. This flap, as an on-lay graft, covers a belt of 1 mm of the denuded eardrum remnant. The cartilage is suspended by the perichondrium and the graft is a special composite island graft (see Chapter 26).

Classification of Tympanoplasty

Cartilage Tympanoplasty

The term *cartilage tympanoplasty* covers any reconstruction of the eardrum with cartilage, either with or without perichondrium. Reconstruction of the superior or of the posterior scutum in connection with the reconstruction of the eardrum with cartilage will also be called cartilage tympanoplasty. Major reconstruction of the ear canal with cartilage will be called cartilage tympanoplasty with cartilage meatoplasty.

Classification of Tympanoplasty in Relation to Ossiculoplasty

Several classifications of tympanoplasty have been devised and used during the last 60 years. They are described and discussed in detail in *Manual of Middle Ear Surgery*, volume 1 (Tos 1993). Here only the classic tympanoplasty classification used internationally will be described. Other classifications are described and discussed in Tos 1993).

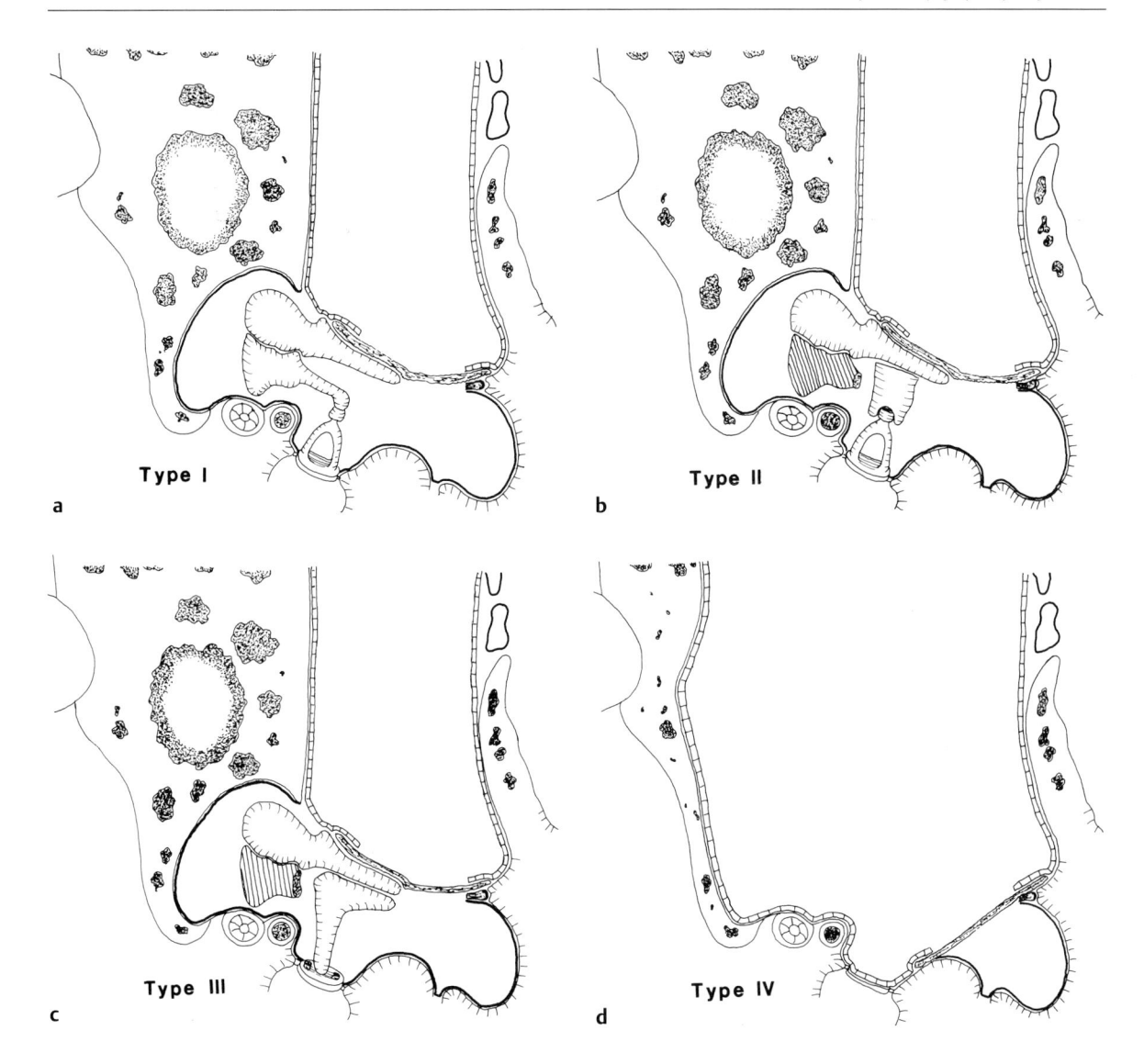

Fig. 2.25a–d The most common classification of tympanoplasty into four types in relation to ossiculoplasty.
a **Type 1,** with intact ossicular chain.
b **Type 2** with interposition of a prosthesis between the stapes and the eardrum and/or the malleus handle.
c **Type 3**, with a columella between the footplate and the eardrum and/or the malleus handle.
d **Type 4**, with a mobile footplate and sound protection of the round window with a graft, and formation of an air space in the hypotympanum and anterior tympanum. The footplate is covered with keratinized epithelium.

Tympanoplasty Type 1

Tympanoplasty type 1 is a procedure resulting in an **intact ossicular chain** at the end of the operation (**Fig. 2.25a**). Such an operation can be very easy (removal of some remnants of previous retraction or some adhesions), but it can also be extremely difficult because the surgeon needs to preserve the ossicular chain. It is my strong opinion that the surgeon should do everything possible to keep the ossicular chain intact. All our clinical studies and others have shown better primary and long-term hearing results with an intact ossicular chain than with an interrupted chain in various conditions such as cholesteatoma (Tos and Lau 1991), bony fixations (Tos 1970), adhesive otitis (Tos 1972), and tympanosclerosis (Tos et al. 1990).

Tympanoplasty Type 2

Tympanoplasty type 2 denotes **interposition** of a prosthesis between the stapes and the eardrum and/or the malleus handle (**Fig. 2.25b**). In cases with a defective long process of the incus, or even with missing stapes head and stapes neck, interposition between the stapes and the eardrum and/or malleus handle is possible with reasonably good results. The interposition graft, such as an autogenous incus, can be placed either onto the head or

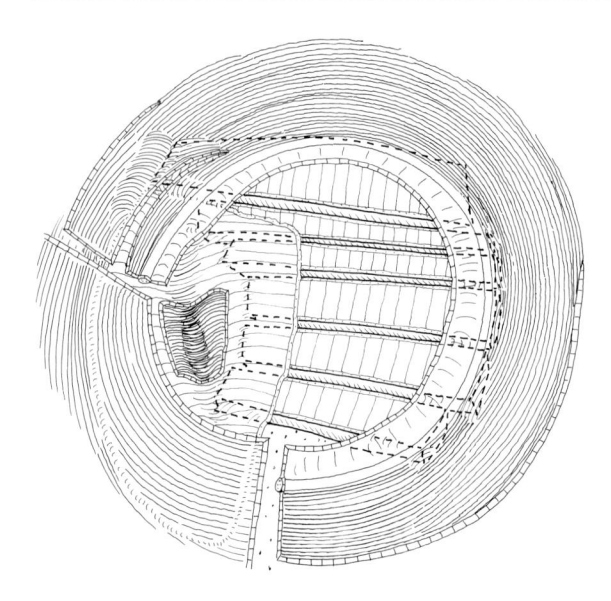

Fig. 2.26 The Heermann cartilage tympanoplasty of type 4 in a case without ossicles. After elevation of a large inferior and a shorter superior flap, the anterior palisade is placed under the bony annulus and onto a piece of cartilage placed onto the eminence of the tensor tympani muscle. The other palisades are placed onto the inferior bony annulus. The superior ends of the palisades are placed onto the medial wall of the tympanic cavity, isolating the anterior and inferior parts of the tympanic cavity with the round window and the entrance of eustachian tube. The superior ends of the palisades are covered with perichondrium; the footplate and the oval window region are covered with a split-skin graft. The epithelium from the eardrum remnants covers the inferior ends of the palisades.

onto the neck of the stapes. The graft may be shaped in different ways: Various grooves may be formed on the incus or malleus head or on cortical bone to accommodate the stapes head or the stapes neck.

Even in partial resorption of the arch of the stapes, the ossicles can be shaped in a special way to interpose the graft between the stapes remnant and the eardrum.

All interposition techniques are described and illustrated in Tos (1993).

Tympanoplasty Type 3

In tympanoplasty type 3, the footplate is connected to the eardrum with a columella (**Fig. 2.25c**). A **columella** is often a shaped autogenous or homogenous incus or autogenous cortical bone. Shaping of columellae is described in detail in Tos (1993).

A columella of cartilage is seldom applied nowadays because it becomes soft after some years (Steinbach and Pusalkar 1981; Steinbach et al. 1992); see Chapter 27.

Columellae of biocompatible materials, such as hydroxyapatite, glass ceramic, or ionomer cement are still used in some countries. They are also described in Tos 1993) and should be covered with cartilage.

Metallic prostheses, in particular the titanium prosthesis, consist of a foot that is placed onto the footplate and a round head that is covered with a separate cartilage plate. Often the round head of the prosthesis is placed under the cartilage disk of the cartilage–perichondrium composite graft; here either the posterior graft (see Chapter 15), the total pars tensa graft (see Chapter 17), or one of the special grafts, such as the annular graft (see Chapter 18), the crown cork graft (see Chapter19), or the cartilage shield T-tube graft (see Chapter 20), can be used.

Although hearing with some columellae may be surprisingly good in some cases, hearing results with columellae of tympanoplasty type 3 are generally poorer than with interpositions in tympanoplasty type 2.

Furthermore, the long-term stability of a tympanoplasty type 3 with a columella is poorer than that of a tympanoplasty type 2 with an interposition. This is logical because the movements of the footplate via the stapes are more physiological than the movements of the footplate via the columella. If the stapes is present, I will accordingly try to perform a tympanoplasty type 2 with an interposition of an autogenous prosthesis rather than with a columella.

Tympanoplasty Type 4

In tympanoplasty type 4, no ossiculoplasty is performed but the round window is protected so that sound pressure is not allowed to act at the same time on the oval and the round windows (**Fig. 2.25 d**). If the footplate is mobile and exposed to sound, and if the round window is protected against sound pressure by creating a ventilated cavity involving the anterior parts of the tympanic cavity, which is connected to the eustachian tube, hearing of 30 dB can be achieved. The surgical steps of a tympanoplasty type 4 are illustrated in Tos (1993). Here only the modification of the classic cartilage tympanoplasty type 4 as performed by Heermann and Heermann (1967) is shown (**Fig. 2.26**).

Tympanoplasty Type 5A and Type 5B

Tympanoplasty type 5A denotes fenestration of the lateral semicircular canal in cases with a fixated footplate and with no ossicles. This type of tympanoplasty is not done nowadays and has no connection with cartilage tympanoplasty. The method is illustrated in Tos (1993).

Tympanoplasty type 5B denotes a platinectomy in cases with fixed footplate and no ossicles. The tympanoplasty type 5B has completely replaced type 5A. In type 5B, removal of the fixed footplate—a platinectomy—is performed. The round window can be covered with fascia or perichondrium and a split-skin graft. The round window has to be protected in a similar way as in a cartilage tympanoplasty type 4 (**Fig. 2.26**).

Another way is to reconstruct the eardrum and to connect it with the open oval window. The safest method is to fill out the oval window niche with fatty tissue and bring the fatty tissue into connection with a vibrating eardrum. This is performed by placement of additional fatty tissue in the posterosuperior part of the tympanic cavity.

Pictorial Key to the Drawings in this Book

To avoid overcrowding of the drawings with repetitive labels, the following section provides a pictorial key to the representation of the different elements and structures that are contained in the drawings (**Figs. 2.27–2.39**).

Pieces of Cartilage and Cartilage Palisades

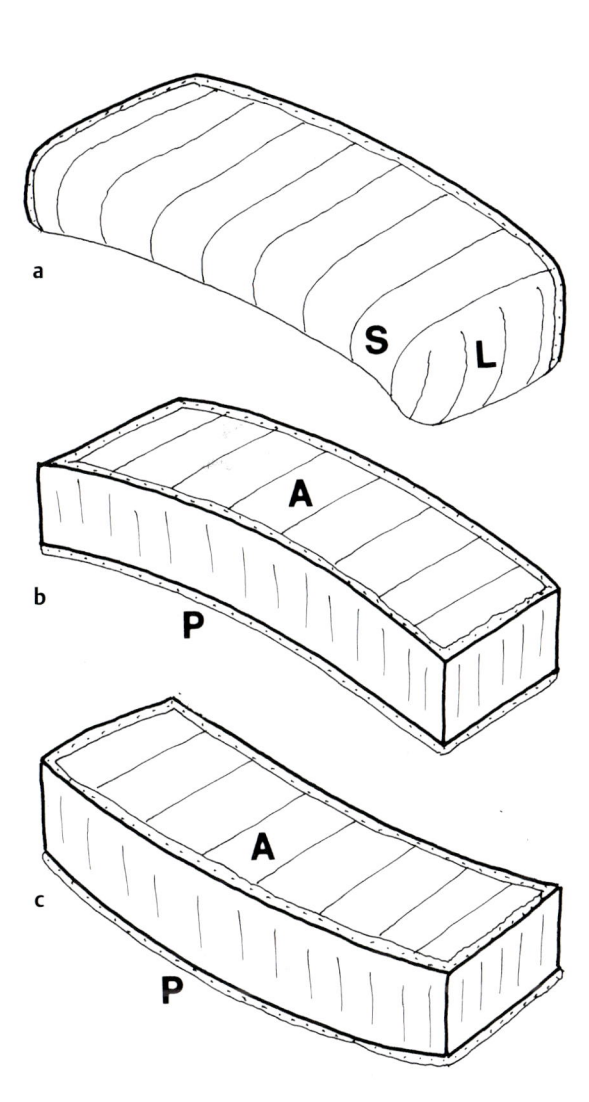

Fig. 2.27a–c Pieces of harvested cartilage.
- **a** Tragal dome: superolateral (S) and lateral (L) edges are covered by perichondrium.
- **b** Tragal cartilage, cut: anterior (A) perichondrium on convex side; posterior (P) perichondrium on concave side.
- **c** Conchal cartilage, cut: posterior (P) perichondrium on convex side; anterior (A) perichondrium on concave side.

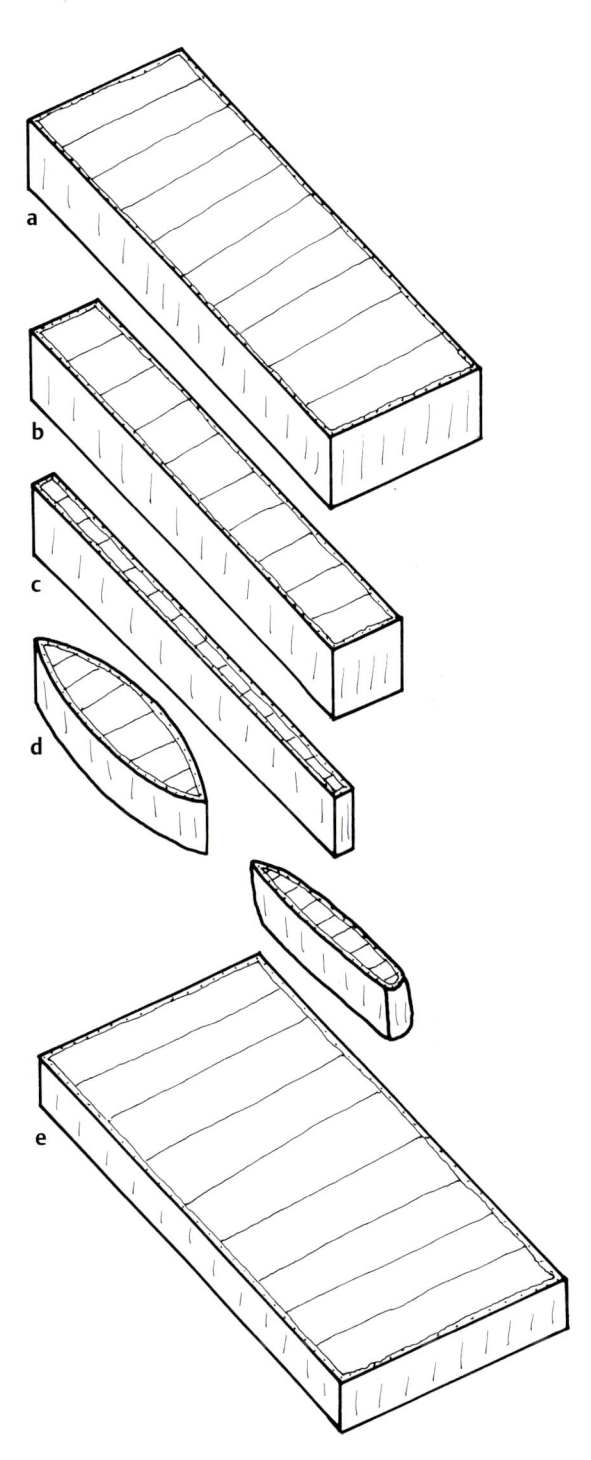

Fig. 2.28a–e Cartilage palisades. Cut rectangular, perichondrium on one side only, turned to the ear canal.
- **a** 2 mm wide.
- **b** 1 mm wide.
- **c** 0.5 mm wide.
- **d** Small palisades.
- **e** Broad palisades, 3–5 mm.

Cartilage Strips, Foils, and Plates

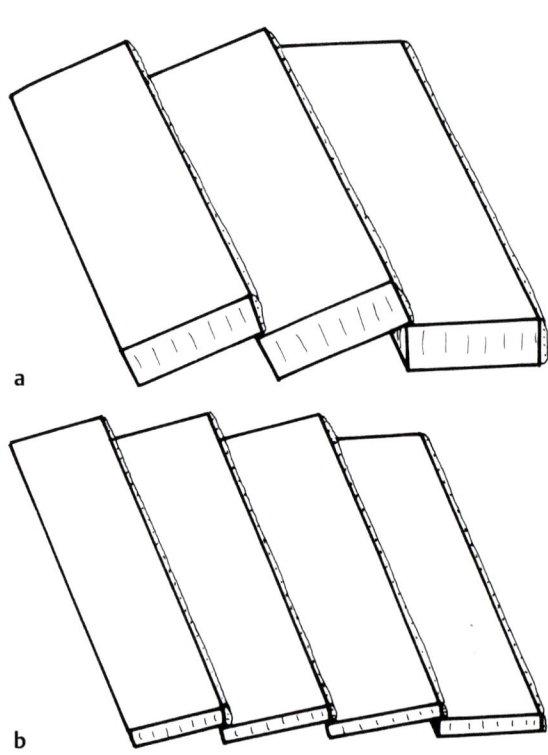

Fig. 2.29a, b Cartilage strips (or slices). Cut obliquely, small belts of perichondrium turned on the ear canal side.
a Thick.
b Thin.

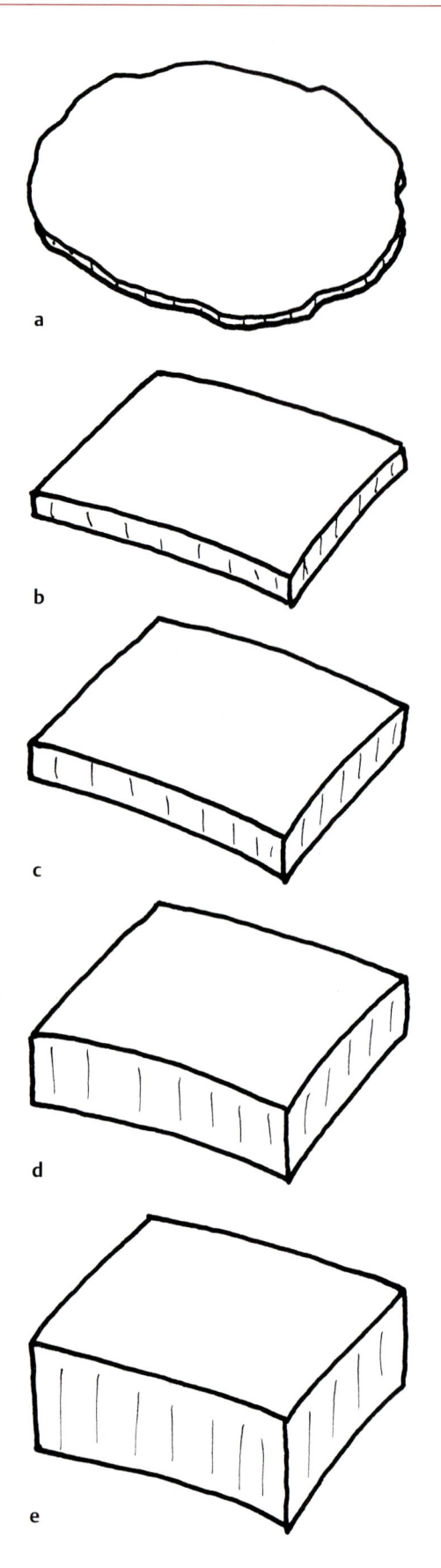

Fig. 2.30a–e Cartilage foils and plates, cut with the chondrotome and not covered with perichondrium.
a Foils, 0.2 or 0.3 mm.
b Thin plates, 0.4 mm.
c Half-thickness plate, 0.5 mm.
d Three-quarter-thickness plate.
e Full-thickness plate.

Composite Cartilage–Perichondrium Grafts

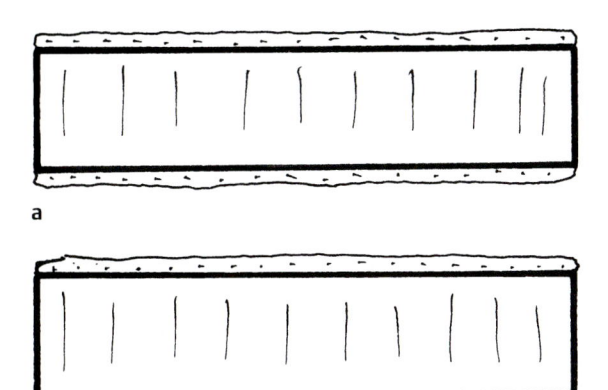

Fig. 2.31a, b Composite cartilage–perichondrium grafts, covered with perichondrium but without perichondrium flaps.
a With perichondrium on both sides.
b With perichondrium on one side.

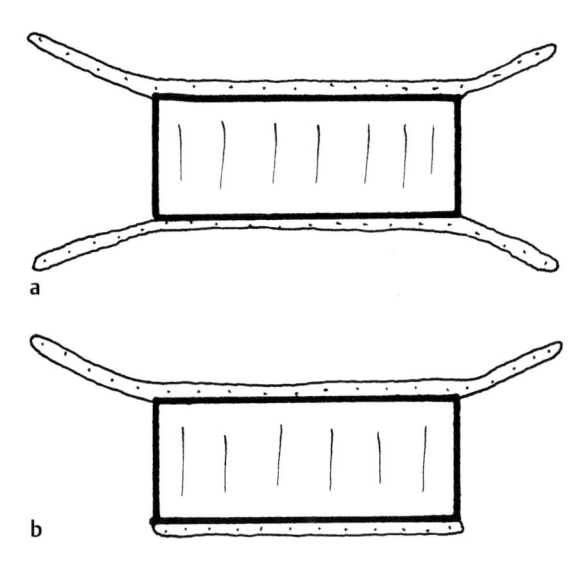

Fig. 2.32a, b Cartilage–perichondrium composite island grafts with perichondrium on both sides.
a With perichondrium flaps on both sides.
b With perichondrium on both sides, but flaps on one side only.

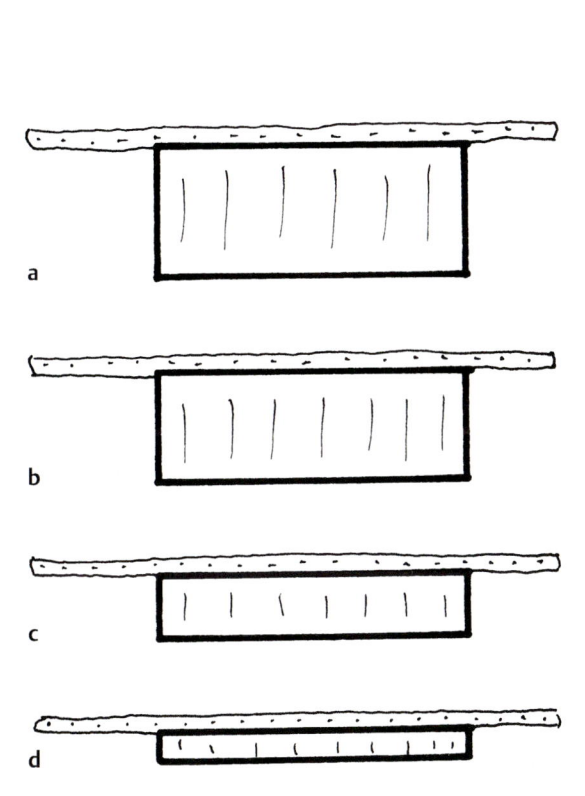

Fig. 2.33a–d Cartilage–perichondrium composite island grafts with perichondrium on one side only—on the ear canal side. Perichondrium flaps are present on at least one edge.
a Full-thickness island graft.
b Three-quarter-thickness island graft.
c Half-thickness island graft.
d One-third-thickness island graft.

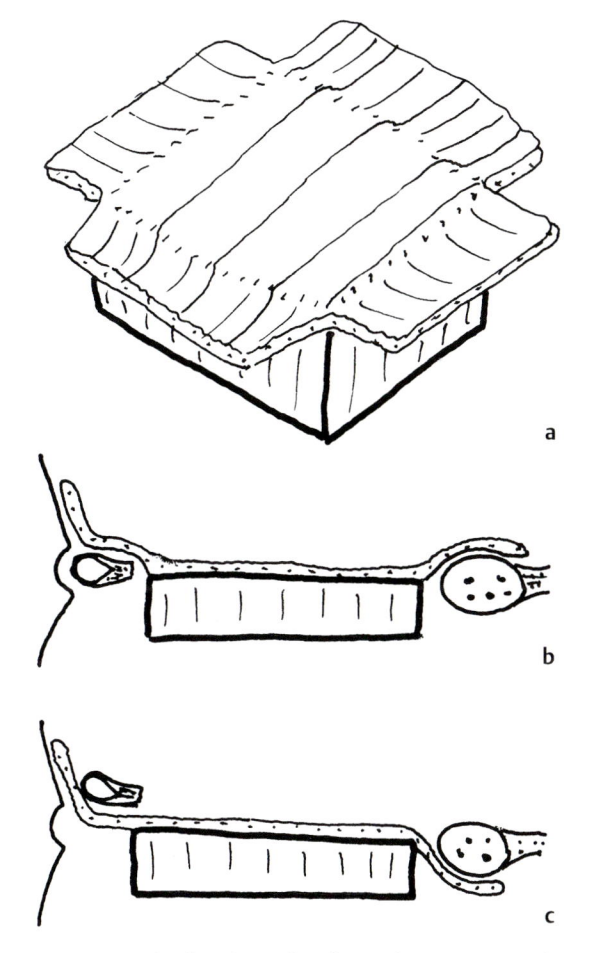

Fig. 2.34a–c Island graft as placed into the tympanic cavity. Perichondrium is on the ear canal side.
a As seen from above.
b Flap onto the malleus handle and onto the fibrous annulus.
c Flap under the malleus handle and under the fibrous annulus and/or bony annulus.

Soft Tissues

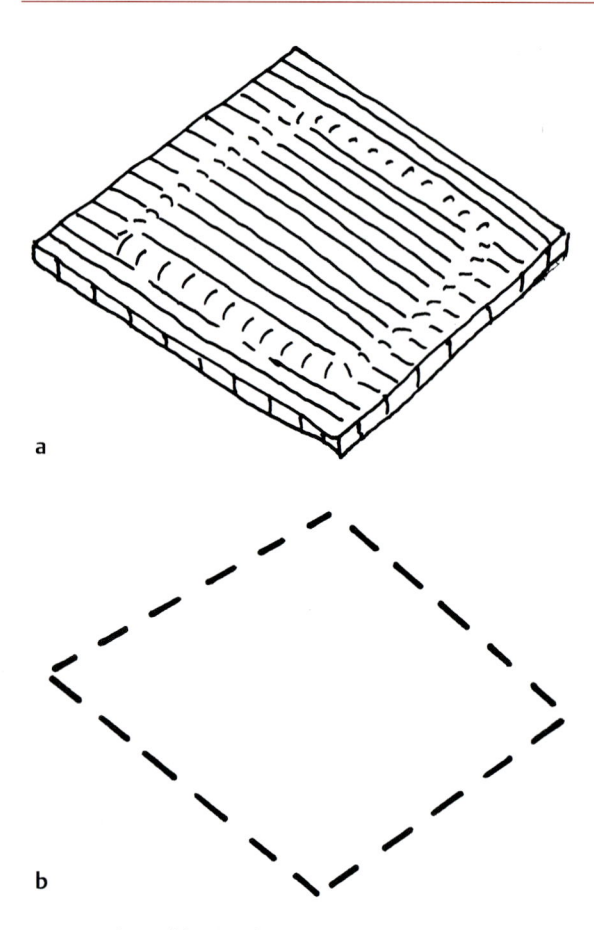

Fig. 2.35a, b Hidden cartilage.
a Hidden under the skin.
b Otherwise hidden cartilage.

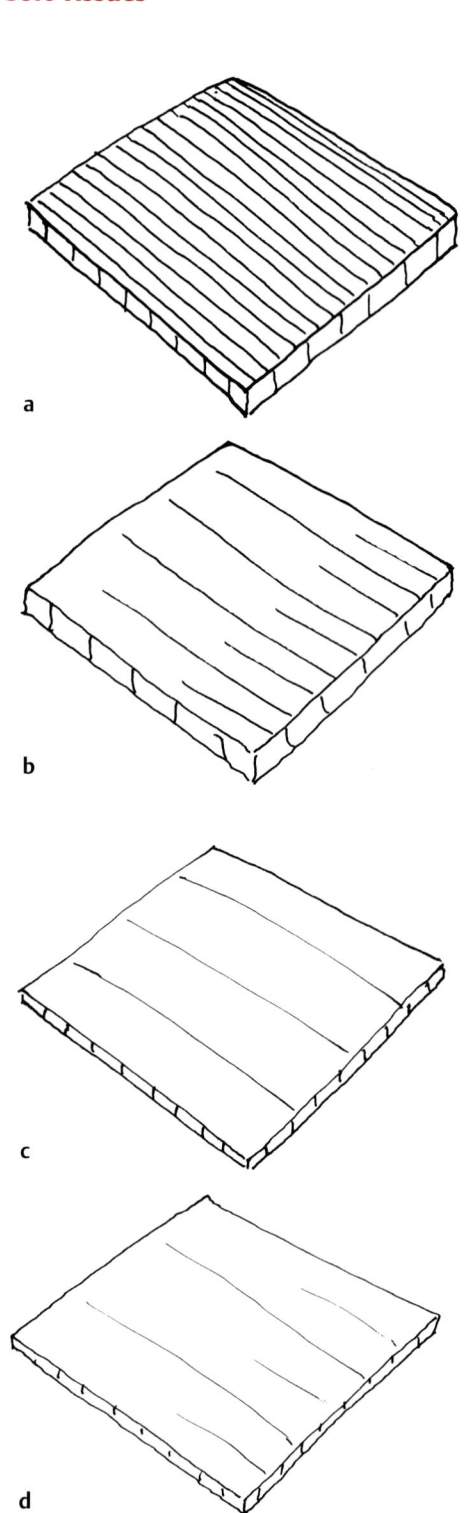

Fig. 2.36a–d Epithelia.
a Epithelium of the ear canal skin, outer side.
b Epithelium of the ear canal skin, inner side, elevated.
c Epithelium of the eardrum, outer side.
d Epithelium of the eardrum, inner side.

Pictorial Key to the Drawings in this Book

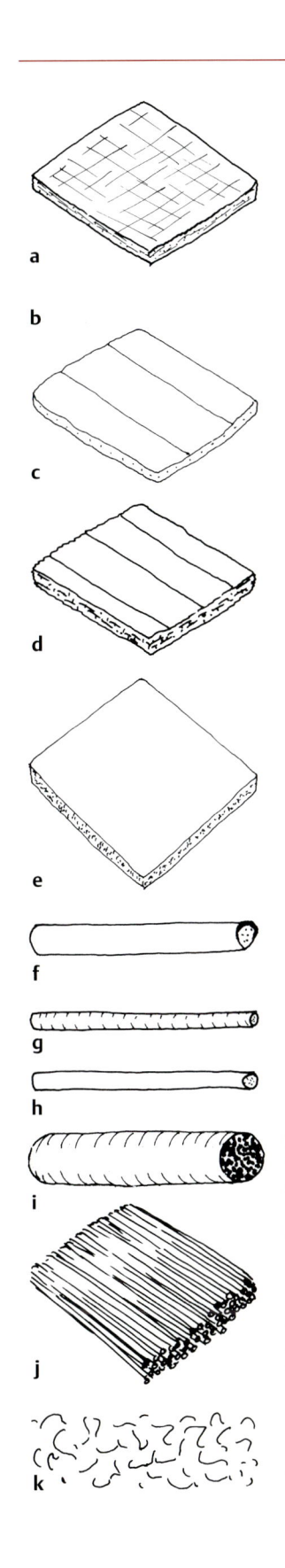

Bony Tissues

Fig. 2.37 a–k Other soft tissues.
- a Lamina propria of the eardrum, outer side.
- b Mucous membrane of the eardrum and of the tympanic cavity.
- c Perichondrium.
- d Fascia.
- e Dura.
- f Fibrous annulus.
- g Tendon.
- h Nerve, chorda tympani.
- i Facial nerve.
- j Muscle.
- k Subcutaneous tissue.

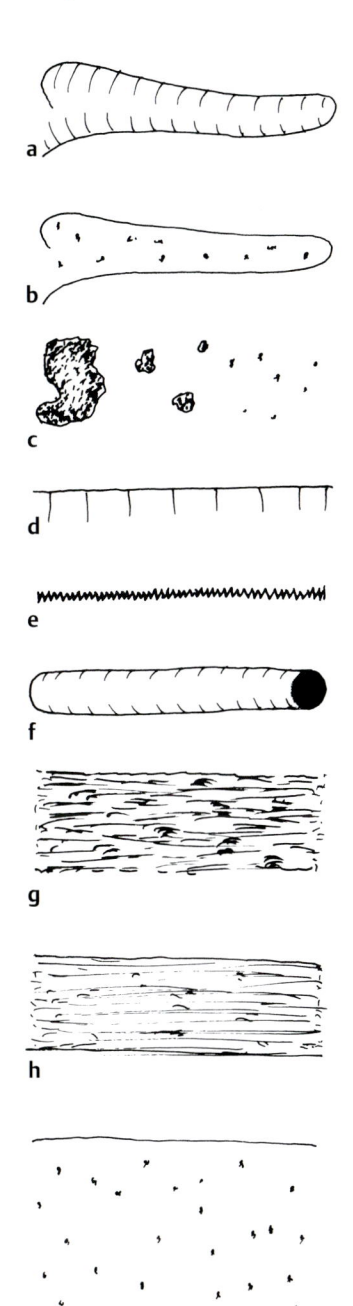

Fig. 2.38 a–i Bony tissues.
- a Malleus handle, natural covering.
- b Malleus handle, denuded.
- c Mastoid process, air cells.
- d Cortical bone, schematic border.
- e Suture, tympanomastoid, tympanosquamous.
- f Sigmoid sinus.
- g Cortical bone drilled with cutting drill.
- h Cortical bone drilled with diamond.
- i Denuded ear canal bone.

Other Elements

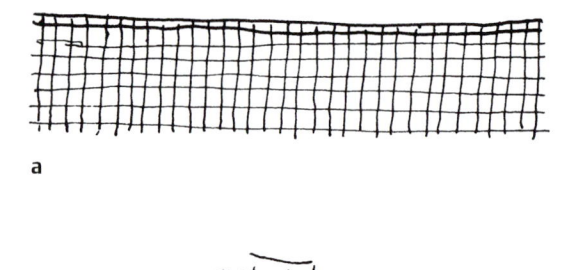

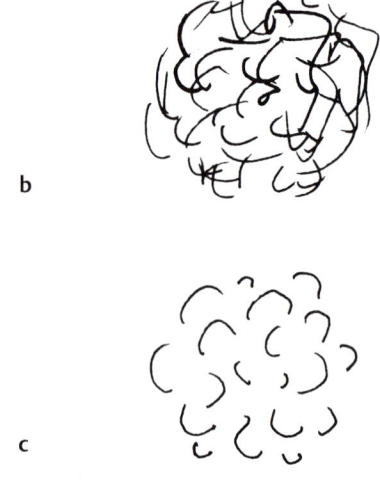

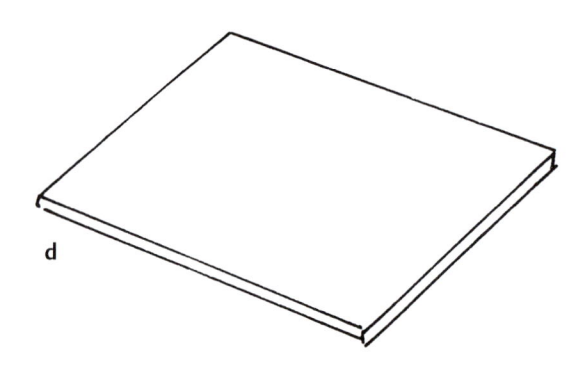

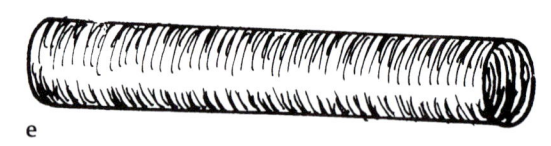

Fig. 2.39a–e Other elements.
a Gauze
b Gelfoam
c Cotton
d Silastic
e Titanium

References

Adkins WY, Osguthorpe JD. Use of composite autograft to prevent recurrent cholesteatoma caused by canal wall defects. Otolaryngol Head Neck Surg 1984;92:319–321.

Amedee RG, Mann WJ, Richelmann H. Cartilage palisade tympanoplasty. Am J Otol 1989;10:447–450.

Andersen J, Caye-Thomasen P, Tos M. Cartilage palisade tympanoplasty in sinus and tensa retraction cholesteatoma. Otol Neurotol 2002;23:825–831.

Andersen J, Caye-Thomasen P, Tos M. A comparison of cartilage palisades and fascia in tympanoplasty after surgery for sinus or tensa retraction cholesteatoma in children. Otol Neurotol 2004;25:856–863.

Bernal-Sprekelsen M, Barberan T. Indicationes, tecnica y resultados anatomicos de la tympanoplastica con cartilago en empalizada. Acta Otorrinolaringol Esp 1997;48:279–286.

Bernal-Sprekelsen M, Barberan TM, Lliso MDB. Resultados funktionales preliminaries de la timpanoplastica con cartilago en empalizada. Acta Otorrinolaringol Esp 1997;48:341–346.

Bernal-Sprekelsen M, Lliso MDR, Gonzalo JJSG. Cartilage palisades in type 3 tympanoplasty: anatomic and functional long-term results. Otol Neurotol 2003;24:38–42.

Danner CJ, Dornhoffer JL. Primary intubation of cartilage tympanoplasties. Laryngoscope 2001;111:177–180.

Dornhoffer JL. Hearing results with cartilage tympanoplasty. Laryngoscope 1997;107:1094–1099.

Dornhoffer JL. Surgical management of the atelectatic ear. Am J Otol 2000;21:315–321.

Dornhoffer JL. Cartilage tympanoplasty. Otolaryngol Clin North Am 2006;39:1161–1176.

Duckert LG, Müller J, Makielski KH, Helms J. Composite autograft "shield" reconstruction of remnant tympanic membranes. Am J Otol 1995;16:21–26.

Eavey RD. Inlay tympanoplasty: cartilage butterfly technique. Laryngoscope 1998;108:657–661.

Ferekidis EA, Nikolopoulos TP, Kandiloros DC, . Chondrotympanoplasty: a modified technique of cartilage graft tympanoplasty. Med Sci Monit 2003;9(2):CR73–CR78.

Fernandes SV. Composite chondroperichondrial clip tympanoplasty: the triple "C" technique. Otolaryngol Head Neck Surg 2003;128: 267–272.

Fleury P, Legent F, Lefevbre C. Techniques chirurgicales de l'oreile. Paris: Masson; 1974..

Ghanem MA, Monroy A, Farmaz SA, Alizade FS, Nicolau Y, Eavey RD. Butterfly cartilage graft inlay tympanoplasty for large perforations. Laryngoscope 2006;116:1813–1816.

Glasscock ME 3 rd, Jackson CG, Nissen AJ, Schwaber MK. Postauricular undersurface tympanic membrane grafting: a follow-up report. Laryngoscope 1982;92:718–727.

Goodhill V. Tragal perichondrium and cartilage in tympanoplasty. Arch Otolaryngol 1967;85:480–491.

Hall LJ. T-tube with tragus cartilage flange in long-term middle ear ventilation. Am J Otol 1990;11:454–457.

Hartwein J, Leuwer RM, Kehrl W. The total reconstruction of the tympanic membrane by the "crowncork" technique. Am J Otolaryngol 1992;13:172–175.

Heermann J. Entwicklung von der Haut-zur Faszien- und zur Knorpeltympanoplastik (Epitympanon-Antrum-Mastoidplastik). Z Laryngol Rhinol 1977;56:267–270.

Heermann J. Auricular cartilage palisade tympano-epitympano-antrum- and mastoid- plasty. Clin Otolaryngol 1978;3:443–446.

Heermann J. Autograft tragal and conchal palisade cartilage and perichondrium in tympanomastoid reconstruction. Ear Nose Throat J 1992;71:344–349.

Heermann J, Heermann H. Sieben Jahre Faszien – Knorpel- Dachschindel -Tympanoplastik und Antrum-Mastoidplastik. Z Laryngol Rhinol Otol 1967;46:370–382.

Heermann J, Heermann H, Kopfstein E. Fascia and cartilage palisade tympanoplasty. Nine years' experience. Arch Otolaryngol 1970; 91:228–241.

Helms J. Moderne Aspekte der Tympanoplastik. Eine Übersicht. Laryngorhinootologie 1995;74:465–467.

Hildmann H, Lockhaupt H, Schmelzer A. Die Verwendung von Knorpel in der Mittelohrchirurgie. HNO 1996;44:597–603.

Jansen C. Cartilage tympanoplasty. Laryngoscope 1963;73: 1288–1302.

Jansen C. The combined approach for tympanoplasty. J. Laryngol Otol 1968;779–793.

Kazikdas KC, Onal K, Boyraz I, Karabulut E. Palisade cartilage tympanoplasty for management of subtotal perforations: a comparison with the temporalis fascia technique. Eur Arch Otorhinolaryngol 2007;264:985–989.

Kleinfeldt D, Vick U, Lübcke P.-F. Zur Verwendung von antologem Ohrmuschelknorpel zur Doppeltransplantatplastik des Trommelfelles. HNO 1975;23: 13–15.

Kleinsasser O, Glanschneider D. Knorpelplättchen zur Befestigung von Collumellen und zur Überbrückung großer Trommelfelldefekte bei der Tympanoplastik. Z. Laryngol Rhinol Otol 1969;48: 590–599.

Levinson RM. Cartilage-perichondrium composite graft tympanoplasty in the treatment of posterior marginal and attic retraction pockets. Laryngoscope 1987;97:1069–1074.

Linde RE. The cartilage perichondrium graft in the treatment of posterior tympanic membrane pockets. Laryngoscope 1973;83: 747–753.

McCleve DE. Tragal cartilage reconstruction of the auditory canal. Arch Otolaryngol 1969;90:35–38.

Martin HO. A propos de la chirurgie de reinforcement du tympan. J Fr Otorhinolaryngol Audiophonol Chir Maxillofac 1979;28(3): 195–196.

Milewski C. Composite graft tympanoplasty in the treatment of ears with advanced middle ear pathology. Laryngoscope 1993;103: 1352–1356.

Mürbe D, Zahnert T, Bornitz M, Hüttenbrink K-B. Acoustic properties of different cartilage reconstruction techniques of the tympanic membrane. Laryngoscope 2002;112:1769–1776.

Neumann A. Die "Knorpelpalisadentympanoplastik" nach Heermann. HNO 1999;47:1074–1088.

Neumann A, Jahnke K. Trommelfellrekonstruktion mit Knorpel. Indikationen Techniken und Ergebnisse. HNO 2005;53:573–586.

Neumann A, Hennig A, Shultz-Coulon H-J. Morphologische und funktionelle Ergebnisse der Knorpelpalisadentympanoplastik. HNO 2002;50:935–939.

Neumann A., Schultz-Coulon H-J, Jahnke J. Type 3 tympanoplasty applying the palisade cartilage technique: a study of 61 cases. Otol Neurotol 2003;24:33–37.

Nitsche O. Tragusperichondrium und -Knorpel bei der Tympanoplastik. Bericht über 2500 Operationen durch niedergelassenen HNO-Arzt. HNO 1985;33:455–457.

Pere P. Erfarungen mit der palisadentechnik zum Trommelfellverschluss. Laryngorhinootologie 1989;68:569–570.

Poe DS, Gadre AK. Cartilage tympanoplasty for management of retraction pockets and cholesteatomas. Laryngoscope 1993;103: 614–618.

Puls T. Tympanoplasty using conchal cartilage graft. Acta Otorhinolaryngol Belg 2003;57:187–191.

Steinbach E, Pusalkar A. Long- term histological fate in ossicular reconstruction. J Laryngol Otol 1981;95:1031–1039.

Steinbach E, Karger B, Hildmann H. Zur Verwendung von Knorpeltransplantaten in der Mittelohrchirurgie. Eine histologische Langzeituntersuchung von Knorpelinterponaten. Laryngol Rhinol Otol (Stuttg) 1992;71:11–14.

Tolsdorff P. Tympanoplastik mit Tragusknorpel-Transplantat: "Knorpeldeckel-Plastik. Laryngol Rhinol Otol (Stuttg) 1983;62:97–102.

Tos M. Bony fixation of the malleus and incus. Acta Otolaryngol 1970;70:95–104.

Tos M. Tympanoplasty in chronic adhesive otitis media. Acta Otolaryngol 1972;73:53–60.

Tos M. Manual of Middle Ear Surgery. Vol. 1: Approaches Myringoplasty Ossiculoplasty Tympanoplasty. Stuttgart–New York: Georg Thieme Verlag; 1993..

Tos M. Cartilage tympanoplasty methods: Proposal of a classification. Otolaryngol Head Neck Surg 2008;139(6):747–758.

Tos M, Lau T. Long-term hearing results in cholesteatoma. In: Charachon R, Garcia Ibanez E, eds. Long Term Results and Indications in Otology and Otoneurosurgery. Amsterdam: Kugler; 1991:95-98..

Tos M, Lau T, Arndal H, Plate S. Tympanosclerosis of the middle ear: Late results of surgical treatment. J Laryngol Otol 1990; 104:685–689.

Tos M, Uzun C, Caye-Thomasen P. Tympanometry after tympanoplasty with cartilage palisades or fascia after surgery for tensa cholesteatoma in children. In: Lim DJ, Bluestone CD, Casselbrandt M. Recent Advances in Otitis Media. New York: Decker; 2005: 321–323..

Uzun C, Cayé-Thomasen P, Andersen J. Tos M. A tympanometric comparison of tympanoplasty with cartilage palisades or fascia after surgery for tensa cholesteatoma in children. Laryngoscope 2003;113:1751–1757.

Wiegand H. [Tympanic membrane repair with cartilage and double tissue-layered grafts (Author's transl.)] HNO 1978;26(7): 233–236.

3 Approaches and Harvesting of Cartilage

Approaches

All three approaches, the transmeatal or transcanal, the endaural, and the retroauricular approach, can be applied in all reconstructions of the eardrum with cartilage. For a tympanoplasty some surgeons employ mainly a retroauricular approach, some mainly an endaural approach with various intercartilaginous incisions, and some mainly a transmeatal approach through the fixed ear speculum. In mastoidectomy, antrotomy, and atticotomy, most surgeons will employ a retroauricular approach and some an endaural approach with intercartilaginous incision.

Transmeatal Approach through Fixed Ear Speculum

Some surgeons still use an expanding and self-retaining Holmgreen–Plester ear speculum with two blades (MMES_1, Fig. 11). The two blades are expanded by a screw arrangement, thus fixing the speculum into place in the meatus. The disadvantage of this speculum is that the intrameatal fixation is neither solid nor stable.

I have always, and with pleasure, used the Richards speculum holder (**Fig. 3.1a**). A small problem of the Richards speculum holder is the relatively short metal arm for fixation to the operating table. To solve this problem, the technical service of our hospital has extended the metal arm of all Richards speculum holders by 22 cm to a length of 38 cm since the early 1970s. It can now can be adjusted even to the largest patients.

Another small problem arose from variation of placement and mode of attachment of the speculum holder to the operating table. To overcome this, we made a 2 mm thick, 32 cm long, and 22 cm wide metal plate that is placed onto the round, head end of the operating table (**Fig. 3.1b**). To one end of the plate is fixed a small metal, sliding-bearing device with a rectangular slot. Through the slot, the elongated metal arm of the speculum holder is placed. After adjustment in the appropriate position, it is fixed with a screw. The mobile plate makes the speculum

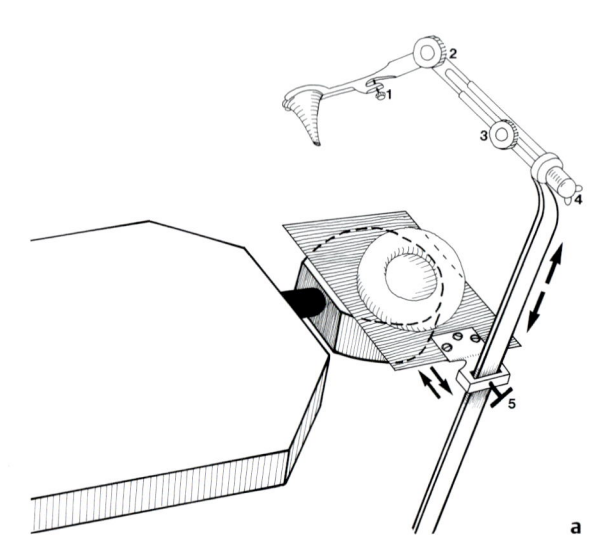

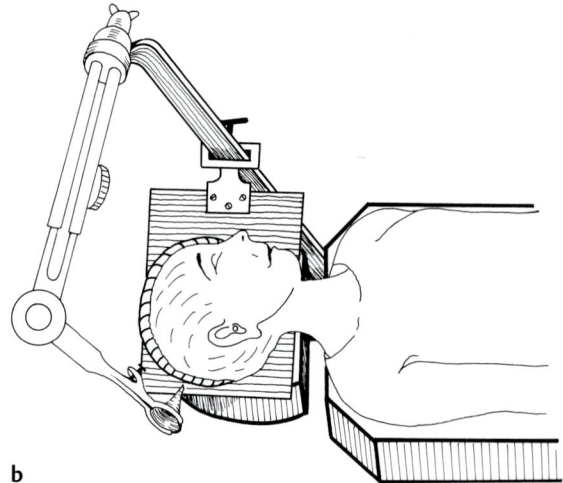

Fig. 3.1a, b Richards speculum holder and plate.
a Richards speculum holder with five screws to accommodate and fix the ear speculum in the appropriate position. The original metal arm is extended by another 22 cm to a length of 38 cm. The first screw (1) fixes the speculum, the second (2) allows in-and-out movement, the third (3) allows greater or shorter distance to the ear, the fourth (4) allows superior–inferior and in–out movement, and the fifth (5) allows higher–lower movement of the metal arm.
b The 22 cm × 32 cm plate of the speculum holder with a sliding-bearing device fixed to the plate. The elongated metal arm of the Richards ear speculum holder is placed through the rectangular hole and fixed with a special screw.

holder completely independent of the operating table. The extended arm makes the holder independent of the size and position of the head of the patient. After these improvements the speculum holder is a tremendous support in transmeatal middle ear surgery and in pediatric middle ear surgery.

Two other well-known ear speculum holders, the Schuknecht and the Treace holder (**Fig. 3.2**), are also too short but can easily be improved in the same manner as the Richards speculum holder. Apart from these best-known instruments, many similar or slightly modified speculum holders are in use worldwide.

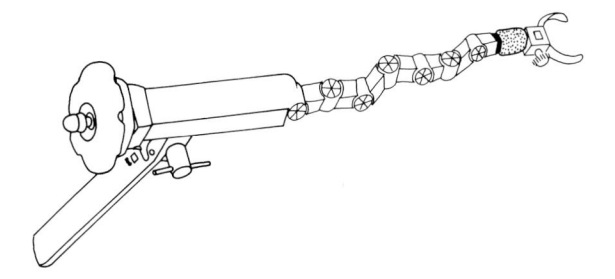

Fig. 3.2 Treace speculum holder with a short metal arm, which can be bowed.

Tilting of the Ear Speculum

A set of Richards specula ranges from the smallest with a diameter of 4 mm, increasing by 0.5 mm to the largest speculum with a diameter of 8 mm. The metal speculum has a special outer edge to accommodate the speculum holder (**Fig. 3.3a**). The largest possible speculum is placed into the ear canal and fixed with the speculum holder (**Fig. 3.3b**). Tilting of the speculum in all four directions is easy if the screws 1 to 3 (see **Fig. 3.1a, b**) do not rigidly fix the speculum. With just a small push of the speculum holder in the superior direction, the inner opening of the speculum will tilt toward the inferior ear canal wall and visualize the superior part of the eardrum (**Fig. 3.4a**). With tilting of the speculum holder in the inferior direction, the inner opening of the speculum tilts toward the superior half of the eardrum and attic region (**Fig. 3.4b**). Tilting of the inner opening of the speculum toward the anterior tympanum (**Fig. 3.4c**) and toward the posterior tympanum (**Fig. 3.4d**) is very important in transmeatal tympanoplasty.

It is not difficult to place even the longest cartilage palisades through the speculum into the tympanic cavity. I have performed transmeatal cartilage palisade tympanoplasty with the fixed ear speculum in almost all children with sinus and tensa retraction cholesteatoma (Andersen et al 2002, 2004) and has good arguments for the transmeatal approach (see Tos 1993).

Transmeatal Cartilage Tympanoplasty Is Minimally Invasive Surgery

A transmeatal cartilage tympanoplasty with a fixed ear speculum is simple and effective surgery without the need for lateral ear canal incisions. In addition to stapes surgery and surgery for hearing loss from any other cause, all sequelae of chronic otitis media with perforations can be and should be managed by surgery via the transmeatal approach. Furthermore, all pars tensa retractions, atelectasis, adhesive otitis, and sinus and tensa retraction cholesteatoma should be operated via the transmeatal approach.

Transmeatal surgery is highly recommended in children. It is advantageous and beneficial to operate in children through the fixed speculum without incision of the

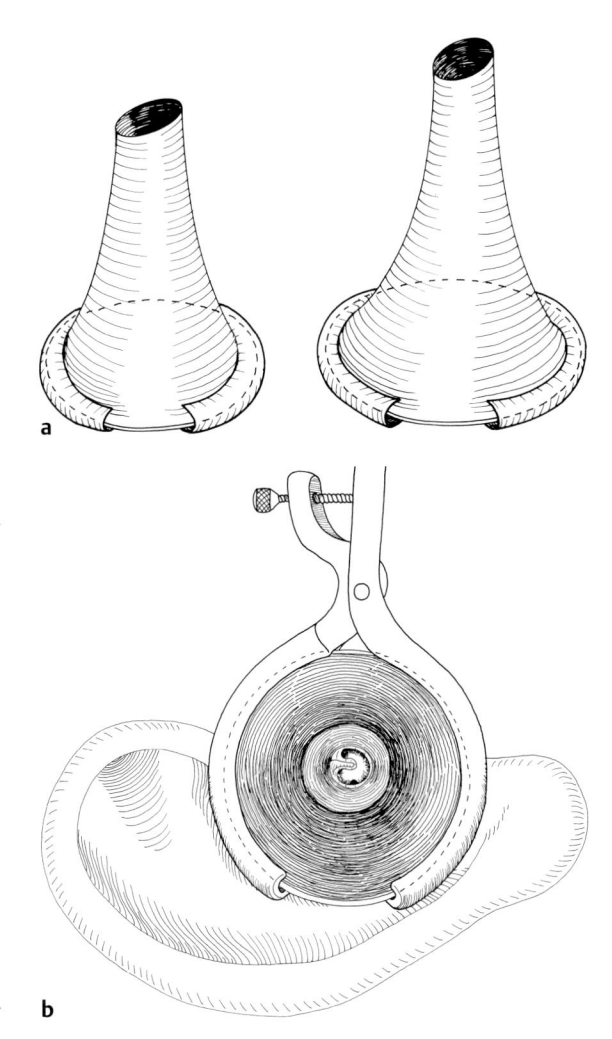

Fig. 3.3a, b Richards metal ear speculum.
a Two Richards metal ear speculums each mounted on the two arms of Richards speculum holder. Left: short speculum with larger lumen; right: long speculum with smaller lumen.
b Fixation of the speculum in the ear canal using a Richards speculum holder with two round arms surrounding the edge of the speculum.

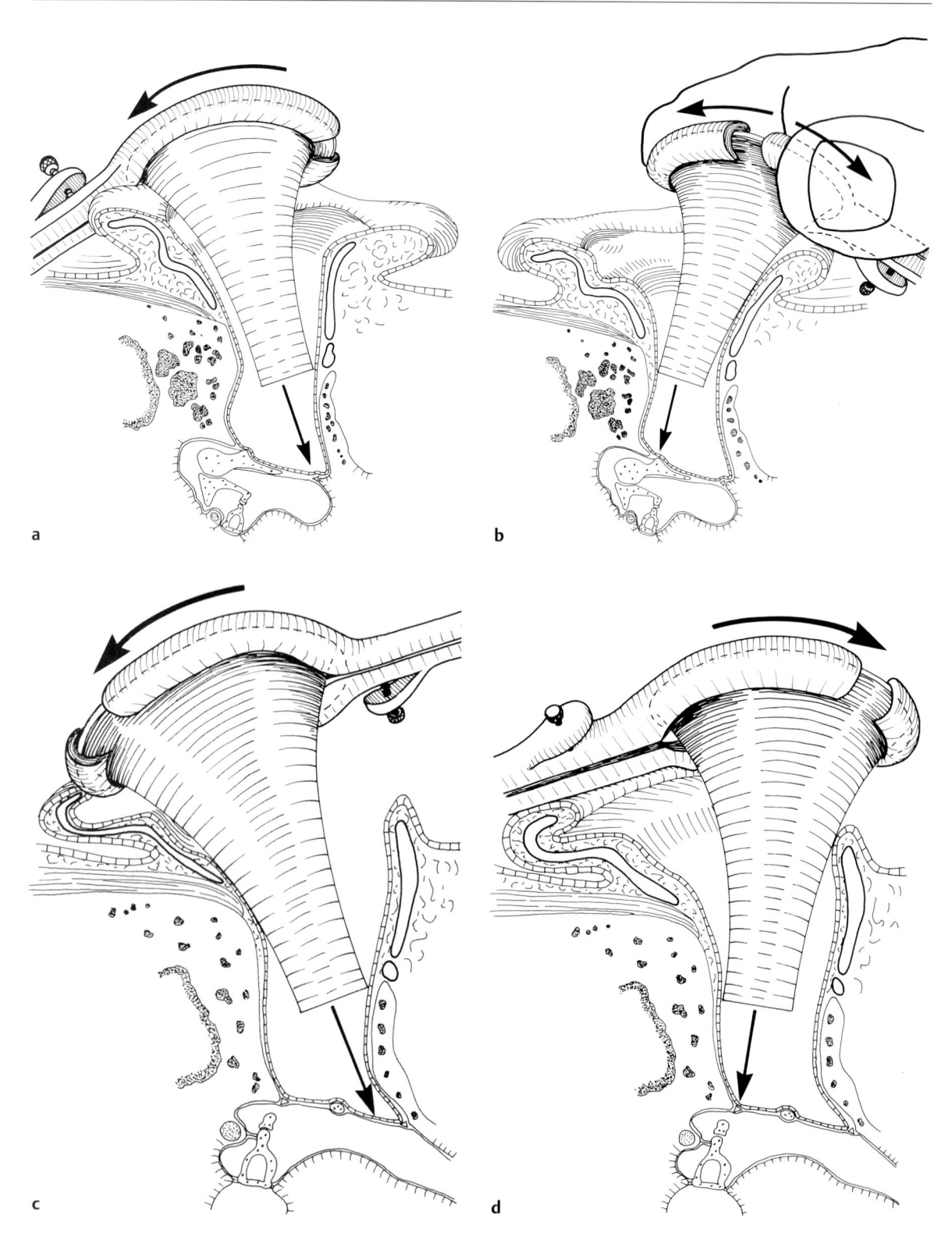

Fig. 3.4a–d Tilting of the speculum holder.
a Tilting toward the inferior ear canal wall.
b Tilting of the speculum holder toward the superior ear canal wall.
c Tilting the speculum in the anterior direction.
d Tilting the speculum in the posterior direction provides better view of the posterior part of the tympanic cavity and tympanic sinuses.

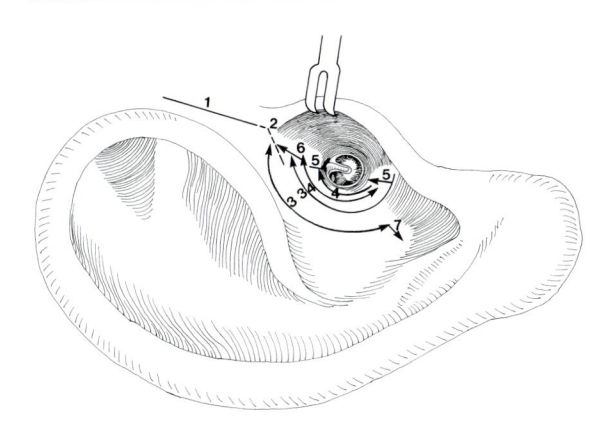

Fig. 3.5 Terminology of ear canal incisions. 1, Vertical; 2, intercartilaginous; 3, lateral circumferential; 4, medial circumferential; 5, medial radial; 6, lateral radial; 7, radial conchal incision.

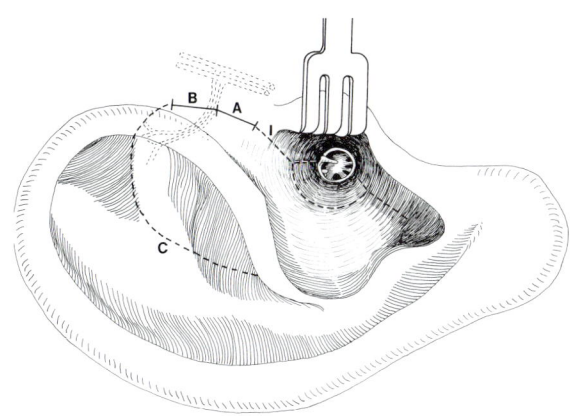

Fig. 3.6 The Heermann A, B, and C endaural incisions. The intercartilaginous incision (I) is dotted.

lateral ear canal skin, which may cause a difficult postoperative period for the child and later lead to stenosis of the introitus of the meatus.

For patients who still need a hearing aid after the operation, the transmeatal approach is also the best solution because it is the most minimal invasive solution. With the increasing age of patients undergoing middle ear surgery, the number of patients with a preoperative and/or postoperative hearing aid is growing. Any surgery of the meatus will delay the fitting of a hearing aid.

Surprisingly, many otosurgeons do not use a fixed ear speculum holder. This is a pity, because surgery through the fixed ear speculum is the most minimally invasive approach with the easiest postoperative care.

Terminology of Ear Canal Skin Incisions

In all three approaches, the many incisions of the ear canal skin have the same terminology (**Fig. 3.5**). The intercartilaginous incision (2) extends in the superior direction as a vertical incision (1). The lateral cicumferential incisions (3) are positioned in the outer half, the medial circumferential incisions (4) in the inner half of the ear canal. Their extension is usually between the 12-o'clock and 6-o'clock positions. The medial radial incision (5) runs from the circumferential incision toward the eardrum; the lateral radial incision (6) runs toward the meatus. The radial conchal incision (7) runs from the lateral circumferential incision toward the concha. The length of the circumferential incisions is denoted clockwise for the right ear: 12-o'clock, 3-o'clock (anterior), 6-o'clock, and 9-o'clock (posterior).

All drawings in this book are made for the right ear. The above terminology will be used throughout in the descriptions of the various cartilage tympanoplasty techniques.

Endaural Approach with Intercartilaginous Incision

The endaural approach with intercartilaginous incision is widely applied in cartilage tympanoplasty. Several variations and modifications of the endaural approach have been published and are still used in modern tympanoplasty. They have been thoroughly described and illustrated in Tos (1993) (MMES_1, Figs. 25–74); here the methods will be briefly shown in **Figs. 3.6–3.11**. The endaural approach with incision is used in particular in cases that in addition to a tympanoplasty need an atticotomy, antrotomy, various types of mastoidectomies, and reconstructive procedures of the mastoid cavity described in Tos (1995), where reconstruction of the ear canal with cartilage is described.

The Heermann Intercartilaginous Incisions

The **Heermann A incision** (**Fig. 3.6**) starts with a scalpel in the bony part of the ear canal at the 12-o'clock position at a point 6 mm lateral to the Shrapnell membrane, and continues laterally on the bone toward the meatus and through the stretched intercartilaginous incisura. After leaving the introitus of the external auditory meatus, it follows the crus of the helix upward for about 10 mm. The Heermann A incision is used by some surgeons in stapedectomy or in myringoplasty of small perforations.

The **Heermann B incision** extends another 15 mm upward, cuts the anterior auricular vein and artery and exposes the temporalis muscle fascia. In the ear canal, a circumferential incision and a radial lateral incision allow displacement of the canal skin outward and exposure of the bone of the ear canal and the mastoid process (**Fig. 3.7**). There are many modifications regarding the tympanomeatal flap (see MMES_1, Figs. 30–47)

The **Heermann C incision** (Heermann and Heermann 1964) extends around the auricle (see **Fig. 3.6**). It is seldom used today.

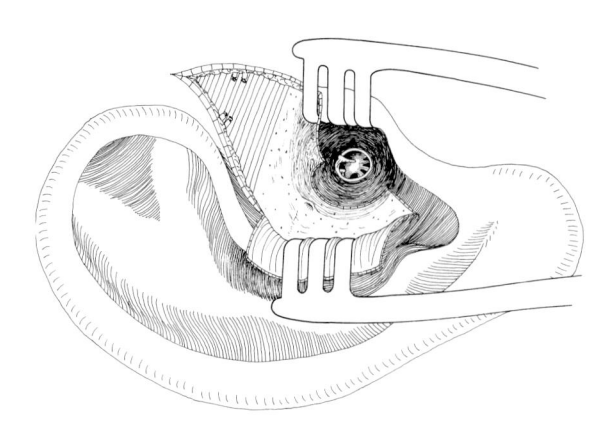

Fig. 3.7 The Heermann B incision with a large tympanomeatal flap and elevated lateral ear canal skin exposing the temporalis fascia and bone of the lateral ear canal and mastoid process.

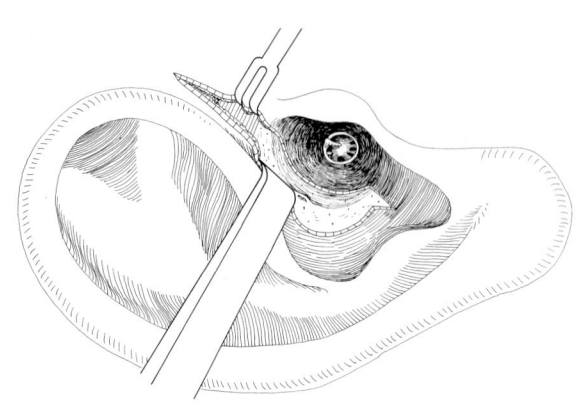

Fig. 3.8 The Shambaugh incision, starting with a lateral circumferential incision, continuing with an intercartilaginous incision and an inferior lateral incision toward the concha.

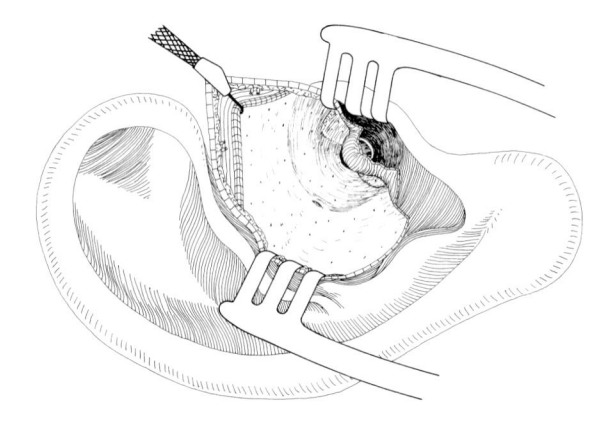

Fig. 3.9 Completed Shambaugh approach, with good exposure of the mastoid process.

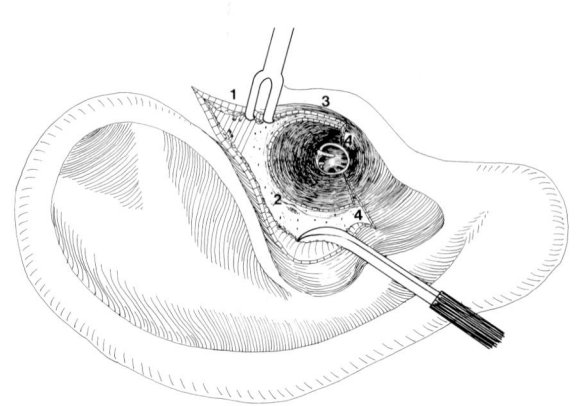

Fig. 3.10 The Lempert incision, with vertical (1), posterior (2), and anterior (3) circumferential incisions and radial incision (4). Elevation of the posterior periosteum has been started.

The Shambaugh Incision

The Shambaugh incision is still popular in the United States. It starts with a lateral circumferential incision and continues with a vertical incision (**Fig. 3.8**), allowing elevation of the periosteum of the lateral part of the ear canal (Shambaugh and Glasscock 1980). The lateral radial incision contributes to good exposure of the mastoid process and the ear canal (**Fig. 3.9**).

The Lempert Incision

The Lempert incision (**Fig. 3.10**) is slightly different from Shambaugh's incision. Lempert elevates the posterior, superior, and anterior skin flaps as far as the fibrous annulus (Lempert 1941). The thinned ear canal skin is supposed to cover the window made on the lateral semicircular canal in Lempert fenestration for otosclerosis. The Lempert approach is also suitable for canal wall down surgery of a cholesteatoma.

Farrior Incision

The Farrior endaural incision is a modification of the Shambaugh and Lempert incisions (Farrior 1968). This interesting approach is suitable for transmeatal anterior atticotomy and transcortical canal wall down mastoidectomy of Farrior (see MMES_2, Figs. 554–567). During opening, Farrior created a subcutis–perichondrium flap (**Fig. 3.11**) attached to the undermined posterior conchal skin flap. This elongated flap serves to anchor the skin flap deep in the mastoid cavity, promoting faster epithelialization of the cavity. Furthermore, resection of the anterior edge of the conchal cartilage widens the lateral part of the ear canal.

Endaural Approaches and Endaural Mastoidectomy Techniques

In all endaural, transmeatal, or retrograde mastoidectomy procedures, drilling starts in the ear canal and follows the disease (most often cholesteatoma) until healthy bone is reached, leaving a cavity that may remain open, may be obliterated, or even may become a total or partly re-ventilated cavity after reconstruction of the ear canal wall. Cartilage plays an important role in the reconstruction of the ear canal wall.

Various endaural approaches are used in the following mastoidectomy techniques:
- Tympanomeatoplasty with preservation of bony bridge (Wigand 1970, 1990) (see MMES_2, Figs. 533–551).
- Transcortical canal wall down mastoidectomy, such as the Bondy operation (see MMES_2, Figs. 568–614).
- Transmeatal canal wall down mastoidectomy (see MMES_2, Figs. 615–644).
- Retrograde mastoidectomy on demand (see MMES_2, Figs. 644–655).
- Endaural canal wall down mastoidectomy (see MMES_2, Figs. 657–717).
- Closure of the bony defects with cartilage or complete reconstructions of the ear canal with cartilage in the above-mentioned endaural mastoidectomies is illustrated in MMES_2, Figs. 561, 563, 565, 567, 576, 577, 649, 650, 653, 686, 690, 692, 694, 696).

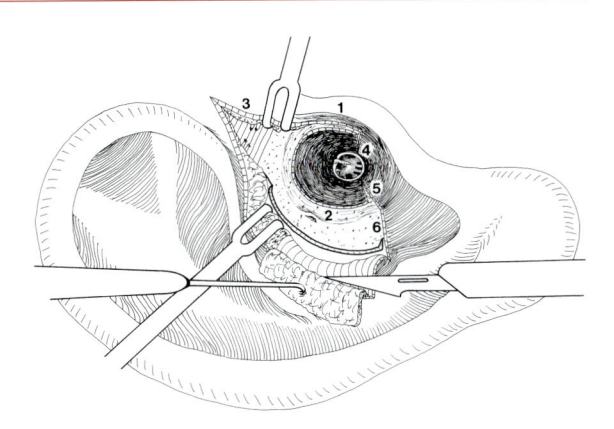

Fig. 3.11 **The Farrior incision** begins with an anterior circumferential incision (1) laterally in the ear canal at the 4-o'clock position and continues with a posterior circumferential incision (2) just medial to the spine of Henle. Then the vertical incision (3) is performed. Anterior (4) and a posterior (5) vertical incision and a lateral incision (6) are made. A posterior skin flap and a periosteum and subcutaneous tissue flaps are also raised and a strip of concha cartilage is cut.

Retroauricular Approach

Many modifications of the retroauricular approach have been published and most of them are still in use. They are systematically described and illustrated in MMES_1, Figs. 76–157). Here only the most commonly used retroauricular approaches are shown.

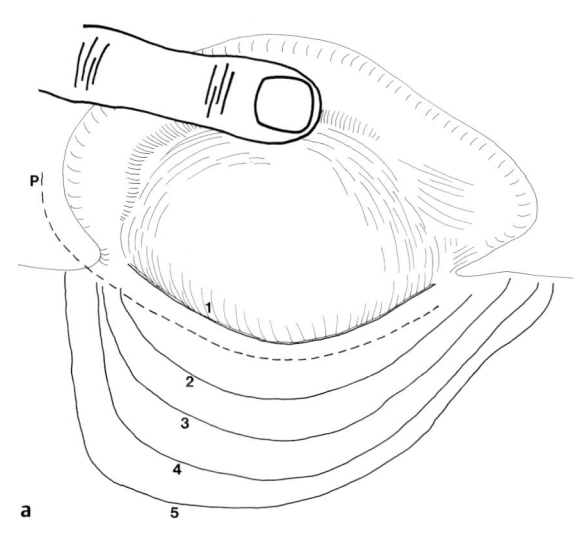

The retroauricular incision may be placed just behind the concha in the retroauricular fold. This is called a **retroauricular fold incision**.

All other incisions made behind the retroauricular fold create musculoperiostal flaps (**Fig. 3.12a, b**). Thus, the incisions are called **retroauricular flap incisions**. They are used in various transcortical mastoidectomies (see MMES_2, Figs. 127–632) and in various cavity obliteration methods with pedicled muscle flaps (see MMES_2, Figs. 867–970). In skull base surgery, in particular in translabyrinthine acoustic neuroma surgery, incisions with large retroauricular flaps are used.

Fig. 3.12a, b The retroauricular incisions.
a Retroauricular fold incision (1) and retroauricular flap incisions (2–5). Posterosuperior (Portmann 1979) incision (P).
b Retroauricular incisions in side view (P and 1–5). Levels of the circumferential incisions of the ear canal skin: (a) lateral, (b) medial incision, (c) elevation of the entire ear canal skin together with the skin of the eardrum remnant, and (d) together with the fibrous annulus and eardrum remnant.

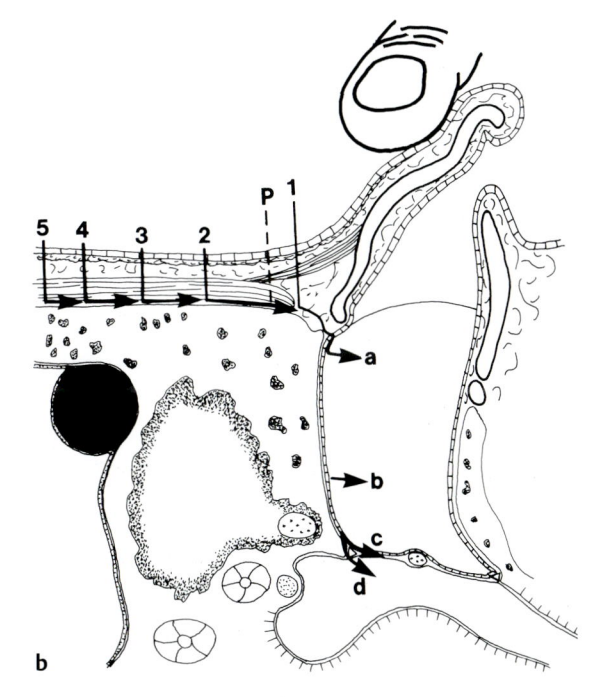

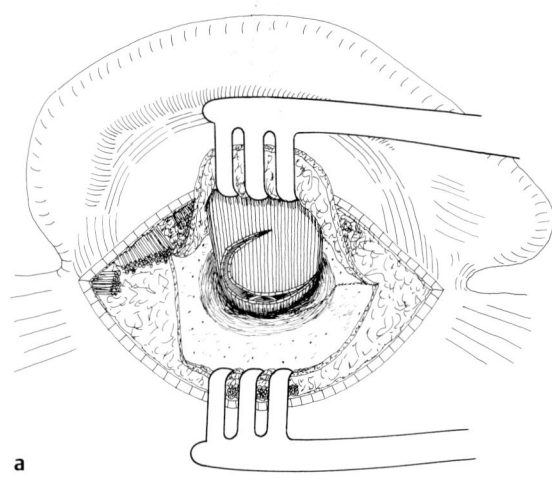

Fig. 3.13a–c The Plester technique.
a Retroauricular fold incision. After drilling of the entrance of the bony ear canal, and exposure of the ear canal skin, a circumferential incision and a superior radial incision running outward from the superior edge of the circumferential incision are performed.
b The triangular skin flap, based inferiorly and laterally in the ear canal, is elevated with a long, self retaining retractor and pulled outward together with the external acoustic meatus.
c Two radial incisions are made and a large tympanomeatal flap with fibrous annulus and eardrum remnant is elevated.

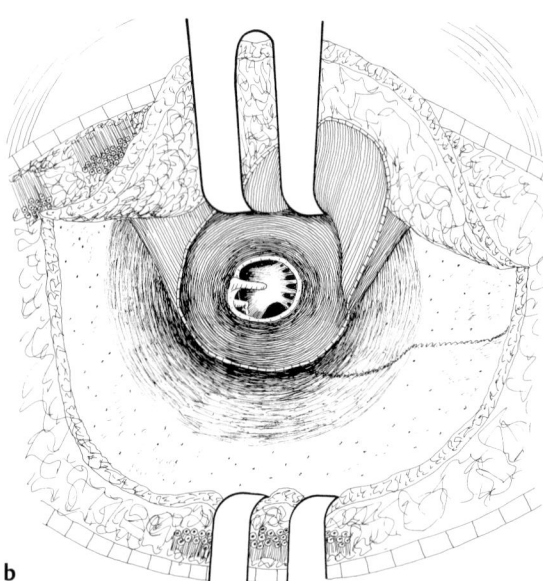

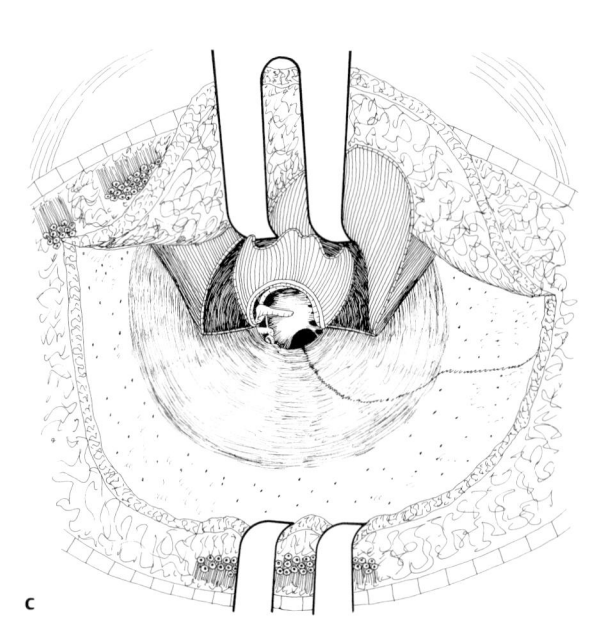

Modifications of the retroauricular approach are related to the level of the circumferential incisions of the meatal skin (**Fig. 3.12b**). They are divided into
- Lateral skin incisions.
- Medial skin incisions.
- No incision, but elevation of the canal skin, with or without elevation of the fibrous annulus.

Plester Technique

After a retroauricular fold incision, an oval subcutaneous–periostal incision on the mastoid process is made. The periosteum flap is elevated with a raspatory, exposing the ear canal skin (**Fig. 3.13a**). Drilling of the entrance of the bony ear canal wall, starting at the suprameatal spine and continuing to the 6-o'clock position, enlarges the exposure of the ear canal skin. At the level of 4–5 mm medially to the suprameatal spine, a circumferential incision of the meatal skin is made from the 12-o'clock to the 6-o'clock position (Plester 1963; Plester et al 1989; Hildmann and Sudhoff 2006). From the superior end of the circumferential incision, a 1–1.5 cm long outward-directed incision is made, allowing elevation of an inferiorly based and laterally based ear canal skin flap (**Fig. 3.13b**). After a superior vertical incision and an inferior vertical incision, a large tympanomeatal flap, together with the fibrous annulus and eardrum, is elevated (**Fig. 3.13c**).

Palva's Swing-Door Technique

From a position as shown in **Fig. 3.13b**, Palva (1963) performed a radial incision at the 9-o'clock position and elevated a large superior and a large inferior tympanomeatal flap, which provides an excellent view of the anterior part of the tympanic cavity and the anterior fibrous annulus (**Fig. 3.14**).

Together with a retroauricular fold incision, other techniques using a lateral circumferential incision of the ear canal skin (see **Fig. 3.12a, b**) and a large tympanomeatal flap are applied:
- **Fisch technique** with a large lateral circumferential incision from the 4-o'clock to the 6-o'clock position, also involving the anterior ear canal wall and temporary removal of all ear canal skin (Fisch 1994; see MMES_1, Figs. 88–92).
- **Farrior technique** with a lateral incision from the 6-o'clock to 3-o'clock position, involving four-fifths of the circumference of the canal skin (Farrior 1968) and temporary removal of all ear canal skin except for an anterior strip (see MMES_1, Figs. 93–95).

Removal of Ear Canal Skin

Surgeons using lateral circumferential incisions with large tympanomeatal flaps often temporarily remove ear canal skin flaps (Sheehy 1972; Plester 1963; Farrior 1968; Plester et al. 1989; Fisch 1994). Reasons for this are the risk of damage to the skin during drilling, or skin flaps being too large and/or too thick and interfering with surgery, and damage during widening of the bony ear canal. The removed skin is replaced and partly covers the fascia and perichondrium grafts.

Surgeons using medial circumferential incisions in the Wullstein–Kley technique seldom remove the skin flaps, mainly because the small flaps do not interfere with surgery. Wullstein (1968) himself often temporarily removed the tympanomeatal flap.

Removal of Ear Canal Skin Flaps in Cartilage Tympanoplasty

It is my experience that temporary removal of the ear canal skin together with the eardrum remnant in a total perforation is advantageous in difficult cases. The tympanic cavity and the removed eardrum can be cleaned more easily and more safely, mainly because of the removal of the fibrous annulus. After placement of the palisades (see Chapter 4), the replaced ear canal skin covers the edges of the palisades, promoting rapid epithelialization of the eardrum (**Fig. 3.15a, b**).

Instead of palisades, the Dornhoffer (2003) cartilage–perichondrium composite island graft can be placed to cover the total perforation (see Chapter 17). The ear canal skin is temporarily removed together with the fibrous annulus and the eardrum remnant, leaving only the anterior strip of skin intact (**Fig. 3.16**). The island graft is easily placed into the tympanic cavity and the perichondrium flap onto the denuded bone, suspending the cartilage disk. The replaced skin will cover the peripheral end of the cartilage and the perichondrium flap.

When a Farrior approach is used (with temporary removal of the ear canal skin together with the epithelium of the ear drum, but leaving the lamina propria and the fibrous annulus intact), the total perforation is easily

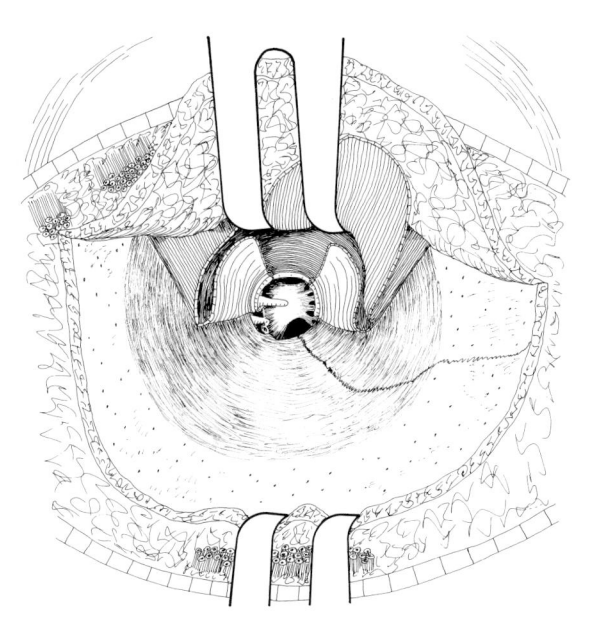

Fig. 3.14 The Palva swing door technique. After a radial incision at the 9-o'clock position, a large superior and inferior flap is elevated together with the cut fibrous annulus and ear drum remnants.

closed with cartilage strip in an on-lay technique (see Chapter 5). The thin strips are positioned onto the denuded eardrum remnant, each strip on the edge of the previous strip so that they overlap slightly like roof tiles (**Fig. 3.17**). The replaced epithelium can easily cover the edges of the cartilage strips.

Medial Circumferential Incision

Medial circumferential incisions can be placed at any level between the eardrum and the middle of the ear canal, but usually they are placed approximately 7 mm lateral to the eardrum. The lateral skin flaps created in a medial circumferential incision are larger than those created with the lateral circumferential incision. The length, elevation, and shape of the lateral flap can differ in various modifications.

After a medial circumferential incision:
- An inferolaterally based flap is created with a superior vertical outward incision (Wullstein 1968).
- A superolaterally based flap is created with an inferior vertical outward incision.
- A laterally based flap is created with superior and inferior vertical outward incisions. This flap is the simplest and most often used in approaches with medial circumferential incisions.

Wullstein–Kley Technique

After a retroauricular fold incision and elevation of the lateral part of the ear and skin, the bony ear canal is widened by drilling for 2–3 mm (**Fig. 3.18**). The ear canal skin is further elevated toward the eardrum. At a level

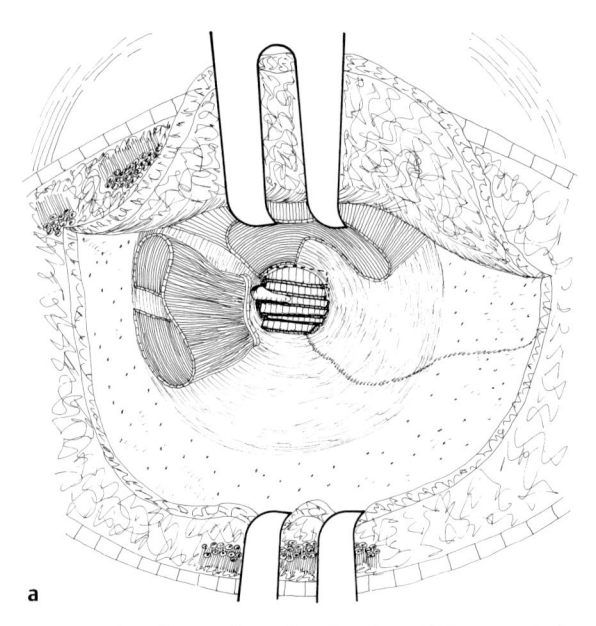

Fig. 3.15a, b Closure of a total perforation with intact ossicular chain, using underlay cartilage palisade technique in Farrior retroauricular approach.

a In the retroauricular fold incision and the lateral circumferential ear canal skin incision, most of the ear canal skin is temporarily removed, together with the fibrous annulus and the eardrum remnant. Gelfoam supports the palisades at the superior and anterior parts of the tympanic cavity, while the inferior ends of the palisades lie on the bony annulus.

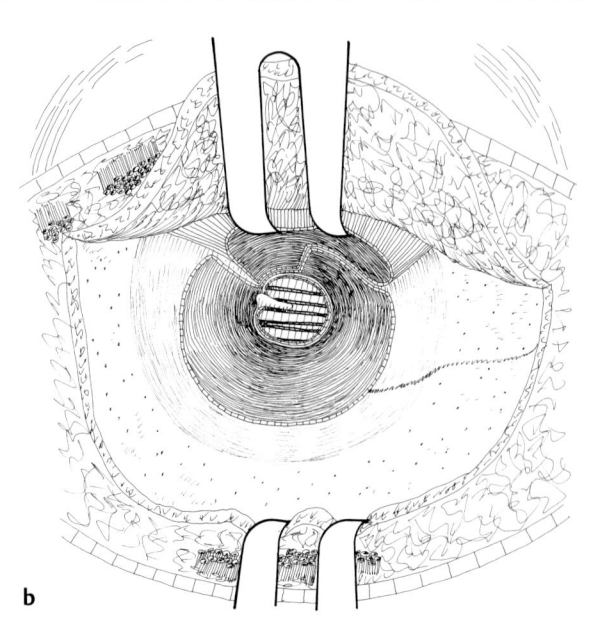

b The skin with the fibrous annulus and the epithelium of the eardrum remnant is replaced, covering the edges of the palisades.

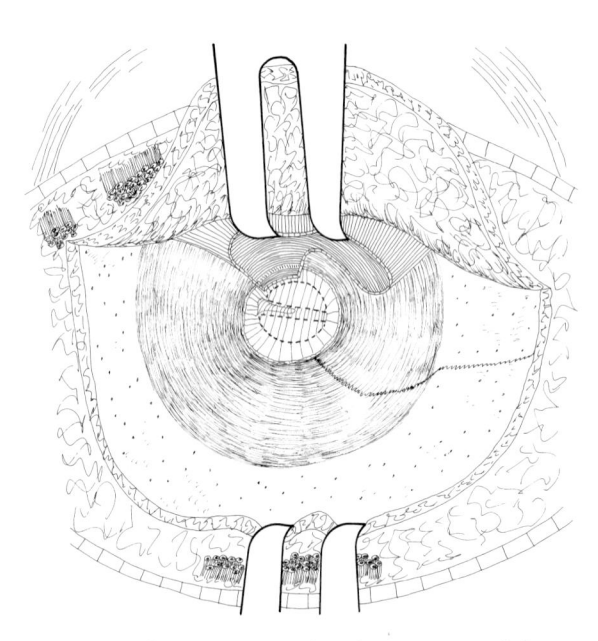

Fig. 3.16 In the Farrior approach with extensive canal skin removal, the total perforation is closed by the Dornhoffer cartilage–perichondrium composite island graft. The fibrous annulus is removed together with the skin, providing good conditions for placement of the island graft into the tympanic cavity at the level of the bony annulus. The perichondrium between the two cartilage disks covers the malleus handle; the peripheral perichondrium covers the bone all around the ear canal, including the attic region. The replaced skin will cover the edges of the grafts as shown in **Fig. 3.15b**.

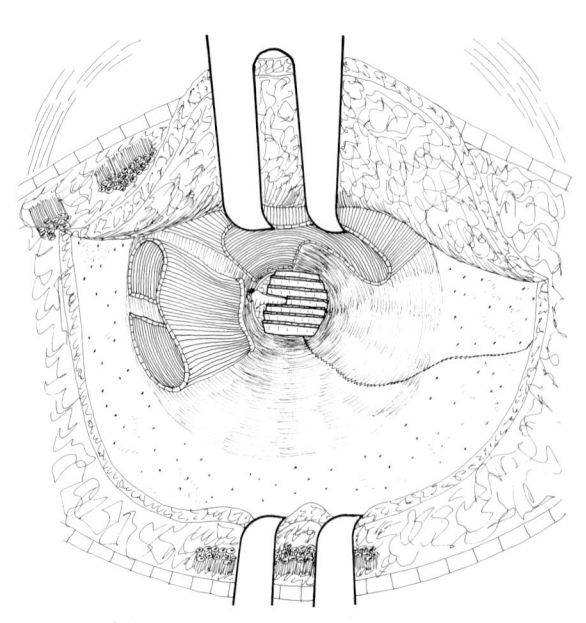

Fig. 3.17 On-lay cartilage strip technique in Farrior retroauricular approach in closure of a total perforation. The fibrous annulus and the denuded lamia propria are covered with thin cartilage strips placed onto the lamina propria and onto the fibrous annulus in a "roof tile" manner: the edge of the previous strip is covered by the next strip. Replacement of the skin is shown in **Fig. 3.15b**.

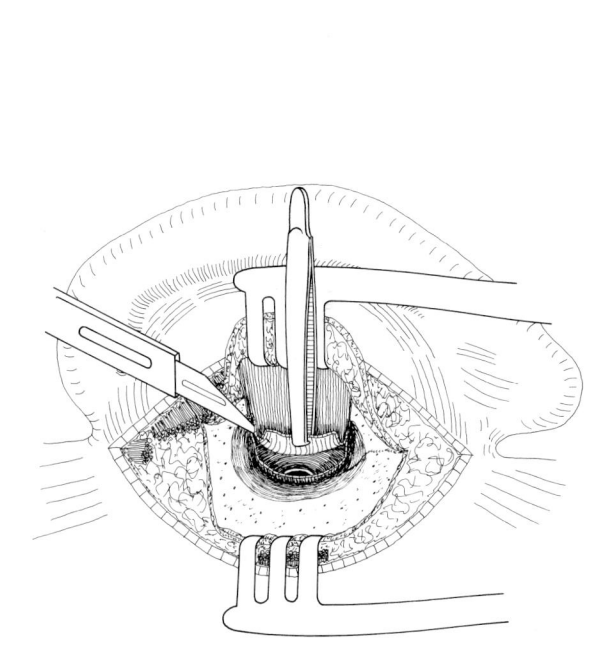

Fig. 3.18 Wullstein–Kley technique. After drilling of the bony ear canal wall, a circumferential incision is made about 10 mm medial to the spine. A small lateral radial incision at the 12-o'clock position and a similar small lateral radial incision at the 6-o'clock position are made. With a pincer a small skin flap is pulled outward and then a superior incision of the skin is continued outward.

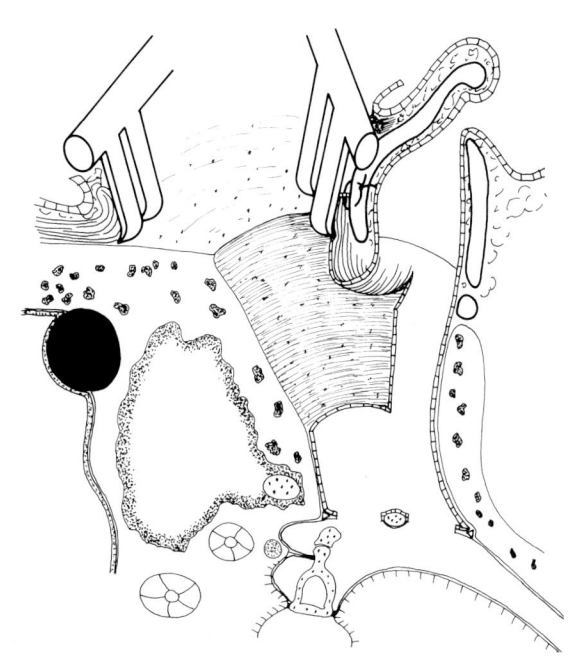

Fig. 3.19 Side view of the completed Wullstein–Kley technique. The inferolateral skin flap is pulled outward and sutured to the concha cartilage. With a long self-retaining retractor the lateral end of the ear canal with the meatus is pulled outward, providing a good view of the tympanic cavity.

about 10 mm medial to the spine of Henle, a circumferential incision between the 12-o'clock and the 6-o'clock positions is performed. Then, a small superior vertical outward incision is started at the 12-o'clock position. A similar small inferior vertical incision is also performed, and a small skin flap is pulled backward and outward, allowing one to proceed with the superior radial outward incision for about 1 cm along the roof of the ear canal (**Fig. 3.18**). The ear canal skin flap is turned backward and sutured to the conchal cartilage. Finally, a self-retaining retractor is used to pull the external meatus outward, providing a good view of the tympanic cavity (**Fig. 3.19**) (Wullstein 1968; Kley 1982; Wullstein and Wullstein 1990).

Management of the Medial Tympanomeatal Flap

- The medial flap can be temporarily removed.
- It can be elevated together with the fibrous annulus and eardrum remnant (see **Fig. 3.13c**). This is suitable for an underlay technique.
- It can be divided with a radial incision at the 9-o'clock position into two parts and elevated as in Palva's swing-door underlay technique (see **Fig. 3.14**).
- Most of the medial ear canal skin, with the fibrous annulus, is temporarily elevated for placement of the palisades (**Fig. 3.15a**) onto the Gelfoam balls and partly onto the bony annulus. The entire skin flap is replaced (**Fig. 3.15b**). Instead of palisades, a total perforation can be covered with the Dornhoffer total cartilage–perichondrium composite island graft (**Fig. 3.16**)
- The medial flap is not elevated (**Fig. 3.20a**), but the skin is incised 0.5–1 mm laterally to the fibrous annulus all the way around the total perforation. Three superior skin/epithelium flaps are elevated and the ear canal skin from the fibrous annulus as well as the epithelium from the eardrum remnant is removed. This technique is suitable for on-lay tympanoplasty (Tos 1980); closure of a total perforation with a cartilage–perichondrium island graft (**Fig. 3.20b**) or with cartilage palisades is easy as well.

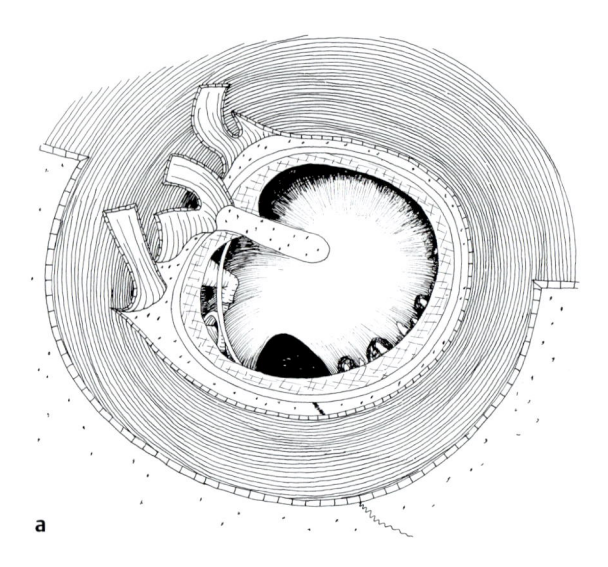

Fig. 3.20a, b Three-flap on-lay technique in retroauricular approach (Tos 1980) with medial tympanomeatal flap technique.
a After a circumferential skin incision close to the annulus, three epithelial flaps are formed and the fibrous annulus and eardrum remnant are cleansed of epithelium.

b The total perforation is closed with a cartilage–perichondrium composite island graft with a U-shaped wedge for the malleus handle. The surrounding perichondrium is placed onto the denuded eardrum remnant, fibrous annulus, and bone. The epithelial flaps are replaced.

Harvesting of Cartilage

Harvesting of cartilage is described in depth in the later chapters and only the general aspects of harvesting the cartilage of the tragus and of the concha will be described here. The illustrations of the harvesting of cartilage that can be found in the later chapters will be cited here.

Harvesting of Tragal Cartilage

Tragal cartilage seems to be used more often than conchal cartilage, mainly because it is harvested along the same route as that of the transcanal and the endaural approaches. Also, tragal cartilage is slightly thinner and less convex than conchal cartilage.

For cosmetic reasons, the incision is most often made 2–3 mm medial to the tragal dome, in one sweep through the skin, posterior perichondrium, cartilage, and anterior perichondrium.

In most cases, with small or medium-sized perforations, only a small piece of tragus or concha cartilage is needed. A small or medium-sized tragus graft can be harvested during the endaural approach by exposing the superior edge of the tragus or the inferior edge of the concha. Nitsche (1985) harvested tragus cartilage through the Heermann B endaural approach (see **Fig. 17.4a–c**).

For the removal of a large piece of tragal cartilage (**Fig. 3.21**), the incision is 15 mm long. Using a pair of scissors, the extraperichondrial plane is created on both sides and the cartilage graft is excised.

Tolsdorff (1983), who was the first to apply the total pars tensa island graft, harvested the tragal graft with an incision placed 2 mm medial from the dome. The cartilage disk was covered with the perichondrium on both sides (see **Fig. 17.6**)

Dornhoffer (1997) made an incision 2 mm medial to the tragus dome, saving the dome. Subcutaneous tissue from the posterior and anterior perichondrium is removed by spreading a pair of sharp scissors, creating a plane as medial as possible. At this point, it is important to make the inferior incision as low as possible. The tragus graft is then grasped and retracted inferiorly, which delivers the superior portion from the incisura area. The superior border is then dissected out while retracting. Along the superior border, all cartilage is removed (see **Fig. 17.5a–c**), which produces a large piece of cartilage, typically 15 mm long and 10 mm wide in children and somewhat larger in adults.

Tragus Dome Cartilage and Perichondrium

Some surgeons perform the skin incision over the dome of the tragus (see **Fig. 26.2a–c**) and remove a piece of tragal cartilage together with the dome, covered on both sides with the perichondrium. Fernandes (2003) used perichondrium from the opposite side of his "triple C" technique graft if the cartilage is not large enough for closure of a perforation(see **Fig. 26.2 d, e**).

In the superior composite graft (see Chapter 14), the tragal dome is widely used in large superior composite grafts with large perichondrial flaps, such as the McCleve graft (see **Fig. 14.4e–f**), the Fleury graft (see **Figs. 14.5, 14.6**), and the Adkins grafts (see **Fig. 14.7a, b** and

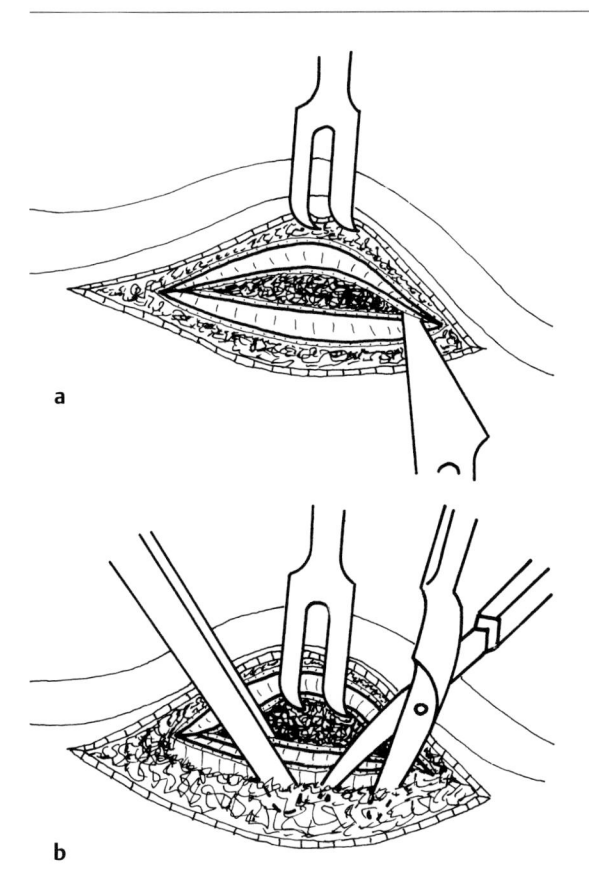

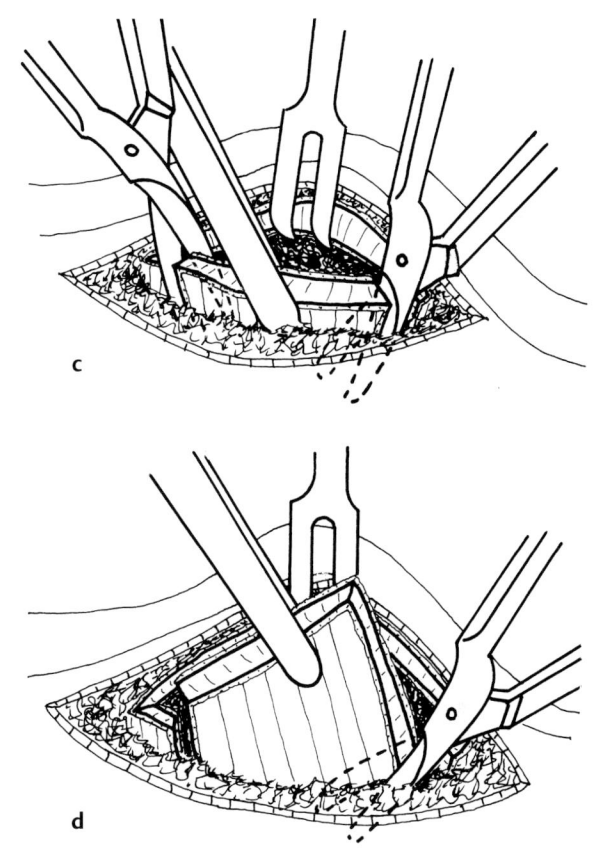

Fig. 3.21a–d Harvesting a large tragal cartilage graft with a 15 mm incision 2 mm medial to the dome.
a The large incision is made in one sweep through the skin and the cartilage with the perichondrium.
b Using a pair of scissors, the extraperichondrial tissue is elevated on both sides of the tragus.
c The tragus is first cut along the superior border and then the inferior cut is made.
d Using pincers the tragus is pulled outward and cut along the medial border.

Fig. 14.9b) (McCleve 1969, 1985; Fleury et al. 1974; Adkins and Osguthorpe 1984; Adkins 1990). The cartilage dome with the dome perichondrium is used to extend the perichondrium from the opposite side of the graft.

In large composite grafts, such as the total pars tensa island graft, a large piece of tragus cartilage is needed. The cartilage dome can be preserved, but the dome perichondrium has to be elevated (**Fig. 3.22**) before the cartilage incision.

To achieve a large perichondrium flap, as needed in some total pars tensa island grafts (see Chapter 17), especially in cases with bony defects in the attic or the posterior scutum, and in particular in crown cork grafts (see Chapter 19), we have introduced a method of in-situ elevation of the perichondrium with reduced removal of the cartilage. This method is described in Chapter 19.

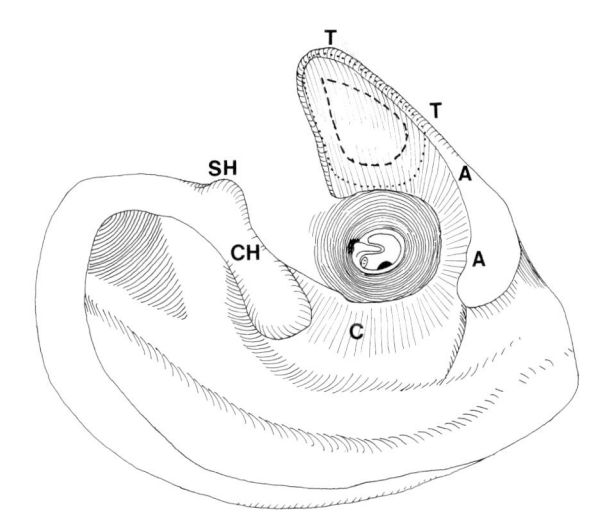

Fig. 3.22 After making the intercartilaginous incision, the entire tragal cartilage is visualized by pulling the tragal cartilage forward. The size of the cartilage and of the incision is shown by a dashed line. The incision of the perichondrium is larger, and is indicated by the dotted line. T, tragus; A, antitragus, C, concha, CH, crus of the helix; SH, spine of the helix.

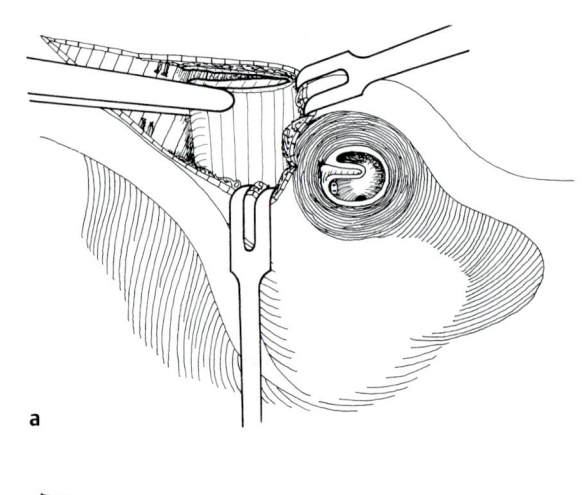

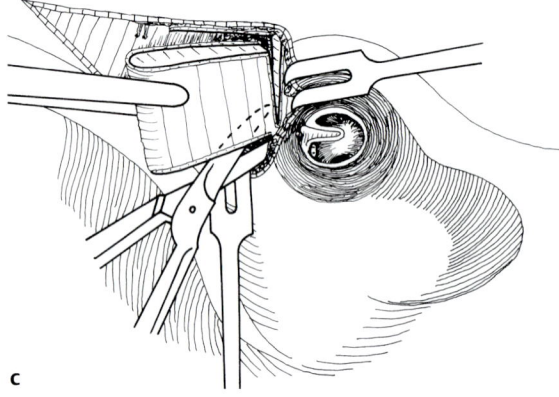

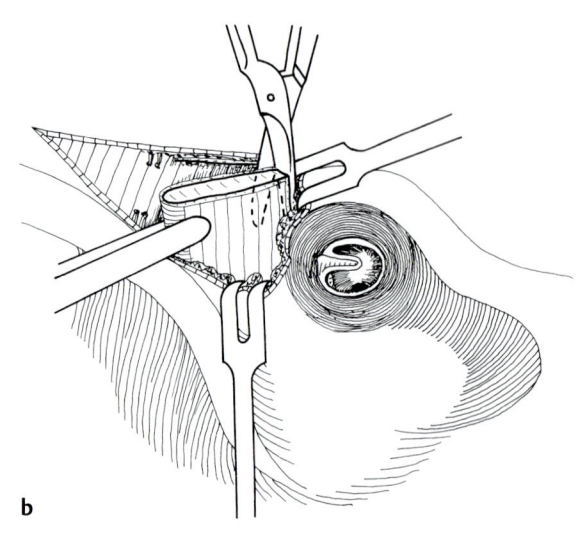

Fig. 3.23a–c Harvesting of tragal cartilage in Heermann B incision and preserving the dome.
a A 15 mm long vertical skin incision at the 12-o'clock position is made in the ear canal. The superior border of the tragus cartilage is identified and the subcutis is separated from the perichondrium on both sides, but the dome is not exposed. A horizontal incision is made through the tragus cartilage, 2 mm medial to the tragus dome.
b The tragus is pulled further in the superior direction, allowing an inferior vertical incision.
c After a medial incision, the tragus cartilage is removed. The tragus dome is intact.

Harvesting Tragal Cartilage Through an Intercartilaginous Incision

Surgeons who frequently perform endaural approaches will often harvest **tragal** cartilage using an intercartilaginous incision, such as the Heermann B incision (see **Figs. 3.6**, **3.7**), the Shambaugh incision (see **Fig. 3.8**), the Lempert incision (see **Fig. 3.10**), or the Farrior incision (see **Fig. 3.11**).

Heermann most often harvested tragal cartilage for his palisades through the intercartilaginous B incision.

In the Hermann B incision, the superior edge of the tragus and the dome are easily palpated with a pair of scissors, grasped with pincers, and pulled outward in the superior direction (see **Fig. 17.4a**). The subcutaneous tissue is cleaned from the perichondrium and either the superior half or the superior two-thirds of tragal cartilage is cut (see **Fig. 17.4b**) and removed (see **Fig. 17.4c**).

Preservation of the dome. The superior border of the tragal cartilage is identified and pulled in the superior direction. Using a pair of scissors, the plane between the perichondrium and the subcutaneous tissue is established on the anterior and posterior side of the tragus. A horizontal incision of the tragus 2 mm medial to the dome (**Fig. 3.23a**) separates the dome from the tragus. An inferior vertical incision mobilizes the tragus, which is then pulled in the superior direction (**Fig. 3.23b**), cut medially, and removed (**Fig. 3.23c**).

Additional illustrations on harvesting tragal cartilage and perichondrium are shown in MMES_1, Figs. 255–266).

Harvesting of Cartilage from the Auricle

Cartilage can be harvested from various sites of the posterior side of the auricle (**Fig. 3.24**):
- Eminence of the concha
- Eminence of the cymba concha
- Eminence of the triangular fossa
- Eminence of the scapha

From the anterior side of the auricle, large parts of the conchal cartilage can be removed in various endaural approaches.

Harvesting of Conchal Cartilage

Conchal cartilage is slightly thicker and more convex than tragal cartilage, but it is always large enough for any composite graft, even for the crown cork graft, which demands the largest perichondrium flaps (see Chapter 19).

Conchal cartilage can be harvested from the posterior side of the auricle through a separate incision in case of a cartilage tympanoplasty via a transmeatal or endaural approach. The incision provides a good view of the eminence of the concha. The convex posterior side of the graft faces the tympanic cavity. Therefore, the perichondrium is removed first from the convex side (see **Fig. 20.5a**), which is followed by removal of the cartilage–perichondrium graft (see **Fig. 20.5b**). The ease of harvesting a large conchal graft is evident, but most surgeons still prefer to use tragal cartilage.

Harvesting of conchal cartilage via a retroauricular approach during a retroauricular cartilage tympanoplasty and mastoidectomy is usually performed at the beginning of the operation with exposure and resection of a large conchal cartilage–perichondrium island graft (**Fig. 3.25**).

Harvesting of large pieces of conchal cartilage (**Fig. 3.26**) is sometimes necessary in cases with total reconstruction of the ear canal wall with cartilage, which may be required during the reconstruction of radical cavities or in other canal wall down procedures. Heermann (1977, 1992) reported harvesting large pieces of concha cartilage.

Further illustrations of the removal of conchal cartilage and perichondrium are included in MMES_1, Figs. 267–290.

Harvesting of Cymba Cartilage

Seen from the anterior side, the concha of the auricle is divided into a larger cavum conchae and a smaller cymba conchae. The cymba is positioned superiorly and posteriorly to the crus of the helix and inferiorly to the inferior crus of the antihelix. Seen from the anterior side, the cymba is very concave; from the posterior side, it is very convex. On the posterior side, the cymba is considerably more convex than the concha. Bernal-Sprekelsen and colleagues (Bernal-Sprekelsen and Barberan 1997; Bernal-Sprekelsen et al. 1997, 2003) used the convex cartilage from the cymba for cutting broad palisades (see Chapter 6). Dornhoffer (2003) also used cartilage from the cymba.

Subcutaneous tissue is elevated in a 2 cm-long skin incision over the superior part of the concha, exposing the perichondrium of the upper part of the eminence of the concha and of the eminence of the cymba, which protrudes the most (**Fig. 3.27**). Its inferior border is the

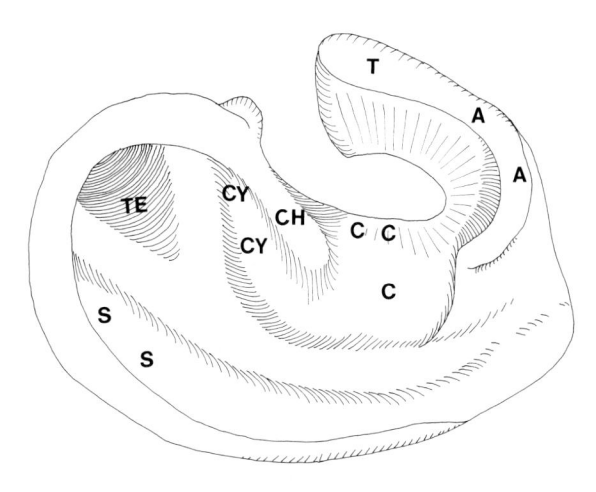

Fig. 3.24 Sites for harvesting the cartilage in the right auricle seen on the front side. C, concha; CY, cymba; TE, triangular eminence; S, scapha; T, tragus; A, antitragus; CH, crus of the helix.

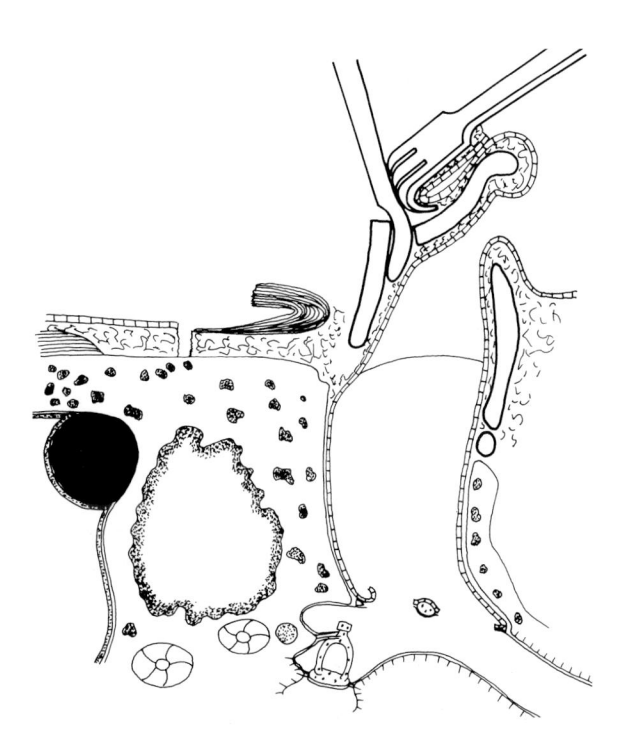

Fig. 3.25 Harvesting of conchal cartilage via a retroauricular approach. Side view of the retroauricular flap approach starting with harvesting a large piece of conchal cartilage. The conchal cartilage is cut and elevated with a rugine.

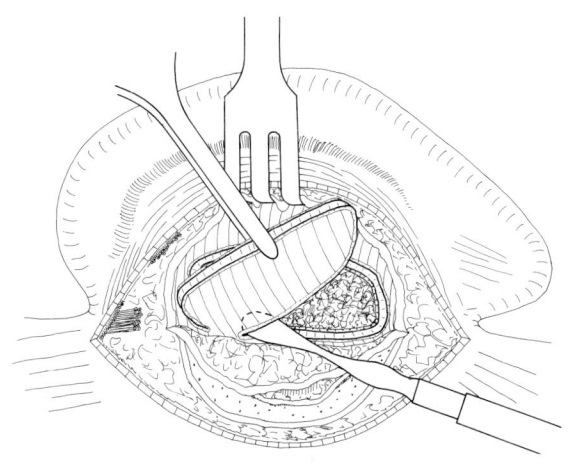

Fig. 3.26 Harvesting of a large piece of conchal cartilage. A large incision is made along the entire conchal eminence; perichondrium is exposed and a large oval-shaped concha including part of the cymba cartilage is excised. Both sides are covered with perichondrium.

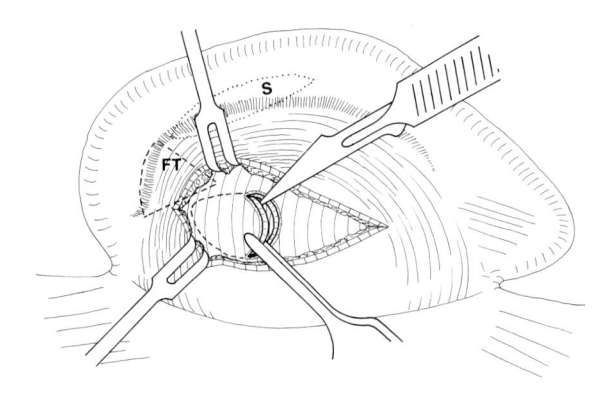

Fig. 3.27 Harvesting of the cymba cartilage and the fossa triangularis cartilage. Incision of the skin is slightly superior to the eminence of the concha. Subcutaneous tissue is elevated and the perichondrium of the superior part of the eminence of the concha and of the cymba is exposed. With a circular incision the most convex part—the cymba cartilage—is cut and removed. The dashed line indicates the eminence of the triangular fossa (FT), the dotted line the eminence of the scapha (S).

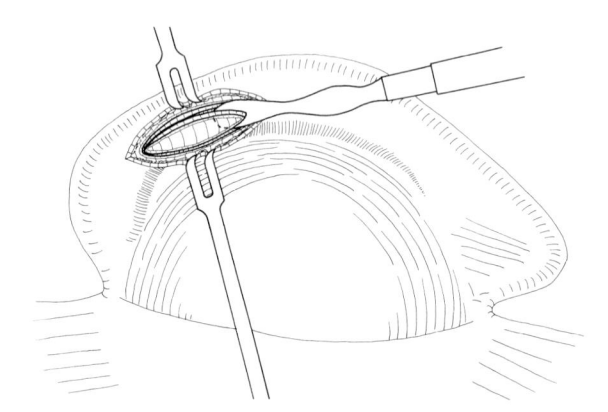

Fig. 3.28 Harvesting of cartilage from the eminence of the scapha. After a 20 mm long skin incision on the eminence of the scapha, the skin and subcutaneous tissue are elevated, exposing an area of 20 mm × 5 mm to allow cutting and removal of a 20 mm × 5 mm piece of cartilage.

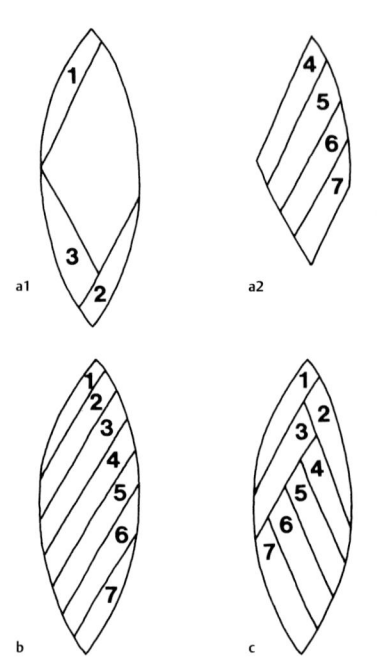

Fig. 3.29a–c Three examples of cutting palisades on a relatively small piece.
a1 The first three palisades are cut along the edges.
a2 The next four palisades are cut in an oblique manner.
b All seven palisades are cut in an oblique manner.
c All seven palisades are cut in an oblique manner, but in various directions.

crus of the helix; its superior border is the crus of the antihelix. An oval piece of cartilage of 1.5 cm × 1 cm is removed.

Harvesting of Fossa Triangularis Cartilage

Moore (2002) showed in a cadaver study that fossa triangularis cartilage is thinner and has less mass than tragal cartilage.

Fossa triangularis cartilage creates a relatively mobile neotympanic membrane with a stiffness that is more resistant than that of fascia.

Seen in the front view, the fossa triangularis has a triangular shape and is bordered by the anterior and posterior crus of the antihelix. The superior border is the helix.

A piece of cartilage with a diameter of 1 cm is harvested from the fossa triangularis through a retroauricular incision. The eminence of the fossa triangularis is positioned superiorly to the cymba (**Fig. 3.27**). It starts at the anterior crus of the antihelix, and ends at the posterior crus of the antihelix. In the same paper, Moore (2002) reported good anatomical and functional results in tympanoplasty of 83 patients with fossa triangularis cartilage in total perforations, but it is not clear whether a perichondrium flap around the cartilage disk was used either as a composite graft or as a thick cartilage plate covered on the ear canal side with perichondrium.

Harvesting of Scapha Cartilage

On the posterior side of the auricle, the eminence of the scapha is a relatively flat and long area between the antihelix and the helix (**Fig. 3.27**). Since 2001, I have often utilized scapha cartilage for the cutting of palisades and strips (see Chapters 4, 5, and 7). The removed piece of cartilage may be very small, but it can be long and is always large enough for cutting sufficient numbers of palisades.

A 2 cm-long skin incision along the eminence of the scapha allows elevation of the subcutaneous tissue and exposes the perichondrium. The perichondrium and cartilage are incised and a 20 × 5 mm piece of cartilage can be removed (**Fig. 3.28**). The cartilage is elevated and removed using a Freer rugine. The cartilage can be cut in various ways with a scalpel to provide up to seven palisades for covering a total perforation (**Fig. 3.29a–c**).

Harvesting of Cartilage in Endaural Approaches

Cartilage removed for various indications from the anterior side of the auricle can be used in tympanoplasty, especially as palisades or as strips. Larger pieces of cartilage can be utilized as composite grafts with peripheral perichondrium flaps.

Lines of Resection of the Cartilage

In addition to harvesting of cartilage for use in endaural approaches, removal of cartilage for other reasons, especially to enlarge the access to the mastoid cavity, dictates various lines of resection and corresponding areas of the conchal cartilage (**Fig. 3.30**):

Lines 1 and 2: Resection of the most anterior 3–4 mm and 4–5 mm, respectively, of the concha, used after canal wall down mastoidectomy to prevent stenosis. Lines 1 and 2 do not involve the crus of the helix.

Lines 3 and 4 are used when treating stenosis after previous canal wall down mastoidectomy. Considerable areas of cartilage are removed, including part of the crus of the helix.

Lines 5a and 5b involve the entire concha, taken as graft material.

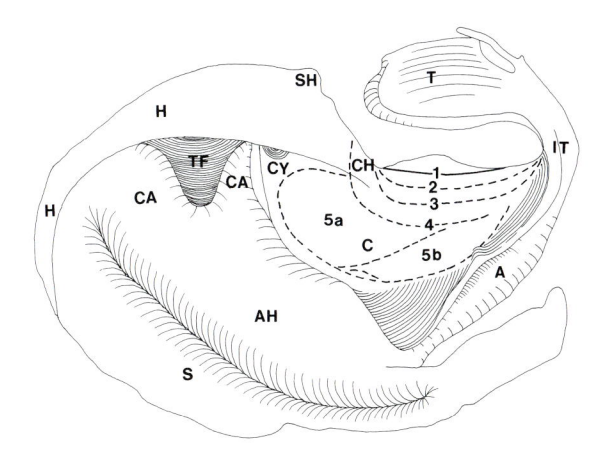

Fig. 3.30 The front side of the auricle showing resection lines 1–4 for widening the ear canal and harvesting the conchal cartilage. The areas 5a and 5b illustrate the possibilities of harvesting conchal cartilage in endaural approaches. T, tragus; IT, intertragal notch; A, antitragus; SH, spine of the helix; CH, crus of the helix; CY, cymba; C, concha; CA, anterior and posterior crus of the helix; TF, triangular fossa; AH, antihelix; S, scapha; H, helix.

Harvesting of Cartilage via an Endaural Approach

The anterior area of the conchal cartilage can easily be harvested in all endaural approaches.

Heermann approach. Using a Heermann B incision, the skin is elevated from the crus of the helix and from the conchal cartilage. A large piece of the cartilage with perichondrium is elevated (**Fig. 3.31**). If a larger piece is needed, a lateral radial skin incision at the 7-o'clock position is performed, allowing further elevation of the conchal skin and cartilage.

Shambaugh and Lempert approaches. Using the Shambaugh incision, the skin from the crux of the helix and concha is elevated, exposing a large area of conchal cartilage. A large piece of conchal cartilage is excised (**Fig. 3.32**). The approach is the same using the Lempert incision.

Farrior approach. In the Farrior approach, a lateral radial incision allows further elevation of the skin, exposing a large piece of conchal cartilage (**Fig. 3.33**).

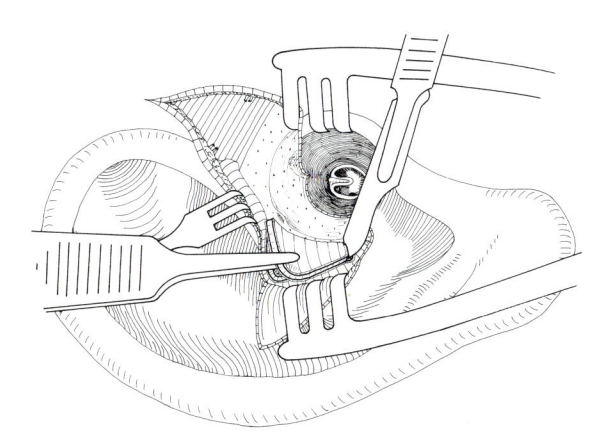

Fig. 3.31 Harvesting conchal cartilage in the endaural approach with the Heermann B incision. The ear canal skin is elevated outward exposing conchal cartilage, which is removed with the perichondrium.

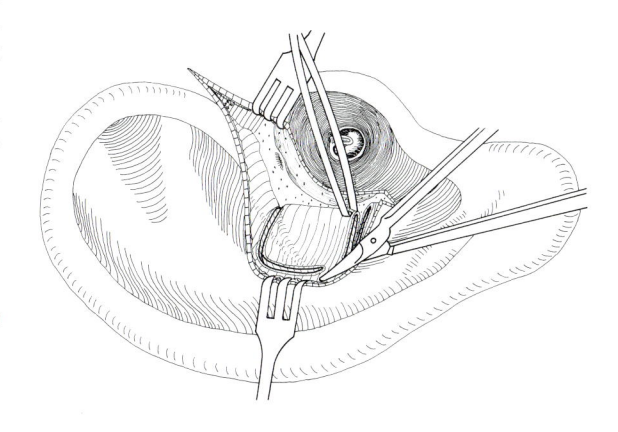

Fig. 3.32 Harvesting conchal cartilage in the Shambaugh endaural approach. The skin is elevated outward from the helix and the conchal cartilage. The lateral radial incision of the conchal skin allows resection of a large piece of the conchal cartilage.

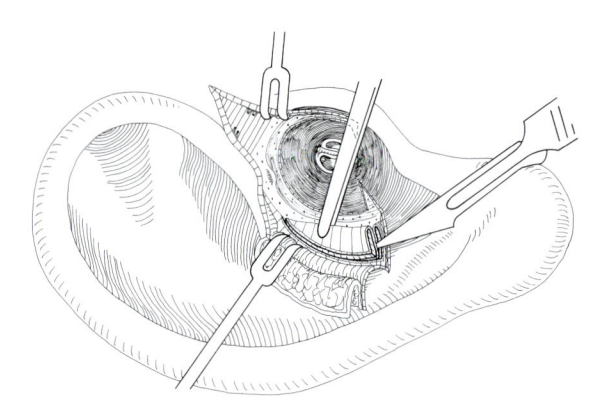

Fig. 3.33 Harvesting conchal cartilage in the Farrior endaural approach. A relatively long lateral radial skin incision and elevation of the lateral ear canal skin allow easy exposure and removal of the conchal cartilage.

Thinning the Cartilage

On 10 tragal cartilages from cadavers, Moore (2002) found a mean thickness of 1.016 mm compared with a mean thickness of 0.775 mm of 10 cartilages from the triangular fossa. Six measurements were performed on each piece of cartilage. It is the general impression of surgeons that the thickness of the tragus is 0.9 mm while the concha cartilage is slightly thicker.

A full-thickness cartilage graft can be thinned to thicknesses of 0.2 mm, 0.3 mm, 0.4 mm, ½ thickness (4–5 mm), ⅔ thickness (6–7 mm) and ¾ (7–8 mm).

Some methods, such as cartilage foil tympanoplasties (Chapter 10), use cartilage foils with a thickness of 0.2 mm, 0.3 mm, or 0.4 mm. Such thin foils or plates have to be cut with the Kurz Precise Cartilage Knife.

In the recent literature, the thickness of grafts is generally specified in tenths of a millimeter, or as full-, half-, one-third-, or two-thirds thickness grafts. These definitions are useful and necessary for comparison of hearing results, but in surgical practice the measurements cannot always be strictly exact. Sometimes the thickness of one edge of the graft is half-thickness while on the other edge it may be one-quarter or three-quarters thickness. Surgeons have to use what material they have and cannot simply abandon it and harvest another total cartilage graft. Use of the Kurz Precise Cartilage Knife enables grafts of exact thickness to be cut.

Thinning Methods and Devices

There are various ways to split a full-thickness graft into two parts.

Holding the graft with two fingers. Most older otosurgeons who started tympanoplasty in the 1960s have presumably tried this method. I have used it sporadically to split a small piece of cartilage with a scalpel (**Fig. 3.34a**).

The Waltner method, holding the tragus cartilage against a wooden tongue depressor with the thumb while slicing the cartilage with a safety razor blade (**Fig. 3.34b**). In this way Waltner (1966) cut 3 mm wide and 12–13 mm long strips for some innovative tympanoplasty methods described in Chapter 1 (see **Figs. 1.4–1.6**).

Grasping the cartilage with flat surgical forceps and using a scalpel to divide the tragal cartilage into two pieces (**Fig. 3.34c**).

Hildmann cartilage clamp. The clamp is a stable and useful tool. It fixates and holds the cartilage, allowing it to be split into two parts with a scalpel (**Fig. 3.35a–d**). The cartilage is placed onto the flat end of the open clump (a), either without or with the perichondrium. The clamp is closed with a screw (b) and the cartilage is cut into two pieces with a scalpel, either from above (c) or from beneath (d). The clamp can also be used in thinning of the cartilage disk of a composite island graft with a surrounding perichondrium flap (c and d). The perichondrium flap remains intact whereas the thickness of the cartilage disk is reduced.

Kurz Precise Cartilage Knife. The cartilage knife (Kurz Medical, Dusslingen, Germany) consists of the two-piece cutting block (**Fig. 3.36a**) and a blade holder with a special blade (**Fig. 3.36b**). In one end of the bottom cutting block is the recess into which the cartilage piece is placed (**Fig. 3.36a**). The rectangular recess is 10 mm × 10 mm and its depth is 0.7 mm. In the center of the bottom cutting block is a threaded post to fixate the upper cutting block (with the Kurz logo) to the lower cutting block. After the cartilage is placed into the rectangular recess, the upper cutting block is turned to align with the bottom part. The nut is placed onto the threaded post and is slightly tightened (**Fig. 3.36c**).

The cartilage knife is now ready for cutting the cartilage and the blade is fixed properly in the blade holder. The cutting block must be stood upright while cutting. The blade holder with the blade is placed into the guiding slots of the cutting block. With slight sawing movements in both directions the blade is moved to the bottom. After the cartilage has been cut through, the cutting block is laid down with the cutting block nut upward. The upper part of the cutting block is removed after unscrewing the nut. This avoids damage to the cartilage slice. Then the blade is removed and the cartilage slice is removed. The resized piece of cartilage will be between the blade and the distance plate.

Distance plates reduce the thickness of the cartilage. The three distance plates of 0.1, 0.2, and 0.3 mm (**Fig. 3.36d**) reduce the thickness of the cut graft in the following way. Maximal thickness of the cut graft is 0.7 mm. With all three plates in place the cut graft will measure only 0.1 mm (0.7–0.6 mm). With a 0.2 mm plate in place the graft will measure 0.5 mm, a thickness that is commonly used. To produce the 0.3 mm thick foils, a 0.1 mm plate and a 0.4 mm plate are needed together.

Figure 3.36e illustrates the following example. The 0.1 mm distance plate was placed first into the recess of

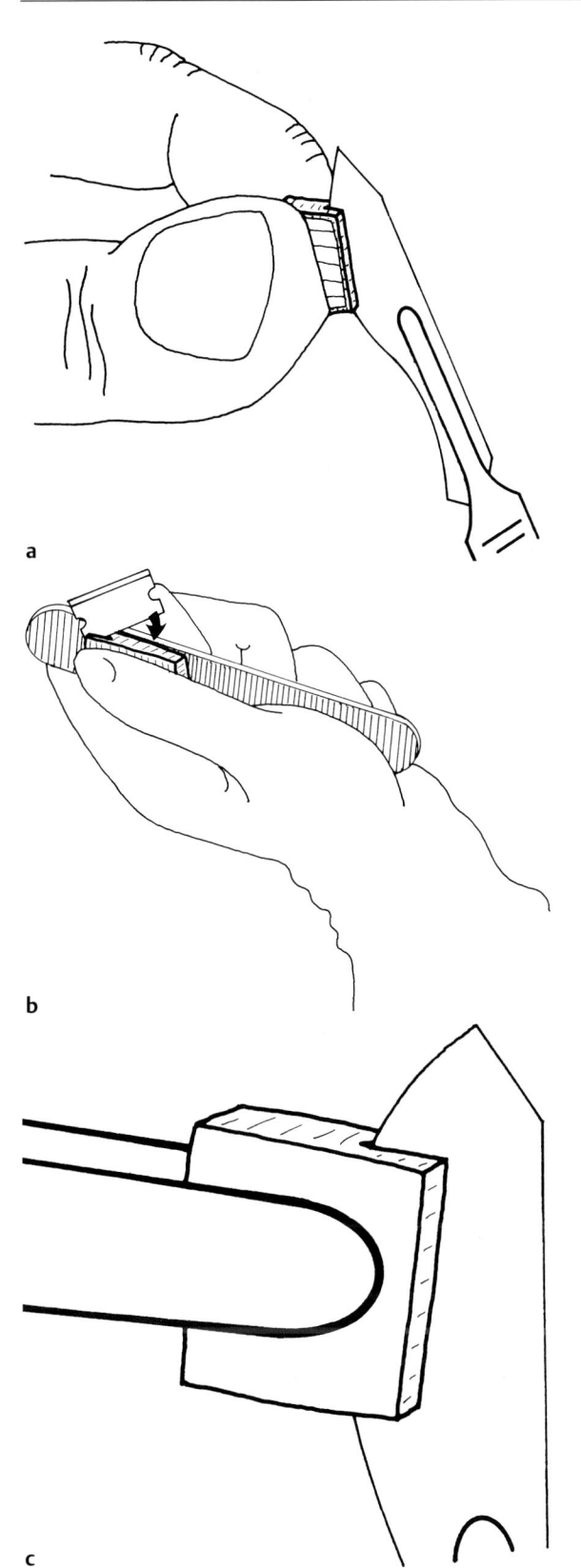

Fig. 3.34a–c Thinning the cartilage.
a Tragal cartilage is held with two fingers and carefully sliced with a scalpel.
b The cartilage is held firm against the wooden tongue depressor and split with a safety razor blade.
c The cartilage is held with a surgical forceps and split with a scalpel.

the lower cutting block, then the cartilage is placed onto the distance plate. After cutting, the result will be a 0.6 mm thick cartilage plate.

Texido Cartilage Cutter. The Microfrance device of Medtronic Xomed Inc. slices cartilage to a standard thickness of 0.3 mm in one swift motion with minimal waste. Working space for trimming and measuring the cartilage is also incorporated to facilitate graft preparation. Slices of 0.3 mm provide 2–3 slices per tragus cartilage graft.

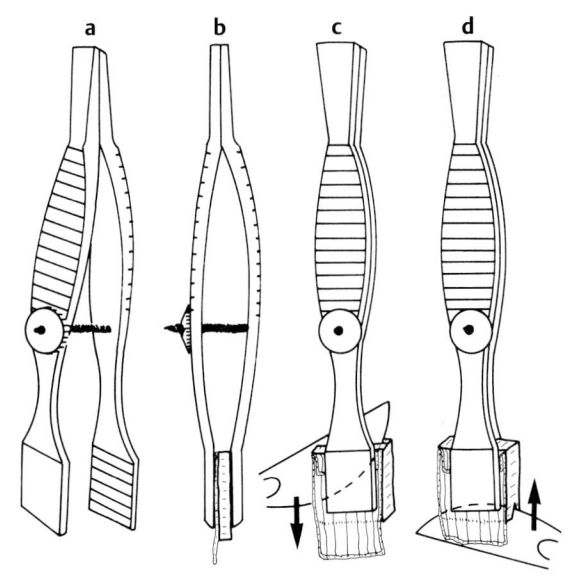

Fig. 3.35a–d The Hildmann cartilage slicing clamp.
a Open clamp.
b The clamp holds the cartilage with the perichondrium to be sliced from above with a scalpel.
c A cartilage island graft with a perichondrium flap is sliced from above.
d The island graft is sliced from below.

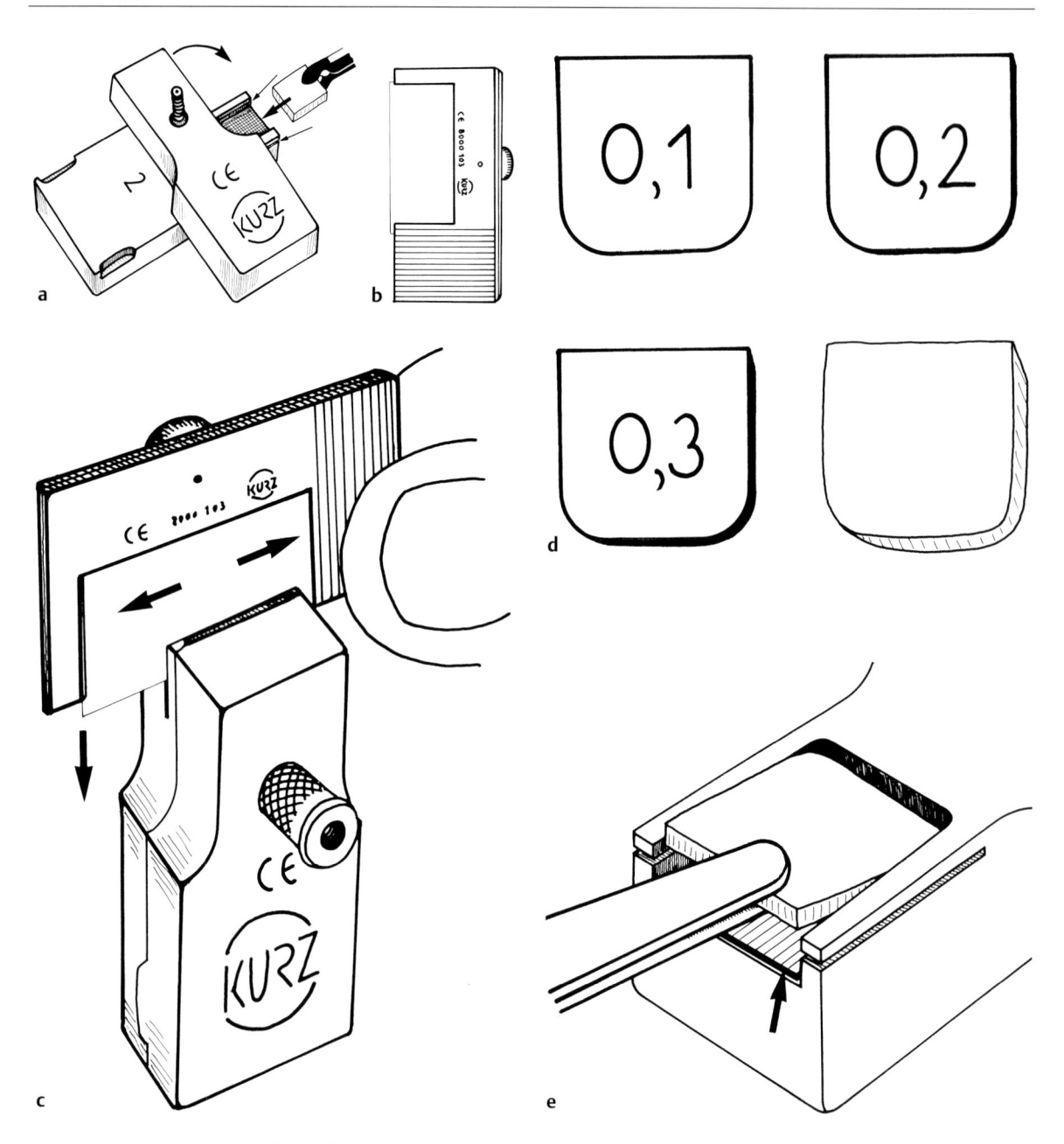

Fig. 3.36a–e Kurz Precise Cartilage Knife.
a The upper part of the two-piece cutting block is positioned at right angles to the lower part, to illustrate the location of the recess of the cutting block into which the cartilage is placed (thick arrow) and the guiding slits (thin arrow) where the razor plate will be placed. After placement of the cartilage, the upper cutting block is turned in the direction of the curved arrow.
b The razor blade is fixed in the blade holder with a screw.
c First the lower and the upper cutting blocks are aligned with each other and the nut is tightened onto the threaded post. Then the blade holder with the blade is placed into the slits of the cutting block. With sawing movements of the blade in directions of the horizontal arrows the cartilage is sliced.
d Distance plates. Metal plates of the same shape and area as the recess of the lower cutting block and of thickness 0.1, 0.2, and 0.3 mm compared with the cartilage of 0.7 mm cut without the use of distance plates.
e The 0.6 mm thick cartilage and a 0.1 mm thick distance plate (arrow) are removed from the recess of the cutting block, after completion of cutting with the distance plate.

The Hüttenbrink Cartilage Guide

Even the optimally fitted columella can be displaced peroperatively by replacement of the tympanomeatal flap, hematoma, strong movement of the malleus handle, or packing of the ear canal, or postoperatively by fluctuations in atmospheric pressure significantly moving the eardrum and by scarring. Dislocation of the prosthesis is the most frequent cause of postoperative hearing loss (Smyth 1983; Hüttenbrink 1994).

The columella is attached to the footplate only through liquid adhesion, and even slight displacements allow the end of the prosthesis to slip and thereby to lose sound transmission. Hüttenbrink (1994) demonstrated that columella prostheses in tympanoplasty type 3 deliver poorer results than interposition prosthesis in tympanoplasty type 2 between the stapes head and the malleus handle. The interposition prosthesis sits much more securely and stably on the stapes head than does the columella on the footplate. In all of our clinical series we found better primary and late results in tympanoplasty type 2 with interposition between the intact stapes and the malleus handle than in tympanoplasty type 3 with a columella placed onto the footplate.

These series involve chronic adhesive otitis media (Tos 1972a), sequelae to chronic otitis media (Tos 1972b), active chronic otitis media with mastoidectomy (Tos 1972c, 1974; Lau and Tos 1986; Tos and Lau 1988), sinus cholesteatoma and tensa retraction cholesteatoma in adults (Lau and Tos 1988, 1989 and in children (Lau and Tos 1987), and middle ear tympanosclerosis (Tos et al. 1990). Thus, our clinical studies strongly support the findings of Hüttenbrink (1994).

To overcome the problems of fixation and stabilization of the columella to the footplate, Fisch (1994) placed a thin spike into the footplate-end of the columella. The spike is attached to a hole made in the center of the footplate, but most surgeons want to avoid the associated opening of the inner ear in the presence of underlying chronic otitis media.

Hüttenbrink and his Dresden group (Hüttenbrink et al 2004) constructed a 0.2–0.3 mm thick, 2.5 mm wide, and 3.5 mm long oval cartilage plate with a 0.8 mm hole. This cartilage guide is placed onto the oval window. Finally the 4.5 mm Kurz titanium columella of Aerial type is placed through the hole of the guide onto the footplate.

The initial hearing results (maximally 1 year after surgery) in 22 patients confirmed the acoustic quality of this stabilization of the columella compared with a matched control group.

Elaboration of the Hüttenbrink Cartilage Guide

With the exact dimensions of the cartilage guide described above, the surgeon can harvest a small piece of tragal or conchal cartilage, remove the perichondrium, cut a 0.3 mm thick plate with a scalpel, and shape it to an oval 2.5 mm ×

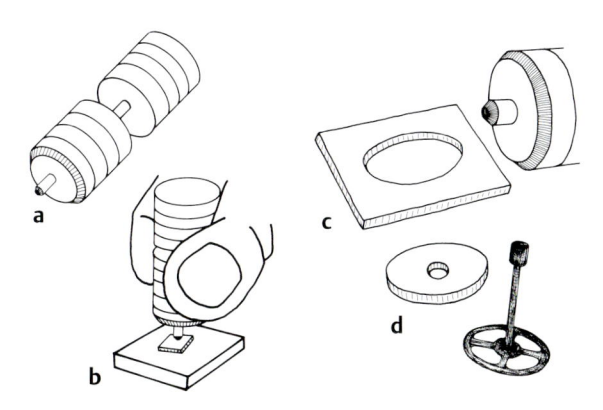

Fig. 3.37a–d Punching out a Hüttenbrink cartilage guide with a special cartilage punch.
a Cartilage punch with two cylinders, one inserted into the other.
b By pressing the upper cylinder downward, both the contour and central hole are punched out.
c Thin cartilage plate, after removal of the cartilage guide, cut with a large oval peripheral punch and a small round punch.
d The 2.5 mm × 3.5 mm oval, 0.3 mm thick guide with a central 0.8 mm hole for the foot of the titanium prosthesis.

3.5 mm plate. Using a small round knife, a 0.8 mm hole can be created in the center of the plate.

The use of the cartilage guide can be made more exact, more sophisticated, and faster as follows.

The piece of cartilage without perichondrium is cut to a thickness of 0.2 or 0.3 mm with a Kurz Precise Cartilage Cutter (see **Fig. 3.36a–d**). Then the thinned cartilage guide is punched out with a special cartilage punch (Kurz Medical, Dusslingen, Germany) that consists of two concentric cylinders (**Fig. 3.37a**), one inserted into the other, a spring maintains some extension of the inner from the outer. The cartilage punch is placed onto the 0.3 mm thick 5 mm × 6 mm piece of cartilage (**Fig. 3.37b**). The lower cylinder has a sharp oval-shaped cutting edge, which punches out a 2.5 mm × 3.5 mm piece of cartilage. In the middle of this oval punch is centered a second rod-shaped punch that is guided by the middle cylinder and has an 0.8 mm diameter. By pressing the upper cylinder downwards, both the contour and the central hole are simultaneously punched out of a cartilage plate (**Fig. 3.37c**). The result is a 2.5 mm × 3.5 mm oval and 0.3 mm thick cartilage plate with a hole of 0.8 mm (**Fig. 3.37 d**). The cartilage guide is placed onto the footplate and the foot of the titanium columella is placed through the hole onto the footplate.

In a recent paper, the Hüttenbrink group in Cologne (Beutner et al. 2008) investigated the validity of the cartilage guide, which is now called the cartilage "shoe," in 52 patients with mobile footplate and missing stapes arch, operated for cholesteatoma (50%) or chronic otitis media (50%). The cartilage shoe with a hole for the prosthesis is placed onto the footplate. The foot of the Kurz titanium TORP prosthesis is placed through the hole of the cartilage shoe onto the footplate. If there are persistent crura remnants, the anterior and posterior poles of the cartilage shoe are cut away.

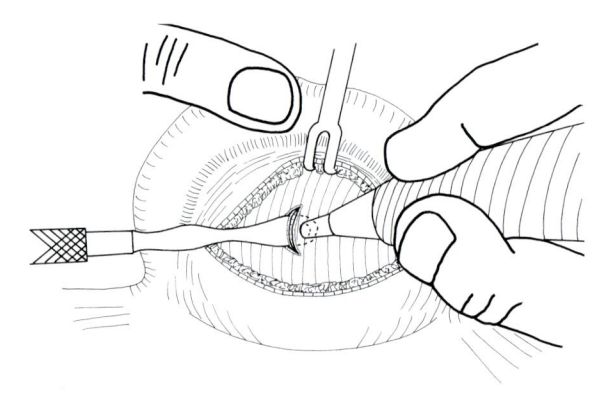

Fig. 3.38 Cutting a round conchal cartilage disk covered on both sides with perichondrium using the Groningen cartilage cutting device. The posterior perichondrium is exposed and cleansed of subcutaneous tissue. A curved incision of the cartilage and the perichondrium on both sides is made. The anterior perichondrium is also cleansed with a Freer. Using a Freer as an anvil and slightly elevating the cartilage, a disk of 4 mm is cut by rotating the cutter.

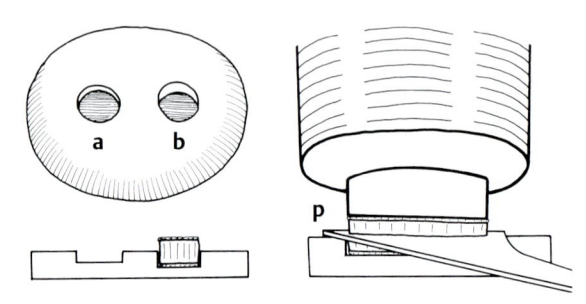

Fig. 3.39a, b Schematic illustration of the cutting block and cutting of the 0.5 mm thick cartilage disk with a diameter of 4 mm.
a The two depressions of the cutting block. In the depression B is placed a full-thickness concha cartilage with perichondrium on both sides
b The removed cartilage disk with the perichondrium on both sides is placed into the round depression of the metallic cutting block. The depression has a diameter of 4 mm and is 0.5 mm deep. The No 11 scalpel blade cuts off the upper part of the cartilage (C).

The mean pure tone average in 52 patients was preoperatively 57.1 dB, postoperatively 42.5 dB. The preoperative mean air–bone gap was 34.4 dB, the postoperative air–bone gap was 21.5 dB.

The Groningen Cartilage Cutting Device

The problem for all synthetic implants is still rejection and extrusion of the prosthesis. Extrusion rates can be lowered by interposing a small cartilage disk between the synthetic implant and the eardrum. Meijer et al. (1999) found in the literature rates of extrusion varying from 15% to 22%. Interposing a cartilage disk between the prosthesis and the eardrum reduces the extrusion rates to 3–6%. Covering the prosthesis with a thick disk may have some negative influence on mechanical properties of the prosthesis, while too thin a cartilage disk may not prevent extrusion. Meijer's group found 0.5 mm thickness optimal, and 0.4 mm to be the minimum thickness required to avoid damage and undesirable changes and instability of the cartilage disk. The Groningen cutting device is constructed on the basis of these figures.

The device consist of a cutter with an external diameter of about 10 mm and an internal diameter of 4.1 mm to cut a cartilage disk of 4.0 mm that covers completely the head of a titanium prosthesis or most other prostheses. The conchal cartilage is used (**Fig. 3.38**). After cleansing the posterior perichondrium, a curved superior incision is made through the cartilage and anterior perichondrium; the anterior perichondrium is cleaned with a Freer and then the 4 mm cartilage disk with the perichondrium on both sides is cut with the cutter. It is sometimes easier to remove a 6 mm × 6 mm piece of tragal or conchal cartilage with the perichondrium and cut the disk on a plastic plate.

The cartilage disk is placed into the 0.5 mm deep depression of the cutting block (**Fig. 3.39a, b**) and pressed with the plastic press and then the outer part of the cartilage disk is cut using a no. 11 blade in the scalpel.

References

Adkins WY. Composite autograft for tympanoplasty and tympanomastoid surgery. Laryngoscope 1990;100:244–247.

Adkins WY, Osguthorpe JD. Use of a composite autograft to prevent recurrent cholesteatoma caused by canal wall defects. Otolaryngol Head Neck Surg 1984;92:319–321.

Andersen J, Cayé-Thomasen P, Tos M. Cartilage palisade tympanoplasty in sinus and tensa retraction cholesteatoma. Otol Neurotol 2002;23:825–831.

Andersen J, Cayé-Thomasen P, Tos M. A comparison of cartilage palisades and fascia in tympanoplasty after surgery for sinus or tensa retraction cholesteatoma in children. Otol Neurotol 2004;25:856–863.

Bernal-Sprekelsen M, Barberan TM. Indications, tecnica y resultados anatomicos de la tympanoplastica con cartilago en empalizada. Acta Otorrinolaringol Esp 1997;48:279–286.

Bernal-Sprekelsen M, Barberan TM, Lliso MDB. Resultados funktionales preliminaries de la timpanoplastica con cartilago en empalizada. Acta Otorrinolaringol Esp 1997;48:341–346.

Bernal-Sprekelsen M, Lliso MDR, Gonzalo JJSG. Cartilage palisades in type 3 tympanoplasty: Anatomic and functional Long-term results. Otol Neurotol 2003;24:38–42.

Beutner D, Luers JC, Huttenbrink KB. Cartilage "shoe": a new technique for stabilization of titanium total ossicular replacement prosthesis at center of stapes footplate. J Laryngol Otol 2008; 122: 682–686.

Dornhoffer JL. Hearing results with cartilage tympanoplasty. Laryngoscope 1997;107:1094–1099.

Dornhoffer J. Cartilage tympanoplasty: indications, techniques, and outcomes in a 1000-patient series. Laryngoscope 2003;113: 1844–1856.

Farrior BJ. Tympanoplasty in 3 D. 3 vols.Tampa, FL: American Academy of Ophthalmology and Otolaryngology; 1968..

Fernandes SV. Composite chondroepithelial clip tympanoplasty: The triple "C" technique. Otolaryngol Head Neck Surg 2003; 128:267–272.

Fisch U. Tympanoplasty and Stapedectomy: A Manual of Techniques. Stuttgart: Georg Thieme Verlag; 1994..

Fleury P, Legent F, Lefevbre C. Techniques chirurgicales de l'Oreile. Paris: Masson; 1974.

Heermann H, Heermann J. Endaurale Chirurgie [Endaural Surgery]. Munich: Urban & Schwarzenberg; 1964..

Heermann J. Entwicklung von der Haut-zur Faszien-und zur Knorpeltympanoplastik (Epitympanon-Antrum-Mastoidplastik). Laryngol Rhinol Otol (Stuttg) 1977;56:267–270.

Heermann J. Autograft tragal and conchal palisade cartilage and perichondrium in tympanomastoid reconstruction. Ear Nose Throat J 1992;71:344–349.

Hildmann H, Sudhoff H. Middle Ear Surgery. Berlin: Springer; 2006: 20–23..

Hüttenbrink K-B. Die operative Therapie der chronischen Otitis media III. HNO 1994;42:701–718.

Hüttenbrink K-B, Zahnert T, Beutner D, Hofmann G. [The cartilage guide: a solution for anchoring a columella prostheses on the footplate] Laryngorhinootologie 2004;83:450–456.

Kley W. Surgical treatment of chronic otitis media and its immediate consequences. In : Neumann HH, ed. Head and Neck Surgery. vol. 3: Ear. Stuttgart: Thieme; 1982:171–265..

Lau T, Tos M. Long- term results of surgery for chronic granulating otitis. Am J Otolaryngol 1986;7:341–345.

Lau T, Tos M. Cholesteatoma in children: Recurrence related to the observation period. Am J Otolaryngol 1987;8:364–375.

Lau T, Tos M. Treatment of sinus cholesteatoma. Arch Otolaryngol Head Neck Surg 1988;114:1428–1434.

Lau T, Tos M. Tensa retraction cholesteatoma: Treatment and long term results. J Laryngol Otol 1989;103:149–157.

Lempert J. Fenestra nova ovalis: a new oval window for improvement of hearing in cases of otosclerosis. Arch Otolaryngol 1941; 34:880–889.

McCleve DE. Tragal cartilage reconstruction of the auditory canal. Arch Otolaryngol 1969;90:35–38.

McCleve DE. Repair of bony canal wall defects in tympanomastoid surgery. Am J Otol 1985;6:76–79.

Meijer AGW, Westerlaken BO, Albers FWJ. The Gronningen cutting device: a new instrument for tympanoplasty. Laryngoscope 1999;109:2025–2027.

Moore GF. Revision tympanoplasty utilizing fossa triangularis cartilage. Laryngoscope 2002;112:1543–1554.

Nitsche O. Tragusperichondrium und -Knorpel bei der Tympanonplastik Bericht über 2500 Operationen durch niedergelassenen HNO-Arzt. HNO 1985;33:455–457.

Palva T. Middle ear surgery in Northern Europe. Arch Otolaryngol 1963;78:363–370.

Plester D. Myringoplasty methods. Arch Otolaryngol 1963;78: 310–316.

Plester D, Hildmann H, Steinbach E. Atlas der Ohrchirurgie. Stuttgart: Kohlhammer; 1989..

Portmann M. The Ear and Temporal Bone. New York: Masson; 1979..

Shambaugh G, Glasscock ME. Surgery of the Ear. 3 rd ed. Philadelphia: Sanders; 1980..

Sheehy JL. Surgery of chronic otitis media. In: English GM, ed. Otolaryngology. Vol. 2 Hagerstown: Harper and Row; 1972:1–86..

Smyth GDL. TORPS—How have they fared after five years? J Laryngol Otol 1983;97:991–993.

Tolsdorff P. Tympanoplastik mit Tragusknorpel-Transplantat: "Knorpeldekkel-Plastik. Laryngol Rhinol Otol (Stuttg) 1983;62:97–102.

Tos M. Tympanoplasty in chronic adhesive otitis media. Acta Otolaryngol 1972a;73:53–60.

Tos M. Assessment of the results of tympanoplasties. J Laryngol Otol 1972b;86:487–500.

Tos M. Results of tympanoplasty with modified radical mastoidectomy. Acta Otolaryngol 1972c;74:61–65.

Tos M. Results of tympanoplasty. *Acta Otolaryngol* 1973;75:286–287.

Tos M. Late results in tympanoplasty. Arch Otolaryngol 1974;100:302–305.

Tos M. Stability of myringoplasty based on late results. ORL J Otorhinolaryngol Relat Spec 1980;42:171–181.

Tos M. Manual of Middle Ear Surgery. Vol.1. Approaches, Myringoplasty, Ossiculoplasty and Tympanoplasty. New York, Stuttgart: Thieme; 1993..

Tos M. 1995 Manual of Middle Ear Surgery. Vol. 2. Mastoid Surgery and Reconstructive Procedures. New York, Stuttgart: Thieme.

Tos M, Lau T. Treatment of cholesteatoma in children. Residual cholesteatoma related to observation time. Adv Otorhinolaryngol 1988;40:142–148.

Tos M, Lau T, Arndal H, Plate S. Tympanosclerosis of the middle ear: late results of surgical treatment. J Laryngol Otol 1990; 104(9):685–689.

Waltner JG. Cartilage tympanoplasty. A new technique in ossicular problems. Ann Otol Rhinol Laryngol 1966;75:1117–1123.

Wigand ME. Transcanal mastoidectomy restoring aerated antrum. Arch Otolaryngol 1970;92:353–357.

Wigand ME. Restitutional Surgery of the Ear and Temporal Bone. Stuttgart: Thieme; 1990..

Wullstein HL. Operation des Gehöres. Grundlagen und Methoden. Stuttgart: Thieme; 1968..

Wullstein HL, Wullstein SR. Tympanoplasty. Osteoplastic Epitympanotomy. Stuttgart: Thieme; 1990..

4 Cartilage Palisades in Underlay Tympanoplasty Techniques

Definition

Cartilage underlay palisade technique is the oldest and the most popular technique in cartilage tympanoplasty. As shown in Chapter 1, during the 1960s and 1970s Heermann gradually developed the method as used today: parallel placement of 0.5–3 mm wide full-thickness cartilage strips in the inferosuperior direction of the tympanic cavity. Palisades are usually cut from pieces of tragal or conchal cartilage covered on the concave side with the perichondrium. Although the palisades are placed side by side and close to each other there will be some distance between the palisades. The edges of the perichondrium on the outer side of the palisade are supposed to stick to each other and close the gaps, facilitating the epithelialization of the eardrum.

Cartilage palisades have most often been used as underlay grafts (Heermann and Heermann 1967; Heermann et al. 1970; Heermann 1977, 1978, 1991, 1992; Wiegand 1978; Milewski 1989, 1991, 1993; Amedee et al. 1989; Péré 1989; Helms 1991, 1995; Hildmann et al. 1996; Velepic et al. 2001; Andersen et al. 2002, 2004; Neumann et al. 2003; Neumann and Jahnke 2005).

The superior ends of the palisades are often supported by the "architrave," a piece of cartilage placed onto the eminence of the tensor tympani muscle (Heermann and Heermann, 1967; Heermann et al. 1970; Heermann 1992). In the posterior part of the tympanic cavity the superior ends of the palisade are supported by the chorda tympani, incudostapedial joint, stapes head, and interposition prosthesis.

The inferior end of the first palisade, the *simmering*, placed under the bony annulus is sometimes supported by a piece of cartilage placed in the anterior part of the hypotympanum. Heermann places the inferior ends of the remaining palisades onto the bony annulus with no need for inferior support by Gelfoam. I often prefer to place the inferior ends at the level of and close to the bony annulus, not onto and not under the bony annulus, and often support the palisades with Gelfoam.

Superiorly, the support by Gelfoam is sometimes needed. In my opinion the "architrave" can often be replaced by Gelfoam. I regularly support the short palisade connecting the undersurface of the umbo with Gelfoam. Some groups and some surgeons never apply Gelfoam within the middle ear, claiming that it causes formation of adhesions in the middle ear. Some other groups and surgeons use always Gelfoam to support the eardrum grafts or interposed ossicles. I frequently use Gelfoam to support the underlay grafts and have not found adhesions caused by Gelfoam.

Indications for Surgery

Heermann considered wide indications for palisade technique and used cartilage palisades in nearly all cases with chronic otitis media and its sequelae.

Since 1995 I have always used underlay techniques in posterior perforation and in total perforation after removal of retractions, in sinus cholesteatoma, after tensa retraction cholesteatoma, and in adhesive otitis media. Primary and late results after surgery of sinus cholesteatoma and tensa retraction cholesteatoma in children have been published. The hearing results and stability of reconstructed eardrum were surprisingly good (Andersen et al. 2002, 2004; Uzun et al. 2003; 2004).

Palisade techniques can be used in endaural approaches, as used by Heermann, or in retroauricular approaches, as used by Milewski, Helms and Hildmann, or—as I prefer—in transcanal approaches with fixed ear speculum.

Generally retractions, atelectasis, adhesive otitis and recurrent surgery cases with poor tubal function or poor tubal patency, expressed in negative preoperative Valsalva test, will be absolute candidates for cartilage palisade technique.

Harvesting and Shaping of Palisades

Harvesting and shaping of palisades is easy (Chapter 3). A piece of conchal or tragal cartilage is removed with the perichondrium attached on both sides. The size for a total perforation is 10 mm × 8 mm. The convex side of the palisade is turned toward the tympanic cavity and should not be covered with perichondrium; the perichondrium is therefore removed from the anterior side of the tragal cartilage, or from the posterior side of the conchal cartilage.

The palisades are cut as 0.5–3 mm wide strips. Even when they are placed close to one another there will always be a small separation between the palisades, but this gap will soon be filled with tissue fluid. The perichondrium on the outer side sticks to the overlying remnant of the eardrum or/and the fibrous annulus. Tissue fluid connects the neighboring strips of perichondrium as well, allowing epithelialization of the new eardrum without any ingrowth of the epithelium around the edges of the palisades into the inner side of the eardrum.

Surgical Techniques

The surgical techniques are adapted to location and size of the perforation as well as the extension of the active disease. The ossicular pathology will also decide the choice of surgical technique.

Posterior Perforation

In posterior perforation the tympanomeatal flap, including the fibrous annulus and the remnants of the eardrum have to be elevated. The tympanomeatal flap may be cut at the 9-o'clock position, resulting in swing-door technique with excellent view of the tympanic sinuses. The technique involving raising a large tympanomeatal flap (MMES_1, Figs. 581–586) is most often used in the retroauricular approach, but can also be used in the endaural approach. The elevation of a tympanomeatal flap is suitable for underlay palisade technique, because the inferoposterior bony annulus is visualized, facilitating placement of the palisades either onto or close to the bony annulus.

Swing-Door Technique

The most popular method is the swing-door technique with a superior and an inferior skin flap providing a good visibility to the tympanic cavity.

Epithelium around the edges of the perforation is removed carefully. A tympanomeatal flap is raised after a medial circumferential incision of the posterior ear canal skin. A medial radial incision divides the flap into a superior and inferior flap (**Fig. 4.1a**). The skin flaps, together with the fibrous annulus and the eardrum remnant, are elevated together with epithelium surrounding the chorda tympani and continuing into the posterior tympanum as a remnant of a retraction. To provide sufficient visibility over the tympanic sinuses, it is often necessary to drill the posterosuperior bony annulus (**Fig. 4.1b**).

The first palisade is placed in the superoinferior direction, slightly posterior to the malleus handle. The second palisade is placed superiorly onto the edge of the bony annulus and onto the chorda tympani (**Fig. 4.1c**). The saved and replaced epithelial flaps will adhere to the palisades (**Fig. 4.1 d**) and it is often not necessary to support the palisades with Gelfoam.

Another option is placement of the palisades at a slightly deeper level. The superior ends of the two palisades just touch the superior bony annulus and the anterior palisade is placed at the level of the malleus handle, but not on it (**Fig. 4.1e**). The palisades rest mainly on the chorda tympani and the long process of the incus (**Fig. 4.1 f**). Inferior ends of the palisades are supported with Gelfoam balls. After replacement of the flaps the palisades will usually remain stable (**Fig. 4.1 g**) because the epithelium sticks to the palisades. It is therefore always advantageous to save all epithelial flaps.

Large Tympanomeatal Flap Technique

This incision provides a good view to the entire posterior tympanum and even to the anterior tympanum when tilting the patient forward. After the edges of the perforation are cleaned, a large posterior tympanotomy incision is performed (**Fig. 4.2a**); the tympanomeatal flap is elevated, and pushed together with the eardrum remnants anterior to the malleus handle (**Fig. 4.2b**). The posterior part of the malleus handle is cleaned of epithelium to provide good contact to the cartilage palisade. The first palisade is placed close to the posterior edge of the malleus handle. Inferiorly, all palisades are placed onto the bony annulus; superiorly, the palisades just touch the superior bony annulus (**Fig. 4.2c**). After replacement of the tympanomeatal flap, good contact with the palisades is established (**Fig. 4.2 d**).

Thus, in posterior perforation there are two options in placement of palisades in relation to the bony annulus: either close to or onto the bony annulus, but we do not know which option is better.

Instead of placing the inferior ends of the palisades onto the bony annulus they can be placed at the level of the bony annulus (**Fig. 4.2e**). Avoiding placement of the palisades onto the bony annulus may increase the vibratility of the palisades.

Inferior Perforation

Application of cartilage palisades in underlay technique in inferior perforation is less common than in posterior or total perforation. However, in reoperation, poor function of the eustachian tube, retraction, and previous cholesteatoma, or in adhesive otitis media, underlay palisade technique can be a good solution. Swing-door technique or large tympanomeatal flap technique can be employed, but even the simple technique without tympanomeatal flaps can be used.

Technique without Tympanomeatal Flap

In this technique the removal of the epithelium around the perforation and scarification of the mucosa under the edges of the perforation are important. This can be achieved with a sickle knife, round knife, curved cup forces, or curved small elevator (**Fig. 4.3a**). Gelfoam balls

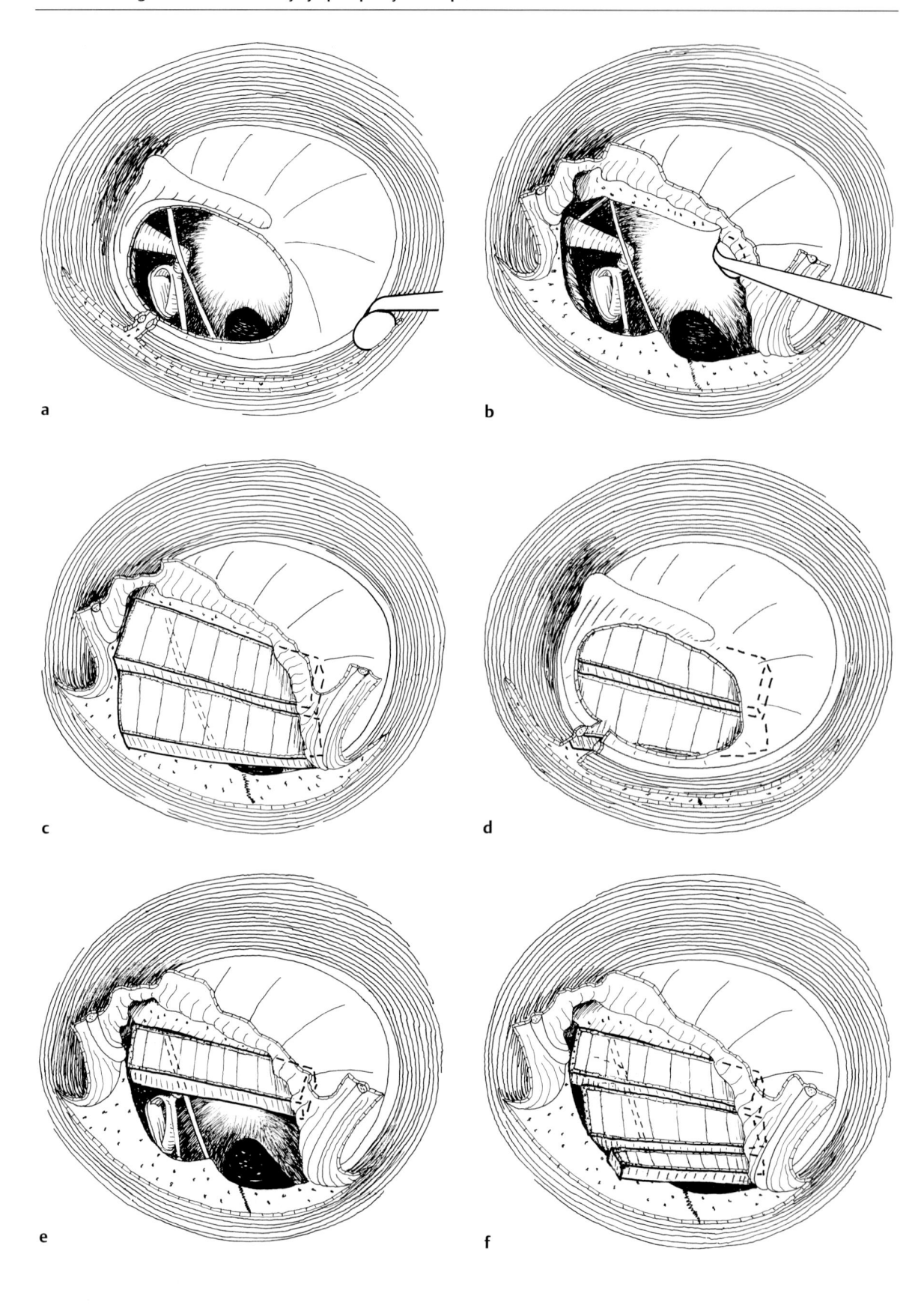

54 4 Cartilage Palisades in Underlay Tympanoplasty Techniques

a

b

c

d

e

f

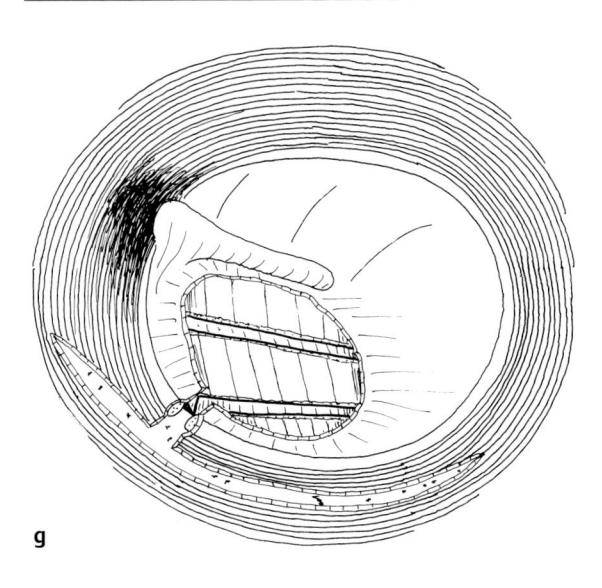

Fig. 4.1a–g Underlay swing-door cartilage palisade technique in a posterior perforation with intact ossicular chain.

a The edges of the perforation are deepithelialized. A posterior circumferential medial incision and a radial incision at the 9-o'clock position are made.

b A superior and an inferior skin flap and all epithelial flaps around the perforation are elevated. Using a round knife, the mucous membrane of the underside of the eardrum is removed around the perforation to facilitate a better attachment of the palisade to the eardrum.

c Two large palisades are placed close to the malleus handle and superiorly onto the bony annulus. Inferiorly, the palisades are most often placed just under the eardrum remnant with the contact to the denuded mucosa.

d All flaps are replaced, but superiorly and anteriorly only small flaps cover the palisades.

e **An alternative placement of the palisades in a slightly deeper level in a posterior perforation.** The first palisade is placed closed to and parallel to the malleus handle, resting on the chorda tympani. The palisade is thus placed slightly deeper.

f The following two palisades are also placed onto the chorda tympani. The palisades may also touch the long process of the incus.

g The epithelial flaps are replaced.

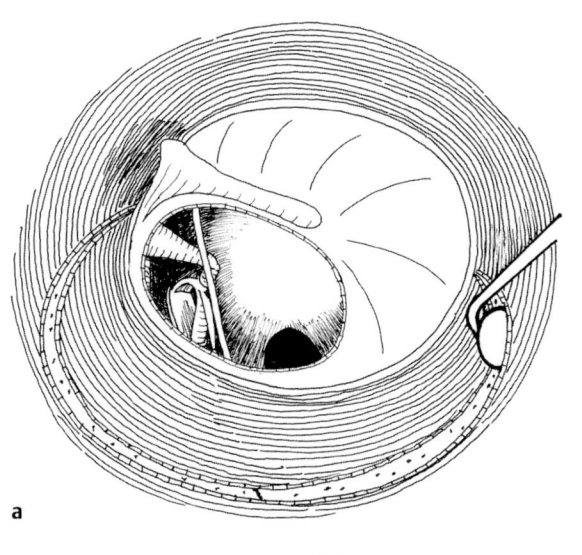

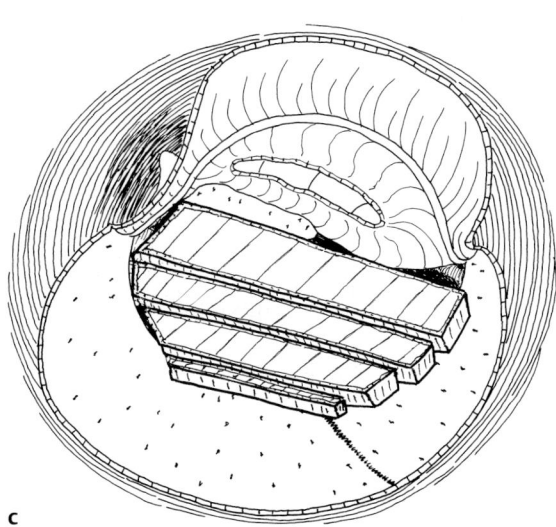

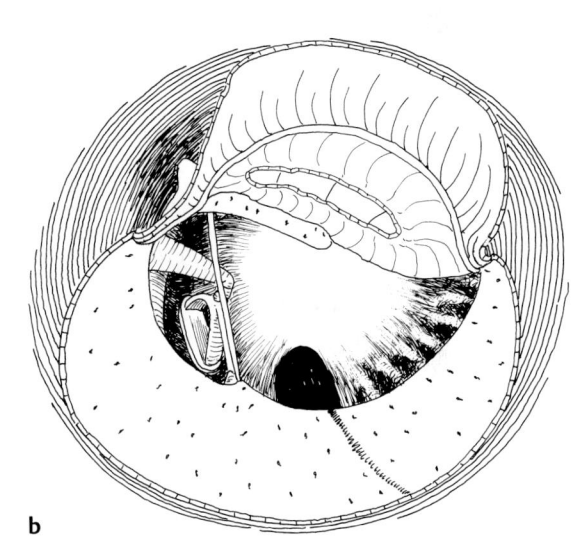

Fig. 4.2a–e Underlay cartilage palisade technique with large tympanomeatal flaps in posterior perforation and intact ossicular chain.

a The edge of the perforation with the keratinized epithelium is excised. The skin incision is placed relatively laterally in the ear canal.

b A large tympanomeatal flap is elevated together with the fibrous annulus and the remnants of the posterior half of the eardrum and the epithelium covering the posterior half of the malleus handle.

c The palisades are placed onto the inferoposterior bony annulus. The first palisade is placed on the posterior edge of the malleus handle. Superiorly, the palisades are placed close, but not onto, the bony annulus.

Fig. 4.2d, e ▷

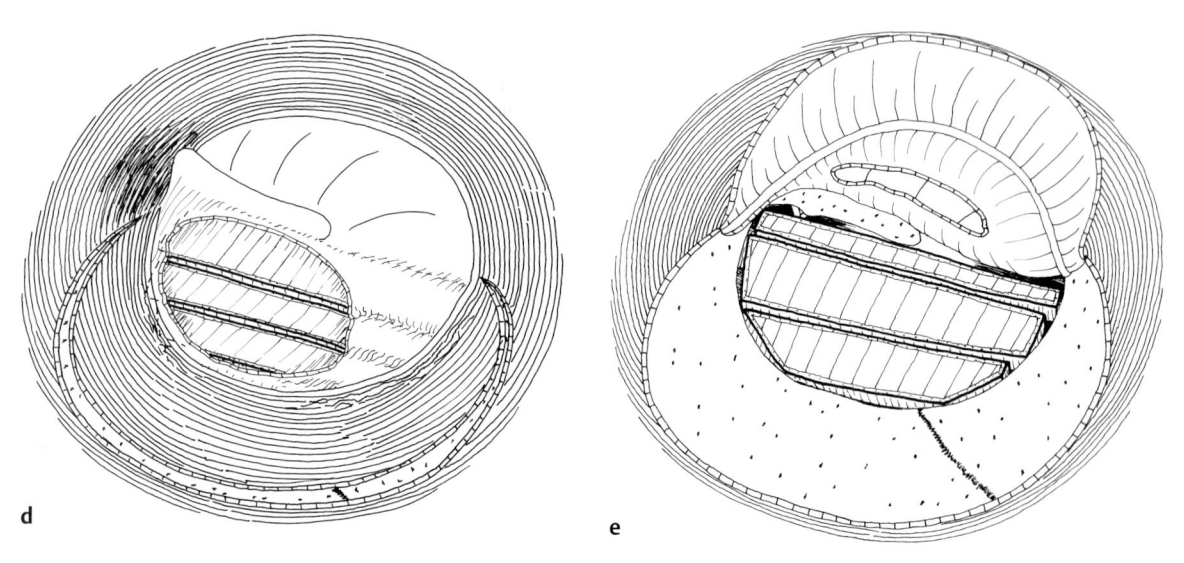

Fig. 4.2d–e
d The tympanomeatal flap with the fibrous annulus and the remnants of the eardrum are replaced.
e Alternative placement of the palisades under the eardrum remnant close to the bony annulus.

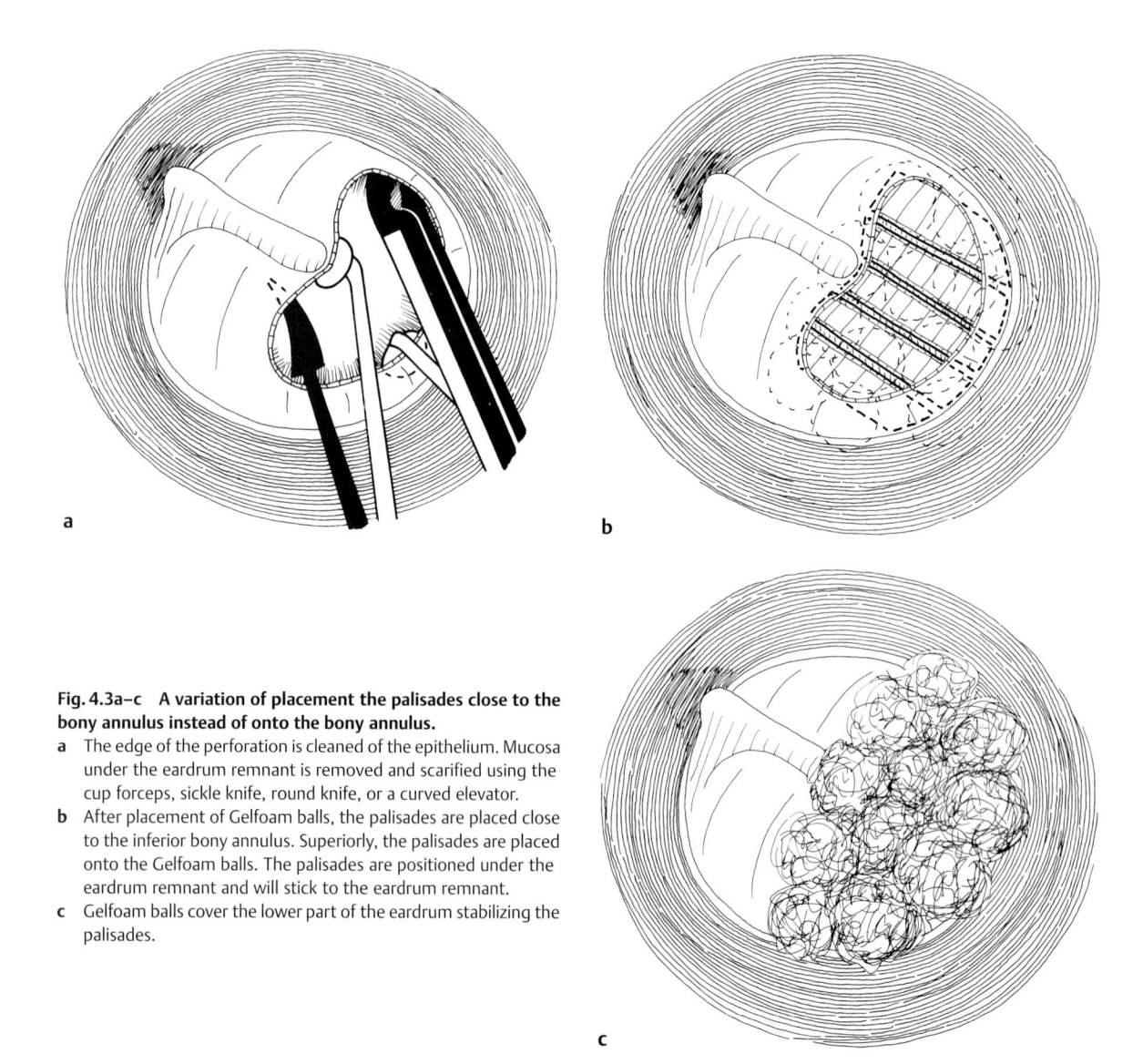

Fig. 4.3a–c A variation of placement the palisades close to the bony annulus instead of onto the bony annulus.
a The edge of the perforation is cleaned of the epithelium. Mucosa under the eardrum remnant is removed and scarified using the cup forceps, sickle knife, round knife, or a curved elevator.
b After placement of Gelfoam balls, the palisades are placed close to the inferior bony annulus. Superiorly, the palisades are placed onto the Gelfoam balls. The palisades are positioned under the eardrum remnant and will stick to the eardrum remnant.
c Gelfoam balls cover the lower part of the eardrum stabilizing the palisades.

Surgical Techniques **57**

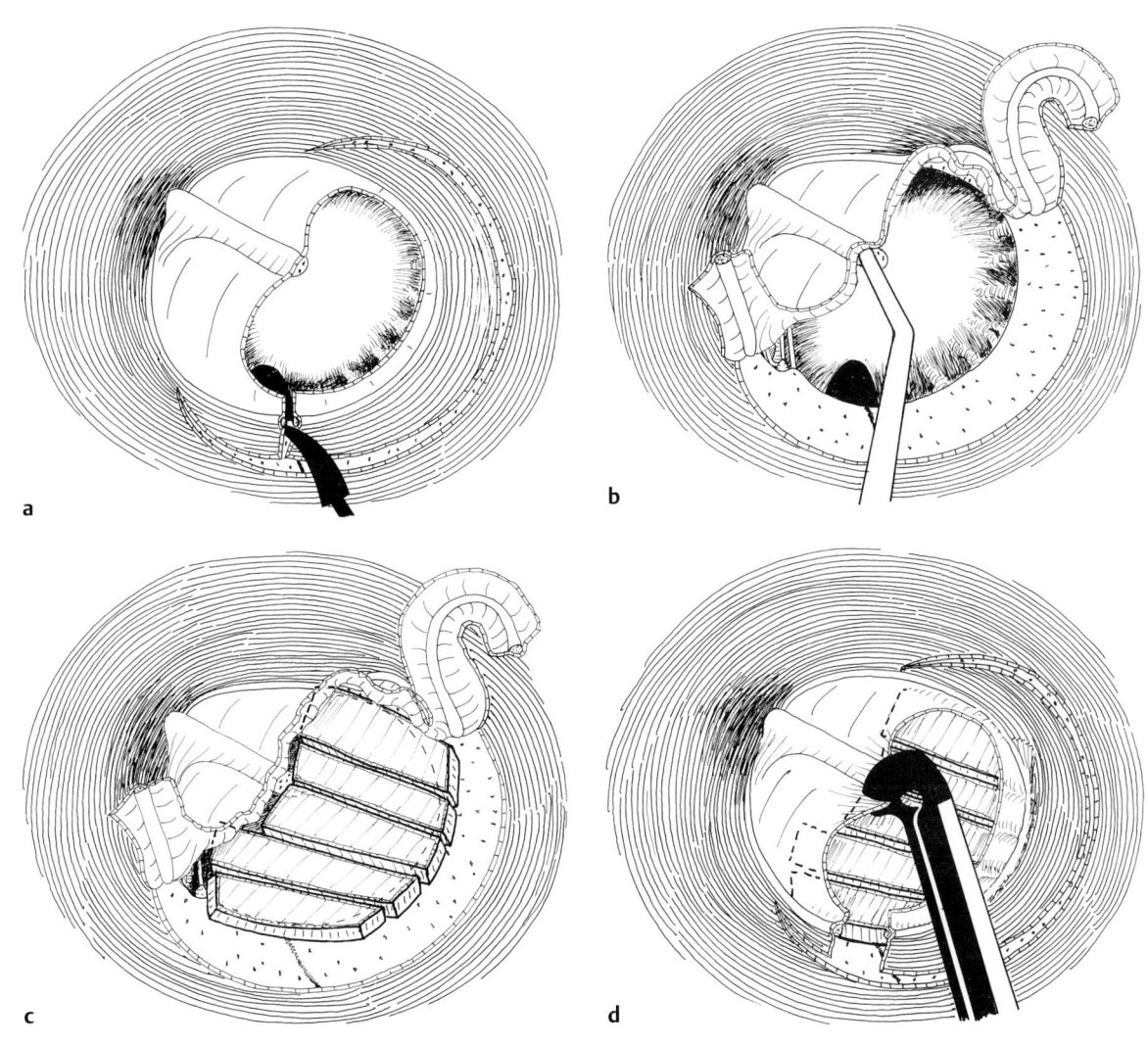

Fig. 4.4a–g Underlay swing-door cartilage palisade technique in a large inferior perforation with intact ossicular chain.
a Epithelium is removed from the borders of the perforation. A circumferential incision and a radial incision are made.
b The superior and inferior flaps are elevated. At the anterior border of the perforation, the fibrous annulus is elevated, exposing the bony annulus. Epithelium from the umbo is elevated and a small epithelial flap is elevated.
c The anterior palisade is placed onto the anterior and inferior bony annulus. The second palisade is placed onto the anterior edge of the umbo. The third palisade is placed onto the posterior edge of the umbo. Inferior ends of the palisades are placed onto the inferior bony annulus.
d The tympanomeatal flaps are replaced.

Fig. 4.4e–g ▷

are placed into the tympanic cavity to support the palisades positioned under the denuded eardrum (**Fig. 4.3b**). Finally, the edges of the perforation are covered with Gelfoam balls for three weeks to fix the palisades (**Fig. 4.3c**)

Swing-Door Technique

The edges of the perforation are cleaned of epithelium. A circumferential incision between the 10-o'clock and 3-o'clock positions and a radial incision at the 9-o'clock positions are made (**Fig. 4.4a**). Two flaps are elevated. Anteriorly, the annulus fibrosis is elevated together with the eardrum remnant. Epithelium from the umbo is elevated and a small epithelial flap is created (**Fig. 4.4b**). Gelfoam balls are placed in the central part of the tympanic cavity to support the superior ends of the palisades. The anterior palisade is placed onto the anterior bony annulus. Two palisades have contact with the umbo. Inferiorly, the palisades lie on the inferior bony annulus (**Fig. 4.4c**). The superior ends of the palisades may be supported by Gelfoam, especially in the umbo region. The tympanomeatal flap and the remnant of the eardrum are replaced (**Fig. 4.4d**). The epithelial flap of the umbo is replaced. The eardrum is covered with several Gelfoam balls (**Fig. 4.4e**).

e

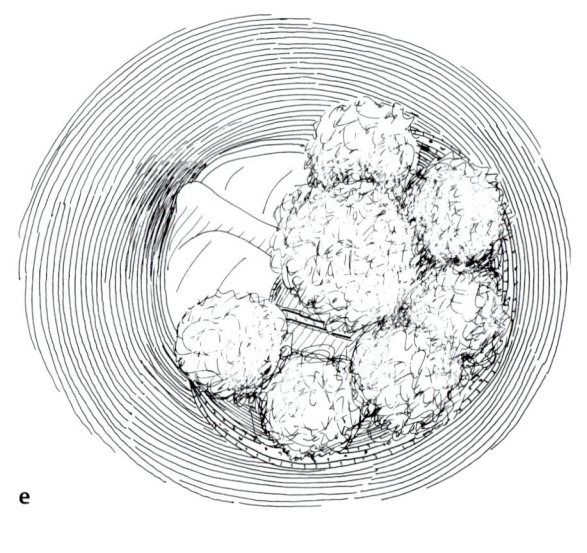

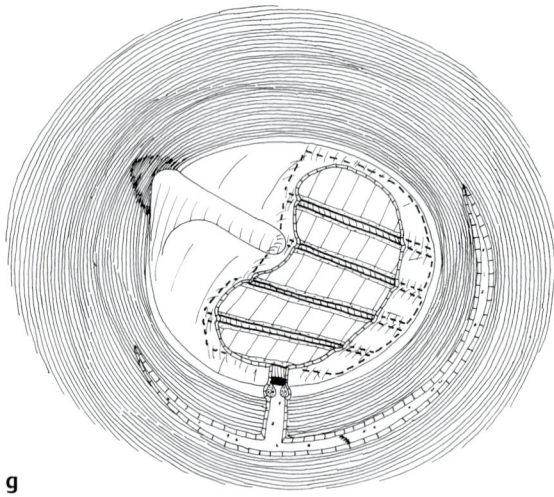

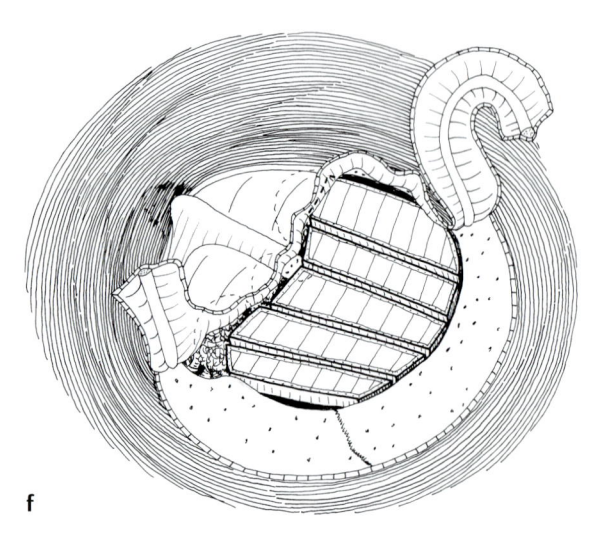

f

Fig. 4.4e–g
e The eardrum is covered with Gelfoam balls.
f Placement of the palisades at the level of the bony annulus. The palisades touch the bony annulus, but they are not placed onto it. The palisades are supported by Gelfoam balls.
g The epithelial flaps are replaced and the eardrum remnant is in good contact with the palisades.

g

The alternative of placing the inferior and posterior ends of the palisades close to and at the level of the bony annulus (**Fig. 4.4f**) requires extensive scarification of the eardrum remnant to promote gluing of the palisades to the undersurface of the denuded eardrum (**Fig. 4.4g**)

Large Tympanomeatal Flap Technique

After removal of the epithelium from the edges of the perforation, an inferior circumferential incision is made (**Fig. 4.5a**). A large tympanomeatal flap is elevated and the umbo is cleaned of epithelium (**Fig. 4.5b**). Gelfoam balls are placed into the tympanic cavity to support the superior ends of the palisades. In this example the most anterior palisade is placed under the bony annulus, but it could be placed onto the bony annulus (**Fig. 4.5c, d**). The short palisade is placed under the umbo, but it can be placed onto the umbo as well. The tympanomeatal flap is replaced (**Fig. 4.5e**) and the eardrum covered with Gelfoam (**Fig. 4.5f, g**).

In inferior perforation, the inferior ends of the palisades are placed onto the bony annulus, but they could be placed close to the bony annulus or even under it. In such cases a support of Gelfoam balls should be applied (**Fig. 4.5h**). After replacement of the tympanomeatal flap the palisades will come into contact with the eardrum remnant (**Fig. 4.5e, f**) and be stabilized.

Total Perforation

Reconstruction of the eardrum with cartilage palisades or cartilage strips is often indicated in total perforation, in particular with signs of previous retraction. Cartilage tympanoplasty is also indicated in cases of previously unsuccessful surgery of a total perforation. In cases with a dry total perforation with negative preoperative Valsalva maneuver, cartilage tympanoplasty is absolutely indicated. Cartilage palisades can also be employed in slightly moist ears with some thickness of the mucosa.

Fig. 4.5a–h Cartilage palisades as underlay grafts with a large inferior tympanotomy in an inferior or subtotal perforation.
- **a** The edges of the perforation are cleaned of the epithelium and a circumferential incision is made.
- **b** The inferior tympanotomy is performed, and a large tympanomeatal skin flap with the fibrous annulus, together with the remnant of the eardrum, are elevated. Than tympanic cavity will be filled with Gelfoam balls.
- **c** The most anterior palisade is placed under the bony annulus and is supported with Gelfoam balls. A short palisade is placed under the umbo.
- **d** The posterior palisades are placed onto the edge of the inferior bony annulus and superiorly under the eardrum.
- **e** The skin flap with the fibrous annulus and the epithelial flaps are replaced.

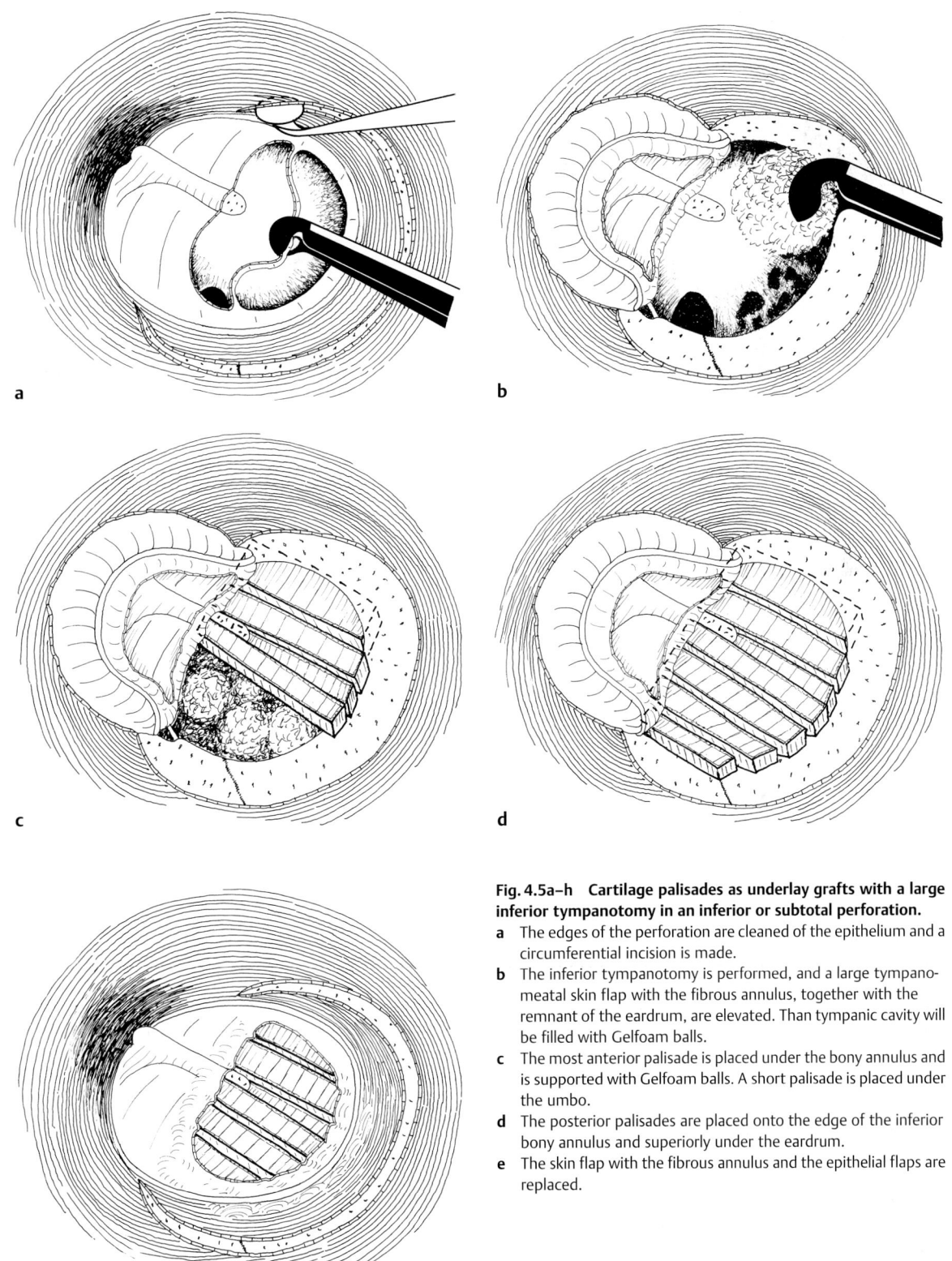

Fig. 4.5f–h ▷

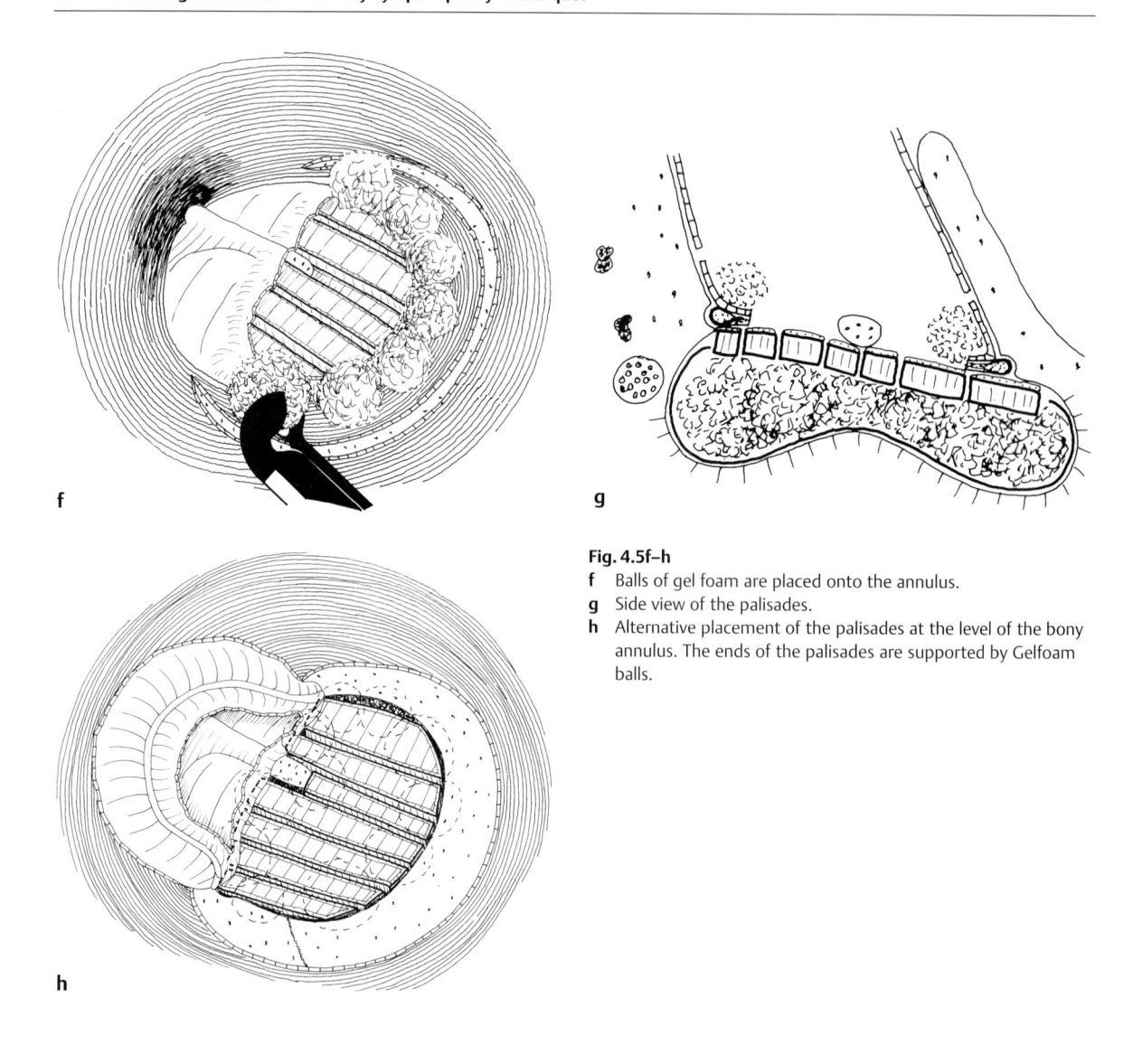

Fig. 4.5f–h
f Balls of gel foam are placed onto the annulus.
g Side view of the palisades.
h Alternative placement of the palisades at the level of the bony annulus. The ends of the palisades are supported by Gelfoam balls.

Swing-Door Technique

A circumferential incision between the 12-o'clock and 5-o'clock positions and a radial incision at the 9-o'clock position (**Fig. 4.6a**) provide a good view of the entire tympanic cavity, after elevation of the two flaps (**Fig. 4.6b**). The anterior and anterosuperior fibrous annulus with the epithelial remnants is scarified and partly elevated, exposing the bony annulus (**Fig. 4.6c–e**). The anterior palisade is placed under the bony annulus, and in the hypotympanum supported by Gelfoam. The next palisade is placed onto the bony annulus (**Fig. 4.6f**). The malleus palisades vary in size in relation to the space between the previous palisade and the malleus handle (**Fig. 4.6g**) The posterior palisades are placed inferiorly onto the bony annulus, superiorly they do not touch the bony annulus. After the epithelial flaps are replaced (**Fig. 4.6h**) many surgeons, especially in Germany, will cover the eardrum with bluish Silastic strips, placed onto the eardrum and ear canal wall (**Fig. 4.6i**). They are fixed with small cotton balls placed mainly along the annulus (**Fig. 4.6j**). Finally the entire ear canal is packed (**Fig. 4.6k**). The bluish Silastic strips are more clearly visible in the ear canal, facilitating their removal.

Instead of placing the inferior ends of the palisades onto the bony annulus, the palisades can be placed at the level of and close to the bony annulus (**Fig. 4.6l**). The palisades are supported in the hypotympanum by Gelfoam.

Large Tympanomeatal Flap Technique

After cleaning the edges of the total perforation of epithelium (**Fig. 4.7a**), a large circumferential incision is made (**Fig. 4.7b**). The skin flap is elevated and the undersurface of the anterior bony annulus is scraped with either a round knife (**Fig. 4.7c**) or a sickle knife. The anterior palisade is placed under the anterior bony annulus (Heermann 1978, 1992). To secure its position an "architrave" is placed onto the eminence of the tensor tympani muscle and another piece of cartilage is placed into the anterior hypotympanum (**Fig. 4.7d**). The other palisades are placed onto the

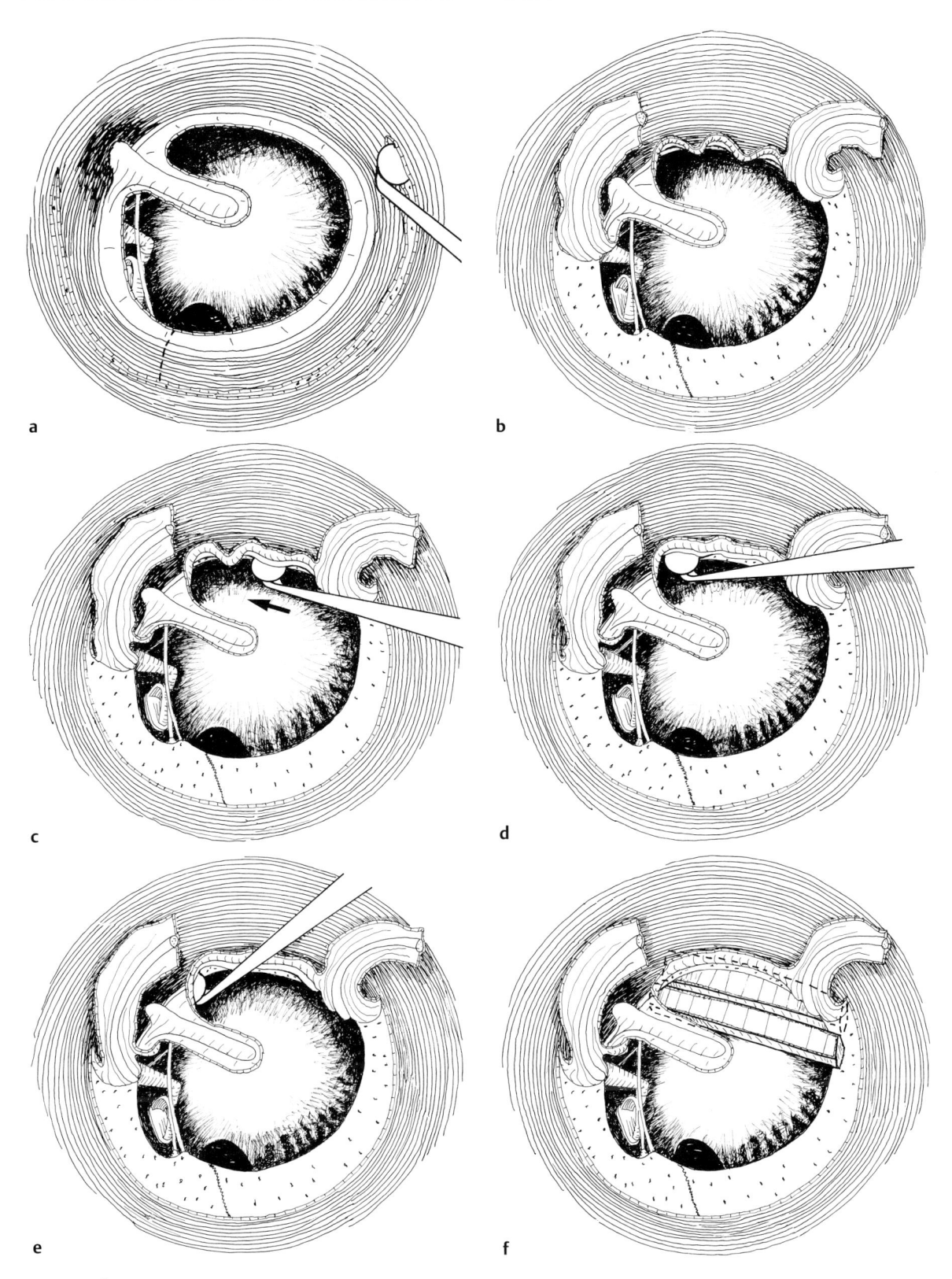

Fig 4.6a–l
Swing-door technique with cartilage palisades placed as underlay graft in a case with total perforation and intact chain.

a A large circumferential incision of the posterior ear canal skin is performed and the edge of the perforation is cleaned of the epithelium. The radial incision is indicated by a dotted line.

b Ear canal skin with the fibrous annulus together with the eardrum remnants is widely elevated as a superior and an inferior flap.

c Further elevation of the anterior fibrous annulus and removal of the mucus under the annulus.

d Further elevation of the anterosuperior fibrous annulus and scraping of the medial site of the bony annulus to prepare the space for the anterior palisade.

e Elevation of the superior fibrous annulus, exposing the bony annulus.

f The most anterior palisade is placed under the fibrous and bony annulus and pressed firmly to the undersurface of the fibrous annulus. The second palisade is placed onto the inferior bony annulus.

Fig. 4.6g–l ▷

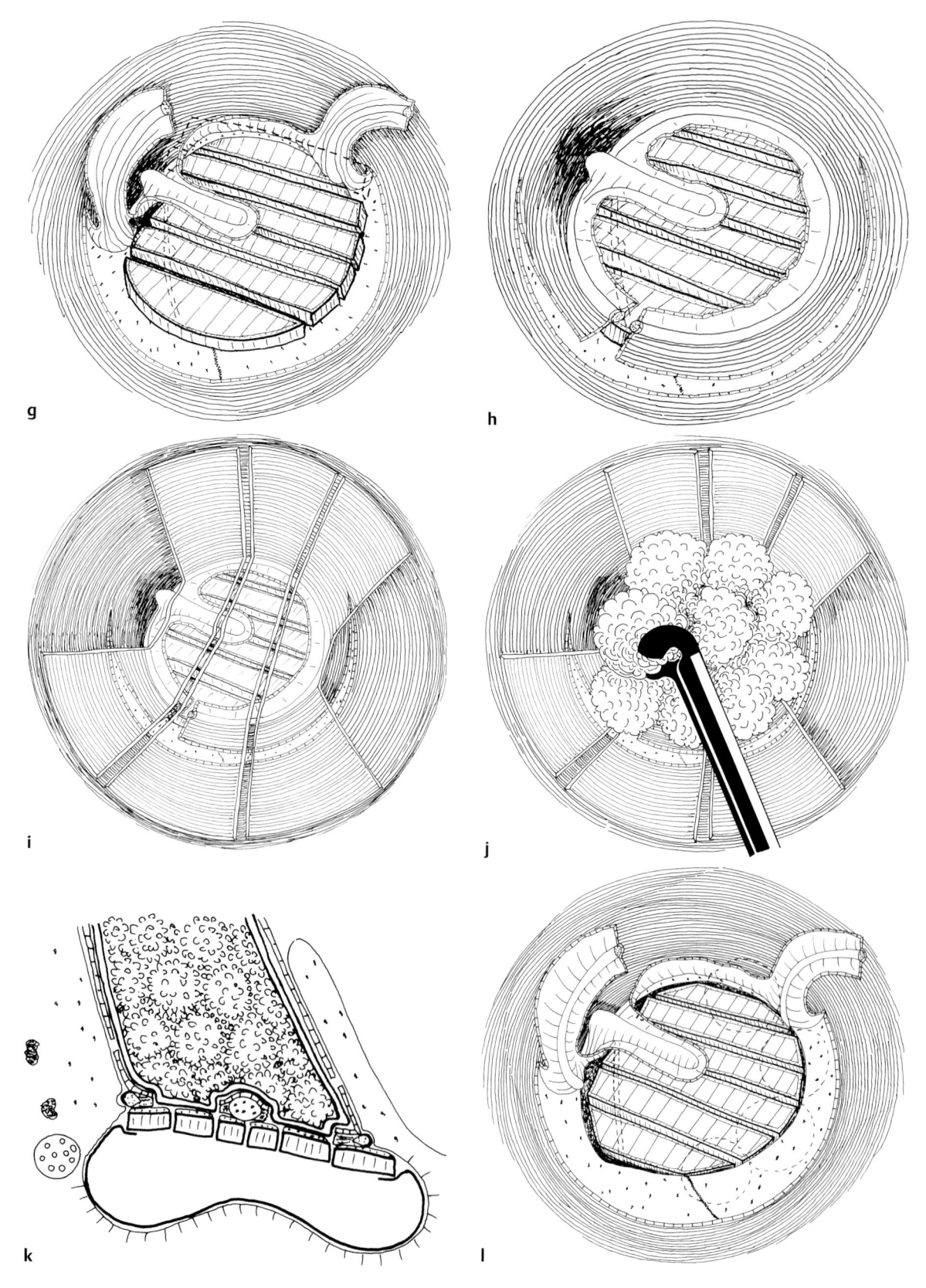

Fig. 4.6g–l

g The palisades along the malleus handle are wider in the inferior half. The upper ends of the palisades are placed on the chorda tympani and onto the long process of the umbo.
h The epithelial flaps are replaced.
i Packing of the ear canal, applying bluish silicone strips. Three silicone strips cover eardrum and ear canal.
j The strips are gently pressed to the fibrous annulus, using small cotton balls.
k Side view of the reconstructed eardrum with underlay cartilage palisade technique and packing of the ear canal with silicone strips and cotton balls.
l A variation of placement of the palisades at the level of the bony annulus instead of onto the bony annulus. The palisades are supported by Gelfoam balls.

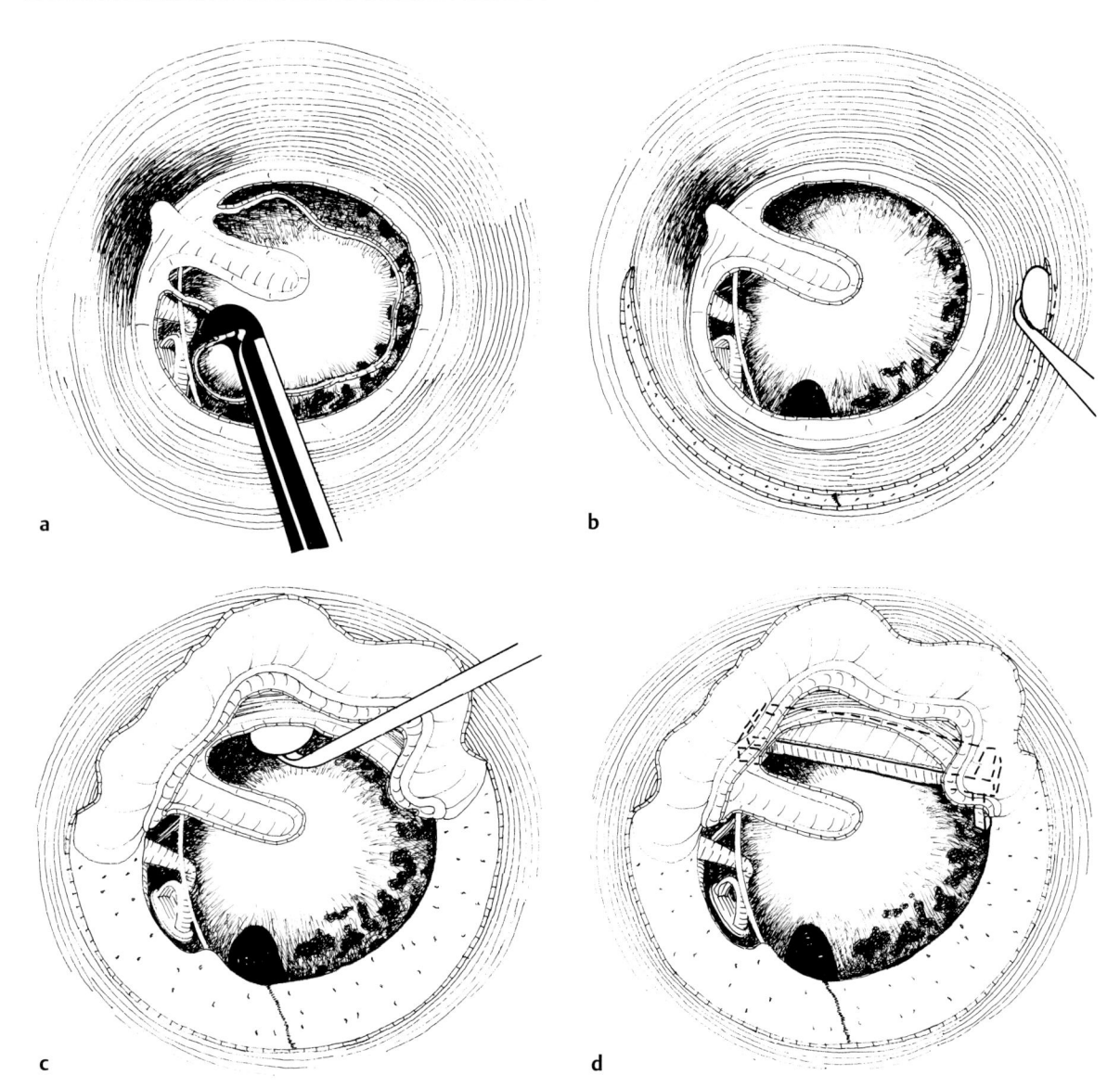

Fig. 4.7a–h Large tympanomeatal flap technique in total perforation. Elevation of large skin flaps with the posterior and inferior fibrous annulus.

a Epithelium along the edges of the perforation is carefully removed.
b A posterior and inferior circumferential incision is made between the 11-o'clock and 7-o'clock positions.
c The skin flap together with the fibrous annulus is elevated. The mucosa under the inferior and anterior annulus is elevated.

d The broad anterior palisade—the *simmering*—is placed under the bony annulus and is superiorly supported by a small rectangular 2 mm × 3 mm piece of cartilage—the *architrave*—placed onto the eminence of the tensor tympani muscle. A similar small piece of cartilage is placed in the anteroinferior part of the tympanum to support the *simmering* palisade.

Fig. 4.7e–h ▷

inferior but not onto the superior bony annulus. Superiorly and under the umbo, the palisades are supported by Gelfoam balls (**Fig. 4.7e**). After replacement of the tympanomeatal flaps (**Fig. 4.7f**), the eardrum is covered with Gelfoam balls or Gelfoam plates (**Fig. 4.7g**) and the ear canal is packed with 1 cm gauze moistened with hydrocortisone/oxytetracycline/polymyxin B ointment for 3 weeks. The packing may vary in different institutions and with different surgeons.

The alternative placement of the palisades under the eardrum close to the bony annulus requires a thorough scarification of the undersurface of the eardrum and placement of Gelfoam balls. The anterior palisade is wide (**Fig. 4.7h**), the other palisades are accommodated to the malleus handle. A short palisade has contact with the undersurface to the scarified umbo. Superiorly, the palisades are supported by the chorda tympani.

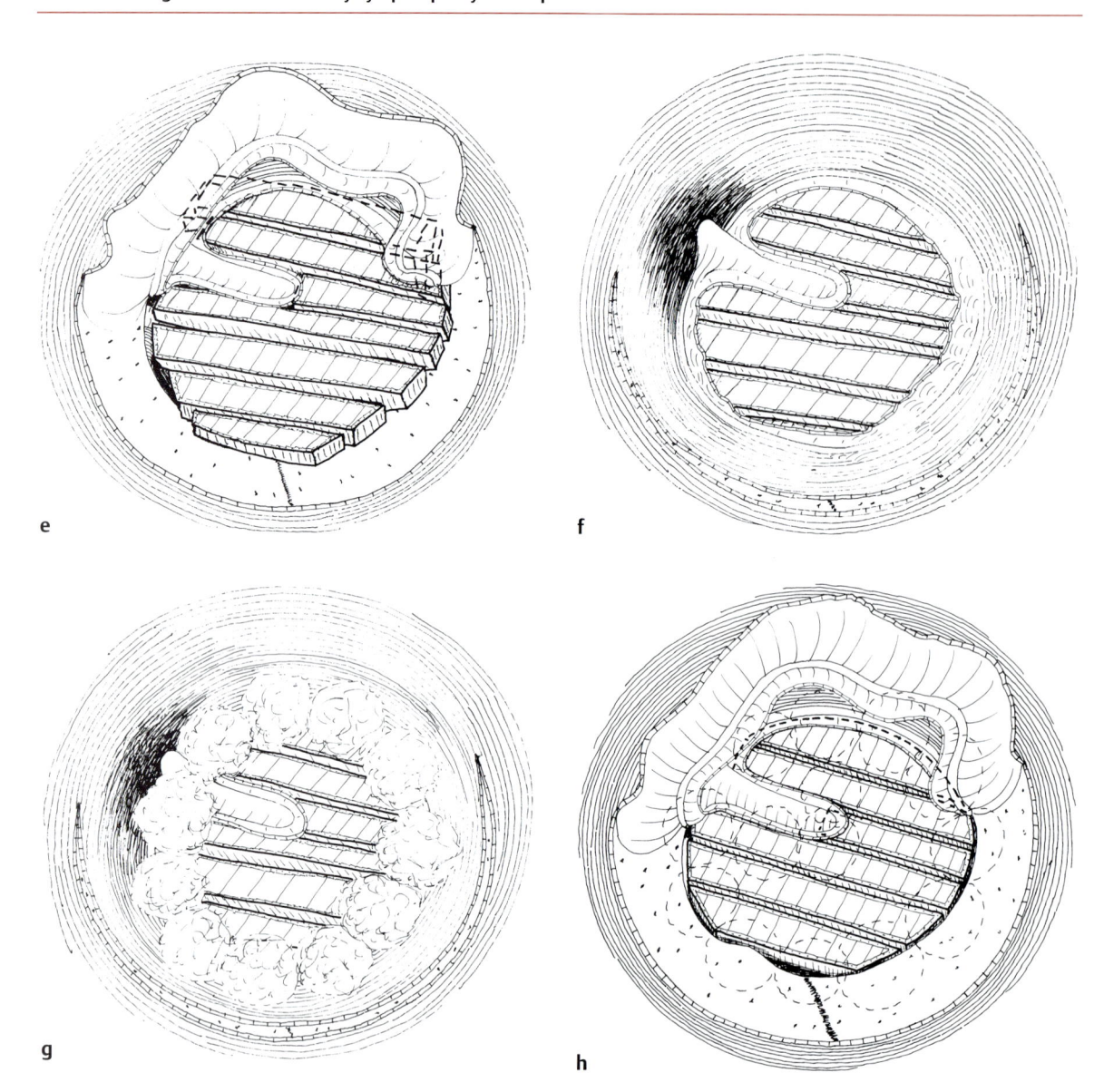

Fig. 4.7e–h

e The posterior palisades are placed onto the inferior bony annulus and close to, but not onto, the superior bony annulus.
f The flaps are replaced.
g The eardrum is covered with Gelfoam balls, first along the annulus.
h The alternative placement of the palisades at the level of the bony annulus. The palisades touch the bony annulus and are supported by Gelfoam balls. The wide anterior palisade is placed under the eardrum remnant and close to the bony annulus.

Underlay Cartilage Palisade Technique and Ossiculoplasty

Reconstruction of the ossicular chain is an important part of cartilage tympanoplasty. Placement of the cartilage palisades must be adapted to the type of ossiculoplasty, the shape, and the material of the prosthesis.

The most commonly used classification of tympanoplasty is illustrated in Chapter 2. The following definitions are used:

— **Myringoplasty:** Closure of the eardrum perforation with normal ossicular chain without any surgical procedures in the tympanic cavity.
— **Tympanoplasty type 1:** Closure of the eardrum perforation with intact ossicular chain at the end of the operation. All procedures illustrated so far in this chapter in **Figs. 4.1 to 4.7** have been tympanoplasties type 1, because the fibrous annulus is elevated and mucosa is partly removed under the eardrum remnant, bony annulus, and malleus handle.

- **Tympanoplasty type 2:** In cases of defective or missing lenticular process and/or long process of the incus, but with stapes present, various interposition techniques between the stapes and the malleus handle or the reconstructed eardrum can be performed. In case of missing head and neck of the stapes, the interposition is performed between the stapedial arch and the malleus handle.
- **Tympanoplasty type 3:** In cases with absent or severely damaged stapes crura, a columella is placed onto the middle of the footplate and under the malleus handle or grafted eardrum.
- **Tympanoplasty type 4:** This type protects the round window in cases of mobile footplate and missing ossicles. No ossiculoplasty is involved but the construction of the hypotympanum and protection of the round window can be carried out with cartilage palisades (see **Fig. 2.26**).
- **Tympanoplasty type 5A:** In cases with no ossicles and fixed footplate, fenestration of the lateral semicircular canal used to be performed. Nowadays, type 5B with stapedectomy and protection of the round window is done. The tympanic cavity can be closed by cartilage tympanoplasty in similar way as in type 4 (see **Fig. 2.26**).

Preservation of an Intact Ossicular Chain

Some surgeons are tempted too early to disrupt an intact ossicular chain in difficult situations such as removal of cholesteatoma from the attic and/or tympanic cavity, tympanosclerosis around the ossicles (see MMES_4, pp. 1–46), or acquired or congenital bony fixations of the ossicles (see MMES_4, pp. 47–82, 212–239). Tympanoplasty type 1 in such situations may be extensive and difficult surgery, but it is also rewarding because the primary and late hearing results are better by far in an intact ossicular chain with tympanoplasty type 1 than with type 2 with interposition.

We report in our publications on primary and late hearing results that hearing results were best in ears with a preserved and intact ossicular chain in the following diseases:
1. Chronic adhesive otitis media (Tos 1972a)
2. Sequelae to chronic otitis media (Tos 1972b, 1974b)
3. Active chronic otitis media after radical mastoidectomy (Tos 1971, 1974b; Lau and Tos 1986)
4. After tympanoplasty for bony ossicular fixation (Tos 1970, 1974a)
5. Cholesteatoma in children (Lau and Tos 1987)
6. Sinus cholesteatoma and tensa retraction cholesteatoma in adults (Lau and Tos 1988, 1989)
7. Middle ear tympanosclerosis (Tos et al. 1990).

Several other authors, cited in these papers, have published similar good hearing results in tympanoplasty type 1 in comparison with tympanoplasty type 2 with interposition. Thus it is worthwhile trying to keep the ossicular chain intact, even in severe cholesteatoma. The incus can nearly always be safely cleaned of cholesteatoma.

Cartilage Palisades and Incus Interposition in Tympanoplasty Type 2

Interposition of the autogenous incus is the most common ossiculoplasty. The incus without its long process can be shaped in many ways (see MMES_1, Figs. 746–763). It can be recued, with a hole or a groove for the stapes head or malleus handle, or it can be placed unshaped onto the stapes head and the short process under the malleus handle (**Fig. 4.8a**). Two long palisades, supported inferiorly by Gelfoam balls are placed behind the incus, and several short palisades are placed around the incus, covering and closing any gaps (**Fig. 4.8b, c**).

The incus may be turned in the opposite direction (**Fig. 4.9a**) and the palisades placed around the incus, leaving no uncovered holes (**Fig. 4.9b, c**).

In total perforation and classic incus interposition (**Fig. 4.10a**), the inferior ends of the palisades are placed onto the bony annulus and partly onto the incus (**Fig. 4.10b**).

The alternative placement of the palisades at the level of the bony annulus (**Fig. 4.10c**) requires the use of some Gelfoam balls in the hypotympanum and scarification of the undersurface of the eardrum. After replacement of the epithelial flaps, the eardrum is covered with Gelfoam balls (**Fig. 4.10 d, e**).

Reduction and shaping of the incus with a hole for the stapes head and the short process firmly positioned under the malleus handle (**Fig. 4.11a**) in a total perforation provides enough space for the palisades (**Fig. 4.11b**). The malleus palisade is placed onto the short process of the incus. Two palisades can even be placed posterior to the incus.

Alternatively, the palisades are placed at the level of the bony annulus after placing Gelfoam balls in the tympanic cavity and thorough scarification of the undersurface of the eardrum remnant. In this case the anterior palisade is placed at the level of the bony annulus (**Fig. 4.11c**), supported by Gelfoam, and will stick to the anterior remnant of the eardrum. The malleus palisade is shaped, and the two posterior palisades are supported by the chorda tympani. Replacement of the tympanomeatal and malleus flaps (**Fig. 4.11 d**) will further stabilize the palisades.

Several other interposition methods with autogenous materials can be applied together with the palisades, such as the head of the malleus (see MMES_1, Figs. 765–770) and shaped cortical bone (see MMES_1, Figs 771–781).

When performing grafting of the perforation with fascia and an interposition of incus, cortical bone or malleus head, the tendency is to shape a relatively large interposition prosthesis to prevent retraction of the fascia along the prosthesis. When applying cartilage palisades, the bony interposition is often small, partly because there is no fear of retraction, partly because the palisades and the interposition graft occupy too much space in the posterior tympanum.

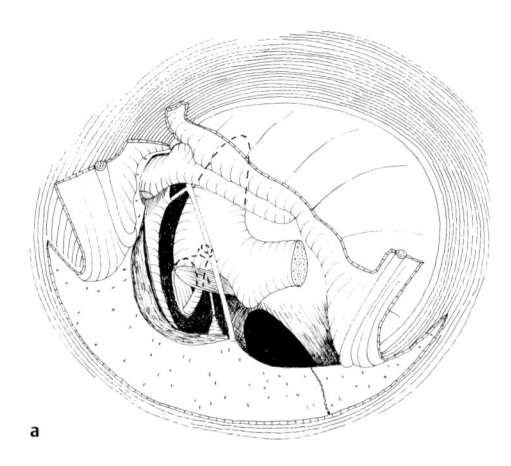

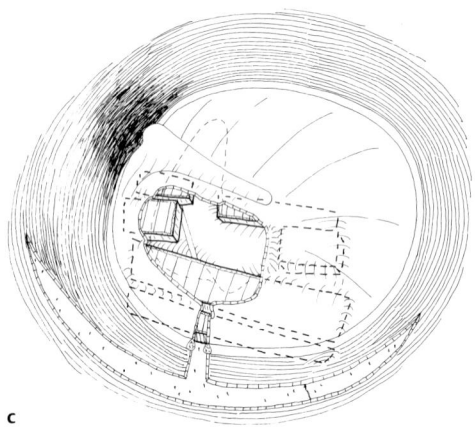

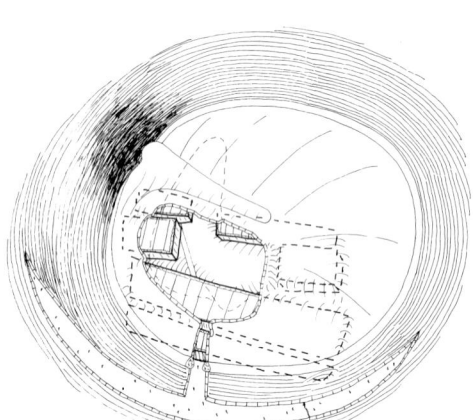

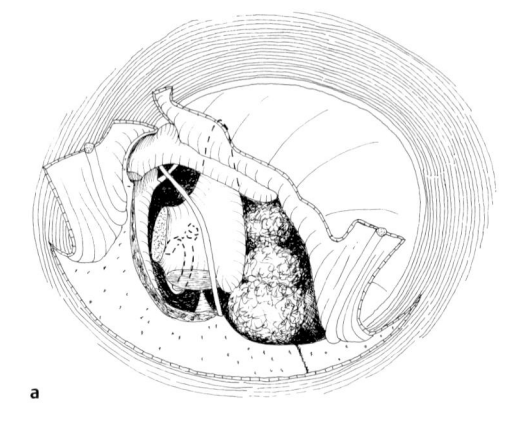

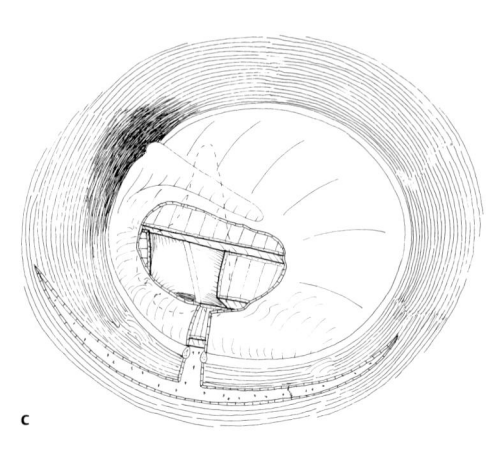

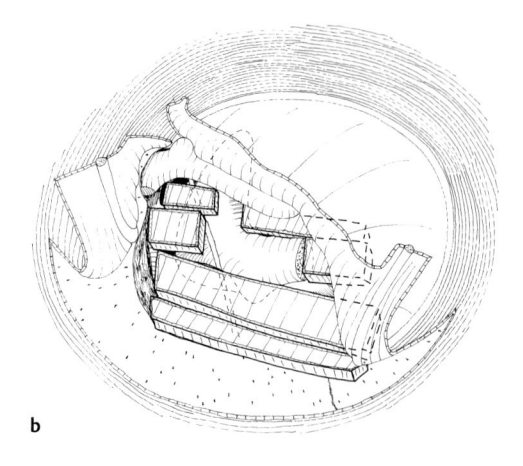

Fig. 4.8a–c Underlay cartilage palisades in posterior perforation and interposition of the incus between the stapes and malleus handle.
a   The posterior tympanomeatal flap is elevated; the defective incus is removed and resituated onto the stapes head with the short process under the malleus handle.
b   Short and longer palisades are placed onto, and behind, the incus body. Inferiorly they are placed under the eardrum.
c   The epithelial flaps are replaced.

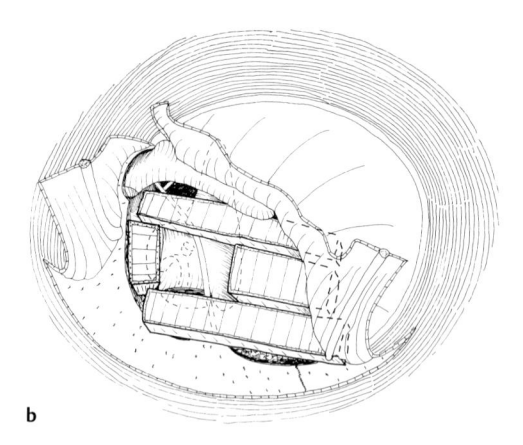

Fig. 4.9a–c Palisades in a posterior perforation with interposed incus onto an intact stapes.
a   Palisades will be inferiorly supported by Gelfoam balls.
b   Palisades are placed onto the incus body and under the eardrum. The posterior palisade is placed onto the posterior bony annulus. A short palisade is placed in the posteroanterior direction
c   The flaps are replaced.

Surgical Techniques   67

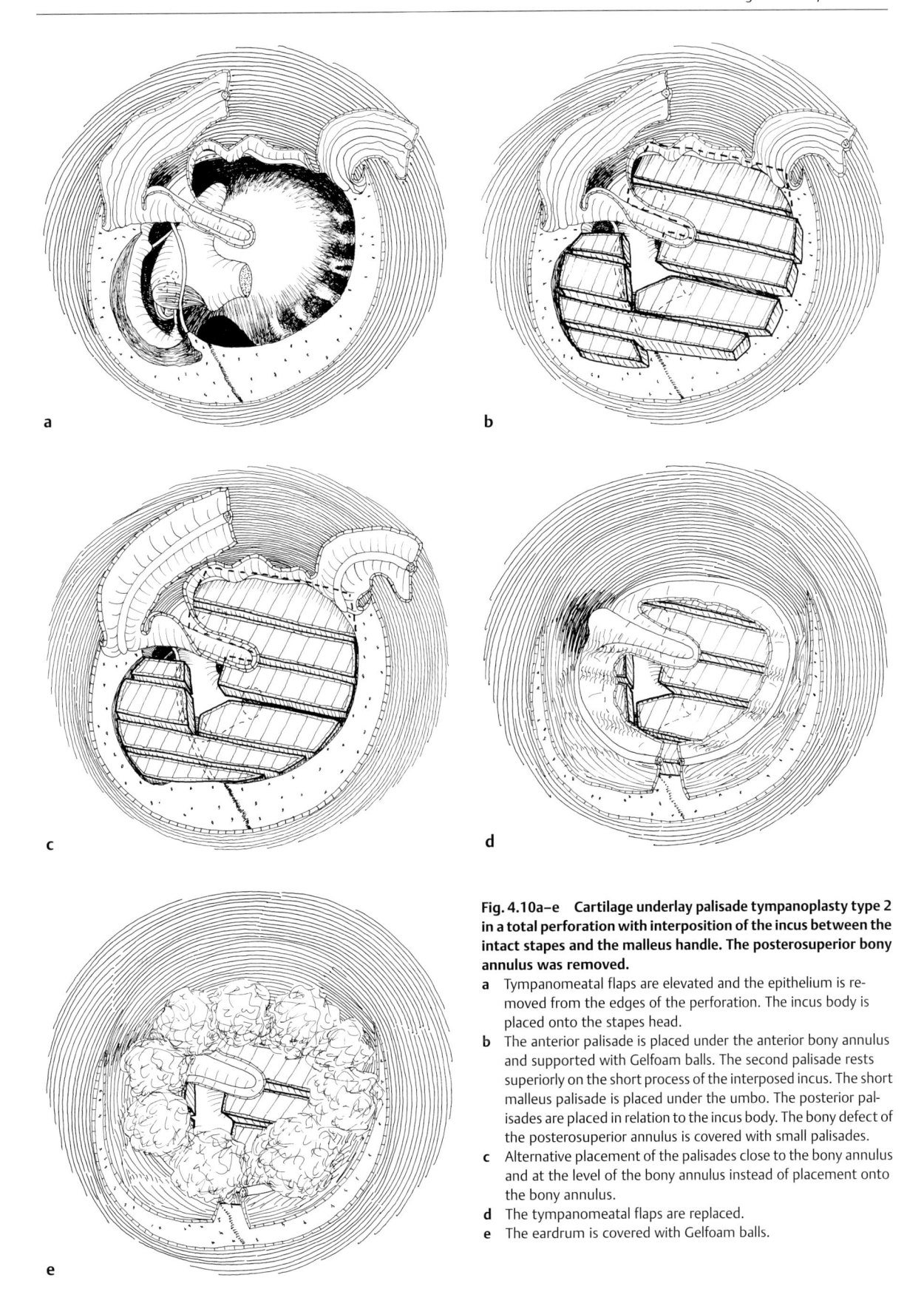

Fig. 4.10a–e   Cartilage underlay palisade tympanoplasty type 2 in a total perforation with interposition of the incus between the intact stapes and the malleus handle. The posterosuperior bony annulus was removed.

a Tympanomeatal flaps are elevated and the epithelium is removed from the edges of the perforation. The incus body is placed onto the stapes head.
b The anterior palisade is placed under the anterior bony annulus and supported with Gelfoam balls. The second palisade rests superiorly on the short process of the interposed incus. The short malleus palisade is placed under the umbo. The posterior palisades are placed in relation to the incus body. The bony defect of the posterosuperior annulus is covered with small palisades.
c Alternative placement of the palisades close to the bony annulus and at the level of the bony annulus instead of placement onto the bony annulus.
d The tympanomeatal flaps are replaced.
e The eardrum is covered with Gelfoam balls.

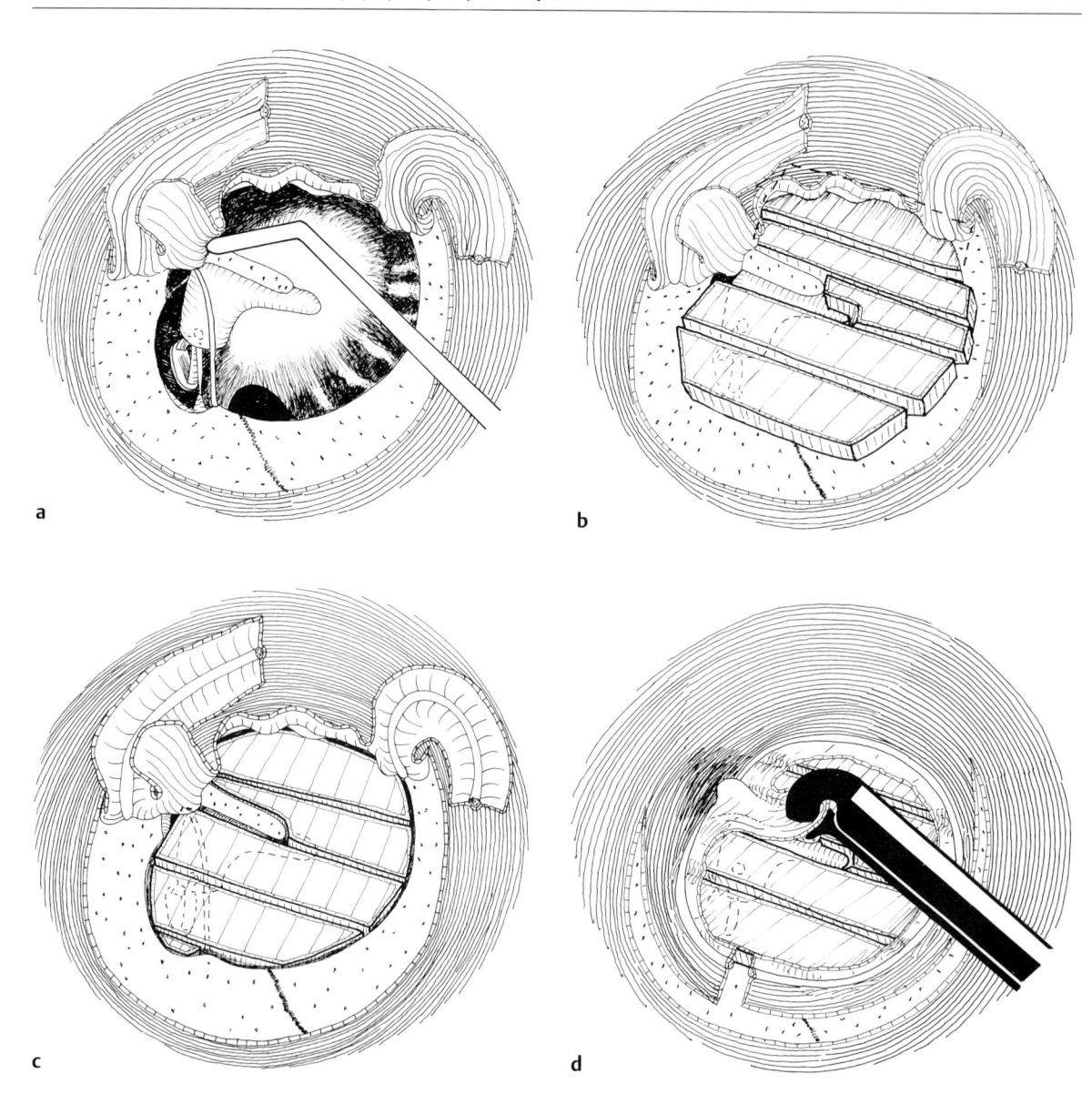

Fig. 4.11a–d Cartilage underlay tympanoplasty in total perforation and missing long process of the incus. Tympanoplasty type 2 with shaped incus.

a The malleus handle is totally cleaned of epithelium and a malleus epithelial flap is raised with the base close to the short process of the malleus. The head of the incus is placed onto the head of the stapes; its shaped long process is placed along the malleus handle. The swing-door technique with widely elevated superior and inferior tympanomeatal flaps provides a good view of the anterior tympanum.

b The first anterior palisade is placed under the anterior bony annulus, the second onto the inferior bony annulus, and both are supported with Gelfoam balls. The short malleus palisade is placed onto the umbo and is shaped to touch the end of the short process of the umbo. The posterior palisades are placed onto the bony annulus.

c Alternative placement of the palisades. The anterior palisade is not placed under the anterior bony annulus but at the level of the bony annulus. The following palisades are also placed at the level of the bony annulus. The malleus palisade is shaped to accommodate the interposed incus.

d The tympanomeatal flaps with the attached eardrum epithelium are replaced. The important malleus epithelial flap is carefully replaced: it will promote fast epithelialization of the central region of the eardrum.

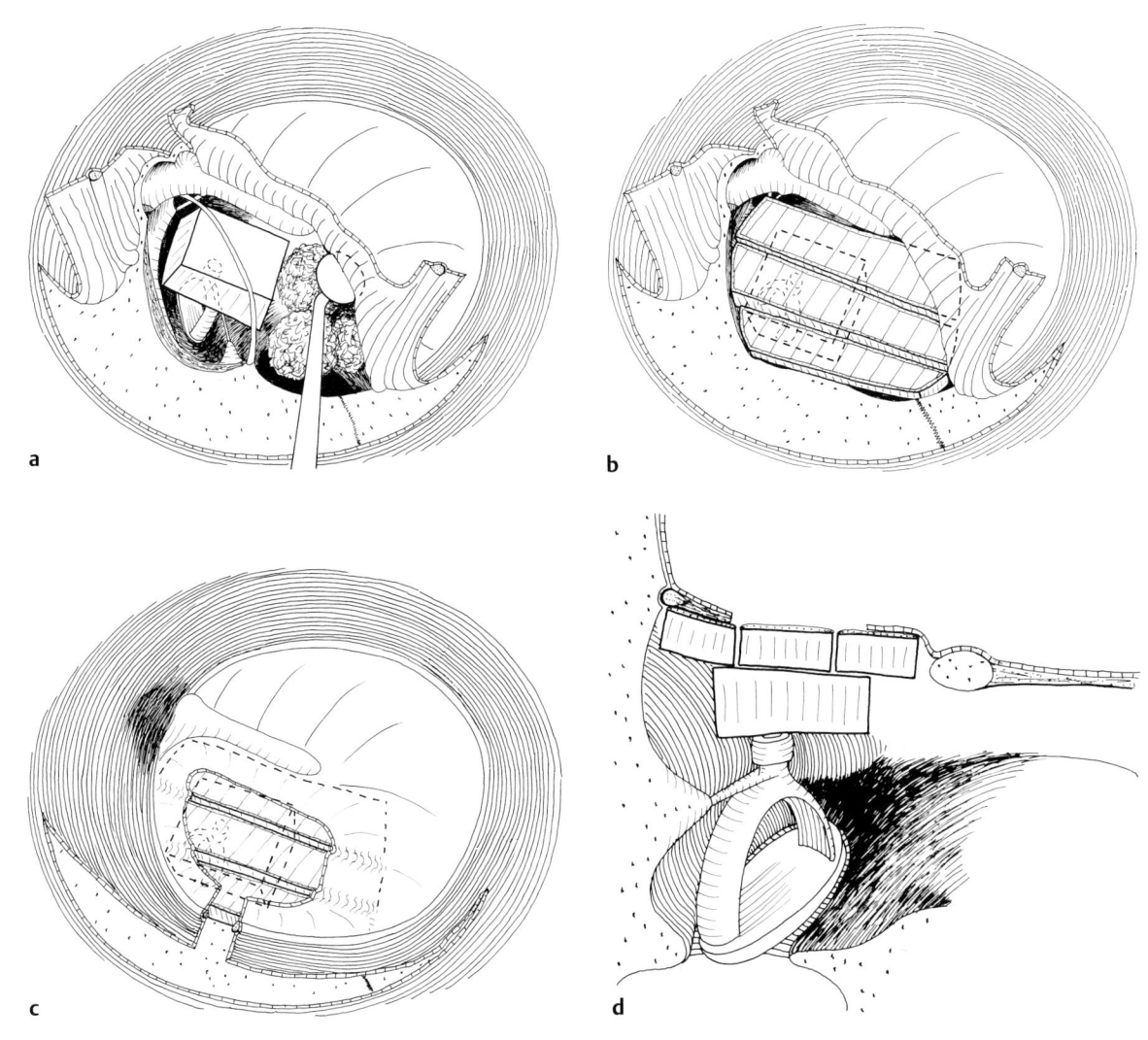

Fig. 4.12a–d Underlay cartilage palisade tympanoplasty type 2 with interposition of a cartilage graft between the head of the stapes and the eardrum in a posterior perforation.
a A swing-door incision is made and the superior and inferior tympanomeatal flaps are raised. A rectangular prosthesis made of a relatively thick piece of tragal cartilage is placed onto the head of the stapes. Inferiorly, Gelfoam balls are placed to support the palisades and the cartilage graft.
b Three palisades are placed onto the cartilage graft, they are not placed onto the bony annulus and have good mobility.
c The epithelial flaps are replaced.
d Side view of the palisades and the cartilage graft.

Interposition with Cartilage Graft and Palisades

As Utech showed in the late 1950s (Utech 1959, 1960), the interposition of cartilage between the stapes head and the eardrum is a good ossiculoplasty method (**Fig. 4.12a**); the cartilage palisades additionally stabilize the prosthesis (**Fig. 4.12b, c**). In the side view (**Fig. 4.12d**) it can be seen that the stabilization of the interposed graft is better with cartilage palisades than with fascia or perichondrium.

Another good cartilage interposition method is the helix spine method (see MMES_1, Figs. 797–799), recommended by Suzuki (1988). The helix spine with the perichondrium is excised using a small skin incision. In the center of the cut area a hole is made for the stapes head and the prosthesis is placed onto the stapes head. The palisades are placed onto the curved surface of the helix spine.

Interposition with Biocompatible Materials and Cartilage Palisades

Since the beginning of the 1960s, many biocompatible materials, such as polyethylene, Teflon, and porous plastic have been used as incus replacement prostheses. The tendency to extrusion was very high and all were abandoned. During the 1980s, various bioinert ceramics such as Frialit were used, with problems of stability and connection to the head of the stapes. Later, bioactive glass ceramics such as Bioglass and Ceravital and calcium phosphate ceramics such as hydroxyapatite became popular. In the 1990s, dense hydroxyapatite and glass-ionomer cement have been popular. These grafts are described and illustrated in MMES_1 (pp. 285–297). In principle the grafts are al-

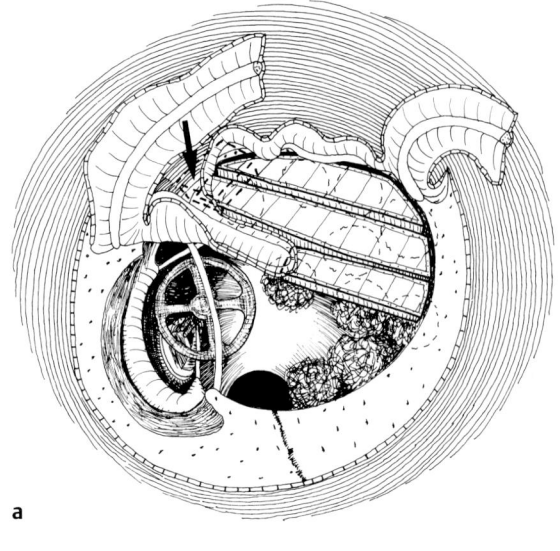

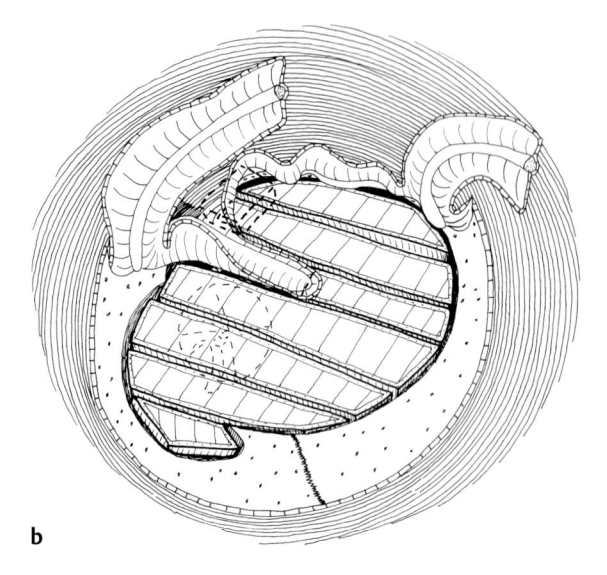

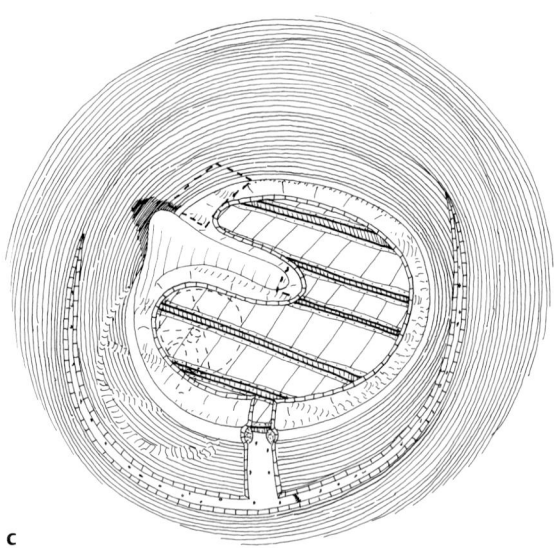

Fig. 4.13a–c Kurz Titanium PORP prosthesis and palisade tympanoplasty type 2.

a The edges of the total perforation are removed and two tympanomeatal flaps are elevated. The posterosuperior scutum, the retraction remnant, and the defective incus are removed. The short titanium prosthesis is placed onto the stapes head. Gelfoam balls support the palisades, which are placed at the level of the bony annulus. The architrave is placed onto the eminence of the tensor tympani muscle (arrow). The palisades are superiorly placed onto the architrave, anteriorly and inferiorly at the level of bony annulus: The short malleus palisade is placed under the denuded umbo

b The head of the titanium prosthesis is covered with three palisades. The small posterior palisade covers the scutum defect.

c The eardrum remnant with the tympanomeatal flap is replaced, stabilizing the palisades.

ways covered with cartilage in any cartilage tympanoplasty and in particular in palisade tympanoplasty.

Interposition with Titanium PORP Prosthesis and Cartilage Palisades

Titanium is nowadays the most commonly used prosthesis, but the round head of the prosthesis has to be covered with cartilage. The Kurz PORP prosthesis with a short shaft is placed onto the head of the stapes; the head of the prosthesis is stabilized by the chorda tympani (**Fig. 4.13a**). After placement of the architrave, the superior end of the anterior palisade is placed onto the architrave with the inferior end close to the bony annulus. The posterior palisades cover the head of the prosthesis (**Fig. 4.13b**). The replaced eardrum remnants stick to the palisades and rapid epithelialization of the new eardrum can take place (**Fig. 4.13c**).

Retracted and Adherent Malleus Handle and Cartilage Tympanoplasty

In cases with total perforation, retracted and adherent malleus handle, and missing long process of the incus, the adhesions are cut, the undersurface of the eardrum is scarified (**Fig. 4.14a**), the malleus handle is elevated, a piece of thin Silastic is placed under the umbo, and the architrave cartilage is placed onto the eminence of the tensor tympani muscle (**Fig. 4.14b**). The incus is removed and placed onto the stapes head (**Fig. 4.14c**). The anterior palisade is placed onto the architrave, and under the bony annulus; the other palisades are placed onto the bony annulus and partly onto the interposed incus (**Fig. 4.14 d**).

The alternative placement of palisades is at the level of the bony annulus after support with Gelfoam balls in the anterior and inferior tympanum and under the umbo (**Fig. 4.14e**). After replacement of the tympanomeatal flap the palisades will stick to the undersurface of the eardrum (**Fig. 4.14 f**).

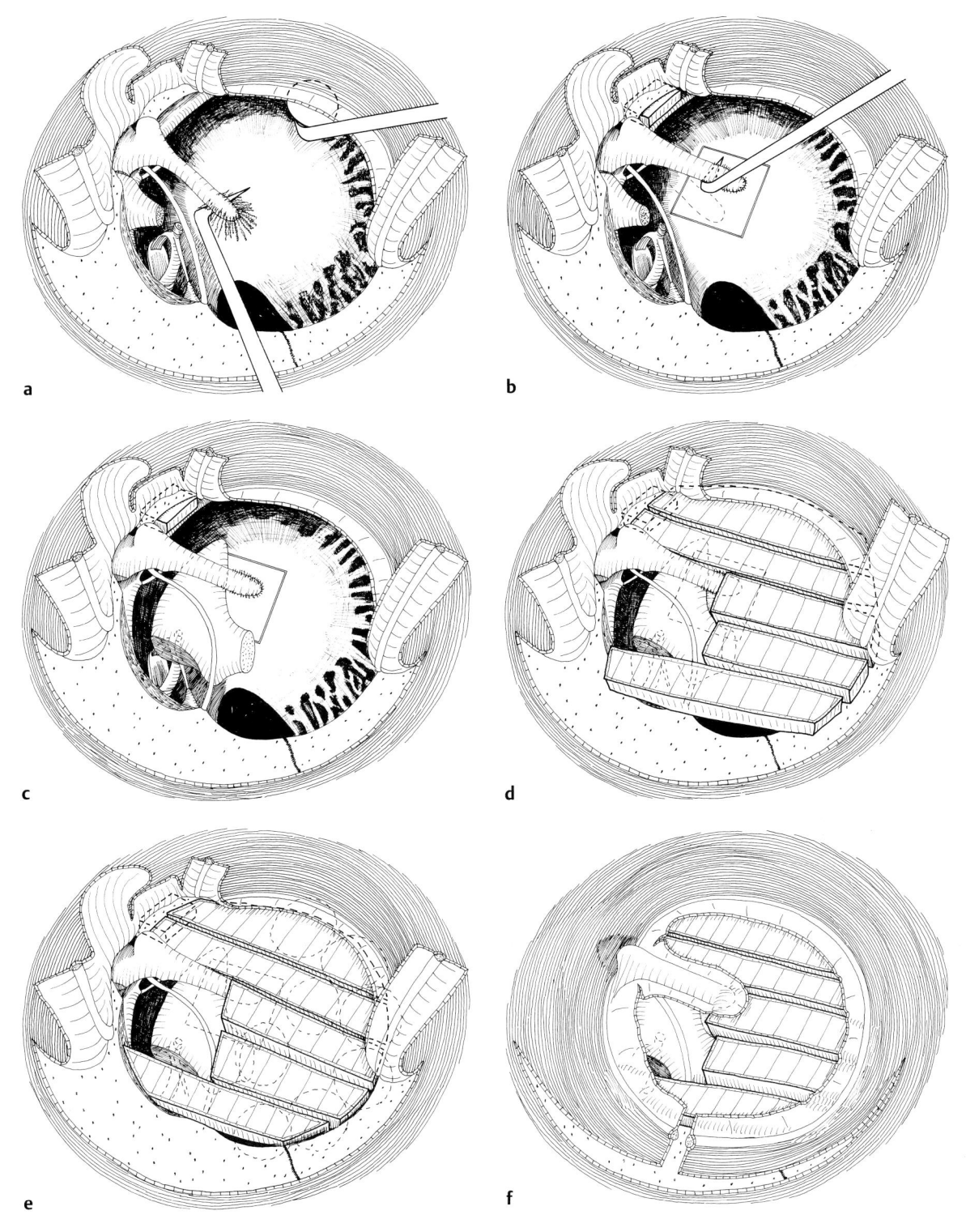

Fig. 4.14a–f Cartilage underlay palisade tympanoplasty in total perforation, missing long process of the incus, retracted and adherent malleus handle.

a Epithelium is removed from the edges of the perforation. A skin flap with fibrous annulus and epithelial remnants is elevated in a swing-door technique. Adhesions to the umbo are removed. Superiorly, the malleus flap is elevated and the eminence of tensor tympani muscle is exposed. The undersurface of the eardrum is scarified.

b The malleus handle is elevated with a hook to its normal level and a piece of cartilage—an architrave—is placed onto the eminence of the tensor tympani muscle to support the anterior palisades. Onto the promontory, at the previous site of the adhesion of the umbo, a 2 mm × 2 mm piece of Silastic sheet is placed.

c The incus is interposed between the stapes head and the malleus handle.

d The anterior palisade is placed under the bony annulus and superiorly onto the architrave. The second palisade is also placed inferiorly under the bony annulus. The malleus palisade and the posterior palisades are placed onto the inferior bony annulus.

e The alternative placement of the palisades at the level of the bony annulus instead of under and respectively on the bony annulus. The palisades are supported by Gelfoam balls.

f The flaps and the eardrum remnant are replaced.

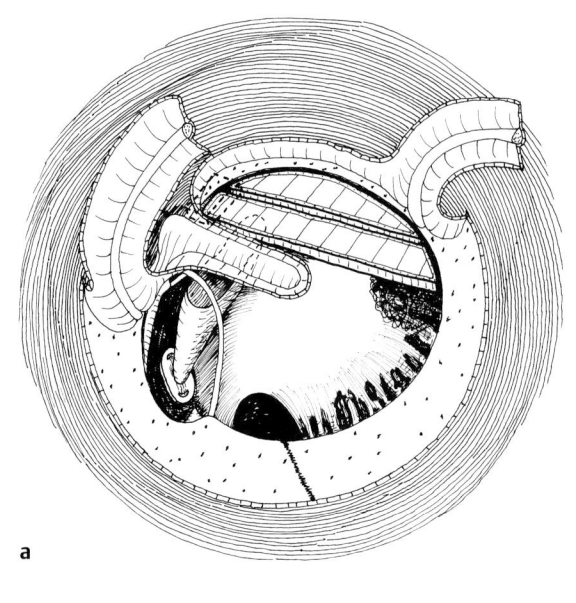

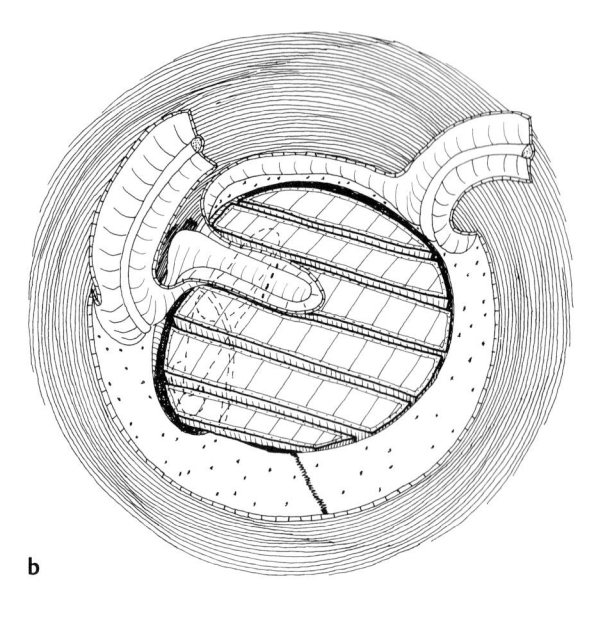

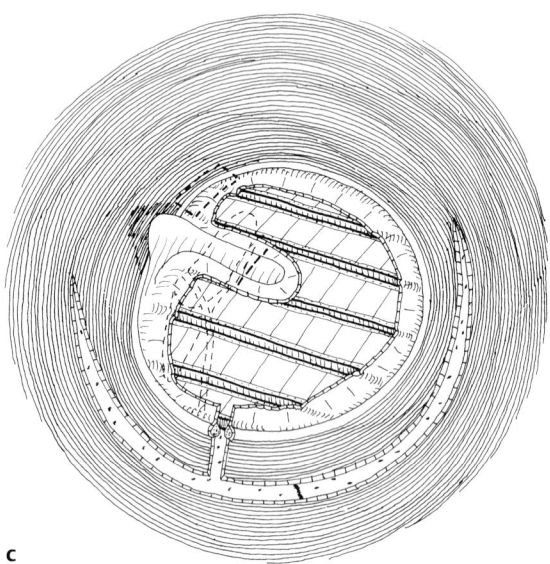

Fig. 4.15a–c Shaped autogenous incus columella in tympanoplasty type 3 with total perforation.
a The incus is placed on the center of the footplate and under the malleus handle. An architrave is placed onto the eminence of the tensor tympani muscle. Two anterior palisades are placed onto the architrave and close to the anterior and inferior bony annulus. The inferior ends of the palisades are supported with Gelfoam balls.
b The posterior palisades are placed onto the incus and onto the chorda. Inferiorly they are in contact with the bony annulus.
c The tympanomeatal flaps with the eardrum remnant are replaced.

Cartilage Palisades and Columella in Tympanoplasty Type 3

In missing stapedial arch and the long process of the incus, a shaped incus columella is placed onto the center of the footplate and under the malleus handle. A small architrave is placed onto the eminence of the tensor tympani muscle to support the two anterior palisades. Gelfoam balls, placed in the inferior and anterior parts of the tympanic cavity, support the palisades, which are placed at the level of and close to the bony annulus (**Fig. 4.15a**). The posterior palisades accommodate the incus columella (see **Fig. 4.15b, c**).

The incus columella can be shaped in various ways, as well as columellae made of cortical bone. They may be T-shaped, L-shaped, or sticklike (see MMES_1, Figs. 979–1002). The palisades should and will accommodate the columellae. Such accommodation is easiest in sticklike columellae (**Fig. 4.16**). The broad palisades rest on each side of the columellae at the level of the malleus handle, the other palisades are placed close to the bony annulus, they are supported by Gelfoam balls.

Cartilage Palisades and Titanium Columella in Tympanoplasty Type 3

The Kurz titanium columella with a large head is very suitable for use with cartilage palisades, which can be positioned onto the head of the prosthesis. After removal of the edges of the total perforation and scarification of the undersurface of the eardrum remnant, the Hüttenbrink cartilage guide (see Chapter 3, **Fig. 3.37**) is placed onto the footplate (**Fig. 4.17a**). The foot of the Kurz titanium columella is positioned onto the footplate through the central hole. To maintain the proper position, the colu-

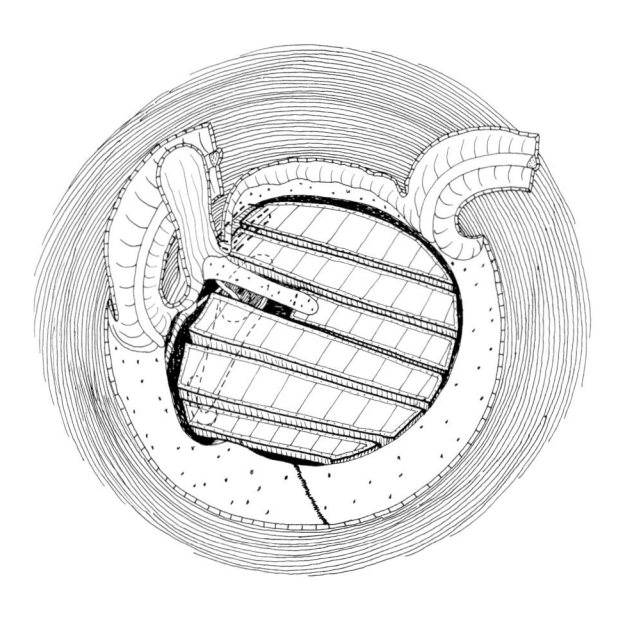

Fig. 4.16 A sticklike columella of cortical bone between the malleus hande and the footplate. The edges of the total perforation are cleaned. In a swing-door technique two tympanomeatal flaps and the malleus flap are elevated. A small architrave is placed onto the eminence of the tensor tympani muscle. The head of the columella is large and flat, allowing placement of the two palisades on both sides of the malleus handle. The remaining palisades are supported by Gelfoam and have contact with the bony annulus.

a

b

c

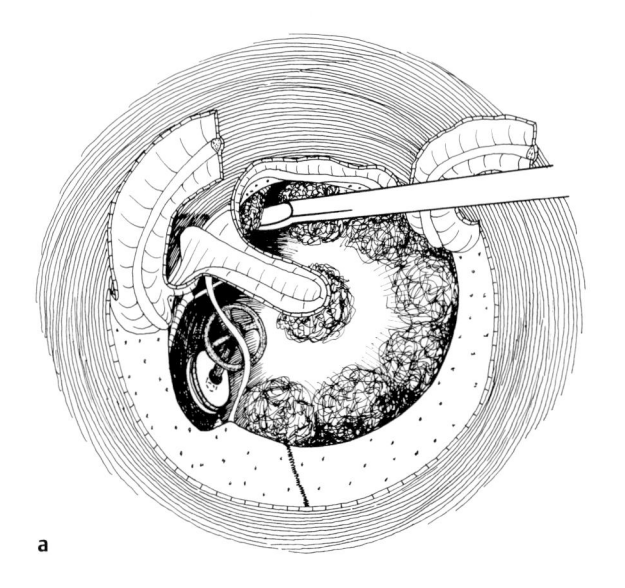

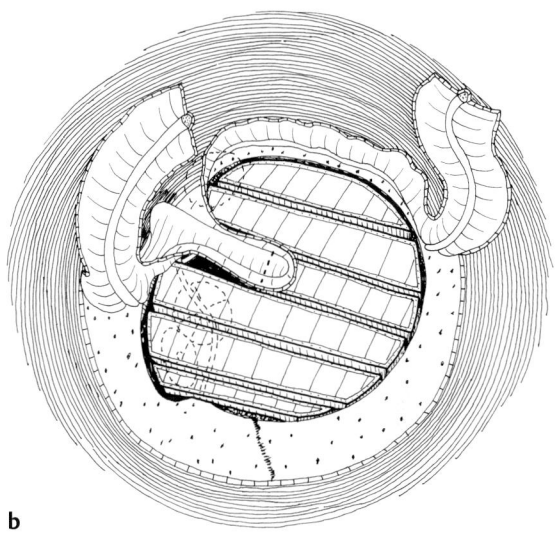

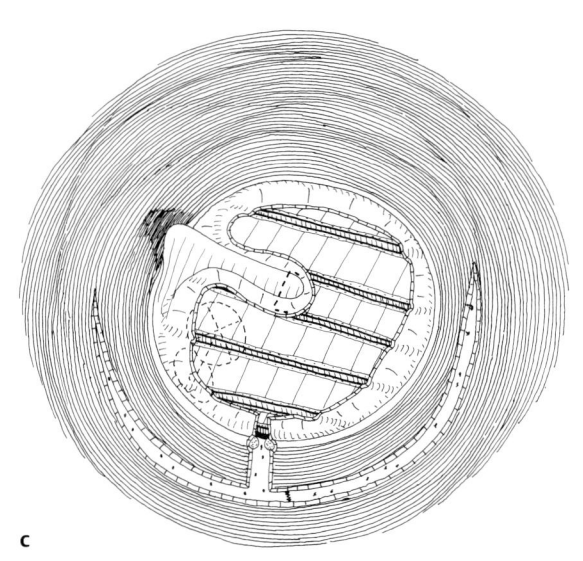

Fig 4.17a–c Kurz titanium columella placed onto the footplate through the hole of the Hüttenbrink Cartilage Guide.
a The 3.5 mm × 2.5 mm oval, 0.2–0.3 mm thick cartilage plate with a central hole of 0.8 mm is first placed onto the footplate; then the 4.5 mm long Aerial type columella is placed through the 0.8 mm hole onto the footplate. Instead of an architrave, a solid ball of Gelfoam is placed onto the eminence of the tensor tympani muscle. Gelfoam supports the palisades.
b The palisades are placed at the level of the bony annulus, onto the head of the titanium columella and onto the chorda tympani. The short malleus palisade is placed under the umbo.
c The tympanomeatal flaps are replaced together with the eardrum remnant, which will adhere to the palisades.

mella may be supported by Gelfoam and a Gelfoam ball is placed onto the eminence of the tensor tympani muscle instead of an architrave. The palisades are placed close to the bony annulus; the posterior palisades onto the head of the columella (**Fig. 4.17b**). After replacement of the tympanomeatal flaps, the perichondrium of the palisades will adhere to the denuded undersurface of the eardrum (**Fig. 4.17c**).

Modifications of Cartilage Palisade Technique

The classic underlay cartilage palisade technique as described and used by Heermann can be and has been modified in various ways:
a) Placement of the palisades exclusively under the bony annulus (Ferekidis chondrotympanoplasty)
b) Covering of the palisades with the perichondrium
c) Covering of the palisades with the fascia

Ferekidis Chondrotympanoplasty

Ferekidis placed all palisades under the bony annulus, both superiorly and inferiorly (Ferekidis et al. 2003). The palisades are supported only by Gelfoam balls.

Chondrotympanoplasty Type 1

In total or subtotal perforation with intact ossicular chain, the following technique is applied by Ferekidis et al (2003).

After removal of the edges of the perforation and cleaning of the umbo the mucosa under the bony annulus all the way around is scarified (**Fig. 4.18a**). The tympanomeatal flap is elevated and the tympanic cavity is filled with Gelfoam (**Fig. 4.18b**). Palisades are placed under the bony annulus, touching the scarified mucosa (**Fig. 4.18c**). The perichondrium, divided into an anterior on-lay graft and a posterior underlay graft covers the lateral side of the palisades. The posterior perichondrium is extended over

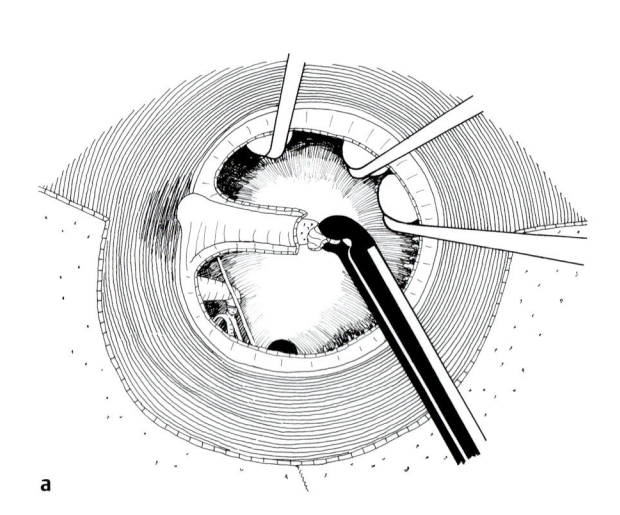

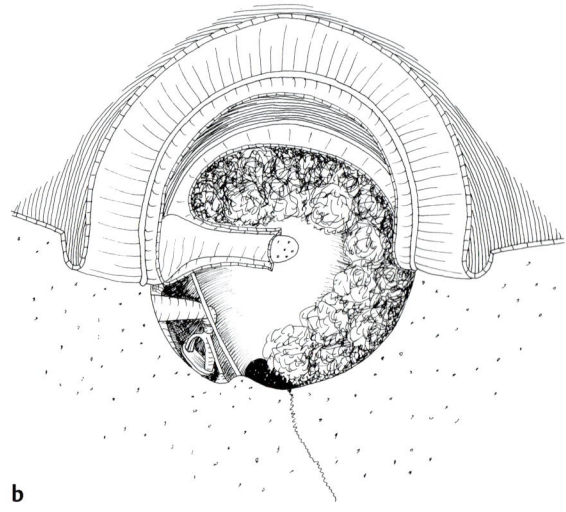

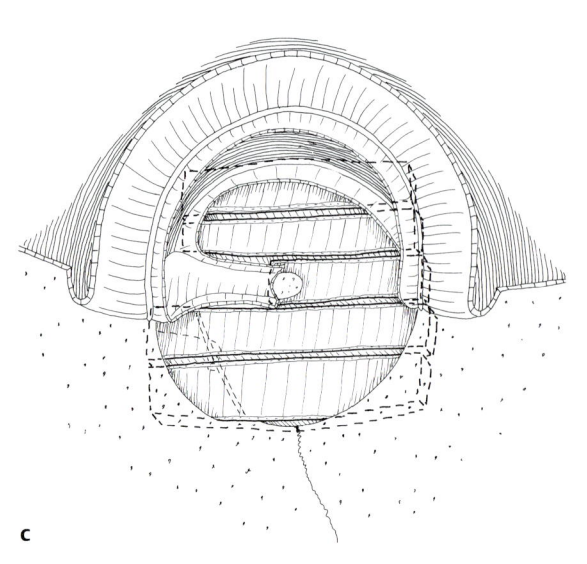

Fig. 4.18a–h Ferekidis type 1 chondrotympanoplasty in a case with total perforation and intact ossicular chain.

a In endaural approach, the edges of the perforation and of the malleus handle are cleaned of epithelium. The umbo is also cleaned of epithelium. Using a round knife, the mucosa of the eardrum remnant, the bony annulus, and the lateral wall of the anterior and inferior tympanum is scarified and partly removed.

b A posterior tympanomeatal flap is elevated and wet Gelfoam balls are placed into the tympanic cavity, in particular in the anterior and inferior part.

c The anterior palisade is placed under the anterior and inferior bony annulus. It is supported by the Gelfoam and will adhere to the undersurface of the eardrum. The second palisade is also placed under the superior and inferior bony annulus. It is supported by Gelfoam. The short malleus palisade is also placed under the bony annulus and umbo, supported by Gelfoam. Both posterior palisades are placed under the bony annulus. Superiorly, they may touch the long process of the incus and are supported by the chorda tympani.

Fig. 4.18 d–h

d The palisades are covered with two pieces of perichondrium removed from the convex side of the cartilage graft. The anterior perichondrium is placed as an on-lay graft and touches the edge of the epithelium of the eardrum. The posterior perichondrium is placed as an underlay graft onto the denuded ear canal bone and under the fibrous annulus and eardrum.
e The tympanomeatal flap with the eardrum remnant is replaced.
f Side view of Ferekidis type 1 chondrotympanoplasty. The palisades are positioned under the bony annulus and are supported by Gelfoam balls. Perichondrium covers the palisades— anteriorly as an on-lay graft, posteriorly as an underlay graft— and extends over the ear canal bone. The short malleus palisade is placed under the umbo.
g Elevation of the malleus epithelial flap and placement of one piece of perichondrium onto the cartilage. Again the anterior perichondrium is an on-lay graft, the posterior an underlay graft.
h The malleus epithelial flap and the tympanomeatal flaps are replaced.

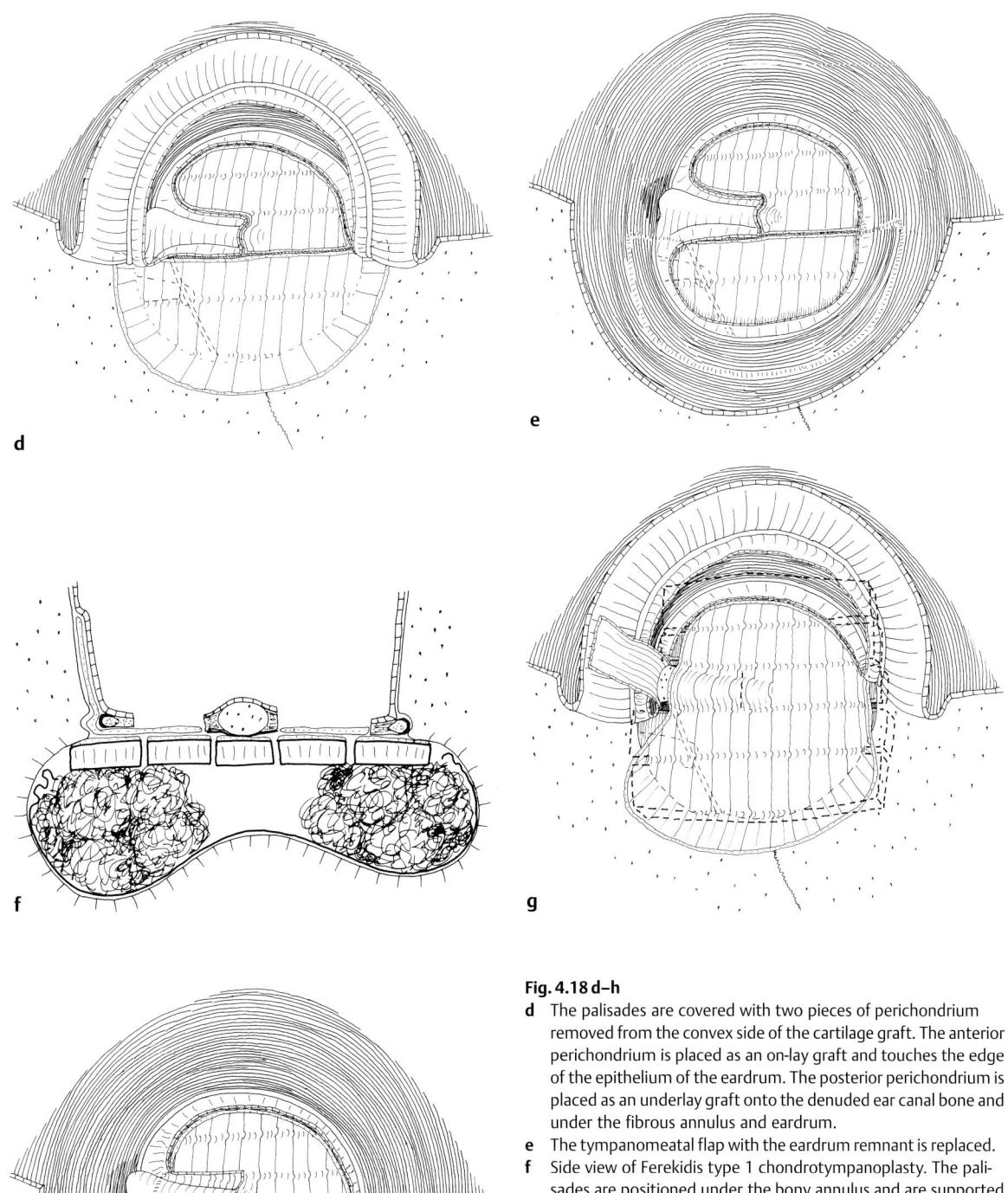

the posterior ear canal wall (**Fig. 4.18 d**) and the epithelial flap is replaced (**Fig. 4.18e**). The palisades are positioned under the bony annulus, both inferiorly and posteriorly (**Fig. 4.18 f**) in contrast to Heermann technique, where only the most anterior palisade is placed under the bony annulus.

With elevation of the malleus epithelial flap, one piece of the perichondrium can cover the palisades (**Fig. 4.18 g, h**).

Chondrotympanoplasty Combined with Ossiculoplasty

Ferekides prefers to call these methods chondrotympanoplasty type 3. In accordance with the nomenclature used in this book, I will call them type 2 in cases with stapes present and type 3 in the absence of the stapes, where a columella is used.

Chondrotympanoplasty Type 2

In type 2 tympanoplasty with stapes present, a bridge with a piece of cartilage is made between the eminence of the Fallopian canal and the head of the stapes and a palisade is placed onto the eminence of the tensor tympani muscle (**Fig. 4.19a**). After placing the Gelfoam balls in the tympanic cavity and under the inferior end of the prosthesis, the first palisade is placed under the bony annulus (**Fig. 4.19b**). The remaining palisades are also placed under the inferior bony annulus. Superior ends of the palisades are placed partly onto the small pieces of cartilage and partly onto the Gelfoam (**Fig. 4.19c**). Perichondrium covers the palisades and the medial attic wall and a small piece of perichondrium closes the anterior attic (**Fig. 4.19 d**). After replacement of the skin flaps, the solid and safe reconstruction will easily be epithelialized.

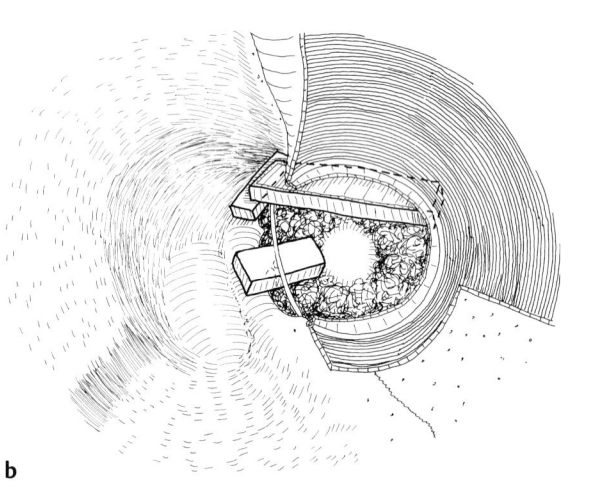

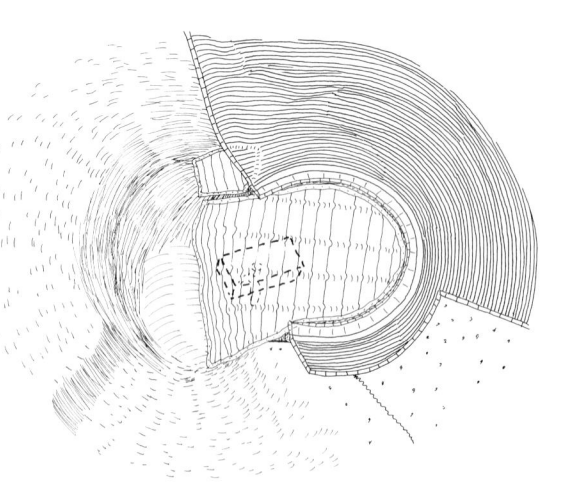

a

b

c

d

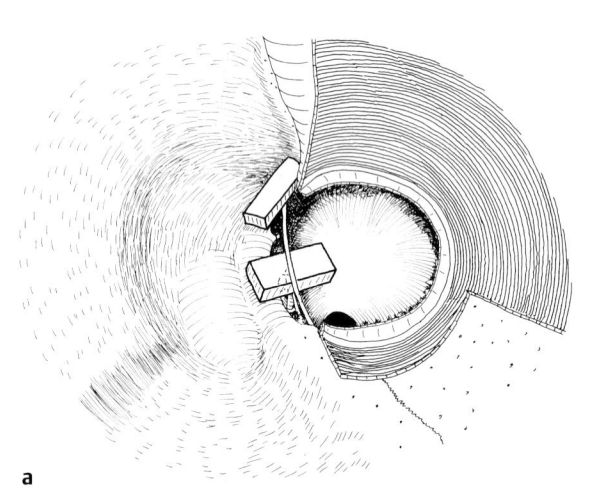

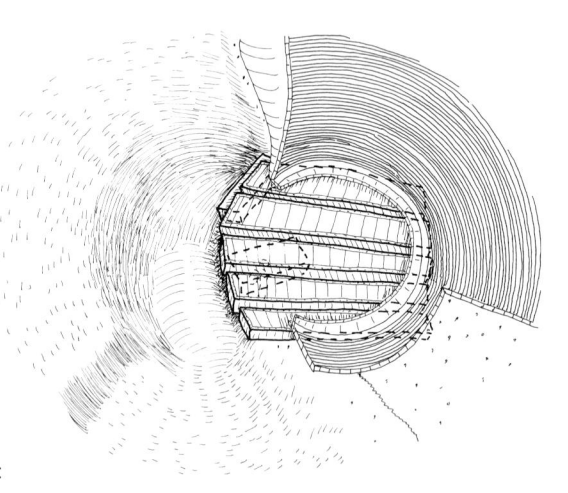

Fig. 4.19a–d Chondrotympanoplasty type 2 in a situation with canal wall down mastoidectomy, total perforation, malleus and incus missing but not the stapes.
- **a** The edge of the perforation is removed, and the mucosa under the bony annulus is scarified. A piece of cartilage is placed on the eminence of the tensor tympany muscle. A wider short palisade is placed onto the fallopian canal and the head of the stapes, providing an ossiculoplasty type 2.
- **b** The tympanic cavity is filled with Gelfoam to support palisades and the first palisade is placed onto the piece of cartilage lying on the eminence of the tensor tympani muscle.
- **c** The palisades are placed inferiorly under the bony annulus. Superiorly, the palisades are placed onto the cartilage forming the ossiculoplasty.
- **d** The palisades are covered with perichondrium as an on-lay graft, tightly closing the connection between the anterior attic and the Eustachian tube in cases with canal wall down mastoidectomy and with open cavity.

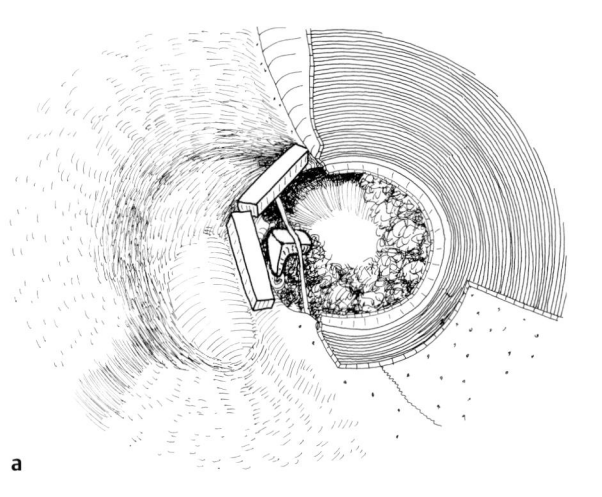

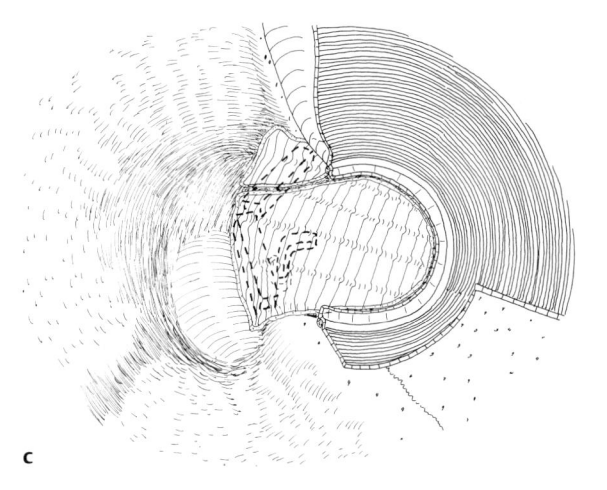

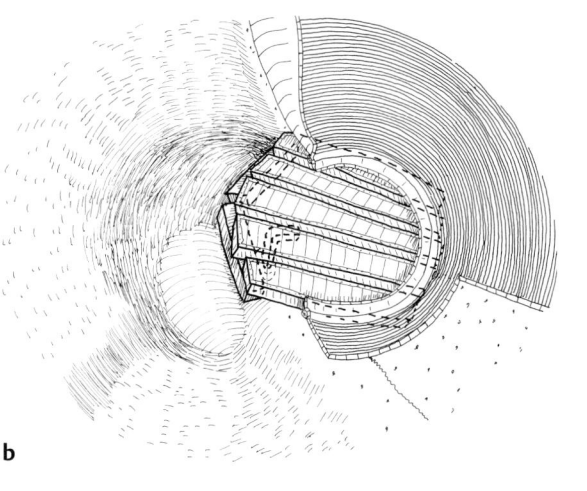

Fig. 4.20a–c Chondrotympanoplasty type 3 with a cartilage columella in a case with canal wall down mastoidectomy, total perforation, and missing ossicles.
a The edge of the perforation is removed and Gelfoam placed into the inferior part of the tympanic cavity. Superiorly, a relatively compact cartilage columella is placed onto the footplate. A palisade is placed onto the eminence of the tensor tympani muscle and another palisade onto the fallopian canal, both to support the superior ends of the palisades, especially of the first palisade.
b All five palisades are placed in the tympanic cavity.
c The palisades are covered with perichondrium, extending onto the attic. The anterior attic is covered with a separate piece of perichondrium or fascia mainly as an on-lay graft.

Chondrotympanoplasty Type 3

In cases of missing ossicles, Ferekidis prefers a solid L-shaped cartilage columella. On the superior border of the tympanic cavity, two cartilage palisades are placed to elevate the eardrum (**Fig. 4.20a**). The inferior ends of the cartilage, placed under the bony annulus, are supported with Gelfoam. The superior ends are laid on the cartilage, firmly closing the tympanic cavity (**Fig. 4.20b**) The perichondrium covers the palisades and the attic wall and the anterior attic (**Figs. 4.20c, 4.21**).

Intratympanal Tubal Chondroplasty

In cases of retraction of the tympanic membrane into the tubal orifice, a tubal plasty can prevent recurrent retraction. After elevation of the retracted part of the thin eardrum, a tubal plasty is made by Ferekidis et al. (2003) in the following way: A 3 mm long piece of cartilage is placed onto the eminence of the tensor tympani muscle. Another piece is placed into the anterior hypotympanum. A broad palisade is placed onto the two cartilage pieces, making a

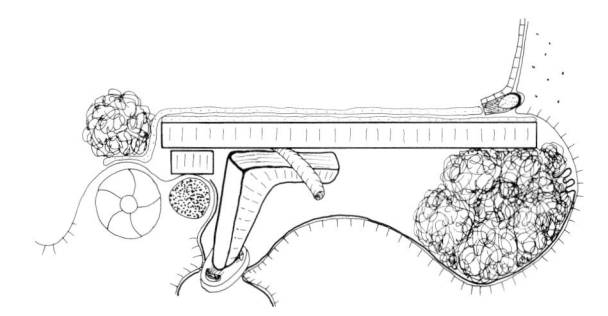

Fig. 4.21 Superoinferior view of the chondrotympanoplasty type 3 with a cartilage columella. A relatively thick columella is covered by a columella supported by Gelfoam balls and a piece of cartilage placed on the eminence of the fallopian canal. Perichondrium covers the palisades.

solid lateral wall of the tubal ostium (**Fig. 4.22**). Further reconstruction is the same chondrotympanoplasty type 3 as already described (**Figs. 4.20, 4.21**).

Covering Palisades with the Perichondrium

In Ferekidis chondrotympanoplasty, at the end of surgery perichondrium is placed onto the palisades as one on-lay graft (**Figs. 4.19 d, 4.20c**), as two on-lay grafts (**Fig. 4.18e**), or partly as an on-lay graft anteriorly and partly as an underlay graft posteriorly (**Fig. 4.18h**).

Cartilage Palisades and the Perichondrium as the Underlay Graft

Dubreuil (personal communication, 2006; Tringali et al. 2008) places the perichondrium as an underlay graft at the beginning of the operation and before placement of the palisades.

First a 1 cm × 1 cm piece of tragal cartilage covered with perichondrium on both sides is harvested. The perichondrium is removed from the convex side and the palisades are cut.

In transcanal approach, the edges of the total perforation are cleaned, and a circumferential incision is made (**Fig. 4.23a**). The tympanomeatal flap with the malleus flap is elevated. The mucosa under the eardrum remnant is scarified (**Fig. 4.23b**). The anterior border of the large perichondrium graft is pushed with a curved elevator under the anterior and inferior eardrum remnant (**Fig. 4.23c**). After placement of the palisades (**Fig. 4.23 d**) the perichondrium will cover the palisades as an underlay graft, the denuded malleus handle, and the bony annulus (**Fig. 4.23e**). After replacement of the malleus flap and the tympanomeatal flap, the conditions for rapid epithelialization are good (**Fig. 4.23 f**).

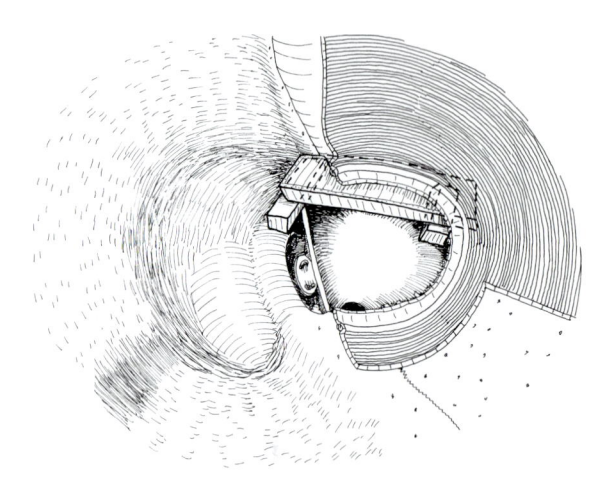

Fig. 4.22 Intratympanal tubal chondroplasty. A small piece of cartilage is placed onto the cochleariform process and at the eminence of the tensor tympani muscle, another in the hypotympanum. A relatively wide palisade is placed as the first palisade, preventing eventual retraction of the eardrum into the eustachian tube.

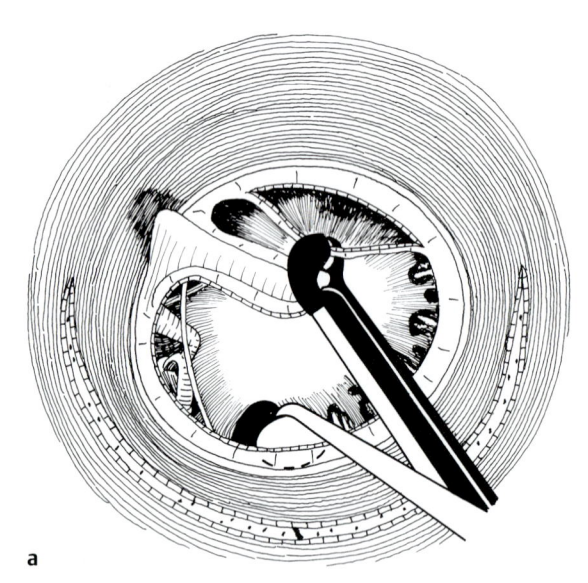

Fig. 4.23a–f Covering the palisades with perichondrium in a total perforation.
a The edges of the perforation are cleaned and the mucosa of the eardrum is scarified. A large circumferential incision is performed.
b The tympanomeatal flap is elevated and also a malleus flap. Further scarification of the mucosa under the anterior eardrum remnant is done.

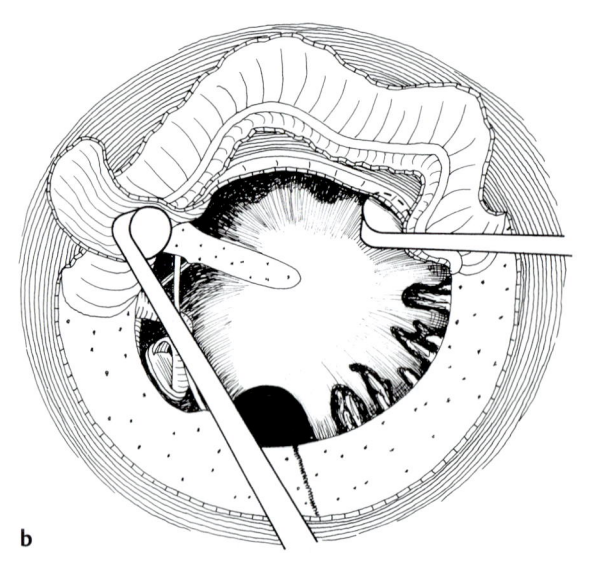

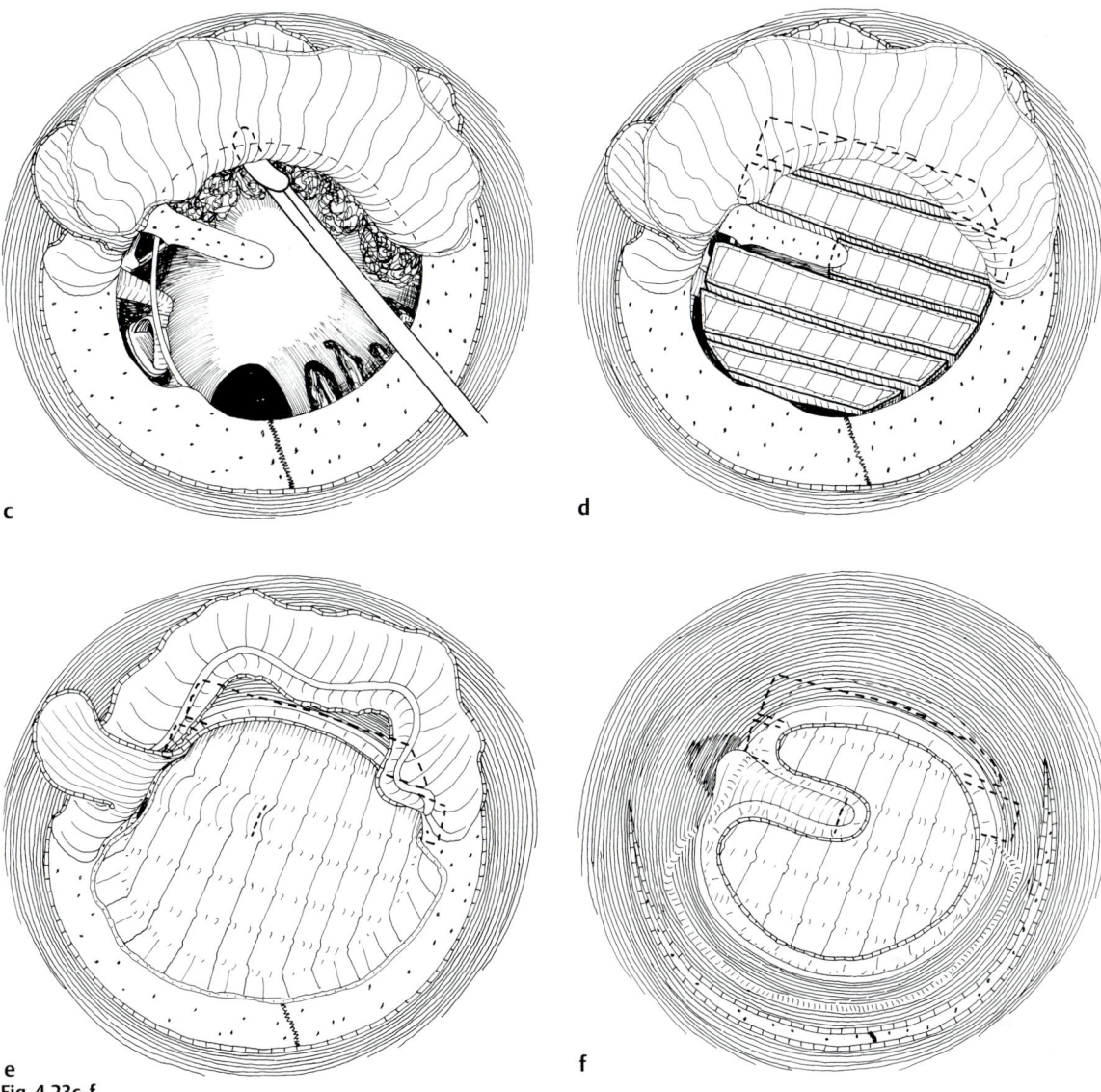

Fig. 4.23c–f

c A large piece of perichondrium is placed and adapted to the undersurface of the eardrum remnant; it is supported with Gelfoam balls.

d The anterior cartilage palisades are placed under the perichondrium. The small palisade is placed under the umbo and supported with Gelfoam. The posterior palisades are placed close to the bony annulus.

e The perichondrium is placed under the denuded annulus and onto the palisades and the posterior ear canal wall.

f The malleus flap and the tympanomeatal flaps are replaced and the epithelialization of the perichondrium begins.

Cartilage Palisades and Fascia

In the early palisade era, from 1960, Heermann used cartilage plates to support the fascia, but in the course of time fascia has increasingly been replaced by cartilage, but fascia was still used to cover the cartilage for a period (Heermann and Heermann, 1967; Heermann et al. 1970; Heermann 1978).

Some surgeons still sometimes use fascia to cover the cartilage palisades. There are no major differences in anatomical results whether the palisades are covered with perichondrium or with fascia. If there is too large a distance between two palisades, the spot can be closed with a small piece of cartilage (see **Fig. 2.1**) or fascia or any fibrous tissue to promote safe epithelialization without ingrowth of the epithelium.

4 Cartilage Palisades in Underlay Tympanoplasty Techniques

Wiegand Palisade Technique Covered with Fascia

This technique is a modification of Heermann technique in several respects.

Harvesting and Elaboration of Palisades

Wiegand (1978) harvests the tragal cartilage through the intercartilaginous incision in Heermann B endaural approach (see **Fig. 17.4**). The large cartilage piece is covered on both sides with perichondrium and so are the palisades (**Fig. 4.24a**). On each end of each palisade, two perichondrium flaps are made to suspend the palisade. Wiegand believes that the presence of perichondrium on both sides of the palisades stabilizes them.

Underlay and On-lay Cartilage–Fascia Tympanoplasty

In endaural approach, a circumferential incision between the 11-o'clock and 7-o'clock positions is made and a posterior ear canal skin flap is elevated outward. The edges of the perforation are removed and the mucosa of the eardrum remnant is scarified (**Fig. 4.24b**). In swing-door technique, the superior tympanomeatal flap is elevated together with the eardrum remnant and the fibrous annulus, as for underlay tympanoplasty flap (**Fig. 4.24c**). The inferior flap is elevated as an on-lay flap, because only the epithelium of the inferior eardrum remnant is elevated, and the fibrous annulus with the lamina propria is left in place. Another innovation is drilling of a groove along the end of the ear canal, just behind the bony annulus. The

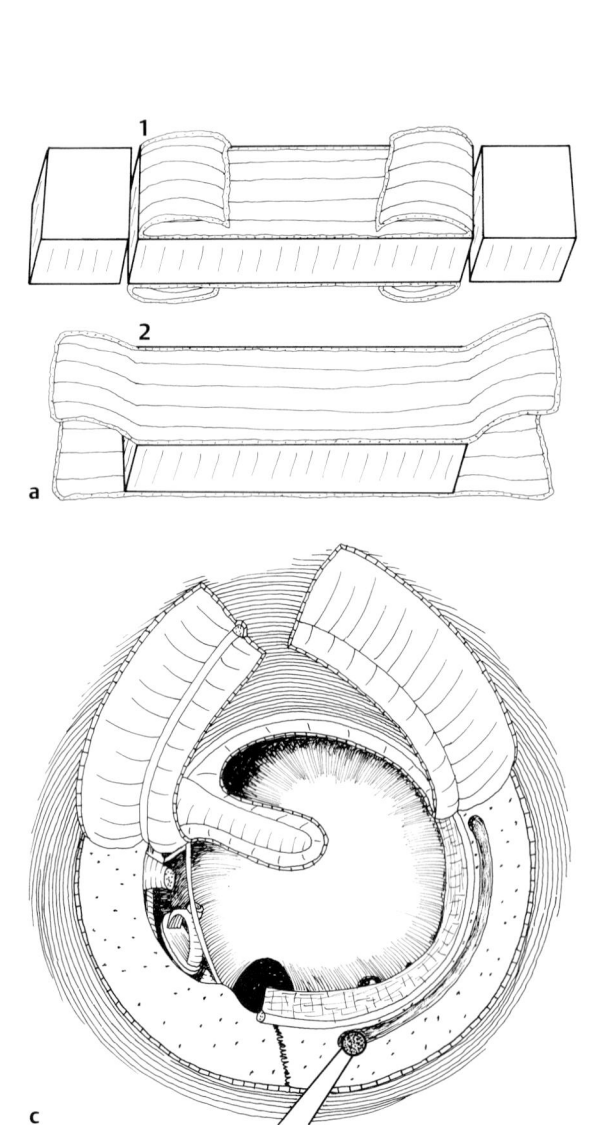

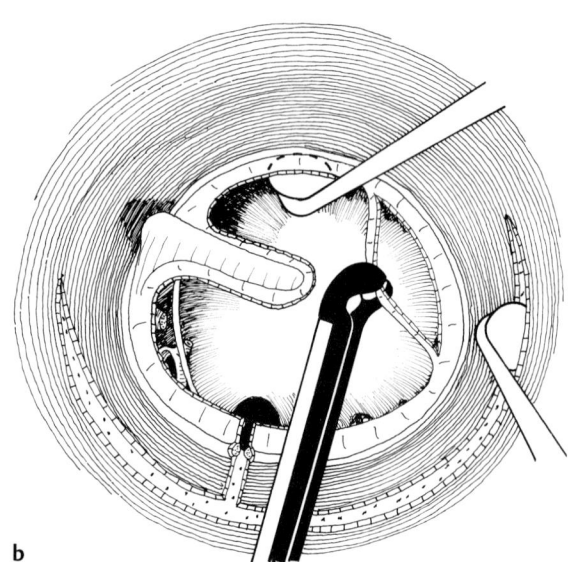

Fig. 4.24a–f Wiegand's on-lay–underlay palisade-fascia technique in a total perforation and missing long process of the incus.

a Elaboration of cartilage palisades with two perichondrium flaps on both ends. **1**, The palisade is covered on both sides with the perichondrium. At each end 2 mm of the perichondrium is elevated and the uncovered cartilage is cut off. **2**, Final palisade with four perichondrium flaps.

b In endaural approach a circumferential incision between the 11-o'clock and 5-o'clock positions and a radial incision at the 9-o'clock position are made and a posterior ear canal skin flap is elevated outward. The edges of the perforation are removed and the undersurface of the anterior eardrum remnant and malleus handle is scarified.

c In a swing-door technique a superior tympanomeatal flap with the fibrous annulus is elevated. The epithelium from the inferior eardrum remnant together with the ear canal skin is elevated as a flap, while the inferior fibrous annulus with the denuded lamina propria is left in place. Using a 0.5 mm diamond drill, a bony sulcus along the inferior bony annulus is drilled out perichondrium flaps of the palisades will be placed into the groove, not the palisade ends. The first palisade is placed under the malleus handle and the two superior perichondrium flaps are pushed upward under the malleus (**Fig. 4.24 d**), stabilizing the palisade. The inferior end of the palisade is placed close to the inferior eardrum remnant, but the outer perichondrium flap is placed onto the lamina propria and onto the fibrous annulus continuing onto the bone of the groove. The superior end of the second palisade is placed onto the head of the stapes. The inferior ends of the remaining palisades are placed close to the lamina propria and the perichondrium flaps are placed onto the lamina propria and onto the fibrous annulus. Wiegand did not close the anterior part of the tympanic cavity with a palisade but with a large piece of fascia placed as underlay graft under the anterior annulus and the onto the cartilage palisades and onto the ear canal bone (**Fig. 4.24e**). After replacement of the tympanomeatal flaps a small round piece of the ear canal skin is placed onto the anterior part of the fascia (**Fig. 4.24 f**).

Thus the Wiegand method involves four tissues—perichondrium, cartilage, fascia, and skin—and the perforation is firmly closed (**Fig. 4.25**).

During the period 1973–1976, Wiegand operated 645 ears by his method and only one primary and three late reoperations were necessitated (Wiegand 1978). There are no reports on hearing.

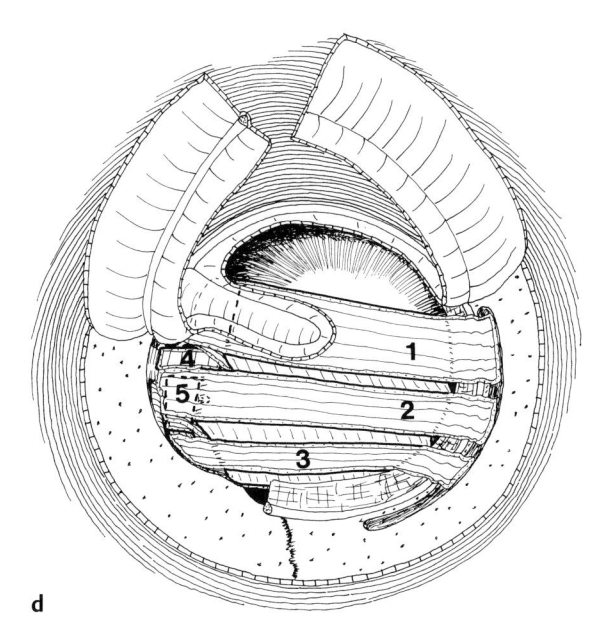

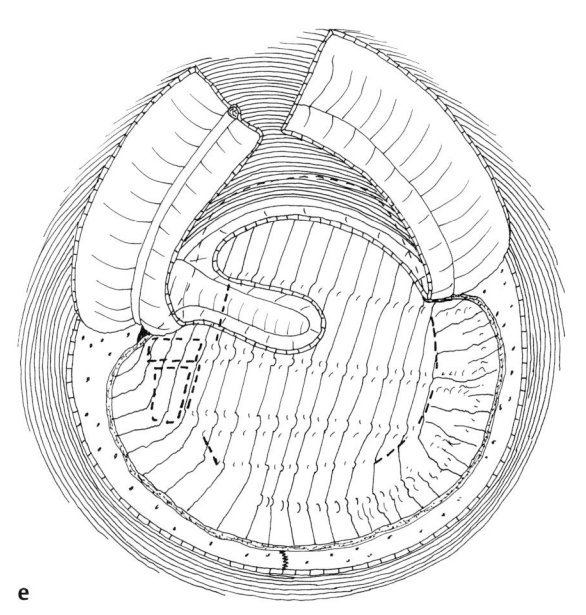

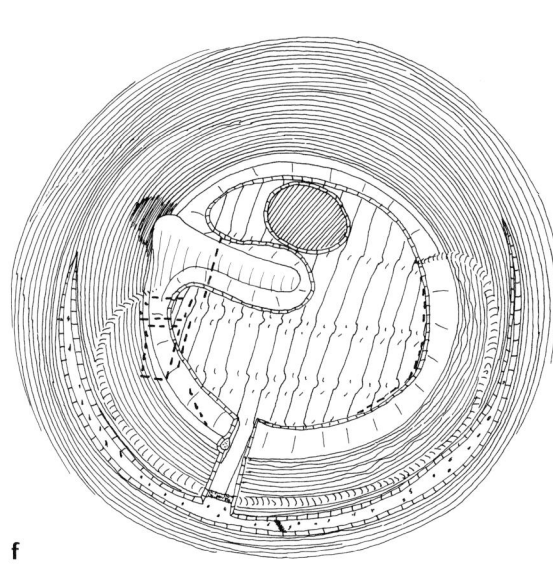

Fig. 4.24d–f
d The first palisade (1) is placed under the malleus handle. The two superior perichondrium flaps are folded out on the undersurface of the malleus. The inferior end of the palisade is placed close to the lamina propria. The outer perichondrium flap (ear canal flap) lies on the lamina propria, fibrous annulus and the bony groove. The inner perichondrium flap is placed under the eardrum remnant. The second palisade (2) is placed onto the head of the stapes. The remaining palisades (3–5) cover the posterior tympanum with the perichondrium flaps placed onto the eardrum remnant, the fibrous annulus, and the groove.
e A round fascia is placed under the anterior eardrum remnant and onto the palisades but under the malleus handle. Posteriorly and inferiorly, the fascia covers the ear canal bone and the groove.
f The epithelial flaps are replaced. Anterior to the malleus handle, a round piece of ear canal skin, taken from the anterior wall, is placed.

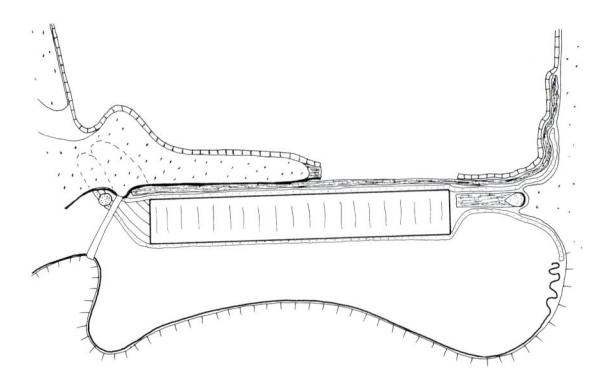

Fig. 4.25 Superoinferior side view of the cartilage palisade–fascia covering of a total perforation. The palisade is placed under the malleus handle and is stabilized by two perichondrium flaps; one is placed under the lamina propria the other onto the lamina propria. Fascia covers the palisades and is placed under the malleus handle. Inferiorly, the fascia is placed onto the perichondrium flaps and onto the ear canal bone.

Results of Surgery with Palisades in Underlay Tympanoplasty Techniques

The Freiburg group (Amedee, Mann, and Riechelmann 1989), were the first to publish results on cartilage palisade tympanoplasties. On 52 ears they achieved 100% eardrum closures. Postoperative hearing 3½ months after surgery was good: in 18 patients with intact ossicles and type 1 tympanoplasty, the mean air–bone gap for frequencies 500–4000 Hz was 20 dB before surgery, and 4 dB 3½ months after surgery.

Péré (1989) found very good hearing results and 100% closure of the perforation in 18 patients. Milewski (1989, 1991) reported cartilage tympanoplasty in 550 cases, half with cartilage palisades, half with composite island graft. There were no major differences in results between the two methods. Among 197 cases with tympanoplasty type 1, 43.6% had an air–bone gap less than 10 dB; 49% had an air–bone gap between 11 and 30 dB; 25% had been operated previously. Eardrum closure was achieved in 95.5%. Among 353 patients with defective ossicular chain, 16% had an air–bone gap less than 10 dB and 63% were in the range 11–30 dB. Eardrum closure was achieved in 96.5%.

Velepic et al. (2001) closed eardrum perforation in three divers; all were able to dive after cartilage palisade tympanoplasties.

In 32 ears with intact ossicular chain Ferekidis et al. (2003) achieved a mean reduction of air–bone gap at 2000 Hz from 20 dB to 8 dB. Only one small "pinhole" perforation was found in one patient. In 44 patients with defective ossicular chain the mean air–bone gap at 2000 Hz was reduced from 25 dB to 10 dB. The results were stable over 2 years.

Results in Pars Tensa Cholesteatoma in Children

From June 1995 to October 2000, 32 children underwent one-stage surgery by me for cholesteatoma and eardrum reconstruction with cartilage palisades at Gentofte Hospital (Andersen et al. 2002). Twenty-one children had sinus cholesteatoma defined as posterosuperior retraction and cholesteatoma mass in the tympanic sinuses, and 11 had tensa retraction cholesteatoma defined as retraction of the entire pars tensa with the cholesteatoma both in the tympanic sinuses and in the hypotympanum. All children were reevaluated at an average of 37 months (range 3–63 months).

Eardrum appearance: All the patients had a dry ear without cholesteatoma, and intact tympanic membrane at the reevaluation, but one small perforation was surgically closed during the observation period. There was retraction behind the interposed incus in two ears; in these cases the palisades were, in error, not placed in the posterosuperior drilling defect behind the interposed incus.

Revisions: Four children underwent reoperation during the observation period: one because of closure of the already mentioned perforation. Two were suspected of cholesteatoma, which was disproved by exploratory tympanotomy. The fourth reoperation was performed for conductive hearing loss caused by bony fixation of the interposed incus, which could also be avoided by placing a small palisade between the incus and the scutum.

Hearing results: In 14 ears with intact ossicular chain, tympanoplasty 1 was done; in 7 ears tympanoplasty type 2 with interposition of the patient's own incus between stapes head and malleus handle was done; and in 5 ears with missing stapes, tympanoplasty type 3 with a columella was done.

Postoperative hearing was good and stable (**Table 4.1**). At the follow-up, pure tone average and speech reception within 0–20 dB was found in 75% of ears; mean absolute hearing was 10–15 dB in tympanoplasty type 1, somewhat poorer in types 2 and 3.

Table 4.1 Mean absolute preoperative, primary, and late and postoperative hearing expressed as pure tone average (PTA), speech reception threshold, and air–bone gap in the palisade group of 32 children operated for cholesteatoma (21 sinus, 11 tensa), expressed as percentages (Andersen et al. 2002)

	Pure tone average		Speech reception threshold		Air–bone gap		
	0–20-dB	0–30-dB	0–20-dB	0–30-dB	0–10 dB	0–20 db	0–30-dB
Preoperative	25	56	41	69	0	44	66
Primary	66	88	66	91	19	66	94
Late	75	81	75	94	41	78	88

Comparing Results of Cartilage Palisades with Fascia

During the same period (1995–2000) and by the same surgeon the eardrum was closed with palisades in 32 children (32 ears) and with fascia in 32 children (33 ears) operated for sinus cholesteatoma (21 ears) and entire tensa retraction cholesteatoma (11 ears). The patients from the fascia group were treated and reevaluated in exactly the same way as the palisade group (Andersen et al. 2004).

Eardrum appearance: In the fascia group there were significantly more retractions (12, or 36%) at the reevaluation ($P < 0.01$; ×2 tests). Six retractions were deep, the other 6 were moderate and minor. The retractions were most frequently localized in the posterosuperior part of the eardrum. Seven of the 12 retractions appeared and developed within the first year after operation.

Revisions: Three patients were reoperated. One patient had a deep sinus retraction and a cholesteatoma was suspected. Adhesive otitis was found during surgery in one patient. Palisades were used for reconstruction. Two patients had a small anterior perforation.

Hearing: At follow-up 58% of the ears had absolute hearing of 20 dB or better. Air–bone gap closure within 10 dB was achieved in 32% at follow-up. At follow-up the mean absolute hearing was 22 dB in the fascia group and 18 dB in the palisade group.

Residual cholesteatoma: In contrast to tympanoplasty with fascia or perichondrium, the opacity of the cartilage palisades compromises the identification of a residual cholesteatoma. This is the only disadvantage of the palisade grafting technique. However, when cholesteatoma is suspected a paracentesis between the two palisades can be performed in the suspected region. When one-stage surgery is performed—as is our practice—the children have to be followed up closely for a long period.

Comparing Functional Results and Tympanometry

The late functional hearing results were better in the palisade group (71% success) than in the fascia group (54% success). This was particularly the case in ears with poor tubal function and an abnormal tympanogram, in which functional success was achieved in 68% in the palisade group, in contrast to 29% in the fascia group. Although only as a trend, the other functional results were also better in the palisade group. Thus the mean hearing gain in the palisade group was 11.5 dB, which was significantly better than the 4.9 dB in the fascia group (Uzun et al. 2003; Tos et al. 2005). We may conclude that hearing results after eardrum reconstruction using cartilage palisades are better than with fascia despite comparable tympanometric findings. Cartilage palisade tympanoplasty seems to provide better functional results, especially in ears with poor tubal function, which is the common situation after cholesteatoma surgery.

Comparison of Underlay Cartilage Palisades with Fascia—Recent Results

Recently Ozbek et al. (2008) published results of comparison of over-underlay tympanoplasty, using either cartilage palisades (on 21 children) or temporalis fascia graft (on 24 children). All 45 children had a dry perforation occupying more than 50% of the eardrum and an intact ossicular chain. At least 12 months after the surgery a 100% acceptance rate was found in the palisade group compared with 70.2% in the fascia group, a significantly poorer anatomical result. Hearing improvement was the same in the fascia group and in the palisade group.

In a Chinese study (Yu et al. 2001), 66 patients with large eardrum perforations were treated with cartilage palisades harvested from the concha. During the same period, 60 patients with similar eardrum perforations were closed by the temporalis fascia. In the palisade group, the perforations were closed in 92.4% of the ears, in the fascia group in 80%. There was no significant difference in postoperative hearing improvement between the two groups. The authors concluded that cartilage palisade tympanoplasty is quite suitable for repairing large perforations and for treatment of adhesive otitis media.

Late Results in Underlay Palisade Technique

Results of Heermann Underlay Palisade Surgery

In 1991, 315 patients were operated in the Otolaryngological Clinic, a part of the A. Krupp Hospital in Essen, using underlay cartilage palisade tympanoplasty. Joachim Heermann himself was most often the surgeon, but senior assistants have also performed the same operation. In 1991, Wielgosz and Mroczkowski (2006) called all 315 patients to a follow up-investigation; 108 patients participated, with a follow-up period of 8.16–9.5 years. The mean age at operation was 46.5 years, range 7–74 years.

In 28 patients with an intact ossicular chain, an ABG (air– bone gap) of 0–10 dB was found in 67.8% and of 11–20 dB in 10% of patients. In 47 patients with tympanoplasty type 2, the corresponding percentages for ABG were 80% and 10%. In 21 patients with tympanoplasty type 3, the corresponding percentages for ABG were 40.4% and 42.5%.

The authors concluded that the cartilage is a good autogenous graft in the long term for reconstruction of the tympanic membrane and the auditory canal on account of stability and absence of secondary perforations. Long-term hearing results were satisfactory.

Ten-year Results of Cartilage Palisades versus Fascia in Eardrum Reconstruction after Surgery for Sinus or Tensa Retraction Cholesteatoma in Children

At the Gentofte Hospital during the period 1995–2000 I operated on a total of 64 children for either sinus or tensa retraction cholesteatoma (mean age 9 years, range 5–15 years). The eardrum was reconstructed using underlay cartilage palisades in 32 children (32 ears) and using fascia or perichondrium in 32 children (33 ears). The patients were followed for at least one year postoperatively and were reevaluated 4 years after surgery (Andersen et al. 2004) and again recently at a mean of 10 years (Cayé-Thomasen et al. 2009).

All but 2 patients in each group attended the 10-year follow-up examination (94% attendance). The mean overall follow-up period was 119 months (115 months in the palisade group and 125 months in the fascia group).

The total number of retractions during follow-up and at the 10-year examination was 6 (19%) for the palisade group and 14 (42%) for the fascia group ($p = 0.03$; chi-squared test). The cumulative numbers for a perforation were 4 (13%) for the palisade group and 7 (21%) for the fascia group (difference not significant). Two residual cholesteatomas, which are not related to the graft material, occurred in the palisade group (6%), whereas both recurrences, which may be related to the graft material, occurred in the fascia group (6%). The hearing acuity for children operated for a sinus cholesteatoma and for children with type 3 tympanoplasty was significantly better when cartilage palisade grafting had been employed.

The cartilage palisade technique is superior in preventing long-term eardrum retraction. The recurrence of eardrum perforation is less in the palisade group, although these results may be due to type 2 error because of low numbers of ears. The length of the observation period was not longer in the fascia group than in the cartilage group, as suggested by Yung (2008). The fascia patients were operated on during the same period, with the same approach, with the same ossiculoplasty, and by the same surgeon as the palisade group. Although the number of patients is small in each group, all patients were children all had sinus or tensa cholesteatoma and attendance at follow-up was high.

Author's Comments and Proposals

Clinical Research on Cartilage Tympanoplasty Is Needed

That the first paper comparing palisades with fascia appeared 40 years after the start of the cartilage palisade technique (Andersen et al. 2004) is astonishing and demonstrates how far behind the clinical research on cartilage palisade surgery is needed. There are many possibilities for good clinical research comparing, prospectively or retrospectively, the outcome of palisade technique with fascia or perichondrium on identical perforations and identical diseases with compatible tubal function. The variations and modifications of the palisade technique should also be compared.

If clinical studies show that palisades bring better results in ears with poor tubal function than does use of the fascia or the perichondrium, then preoperative tubal function testing should be carried out in all cases, and ears with poor tubal function or negative preoperative Valsalva test should be treated by cartilage tympanoplasty. In fact, our studies indicate that results are better in ears with poor tubal function when closed by palisades than when closed by fascia (Uzun et al. 2004; Tos et al. 2005).

If the hearing in comparable series with total perforation is the same after use of cartilage palisades as after use of fascia or perichondrium, then the indications for palisades can and should be extended.

Placement of the Palisades

Working with underlay cartilage palisade technique, I believe that it is not necessary to follow strictly the original methods of Heermann related to placement of the palisades.

Placement of the *simmering*, the most anterior palisade, under the anterior bony annulus seems not always to be necessary; this palisade can be placed inferiorly at the level of and close to the bony annulus. It will be in contact with the denuded anterior eardrum remnant and can be supported by Gelfoam. Inferoanterior postoperative retractions are very rare.

Placement of the architrave can also often be supported by Gelfoam, together with extensive scarification of the undersurface of the anterosuperior remnant of the eardrum.

Placement of inferior ends onto the bony annulus, as practiced by Heermann, definitively prevents retraction along the inferior bony annulus, but such retractions appear very seldom after surgery, presumably because of the depth of the hypotympanum. It is possible that such solid prevention of the retraction is not necessary and can even decrease the vibratility of the palisades. For these reason I prefer to place the inferior ends at the level of the bony annulus, but close to the annulus with the support of Gelfoam balls (see **Figs. 4.5h, 4.6e, 4.7h, 4.10c, 4.14e**).

A further problem might be that the full thickness of the palisades when placed onto the bony annulus occupies too much space in the inferior tympanomeatal angle. Drilling a groove, as performed by Wiegand (1978) may be a solution (see **Fig. 4.24**).

Gelfoam in the Tympanic Cavity or Not?

Many surgeons, especially in the United States, influenced by the House Clinic, use Gelfoam in the tympanic cavity to support a graft; many other ear surgeons, especially in Germany, influenced by the Plester school, never place Gelfoam into the tympanic cavity. I have not found any convincing studies against placement of gel foam in the tympanic cavity and have during the 40 years used Gelfoam in the tympanic cavity when needed to support fascia, and cartilage palisades and have in my many studies on postoperative results not found any evidence that surgical failures were caused by Gelfoam.

Small On-lay Perichondrium Grafts

It is always a good idea to harvest the cartilage with the perichondrium attached on both sides and remove it from the convex side for possible use as a reserve to be placed as small on-lay grafts either just before or after replacing the tympanomeatal flap. Relevant situations include:
- A larger distance between two palisades than can be covered by small pieces of perichondrium.
- Dehiscence of an end of the palisade
- Too short a palisade, creating a small perforation.

When performing ossiculoplasty with autogenous incus, small palisades cover parts of the incus, supported by small pieces of perichondrium.

Why Not Perichondrium Covering on Both Sides of the Palisade?

The immediate advantage of the perichondrium should be to support a contact with the perichondrium of neighboring palisades and, via tissue fluid, to close the space between the two palisades, before the epithelium has reached this space. Later the perichondrium plays a role in nutrition of the cartilage and stabilization of the palisade to the surroundings. Covering of the palisade by the mucous membrane will also be facilitated.

A disadvantage can be the adherence of the perichondrium of a retracted palisade to the medial wall of the tympanic cavity. However, retraction of the palisades down to the bottom of the tympanic cavity occurs extremely rarely and the anatomical results are usually good in the papers cited and discussed above.

I tend to believe that eventual improvement and maintenance of the nutrition of the palisade may be more important in the long term than possible retraction and do not stipulate that perichondrium on the inner side of the palisade should be avoided.

The covering of the palisades on both sides will in my opinion do more good than harm.

References

Amedee RG, Mann WJ, Riechelmann H. Cartilage palisade tympanoplasty. Am J Otol 1989;10:447–450.

Andersen J, Caye-Thomasen P, TosM. Cartilage palisade tympanoplasty in sinus and tensa retraction cholesteatoma. Otol Neurotol 2002;23:825–831.

Andersen J, Caye-Thomasen P, Tos M. A comparison of cartilage palisades and fascia in tympanoplasty after surgery for sinus or tensa retraction cholesteatoma in children. Otol Neurotol 2004;25:856–863.

Cayé-Thomasen P, Andersen J, Usum J, Hansen S, Tos M. 10-year results of cartilage palisades versus fascia in eardrum reconstruction after surgery for sinus or tensa retraction cholesteatoma in children. Laryngoscope 2009; 119(5):944–952.

Ferekidis EA, Nikolopoulos TP, Kandiloros DC, . Chondrotympanoplasty: a modified technique of cartilage graft tympanoplasty. Med Sci Monit 2003;9:73–78.

Heermann J. Entwicklung von der Haut-zur Faszien-und zur Knorpeltympanoplastik (Epitympanon-Antrum-Mastoidplastik). Z Laryngol Rhinol 1977;56:267–270.

Heermann J. Auricular cartilage palisade tympano-epitympano-antrum- and mastoid- plasty. Clin Otolaryngol 1978;3:443–446.

Heermann J. Thirty years autograft tragal and conchal cartilage perichondrium palisade tympanum, epitympanum, antrum and mastoid plasties: 13,000 cases. In: Charachon R Garcia-Ibanez E. eds. Long Term Results and Indications in Otology and Otoneurology. Amsterdam: Kugler Publications; 1991:159–164..

Heermann J. Autograft tragal and conchal palisade cartilage and perichondrium in tympanomastoid reconstruction. Ear Nose Throat J 1992;71:344–349.

Heermann J, Heermann H. Sieben Jahre Faszien – Knorpel- Dachschindel –Tympanoplastik und Antrum-Mastoidplastik. Z Laryngol Rhinol Otol 1967;46:370–382.

Heermann J, Heermann H, Kopfstein E. Fascia and cartilage palisade tympanoplasty. Nine years' experience. Arch Otolaryngol 1970; 91:228–241.

Helms J. Results after surgery of atelectated ears with palisade cartilage. In: Sade J, ed. The Eustachian Tube and Middle Ear Diseases: Clinical Aspects. Amsterdam: Kugler Publications; 1991; 329–330..

Helms J. Moderne Aspekte der Tympanoplastik. Eine Ôbersicht. Laryngorhinootologie 1995;74:465–467.

Hildmann H, Luckhaupt H, Schmelzer A. Using cartilage in middle ear surgery. HNO 1996;44:597–602.

Lau T, Tos M. Long- term results of surgery for chronic granulating otitis. Am J Otolaryngol 1986;7:341–345.

Lau T, Tos M. Cholesteatoma in children: recurrence related to the observation period. Am J Otolaryngol 1987;8:364–375.

Lau T, Tos M. Treatment of sinus cholesteatoma. Arch Otolaryngol Head Neck Surg 1988;114:1428–1434.

Lau T, Tos M. Tensa retraction cholesteatoma: treatment and long term results. J Laryngol Otol 1989;103:149–157.

Milewski C. Fascia or perichondrium/cartilage in tympanoplasties. A comparative study regarding hearing results and recurrence of perforations in 1529 cases. In: Tos M, Thomsen C, Peitersen E, eds. Cholesteatoma and Mastoid Surgery. Amsterdam: Kugler & Ghedini Publications; 1989:1201–1204..

Milewski C. Ergebnisse der Tympanoplastik nach Verwendung von Knorpel-Perichondriumtransplantaten zum Trommelfellersatz unter ungünstigen Bedingungen. Laryngorhinootologie 1991; 70:402–404.

Milewski C. Composite graft tympanoplasty in the treatment of ears with advanced middle ear pathology. Laryngoscope 1993; 103:1352–1356.

Neumann A, Jahnke K. Trommelfellrekonstruktion mit Knorpel. Indikationen, Techniken und Ergebnisse. HNO 2005;53:573–586.

Neumann A, Schultz-Coulon H-J, Jahnke K. Type 3 tympanoplasty applying the palisade cartilage technique: a study of 61 cases. Otol Neurotol 2003;24:33–37.

Ozbek C, Ciftci O, Tuna EE, Yazkan O, Ozden C. A comparison of cartilage palisades and fascia in type 1 tympanoplasty in children: anatomic and functional results. Otol Neurotol 2008;29:679–683.

Péré P. [Experiences with the palisade technic of tympanoplasty] [Article in German] Laryngorhinootologie 1989;68:569–570.

Suzuki JI. Complications of ear surgery, immediate and delayed. In: Alberty PW, Ruben RJ, eds. Otologic Medicine and Surgery. Vol. 2. Edinburgh: Churchill Livingstone; 1988:1363–1387..

Tos M. Bony fixation of the malleus and incus. Acta Otolaryngol 1970;70:95–104.

Tos M. Results of tympanoplasty with modified radical mastoidectomy. Acta Otolaryngol 1971;74:61–65.

Tos M. Tympanoplasty in chronic adhesive otitis media. Acta Otolaryngol 1972a;73:53–60.

Tos M. Assessment of the results of tympanoplasty. J Laryngol Otol 1972b;5:487–500.

Tos M. Late results in tympanoplasty. Arch Otolaryngol 1974a;100:302–305.

Tos M. Tympanoplasty for bony ossicular fixation. Arch Otolaryngol 1974b;99:422–427.

Tos M, Lau T, Arndal H, Plate S. Tympanosclerosis of the middle ear: Late results of surgical treatment. J Laryngol Otol 1990; 104:685–689.

Tos M, Uzun C, Caye-Thomasen P. Andersen J. Tympanometry after tympanoplasty with cartilage palisades or fascia after surgery for tensa cholesteatoma in children. In: Lim DJ, Bluestone CD, Casselbrant M, eds. Recent Advances in Otitis Media. Fort Lauderdale FL: Decker; 2005:321–322..

Tringali S, Dubreuil C, Bordure P. [Tympanic membrane perforation and tympanoplasty] [Article in French] Ann Otolaryngol Chir Cervicofac 2008;125(5):261–272.

Utech H. Über diagnostische und therapeutische Möglichkeiten der Tympanotomie bei Schalleitungsstørungen. Z Laryngol Rhinol Otol 1959;38:212–221.

Utech H. Endhörergebnisse bei der Tympanoplastik durch Veränderungen bei der Operationstechnik. Z Laryngol Rhinol Otol 1960;39:367–371.

Uzun C, Cayé-Thomasen P, Andersen J, Tos M. A tympanometric comparison of tympanoplasty with cartilage palisades or fascia after surgery for tensa cholesteatoma in children. Laryngoscope 2003;113:1751–1757.

Uzun C, Cayé-Thomasen P, Andersen J, Tos M. Eustachian tube function in tympanoplasty with cartilage palisades or fascia after cholesteatoma surgery. Otol Neurotol 2004;25:864–872.

Velepic M, Bonifacic M, Manestar D, Velepic M, Bonifacic D. Cartilage palisade tympanoplasty and diving. Otol Neurotol 2001; 22:430–432.

Wiegand H. Knorpelpalisaden und doppelschichtiges Transplantat als Trommelfellersatz. HNO 1978;26:233–236.

Wielgosz R, Mroczkowski E. Assessment of the hearing results in tympanoplasties with the use of palisade-technique. [In Polish.] Otolaryngol Pol 2006;60(6):901–905.

Yu L, Han C, Yu H, Yu D. [Auricular cartilage palisade technique for repairing tympanic membrane perforation]. [In Chinese.] Zhonghua Er Bi Yan Hou Ke Za Zhi 2001;36(3):166–168.

Yung M. Cartilage tympanoplasty: literature review. J Laryngol Otol 2008;122:663–672.

5 Cartilage Palisades in On-lay Tympanoplasty Techniques

Definitions

The original Heermann cartilage palisade technique was, and still is, exclusively an underlay technique (Heermann and Heermann 1967; Heermann et al. 1970; Heermann 1977).

On-lay technique is defined as placement of the graft (fascia, perichondrium, or cartilage) onto the denuded lamina propria of the eardrum and onto the fibrous annulus. A belt of squamous epithelium around the perforation is (1) totally removed, or (2) partly removed, partly elevated (see **Figs. 5.6b, 5.9c, 5.14a**), or (3) totally elevated (see **Figs. 5.5c, 5.7b, 5.11a, 5.16a**). Details of elevation and removal of the epithelium in on-lay tympanoplasty are described in MMES_1, Figs. 363–403 and 431–532.

There are currently no publications in the literature on on-lay cartilage tympanoplasty. I have elaborated and performed the methods presented in this chapter in recent years.

Full-Thickness Palisades

Full-thickness palisades covered with perichondrium on the ear canal side and of the shape as used in underlay technique can be used in on-lay technique, especially in total perforation, atelectasis, and ears with poor tubal function.

Several innovations in on-lay cartilage palisade tympanoplasties are presented below.

Half-Thickness Palisades and Perichondrium Flaps

In small perforations, such as anterior and inferior perforation, placement of full-thickness cartilage palisades onto the denuded lamina propria will considerably enlarge the thickness of the eardrum and elevate the eardrum at the site of the previous perforation. Use of thinner cartilage and placement of the cartilage at the level of the lamina propria, with some protrusion of the cartilage into the tympanic cavity, will diminish the outer thickness of the eardrum.

Half-thickness palisades will be thick enough to safely cover small perforations (**Fig. 5.1a**). The palisade is placed onto the lamina propria.

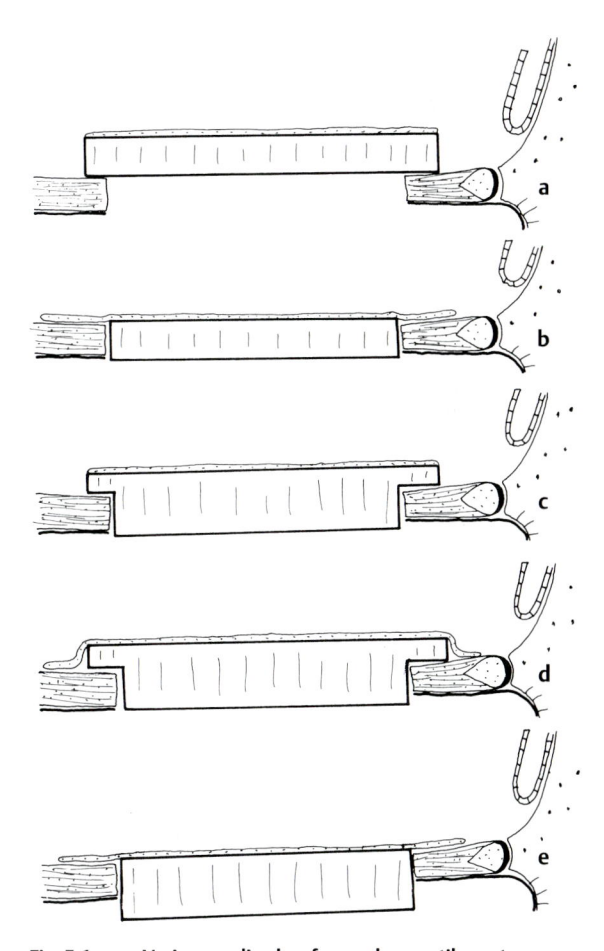

Fig. 5.1a–e Various palisades for on-lay cartilage tympanoplasty.
a   Half-thickness palisade placed on the denuded lamina propria. Epithelium is elevated and will be replaced.
b   Half-thickness palisade with small perichondrium flaps placed onto the lamina propria. The cartilage is placed at the level of the lamina propria.
c   Full-thickness cartilage palisade thinned at the two ends to accommodate the lamina propria and to diminish the outer part of the palisade.
d   The same graft as in **c**, but with perichondrium flaps positioned onto the lamina propria.
e   Full-thickness palisade with perichondrium flaps placed onto the lamina propria. Half of the cartilage palisade is placed at the level of the lamina propria, the remaining part protrudes into the tympanic cavity.

A perichondrium flap at the two ends of half-thickness and full-thickness palisades (**Fig. 5.1b, e**) allows placement of the palisade at the level of the lamina propria. The palisade is suspended from the lamina propria by the perichondrium flap, with good vibratility. Placement of the cartilage into the perforation is partly similar to the on-lay–in-lay composite graft described in Chapter 23.

Shaping the ends of full-thickness palisades to accommodate the lamina propria (**Fig. 5.1c, d**). Half of the palisade thickness rests on the lamina propria, the other half is at the level of the lamina propria.

Harvesting and Shaping of the Palisades

Harvesting of the Palisades

The palisades used in on-lay cartilage tympanoplasty are most often harvested from tragal or conchal cartilage.

Tragal cartilage is used in transcanal approach or endaural approach. When using cartilage palisades to close a total perforation, a 10 m × 10 mm large piece of cartilage, covered on both sides with perichondrium, is sufficient. For anterior and inferior perforation, the area of the cartilage can be smaller.

For cosmetic reasons, the incision is made 2 mm medial to the tragal dome in one sweep through the skin, cartilage, and perichondrium, as illustrated in **Fig. 3.21**. The extraperichondrial tissue is elevated on both sides of the tragus, and the tragus is first cut along the superior and then along the inferior border. Finally, the cartilage is pulled outward with surgical forceps and cut along the medial border.

When using the endaural approach with the intercartilaginous incision, the tragal cartilage is removed through this incision (see **Fig. 3.23**). The superior border of the tragus is identified and saved. A horizontal incision is made 2 mm medial to the bone and the cartilage is pulled in the superior direction, allowing an inferior incision. After the medial incision, the cartilage is removed.

Conchal cartilage will be harvested in retroauricular approach, by exposing the eminence of the concha, cleaning the posterior perichondrium, and making a round incision with a diameter of 10 mm through the posterior perichondrium, cartilage, and the anterior perichondrium (see **Fig. 20.5a, b**).

Scaphal cartilage, harvested from the eminence of the scapha, on the posterior aspect of the auricle, between the helix and the antihelix, has been used by me for on-lay cartilage tympanoplasty. In a 2 cm long incision, a 5 mm wide oval piece of cartilage with the perichondrium is removed (see **Fig. 3.27**). Several palisades of various sizes can be cut in oblique directions. Scaphal cartilage used for minor perforations can easily be harvested from the eminence of the scapha (see **Fig. 3.28**).

Shaping of the Palisades

For on-lay technique in closure of anterior and inferior perforations, the palisades may be thinner than the full thickness of the tragal and conchal cartilage. A reduction of the thickness by a third or a half of the original thickness of the cartilage does not cause a weakness of the short palisades but makes the placement easier and presumably the epithelialization faster.

Reduction of the thickness of the entire harvested piece of the tragal or conchal cartilage is done after removal of the perichondrium from the convex side.

Thinning of the cartilage. Using the Hildmann cartilage clamp (see **Fig. 3.35a**), a large piece of cartilage can be held and the cartilage can be sliced with a scalpel from above into two pieces. More accurate slicing of the large piece of cartilage is achieved using Kurz Precise Cartilage Knife (see **Fig. 3.36a–d**). A small piece of cartilage with a diameter of 5 mm can be thinned by holding the cartilage with two fingers (see **Fig. 3.34a**) or with surgical forceps (see **Fig. 3.34c**) and slicing with a scalpel or a razor blade.

Thinning and shaping of the ends of the palisades. The thickness of the palisades may be reduced at their ends, either on one end only or on both ends (**Fig. 5.2a–c**). A 1 mm deep horizontal incision is made at each end of the cartilage palisade (**Fig. 5.2a**). The palisade is turned so that the perichondrium is at the bottom, contacting the table, and a 1 mm wide piece of cartilage is cut off (**Fig. 5.2b, c**). The adaptation of a thinned palisade to the eardrum remnant or the fibrous annulus is easier than that of a thick palisade.

Trimming of the perichondrium flaps. In total perforation, a large piece of cartilage with the perichondrium on the convex side is required. Along the superior and inferior borders, two 1–1.5 mm belts of cartilage are removed leav-

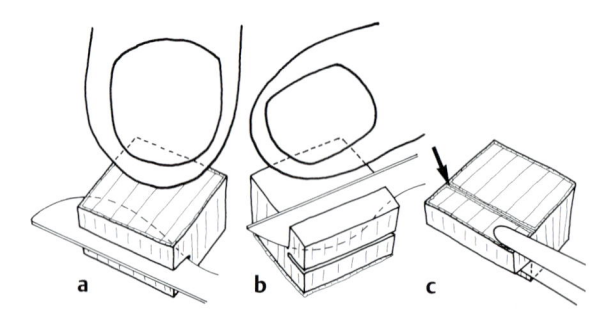

Fig. 5.2a–c Shaping the end of a full-thickness palisade.
a Using a 23-blade scalpel, a 1 mm long horizontal cut is made at half-thickness level of the palisade.
b The palisade is turned so that the perichondrium is facing the table. The knife cuts off a rectangular piece of the cartilage.
c The shaping of one end of the palisade is completed and the small rectangular piece of cartilage is removed. The thinned end of the palisade is placed onto the denuded edge of the lamina propria. To prevent curling of the thinned end of the palisade, the perichondrium is incised (arrow).

ing the perichondrium intact. A round knife or a scalpel cuts the palisades longitudinally (**Fig. 5.3**).

The perichondrium is elevated from individual palisades together with the shaping of the ends (**Fig. 5.4a–c**).

Curling of the Cartilage Grafts

The procedure denoted by the term "curling" is difficult to describe: it is an outward turning of the thin cartilage when covered with the perichondrium. The best demonstration of its existence is the in-lay butterfly cartilage tympanoplasty of Eavey (1998), described in Chapter 25. On cutting a round piece of cartilage parallel to the perichondrium (see **Fig. 25.5**), the cartilage will curl outward on both sides. The curling is caused by the attached perichondrium on each side. However, very little is known about curling and no studies on curling of cartilage have been published.

When cutting the full-thickness tragal or conchal cartilage graft covered on one side with the perichondrium to a half-thickness graft, there is some small peripheral elevation of the graft. This does not seem to cause any disturbance when it is placed onto the eardrum. To prevent the curling, a circumferential incision of the perichondrium 1 mm central to the border is made. In palisades thinned at their ends, an incision of the perichondrium can be made (see **Fig. 5.2b**). The perichondrium of half-thickness palisades is cut at the superior and inferior ends of the palisades (as demonstrated in **Fig. 5.2c**).

Thinning of the cartilage grafts with the perichondrium is a relatively new procedure and there is little experience with curling.

Indications for On-lay Palisade Technique

Indications for on-lay technique are the same as in underlay techniques. These are reoperations, cholesteatoma in adults and children, retractions, adhesive otitis media, thick and secretory middle ear mucosa, ears with poor tubal function, and ears with negative Valsalva maneuver.

Surgical Techniques with On-lay Placement of Palisades

Posterior perforation is best treated in underlay technique with elevation of the tympanomeatal flaps together with the fibrous annulus. Anterior perforation is in my opinion best treated in on-lay technique with several good methods. Inferior, subtotal, and total perforations can equally be treated by underlay and on-lay techniques.

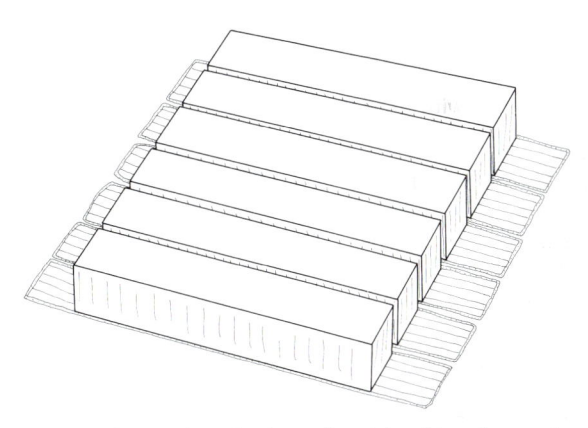

Fig. 5.3 Shaping the palisades with perichondrium flaps at the two ends. Along the superior and inferior parts of the rectangular piece of tragal cartilage two 1–1.5 mm belts of cartilage are removed, leaving perichondrium intact. In inferosuperior direction the palisades with the perichondrium flaps are cut using a 23-blade scalpel.

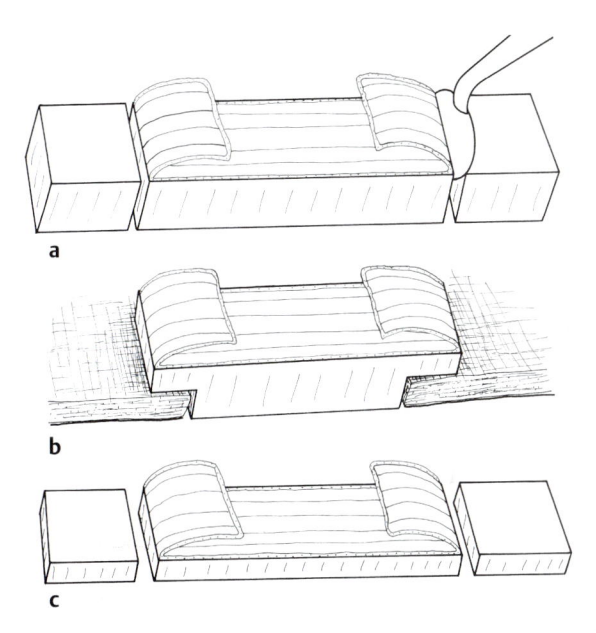

Fig. 5.4a–c Shaping the perichondrium flaps on the ends of the individual palisades.
a From the two ends of a full-thickness palisade, two 1–1.5 mm long perichondrium flaps are elevated and the denuded ends of the cartilage are cut off.
b The full-thickness palisade with the perichondrium flaps has been further shaped as shown in **Fig. 5.2**, and placed onto the denuded lamina propria.
c A half-thickness palisade with elevated perichondrium flaps.

Anterior Perforation

Technique with Small Epithelial Flaps

After excision of the keratinized epithelium from the edges of the perforation (see MMES_1, Figs. 356–362), the epithelium flap is elevated from the malleus handle, using either a sickle knife or an incudostapedial knife (**Fig. 5.5a**). Incision and elevation start on the malleus handle, continuing downward around the perforation and upward along the malleus handle (**Fig. 5.5b**). Anteriorly, close to the fibrous annulus, a small circumferential incision is made. The skin flap is cut at the 3-o'clock position, creating and elevating a larger superior and a smaller inferior skin flap (**Fig. 5.5b**). After completion of elevation and removal of keratinized epithelium (**Fig. 5.5c**) and measurement of the size of the perforation, using a 4 mm hook, the palisades are prepared. To cover an anterior perforation, three thin palisades are needed, each 1 mm wide and 5–6 mm long. The first palisade is placed onto and along the anterior part of the fibrous annulus using a double cup forceps. The first palisade may be stabilized by placing a small ball of Gelfoam. After covering the entire perforation with thin palisades, the posterior edge of the last palisade lies along the anterior edge of the malleus handle (**Fig. 5.5 d**). The epithelial flaps are replaced (**Fig. 5.5e**). The palisades are covered with Gelfoam balls and small pieces of gauze moistened with hydrocortisone–oxytetracycline ointment.

Technique with Partial Removal of the Epithelium

It is my impression that the removal of the epithelium around the edge of the perforation does not have to be so extensive when using cartilage palisade as when using the fascia or the perichondrium. The palisades can be placed piece by piece onto the denuded and cleaned lamina propria of the eardrum. Removal of the epithelium starts at the malleus handle (**Fig. 5.6a**). Using a sickle knife or the cup forceps, the epithelium is gradually removed. Superiorly, a skin flap and a small malleus flap are elevated (**Fig. 5.6b**). Three half-thickness palisades are placed onto the denuded epithelium (**Fig. 5.6c**) and the flaps are replaced (**Fig. 5.6 d**).

Technique with Elevation of a Large Anterior Skin Flap

A medial circumferential incision between the 1-o'clock and 5-o'clock positions is performed and a relatively large skin flap is elevated, down to the annulus (**Fig. 5.7a**). Elevation of the epithelium is continued forward to the anterior and inferior border of the perforation. The epithelium is further elevated along the posterior border of the perforation and the malleus handle (**Fig. 5.7b**). Three palisades are placed onto the edges of the perforation, first anteriorly and then posteriorly (**Fig. 5.7c**). The epithelium and the skin flap are replaced (**Fig. 5.7 d**). The epithelium is covered with Gelfoam balls and small pieces of gauze moistened with hydrocortisone–oxytetracycline ointment.

I have nearly always used on-lay technique to close an anterior perforation in minimally invasive transcanal surgery, without raising a posterior tympanomeatal flap. Hardly ever is the anterior perforation connected to cholesteatoma or does it have squamous epithelium in the medial side of the perforation. The take rate is higher in anterior perforation than with other perforations, with both fascia and perichondrium grafts. Tubal function is also better in anterior perforation than in other perforations. Therefore, results in on-lay cartilage palisade technique can hardly be expected to show significantly better results than achieved with the on-lay technique using fascia- or perichondrium grafts, or in any underlay technique.

Anterior Perforation and Bulged Ear Canal. On-lay Underlay Technique

In anterior perforation with limited view of the anterior annulus, the bony protrusion can be removed by drilling in an endaural or retroauricular approach or even in the transcanal approach. I have used a new minimally invasive on-lay-underlay technique in the transcanal approach, placing the palisades in the anteroposterior direction.

The edges of the perforation are cleaned, using a cup forceps and suction tip, ensuring that there is no squamous epithelium under the edge of the perforation. Epithelium inferior and superior to the perforation is elevated, creating small epithelial flaps (**Fig. 5.8a**). The epithelium in the anterior tympanomeatal angle is not touched. The undersurface of the anterior edge of the perforation is cleaned blindly by placing a round knife under the annulus and pulling the mucosa outward (**Fig. 5.8b**). This procedure is repeated in the inferior and superior parts of the annulus, removing all epithelium of the anterior edge of the perforation (**Fig. 5.8c**). Using a cup forceps, the palisades are pushed in the anterior direction under the anterior fibrous annulus (**Fig. 5.8 d**). The posterior ends are placed onto the denuded lamina propria of the posterior end of the perforation (**Fig. 5.8e**) and the epithelial flaps are replaced (**Fig. 5.8 f**). A thin Silastic foil covers the anterior tympanomeatal angle and the eardrum (**Fig. 5.8 g**).

If the anterior tympanomeatal angle is too small, the skin is elevated outward and part of the anterior bone is removed using a diamond drill.

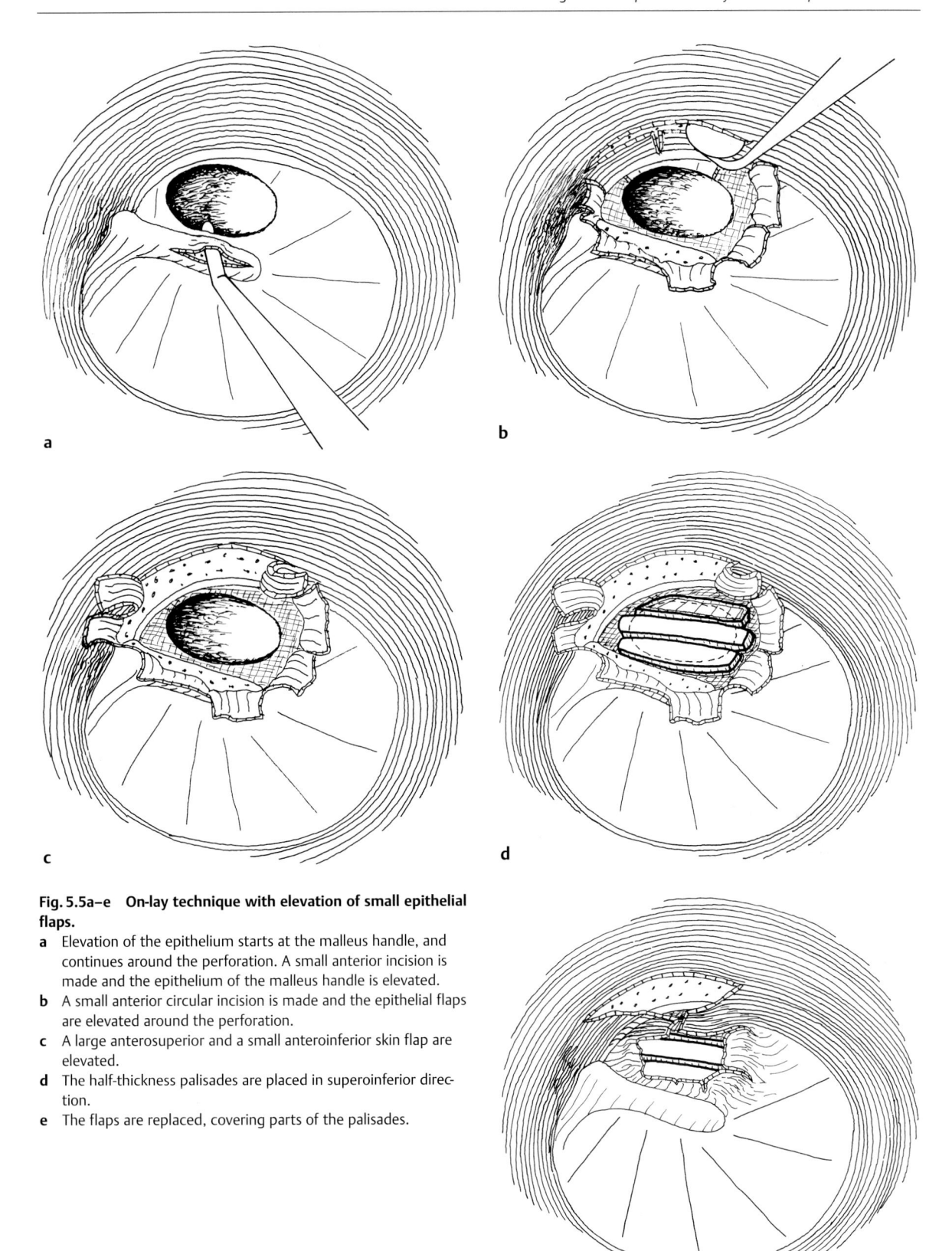

Fig. 5.5a–e On-lay technique with elevation of small epithelial flaps.
a Elevation of the epithelium starts at the malleus handle, and continues around the perforation. A small anterior incision is made and the epithelium of the malleus handle is elevated.
b A small anterior circular incision is made and the epithelial flaps are elevated around the perforation.
c A large anterosuperior and a small anteroinferior skin flap are elevated.
d The half-thickness palisades are placed in superoinferior direction.
e The flaps are replaced, covering parts of the palisades.

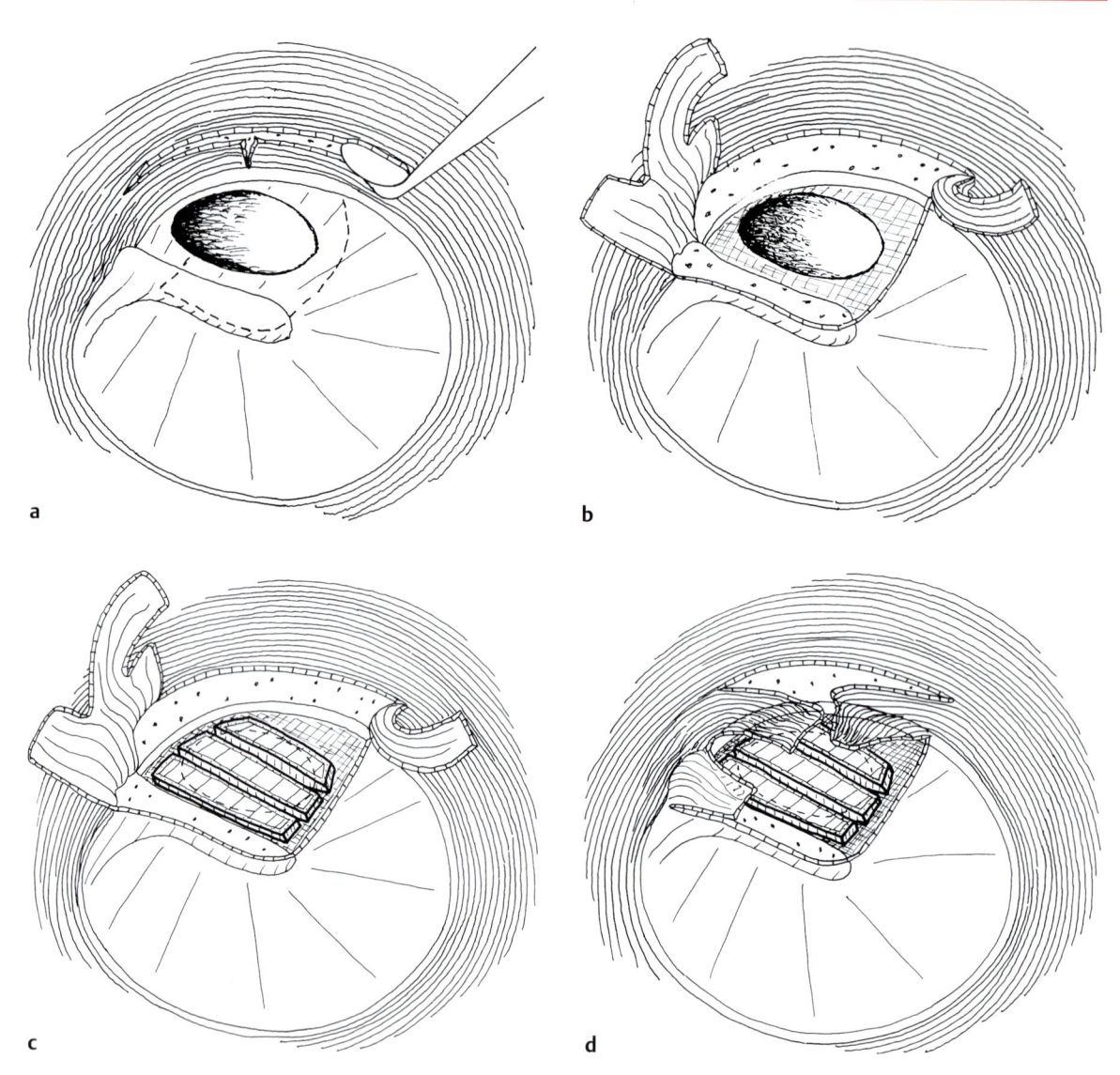

Fig. 5.6a–d Technique with partial removal of the epithelium.
a An anterior circumferential incision is performed. Epithelium will be removed within the dotted line.
b A small superior malleus flap and a small anterosuperior skin flap are elevated and the epithelium around the perforation is removed.
c Half-thickness cartilage palisades are placed onto the cleaned edges of the perforation.
d The flaps are replaced.

Inferior Perforation

Inferior perforation is, in my opinion, very suitable for the on-lay cartilage tympanoplasty in transcanal approach. Because the palisades can be placed accurately onto the deepithelialized edges of the perforation, the removal of the epithelium does not need to be as extensive in palisade techniques as in on-lay techniques using fascia or perichondrium.

Four methods will be illustrated here in a large inferior perforation:

- Partial elevation of superior epithelial flaps
- Elevation of a large tympanomeatal flap together with the epithelium surrounding the perforation
- Outward elevation of the epithelium and skin
- Palisades with perichondrium flaps on both ends

To safely close an inferior perforation, half-thickness palisades can be used. To prevent curling of the cartilage, small incisions of the perichondrium can be made at the ends of palisades.

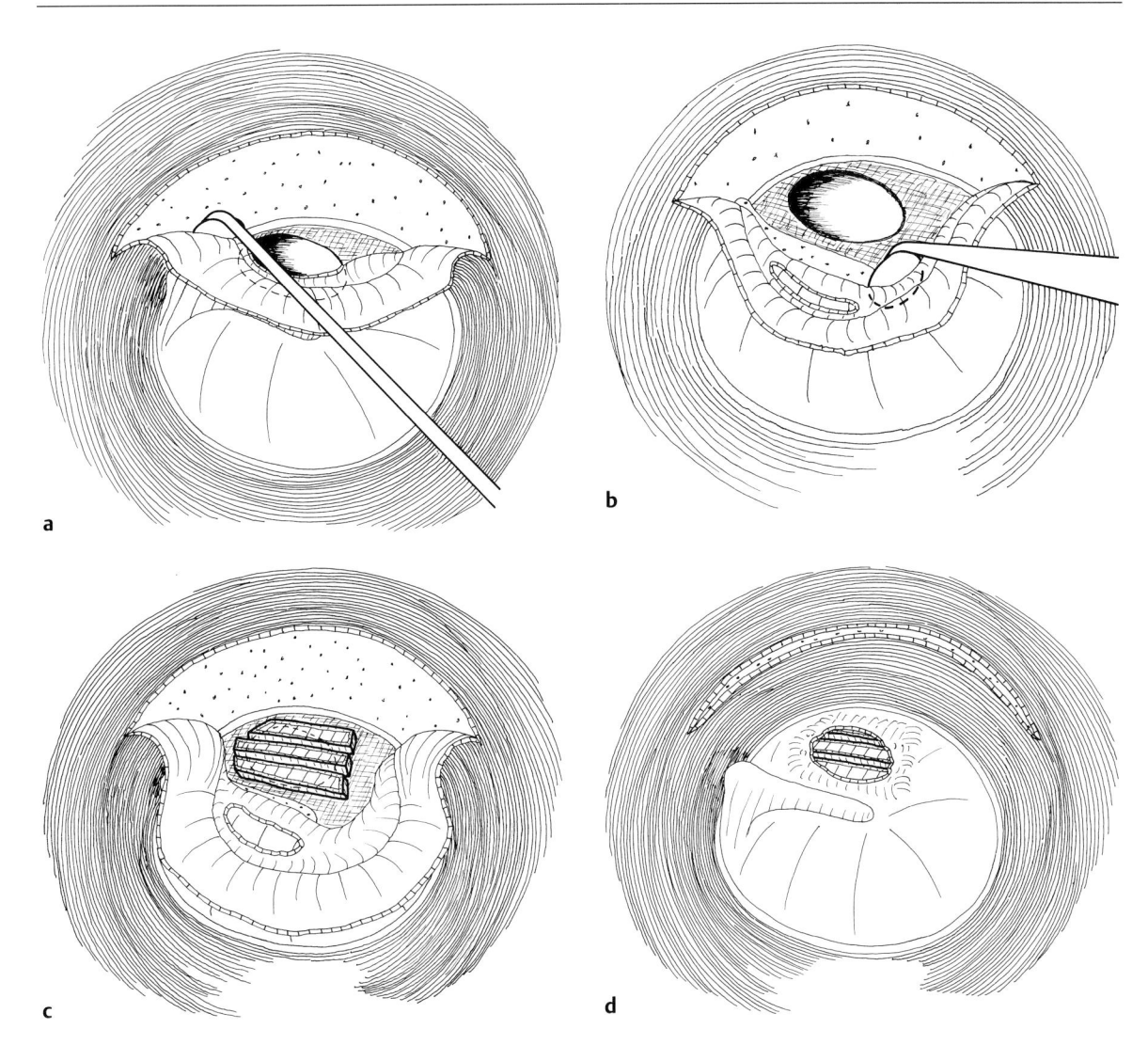

Fig. 5.7a–d Technique with elevation of a large anterior skin flap.
a The ear canal skin flap and the eardrum epithelium at the anterior border of the perforation are elevated.
b The epithelium surrounding the perforation are elevated.
c Three half-thickness palisades are placed onto the denuded edges of the lamina propria.
d The epithelial flaps and the ear canal skin flap are replaced,

Partial Elevation of Superior Epithelial Flaps

A circumferential incision is made at the 3-o'clock to 9-o'clock position, close to the fibrous annulus. The annulus and the edge of the perforation are cleaned of any epithelium (**Fig. 5.9a**). Posterosuperiorly, the epithelium of the eardrum is elevated by placing an incudostapedial knife under the epithelium and by carefully moving the knife toward the edges of the perforation (**Fig. 5.9b**) and toward the malleus handle. (**Fig. 5.9c**) After further elevation, all flaps are elevated and the anterior half-thickness palisades are placed onto the denuded edges of the perforation (**Fig. 5.9 d**). After placement of the posterior palisades (**Fig. 5.9e**), the epithelial flaps are replaced (**Fig. 5.9 f**).

I prefer the described method of partial elevation of the epithelial flaps in most large and small inferior perforations.

Elevation of a Large Tympanomeatal Flap together with the Epithelium Surrounding the Perforation

A circumferential incision between the 9-o'clock and 3-o'clock positions is made about 5 mm lateral to the annulus and a large tympanomeatal flap is elevated together with the epithelium surrounding the large inferior perforation. This elevation can be difficult in some cases around the umbo. Half-thickness palisades are placed in superoinferior direction (**Fig. 5.10a**) and the tympanomeatal flaps are replaced (**Fig. 5.10b**).

Palisades can be placed in a posteroanterior position as well (**Fig. 5.11a, b**)

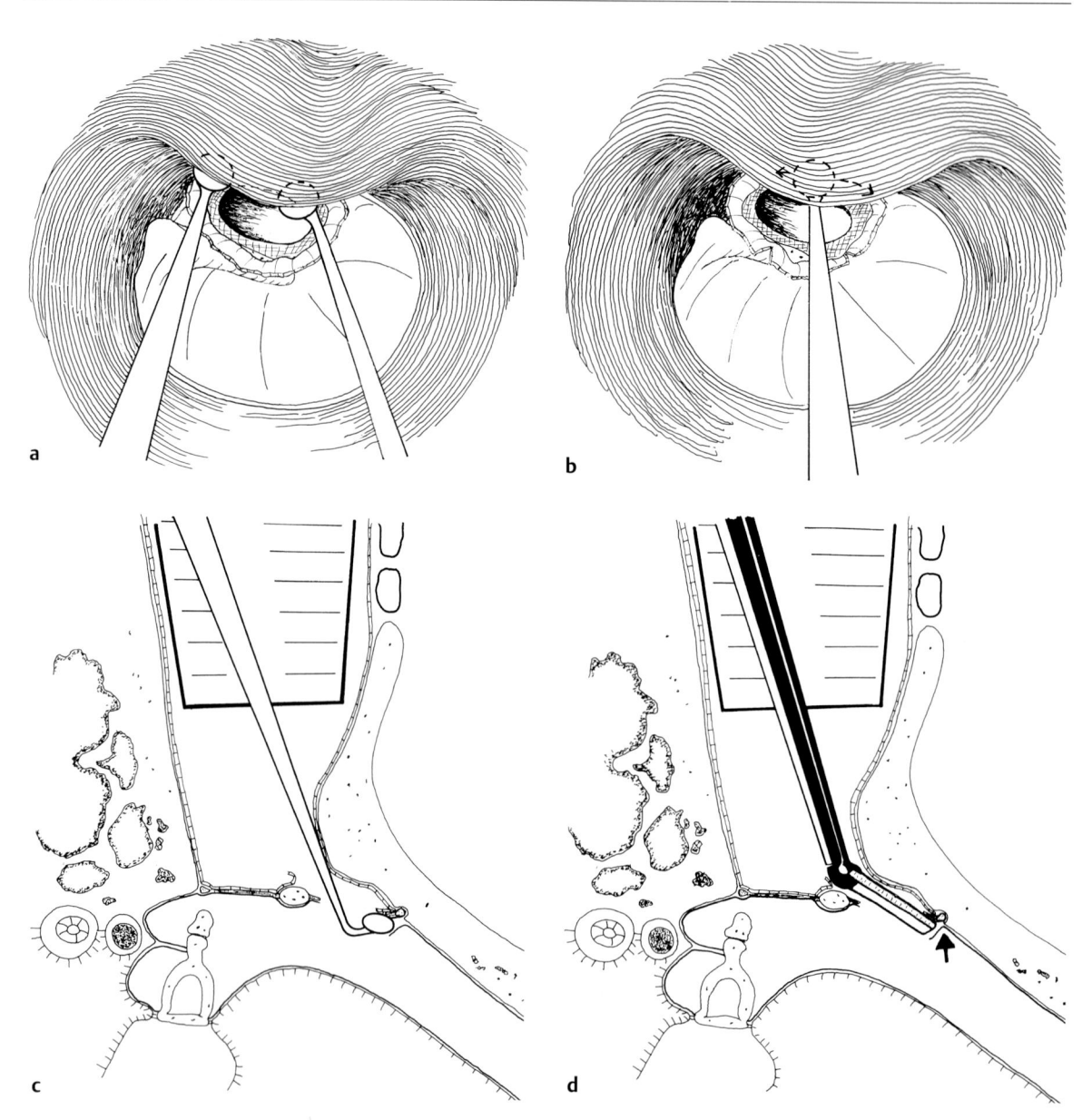

Fig. 5.8a–g On-lay and underlay technique in the anterior perforation with bulged anterior ear canal wall.

a First the ear drum epithelium from the inferior and superior parts of the perforation is elevated, creating small flaps. Then the epithelium of the anterior edge of the perforation is elevated, by placing a round knife in the cleavage plane between the lamina propria and the epithelium.

b Cleaning the undersurface of the anterior edge of the perforation with a round knife.

c Side view of the bulged anterior ear canal wall and the perforation. Anteroposterior manipulation with a round knife elevates or cleans the mucosa and epithelial remnants.

d Using a cup forceps, a palisade is pushed in the posteroanterior direction under the anterior fibrous annulus (arrow) and onto the eardrum remnant, close to the malleus handle.

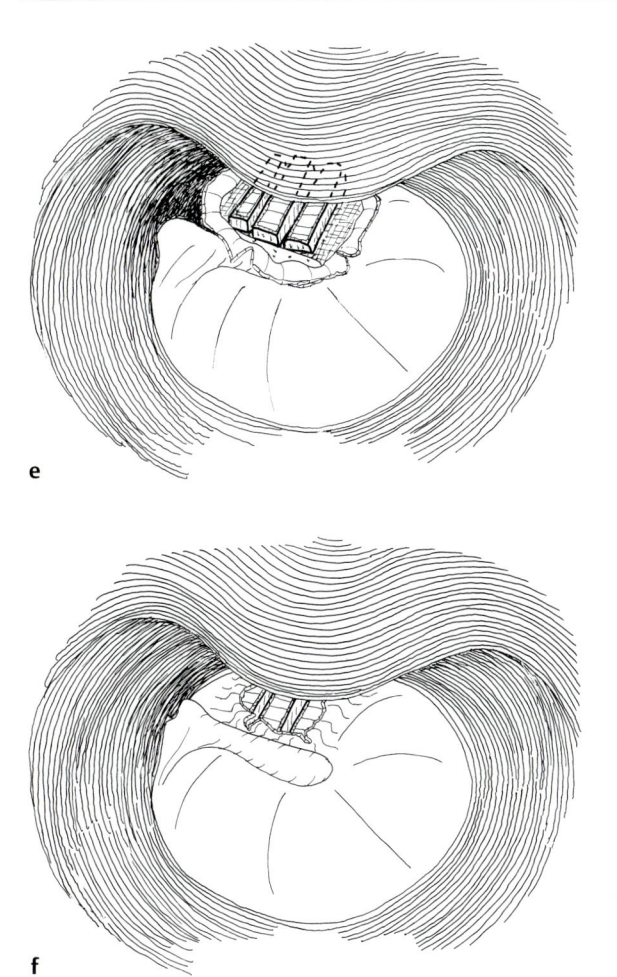

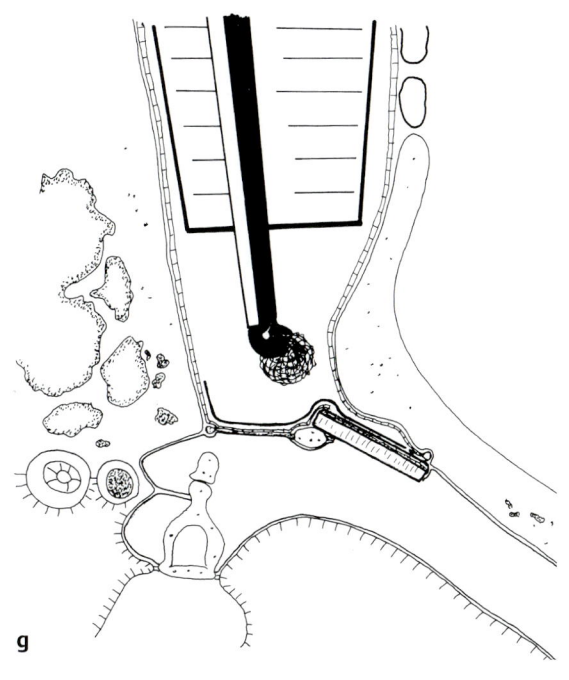

Fig. 5.8e–g
e Three half-thickness palisades are placed in posteroanterior direction. The anterior ends lie under the anterior annulus; the posterior ends, on the remnant of the eardrum.
f The epithelial flaps are replaced and cover the posterior ends of the palisades.
g Side view of the final situation. A thin Silastic foil is placed in the anterior tympanomeatal angle and on the eardrum. Small Gelfoam balls are placed on the posterior ends of the palisades. Finally, balls and strips of gaze moistened with hydrocortisone–oxytetracycline ointment will be placed in the ear canal.

Outward Elevation of the Epithelium and Skin

After three radial incisions of the epithelium around the perforation, the epithelial flaps are gradually elevated, first superiorly, then inferoposteriorly (**Fig. 5.12a**) and inferoanteriorly. After completion of elevation of the flaps, cartilage palisades are placed onto the edges of the perforation (**Fig. 5.12b**) and the epithelium flaps are replaced (**Fig. 5.12c**).

Again it is evident that elevation of the skin is less extensive with cartilage palisades than with fascia or perichondrium.

Palisades with Perichondrium Flaps on Both Ends

In a similar inferior perforation, full-thickness palisades with small perichondrium flaps at the ends can be placed, fixing the palisades to the lamina propria and promoting rapid epithelialization (**Fig. 5.13a**). The perichondrium flaps close the fissures between the ends of the palisades and guide the epithelialization after replacement of the epithelial flaps (**Fig. 5.13b**).

Total Perforation

There are three on-lay techniques wherein cartilage palisades can be used to close a total or subtotal eardrum perforation:
- On-lay technique with elevation of three superior epithelial flaps (as I prefer).
- On-lay technique with elevation of a large tympanomeatal skin flap and epithelial flaps.
- Technique with outward elevation of the epithelium and the skin flaps (illustrated for inferior perforation in **Fig. 5.12a–c**). For total perforation, the outward skin elevation will be illustrated in Chapter 8.

On-lay Technique with Elevation of Three Superior Epithelial Flaps

The principle of this technique (Tos 1980) is to perform a circumferential incision, close to the annulus, starting posteriorly at the 11-o'clock position and 2 mm laterally to the fibrous annulus. The incision continues in inferior and anterior direction close to the fibrous annulus and ends

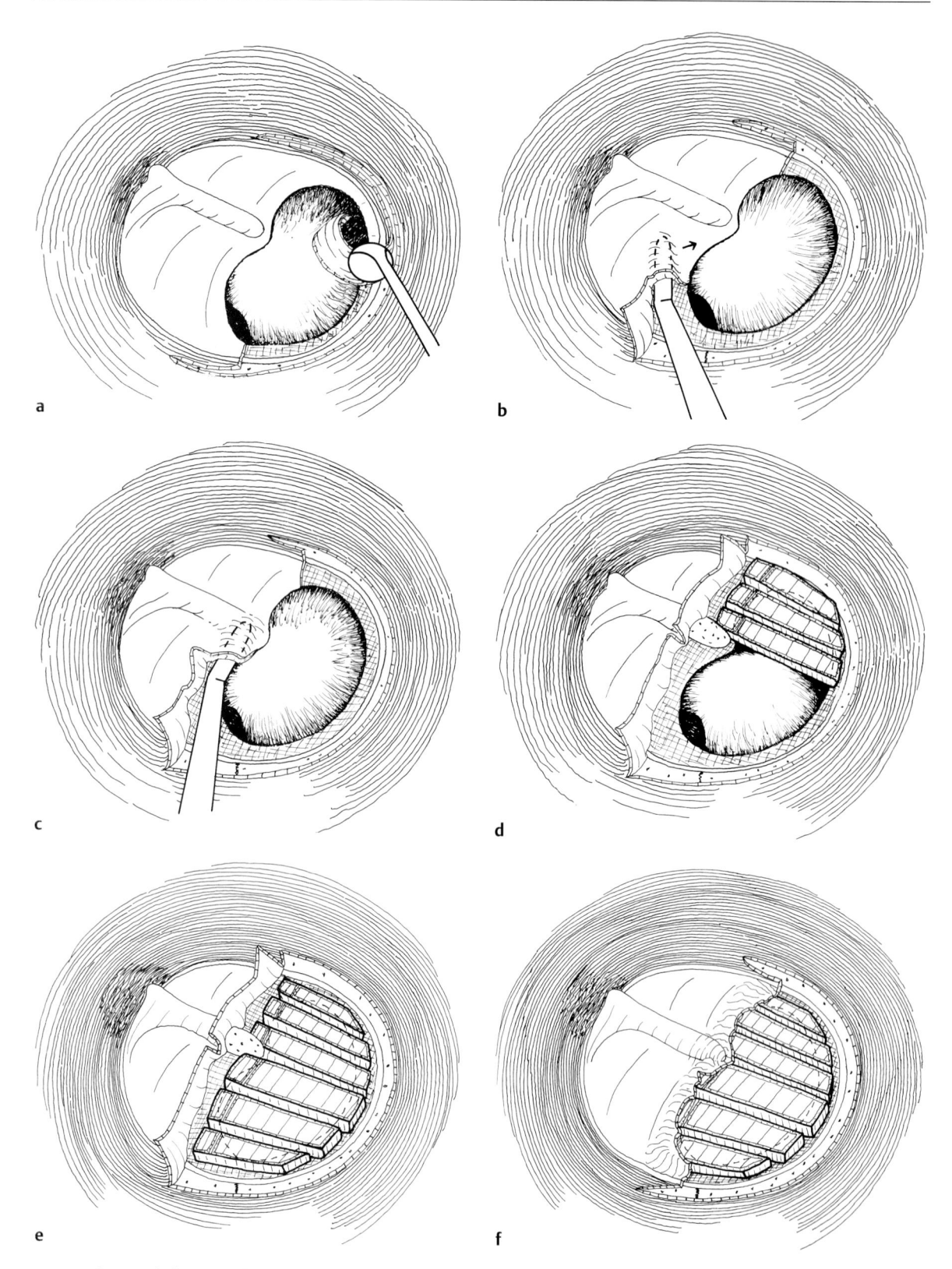

5 Cartilage Palisades in On-lay Tympanoplasty Techniques

Fig. 5.9a–f Partial elevation of the superior epithelial flaps in closure of inferior perforation.

a An inferior circumferential medial incision is made between the 9-o'clock and 3-o'clock positions. All epithelium from the inferior edge of the perforation and from the fibrous annulus is removed.
b A superior epithelial flap is elevated by placing the incudostapedial knife between the lamina propria tynd the epithelium. The knife is moved toward the edge of the perforation.
c Continuing elevation of the epithelium from the umbo by moving the incudostopedial knife downward to the end of the umbo.
d The superoanterior flap is elevated and the anterior half-thickness palisades are placed on the cleaned edge of the eardrum.
e All six palisades are placed and the perforation is closed. The perichondrium is cut to prevent curling before placement onto the eardrum.
f Epithelial flaps are replaced.

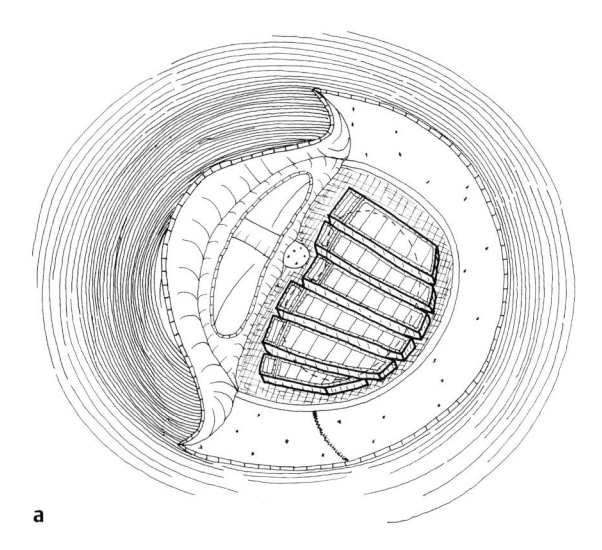

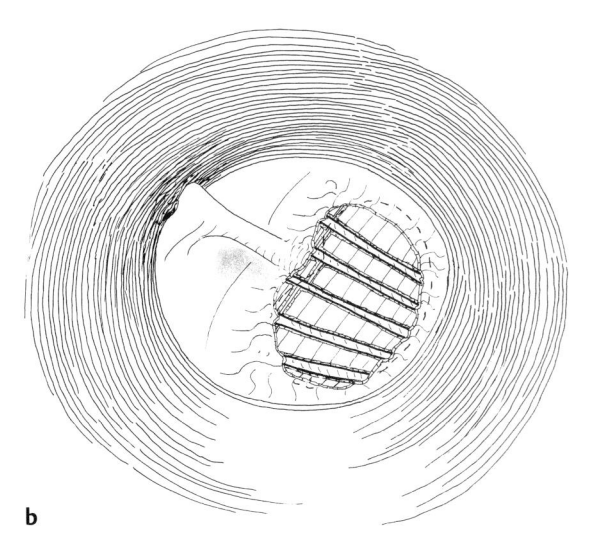

Fig. 5.10a, b Elevation of a large tympanomeatal flap and the epithelium surrounding an inferior perforation.
a After completing a circumferential incision, elevation of the flap and the epithelium is completed. Cartilage palisades are placed on the edges of the perforation in superoanterior position, closing the perforation.
b The flap is replaced and the epithelium covers part of the palisades.

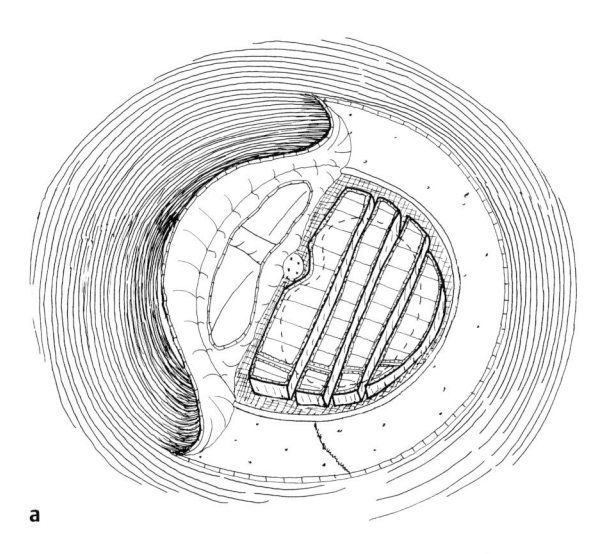

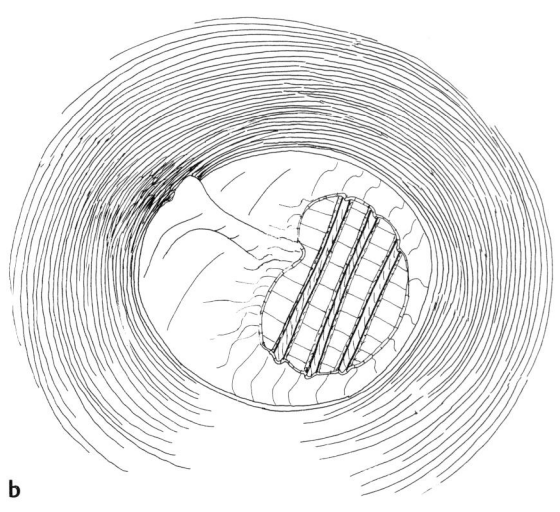

Fig. 5.11a, b The posteroanterior placement of half-thickness cartilage palisades in an inferior perforation.
a A small wedge is made to accommodate the umbo.
b The tympanomeatal and epithelial flaps are replaced.

anterosuperiorly at the 2-o'clock position, again 2 mm lateral to the annulus. Superiorly, a posterosuperior skin flap, a malleus flap, and an anterosuperior skin flap are elevated (**Fig. 5.14a**). The malleus handle is cleaned of the epithelium and so is the remnant of the eardrum surrounding the perforation. Full-thickness palisades are placed onto the eardrum remnant, covering the total perforation. A shorter palisade is placed onto the umbo (**Fig. 5.14b**). Finally, the three elevated superior epithelial flaps are replaced (**Fig. 5.14c**).

Thinned Palisades; Shaped and Thinned Ends of the Palisades

To place the inner half of the palisade at the level of the lamina propria, the ends of the palisade are shaped and thinned (see **Figs. 5.1, 5.2**). Such palisades lie with the thinned end onto the lamina propria (**Fig. 5.15a**). The ends of the palisade are half-thickness, the remaining palisade is of full thickness. The covering with epithelium is more effective (**Fig. 5.15b**) and the epithelialization is faster.

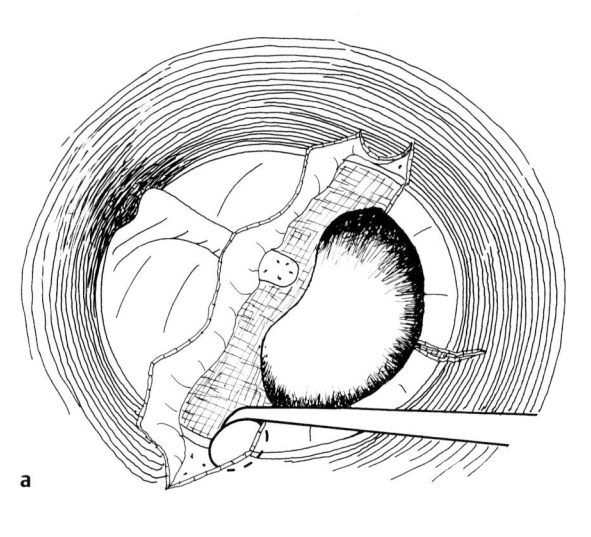

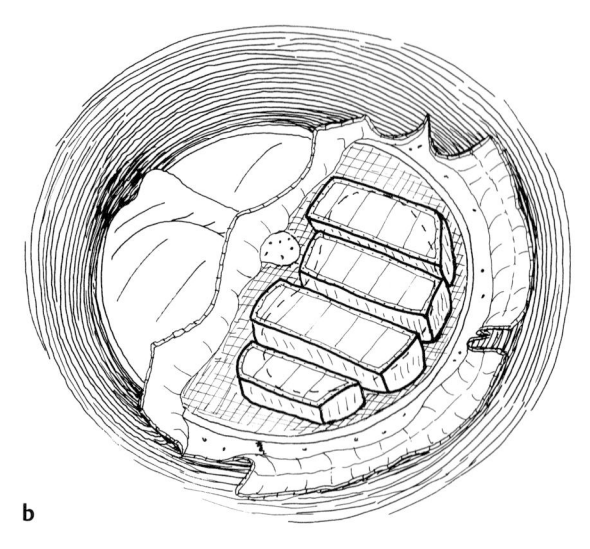

Fig. 5.12a–c Outward elevation of the epithelium in an inferior perforation.
a After three small radial incisions and elevation of the superior flaps, the posteroinferior epithelial flap is elevated.
b After elevation of the inferoanterior flap, four full-thickness cartilage palisades are placed onto the border of the perforation.
c The epithelial flaps are replaced.

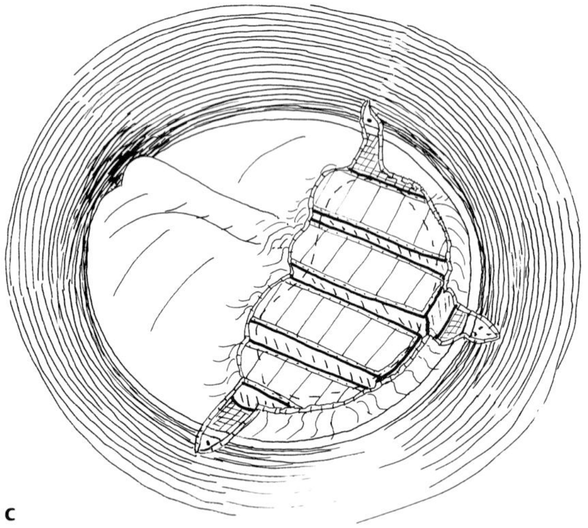

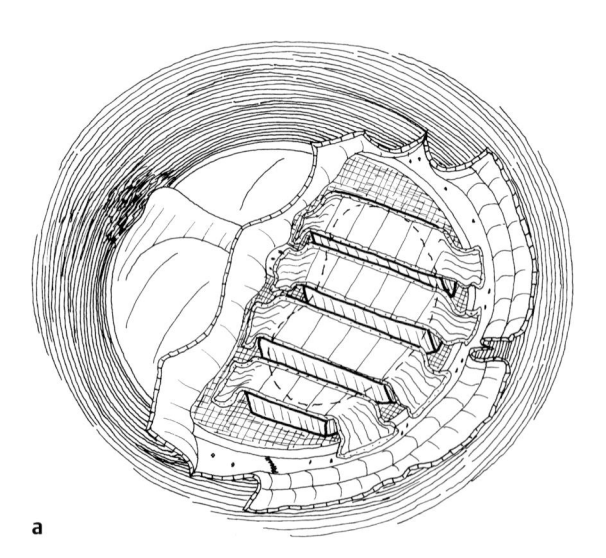

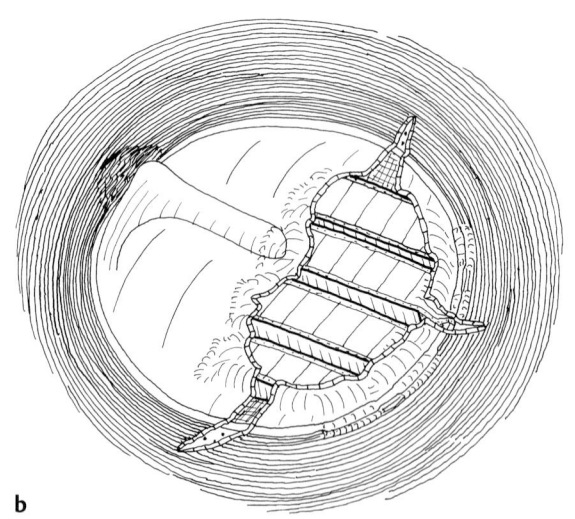

Fig. 5.13a, b Full-thickness cartilage palisades with the perichondrium flaps on both ends cover the inferior perforation.
a Four palisades are placed on the edge of the denuded lamina propria. Each inferior perichondrium flap covers the cartilage ends, the remaining lamina propria, the inferior fibrous annulus, and the denuded bone. Each superior perichondrium flap covers the cartilage and the lamina propria.
b The epithelial flaps are replaced.

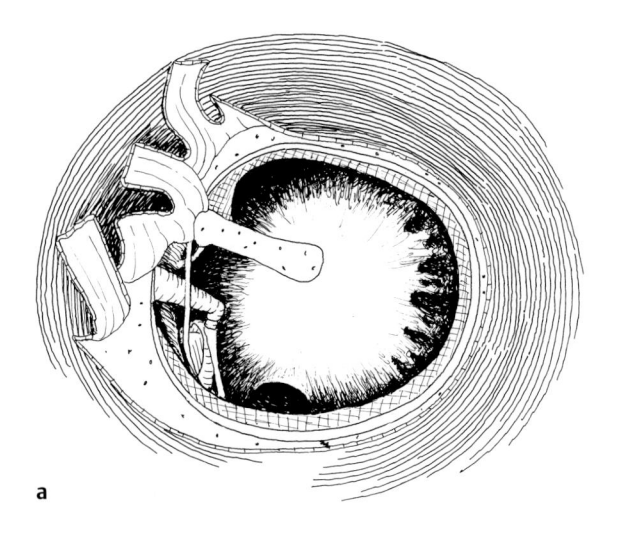

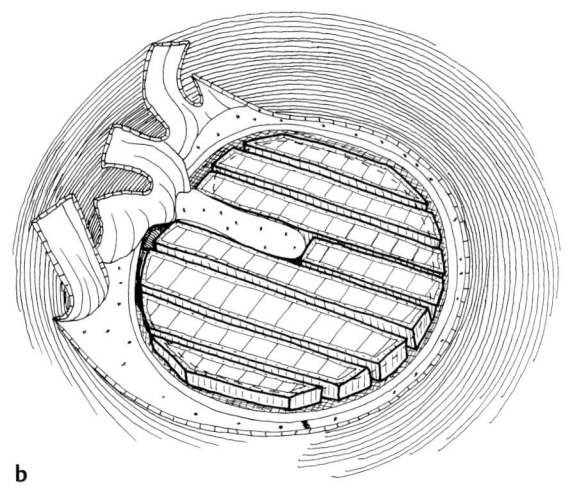

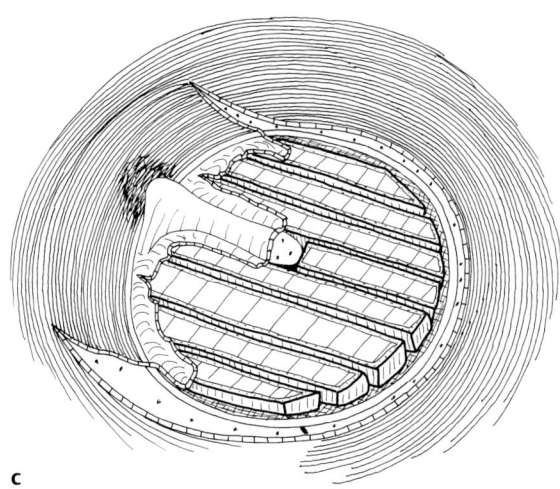

Fig. 5.14a–c On-lay technique with elevation of epithelial flaps in total perforation.
a A circumferential incision is made from the 11-o'clock position to the 2-o'clock position, near the annulus. The superoposterior flap, malleus flap, and anterosuperior skin flap are elevated.
b Eight palisades are placed onto the remnant of the eardrum. One small palisade is placed at the umbo.
c The flaps are replaced.

On-lay Technique with Elevation of a Large Tympanomeatal Skin Flap and Epithelial Flaps

This technique can be performed in the transcanal, endaural, and retroauricular approaches. After a circumferential incision from the 10-o'clock position, a large skin flap is elevated all the way around, together with the epithelium of the annulus and of the eardrum remnant (**Fig. 5.16a**) Epithelium of the inferior part of the malleus handle is removed. The epithelium of the superior part of the malleus handle is elevated up to the short process (**Fig. 5.16a**). Six palisades are placed in inferosuperior direction onto the remnant of the eardrum; the short palisade is placed onto the umbo (**Fig. 5.16b**). The epithelium and the canal skin are carefully replaced (**Fig. 5.16c**).

On-lay Technique with Placement of Palisades with Perichondrium Flaps

In total perforations, a large tympanomeatal flap is elevated together with a large malleus flap (**Fig. 5.17a**). Full-thickness palisades with perichondrium flaps at both ends are placed onto the denuded lamina propria. The perichondrium flaps are adapted onto the ear canal bone (**Fig. 5.17a**). The tympanomeatal flap and the malleus flap are replaced (**Fig. 5.17b**). In this way I attempt to improve the Wiegand perichondrial flap methods in underlay palisade technique.

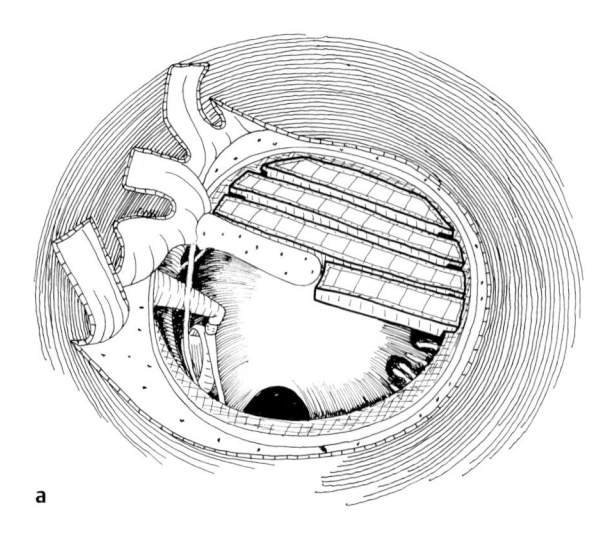

Fig. 5.15a, b Full-thickness cartilage palisades with thinned ends placed as on-lay grafts to cover a total perforation.
a Three superior epithelial flaps are elevated and the epithelium around the inferior part of the perforation is removed. Full-thickness palisades with thinned ends are placed onto the denuded lamina propria. The palisades are positioned at a deeper level than the lamina propria and the palisades do not protrude into the ear canal. Gelfoam balls will be placed under the umbo to support the short umbo palisade.
b The epithelial flaps are replaced.

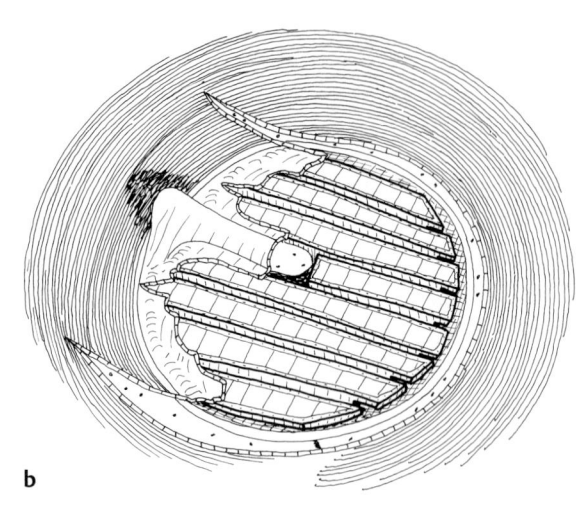

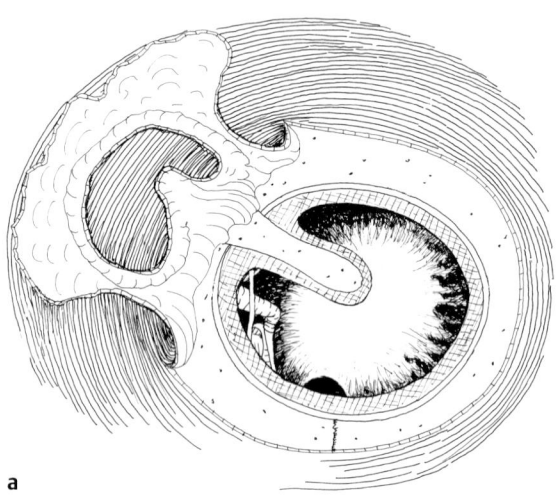

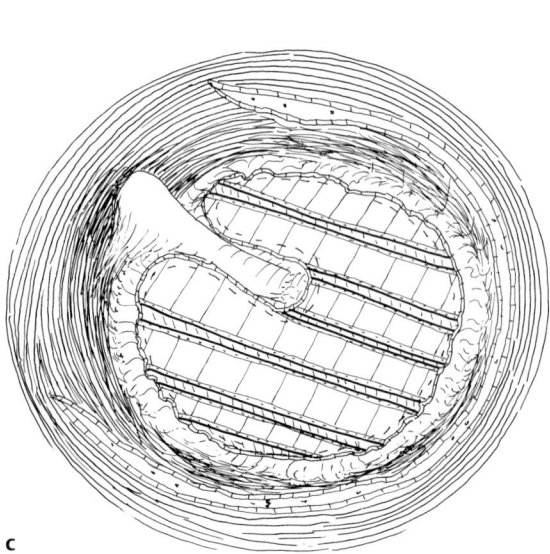

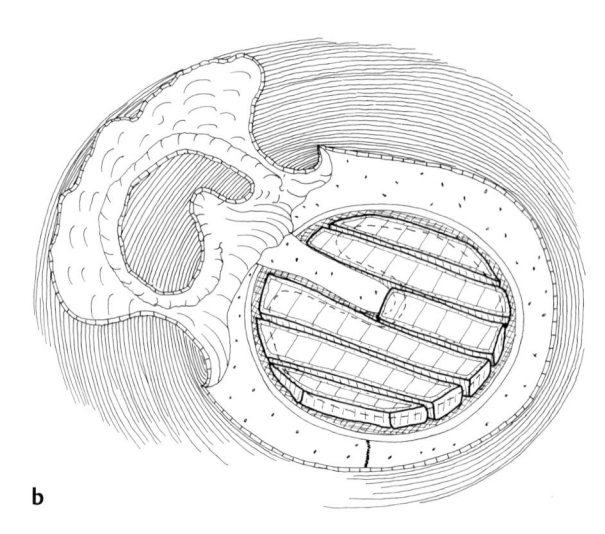

Fig. 5.16a–c Technique with a large epithelial flap.
a A circumferential incision is made from the 10-o'clock to the 2-o'clock position, about 20 mm laterally to the annulus. The ear canal skin is elevated together with the epithelium covering the annulus and the eardrum remnant. A malleus flap is elevated up to the short process. The inferior part of the malleus is cleaned of epithelium.
b Two palisades are placed onto the anterior eardrum remnant. A short palisade is placed onto the umbo and three palisades are placed onto the posterior part of the perforation.
c The ear canal skin and the epithelium are replaced.

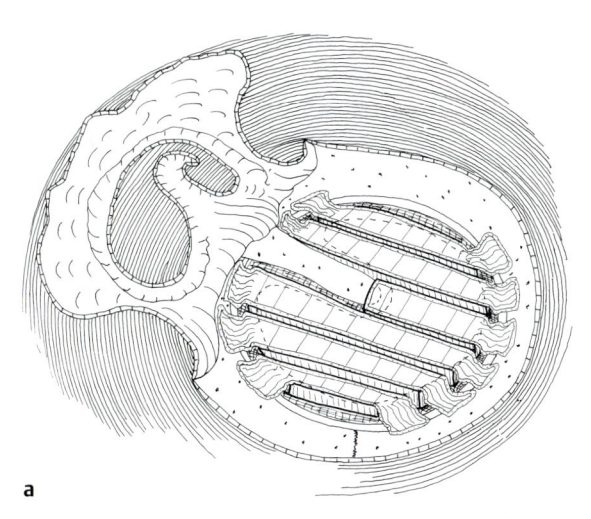

Fig. 5.17a, b Cartilage palisades with perichondrium flaps at the superior and inferior ends cover a total perforation.
a The perichondrium flaps cover the ends of the palisade, the fibrous annulus, and the ear canal bone.
b Epithelial flaps are replaced.

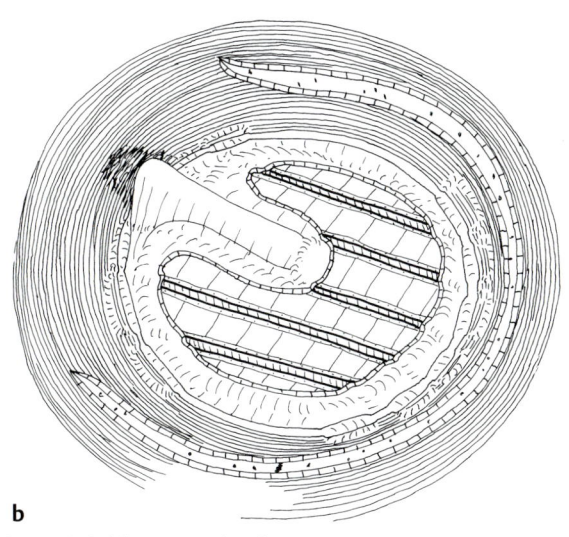

Results of On-lay Cartilage Tympanoplasty Techniques

An intensive search of the literature retrieved no studies on on-lay cartilage tympanoplasty techniques, either on methods or on results. In recent years I have performed about 30 tympanoplasties with on-lay cartilage palisade technique. The surgery was performed at various geographical locations and the primary results were good. No primary re-perforations were observed during the first two months after surgery and the epithelialization of the eardrum was complete. A systematic follow-up study has not been performed on these patients.

The methods described in this chapter have been applied in anterior, inferior, subtotal, and some total perforations, mostly on dry ears without any signs of cholesteatoma.

Author's Comments on On-lay Palisade Techniques

Since the early 1960s, I have performed myringoplasty and tympanoplasty with minimally invasive techniques, whenever possible using a transcanal approach with a fixed ear speculum and fascia or perichondrium as graft materials. In posterior perforation or retraction, underlay techniques with elevation of the posterior tympanomeatal flap and fascia grafting were used exclusively until 1995. Since 1995, the underlay cartilage palisade technique has been used in children with sinus cholesteatoma and entire tensa retraction cholesteatoma as well as in adhesive otitis media and retractions (Andersen et al. 2002). The palisade technique showed better results than fascia (Andersen et al. 2004). Because of the good results with cartilage palisades, since 1995 I have increasingly used on-lay cartilage palisade techniques in anterior, inferior, subtotal, and total perforation, with good primary results.

The advantage of the on-lay technique is avoidance of the need for support of the palisades. The palisades are placed onto the edge of the denuded lamina propria and cannot move into the tympanic cavity. The disadvantage is their full thickness at the inferior ends, because the edges cannot be totally covered by the epithelial flaps. I therefore propose reduction of the thickness at the end of the palisade and/or covering the ends of the palisades with the perichondrium flaps.

Clinical Research in On-lay Cartilage Technique is Needed

Comparison of postoperative hearing in similar total perforations covered either with underlay palisade technique or with on-lay technique is desirable. Results achieved with fascia should be compared with results achieved with on-lay palisade grafting in comparable series.

Furthermore, the postoperative hearing after closure of inferior or anterior perforations with on-lay cartilage palisade technique should be compared with results achieved after closure of comparable series grafted with fascia. Hearing results after placement of the palisades onto the lamina propria in on-lay technique should be compared with placement of the palisades onto the ear canal bone in underlay technique.

References

Andersen J, Cayé-Thomasen P, Tos M. Cartilage palisade tympanoplasty in sinus and tensa retraction cholesteatoma. Otol Neurotol 2002;23:825–831.

Andersen J, Cayé-Thomasen P, Tos M. A comparison of cartilage palisades and fascia in tympanoplasty after surgery for sinus or tensa retraction cholesteatoma in children. Otol Neurotol 2004;25:856–863.

Eavey RD. Inlay tympanoplasty: cartilage butterfly technique. Laryngoscope 1998;108:657–661.

Heermann J. Entwicklung von der Haut-zur Faszien-und zur Knorpeltympanoplastik (Epitympanon-Antrum-Mastoidplastik). Laryngol Rhinol Otol (Stuttg) 1977;56:267–270.

Heermann J, Heermann H. Sieben Jahre Faszien – Knorpel – Dachschindel – Tympanoplastik und Antrum-Mastoidplastik. Z Laryngol Rhinol Otol 1967;46:370–382.

Heermann J, Heermann H, Kopfstein E. Fascia and cartilage palisade tympanoplasty. Nine years' experience. Arch Otolaryngol 1970;91:228–241.

Tos M. Stability of myringoplasty based on late results. ORL J Otorhinolaryngol Relat Spec 1980;42:171–181.

6 Tympanoplasty with Broad Cartilage Palisades

Definition

In the cartilage palisade technique of Heermann, 5–8 palisades are used for closure of a total perforation (Heermann 1992). Bernal-Sprekelsen and co-workers modified the cartilage palisade technique of Heermann by using broad palisades, thereby reducing the number of palisades from six to three for closure of a total perforation (Bernal-Sprekelsen and Barberán 1997; Bernal-Sprekelsen et al. 1997; Menéndez-Colino and Bernal-Sprekelsen 2002; Bernal-Sprekelsen et al. 2003). Those authors believe that the broad palisades enhance transmission of the sound waves because of the increased width of the palisades and the improved contact with the prosthesis.

Harvesting and Shaping of Broad Palisades

Cartilage used for broad palisades can be harvested from the tragus, when using an endaural approach, or from the concha, usually from the cymba region (see **Figs. 3.24, 3.25**), when using a retroauricular approach. The cymba cartilage is relatively thick and convex toward the posterior side. It is usually possible to harvest a round piece of cartilage with a diameter of 11 mm (see **Fig 3.27**). On the convex (posterior) side, the cartilage is covered with perichondrium (**Fig. 6.1a**). The cartilage side of the palisades will face the promontory; the side with the perichondrium will face the ear canal.

Two 4 mm wide palisades with a semilunar shape are made to cover the anterior and the posterior halves of the tympanic cavity. Small palisades are placed along the malleus handle. Usually three palisades are sufficient to close a total perforation (**Fig. 6.1b**). The two semilunar palisades are placed in the tympanic cavity as underlay grafts, first anteriorly and then posteriorly. The small palisade can be placed along the malleus handle or as a prolongation of the malleus handle. In case of a missing malleus handle, the smaller palisade is placed in the middle of the tympanic cavity instead of the malleus handle.

Sometimes the harvested cartilage graft is too short for sufficiently long palisades to be cut. In this case the graft is cut in various directions, resulting in short, broad palisades. When such palisades are placed into the tympanic

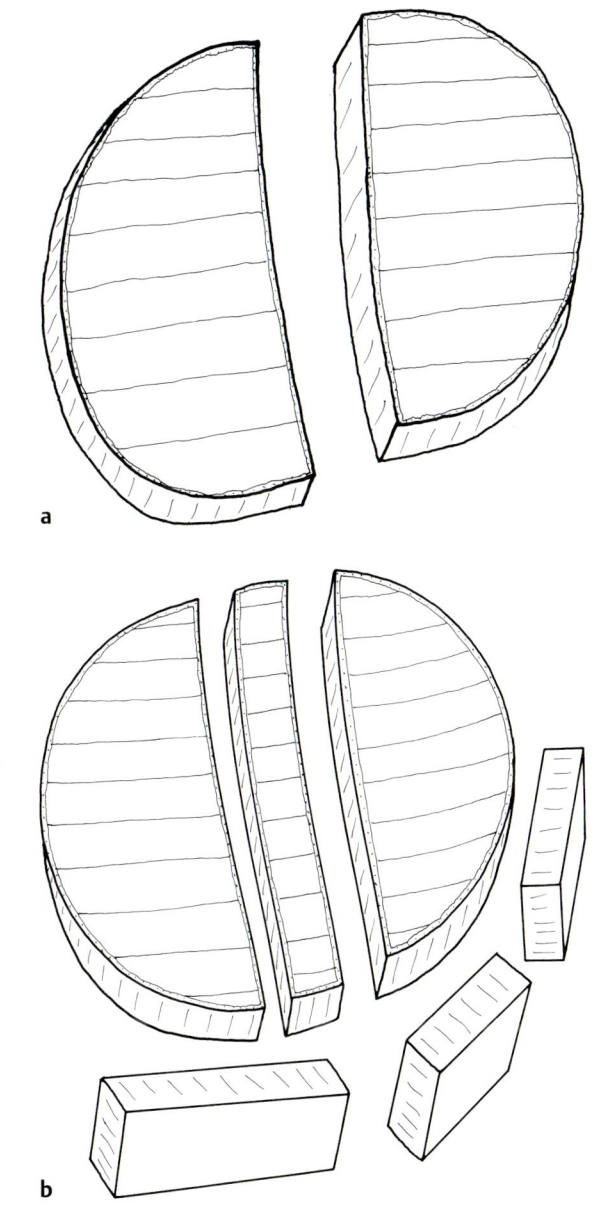

Fig. 6.1a, b Broad palisades.
a Two broad semilunar cartilage palisades are sufficient to cover the tympanic cavity when the malleius handle is present.
b Two broad palisades covered with perichondrium on the convex side (ear canal side) and the small palisade (often used in the middle of the ear drum when the malleius handle is missing). Three small pieces of cartilage without perichondrium are intended for supporting the palisades.

cavity, the reconstructed eardrum has a mosaic appearance (see Chapter 7).

Indications for Tympanoplasty with Broad Cartilage Palisades

Based on nine years of experience with broad palisades, Bernal-Sprekelsen and co-workers (2003) recommend the following indications for tympanoplasty with broad palisades:
- Total and subtotal perforations
- Perforations with tympanosclerotic plaques
- Perforation with atrophic membranes
- Revision surgery for failed myringoplasty or tympanoplasty type 1
- Anterior and inferior perforation with tubal discharge
- Retraction pockets
- Partially or completely atelectatic tympanic membranes
- Tympanic adherences
- Revision surgery for failed tympanoplasties of type 2 and type 3 as well as tympanomastoidectomies.

The Bernal-Sprekelsen Broad Palisade Techniques

Broad palisades are mainly used in total and subtotal perforation as underlay graft. They are supported by 2 mm × 3 mm pieces of cartilage placed vertically into the hypotympanum or into other regions such as the eminence of the tensor tympani muscle (**Fig. 6.1b**).

Total Perforation with Intact Ossicular Chain

The tympanoplasty may be performed in a transcanal, endaural, or retroauricular approach. The supports for the palisades are two or three 2 mm × 3 mm pieces of cartilage. Gelfoam can be used as well. The posterosuperior end of the palisade can rest on the chorda tympani and/or on the long process of the incus.

In an endaural approach, the edges of the perforation and around the malleus handle are cleaned. A medial circumferential incision with a radial incision is performed and two tympanomeatal flaps are elevated (**Fig. 6.2a, b**). The fibrous annulus is further elevated, exposing the bony annulus (**Fig. 6.2c**). Two sufficiently small pieces of cartilage are placed into the hypotympanum and along the eminence of the tensor tympani muscle to support the palisades (**Fig. 6.2d**). An anterior semicircular palisade and a posterior palisade are placed onto the small pieces of cartilage (**Fig. 6.2e**). A small palisade is placed between the two large palisades close to the umbo and is supported with Gelfoam balls (**Fig. 6.2f**). The tympanomeatal flaps with the eardrum remnant are replaced (**Fig. 6.2g**).

Bernal-Sprekelsen and his group use several thin bluish silicone foils to cover the eardrum and the ear canal. After packing the ear canal with Gelfoam, the outer ends of the foils are turned inward (**Fig. 6.2h**), to stabilize the reconstructed eardrum and promote its epithelialization. When suturing the skin incisions laterally in the ear canal, the silicone foils are turned outward to cover the sutures and prevent formation of granulations.

Total Perforation with Missing Ossicles

Even if the entire malleus is missing, the reconstruction of the eardrum will be the same as when the malleus head is present.

The support for the superior ends of the palisades will be a 1 mm × 3 mm piece of cartilage positioned partly onto the eminence of the facial nerve, partly onto the eminence of the tensor tympani muscle. In the hypotympanum a similar piece of cartilage is placed to support the broad anterior palisade (**Fig. 6.3a**). Onto the footplate an oval cartilage guide 0.3 mm thick is placed with a hole for the foot of the TORP prosthesis (see **Fig. 3.37**). The second palisade is placed at the site of the malleus and is supported in the same manner as the anterior palisade. The second palisade rests partly on the head of the TORP prosthesis. The posterior semilunar palisade is supported partly by the TORP and partly by the superior small piece of cartilage (**Fig. 6.3b**). The tympanomeatal flaps and eardrum remnants are replaced (**Fig. 6.3c, d**).

Total Perforation with Missing Long Process of Incus

Tympanoplasty type 2 with interposition of a partial ossicular replacement prosthesis (PORP) of various materials and shapes is illustrated in numerous chapters of this book (see Chapters 4, 5, 7, 8, 9; see also MMES_1, pp. 245–329). Here only an example of the most common ossiculoplasty, the incus interposition, will be shown in connection with cartilage tympanoplasty with broad palisades, in particular to illustrate the need for reduction and careful shaping of the incus to accommodate the broad palisades.

In endaural approach the edges of the total perforation are cleaned. Using a swing-door technique, two tympanomeatal flaps are elevated, and the defective incus is extruded, reduced, and shaped to accommodate the undersurface of the broad palisade. First the anterior semilunar palisade is placed in the anterior tympanum, then the shaped incus is interposed between the head of the stapes and the malleus handle (**Fig. 6.4a**). Inferiorly, the palisade is supported by a piece of cartilage, placed into the hypotympanum, superiorly it is supported by an architrave. A palisade is adapted to the malleus handle and a semilunar broad posterior palisade is placed at the level of the bony

Fig. 6.2a–h Cartilage tympanoplasty with broad palisades harvested from the cymba in a case with total perforation and intact ossicular chain.

- **a** The edges of the perforation and around the malleus handle are cleaned and the epithelium is removed all the way around the entire edge. A medial circumferential incision is made. At the 9-o'clock position, a small radial incision separates the tympanomeatal flap into a superior and an inferior flap.
- **b** Both flaps are elevated together with the fibrous annulus, exposing the bony annulus.
- **c** Further elevation of the remnants of the eardrum and the inferior fibrous annulus.
- **d** Further elevation of the anterior fibrous annulus and the eardrum remnant. Placement of a small piece of cartilage in the hypotympanum and one along the eminence of tensor tympani muscle to support the palisades.
- **e** The first palisade is placed onto the piece of the cartilage previously placed into the hypotympanum and onto the cartilage placed along the eminence of the tensor tympani muscle. The palisade is placed at the level of the bony annulus and beside the malleus handle under the small eardrum remnant. The posterior broad palisade is placed onto the small inferior and superior cartilage supports. The palisades are positioned at the level of the bony annulus and along the malleus handle.

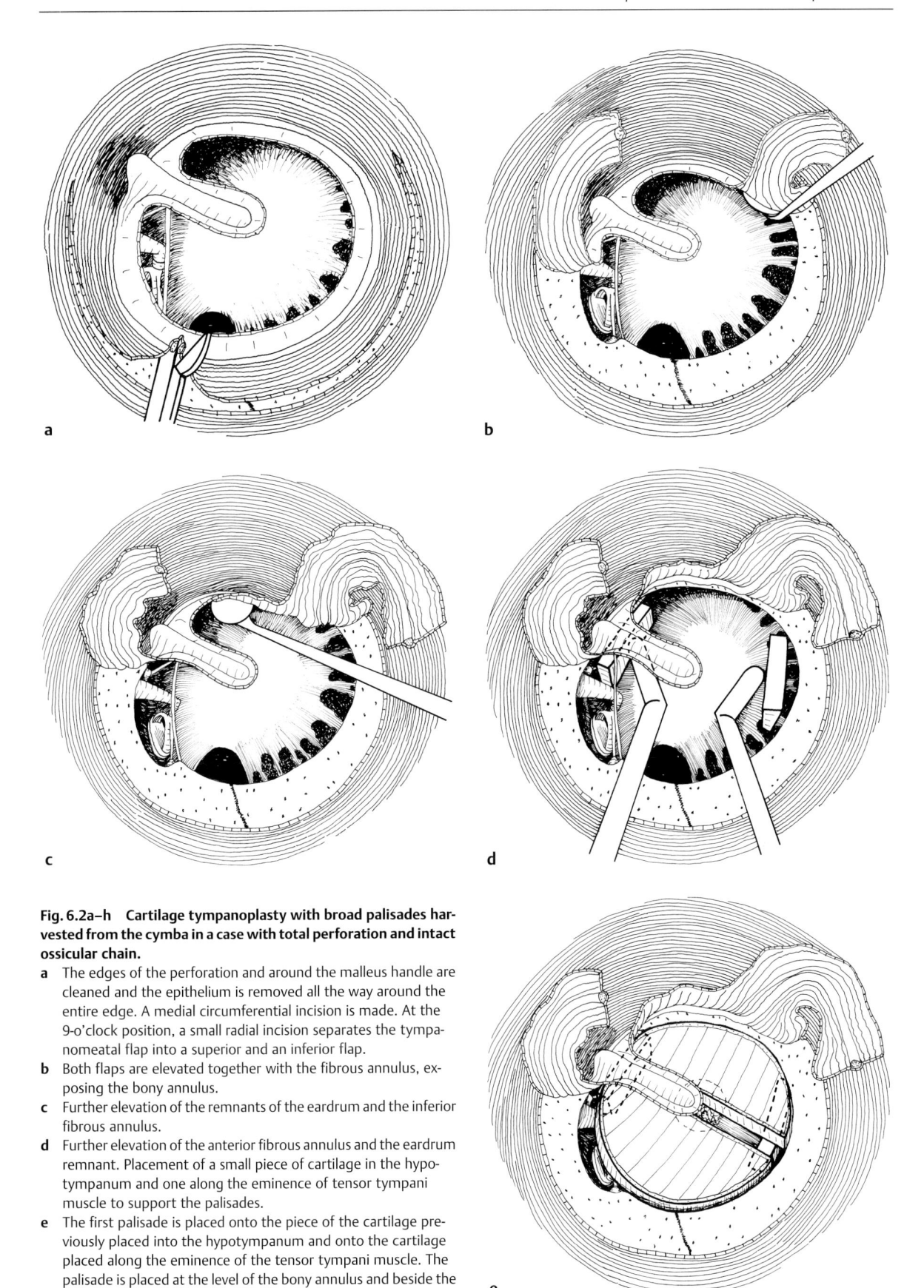

Fig. 6.2f–h ▷

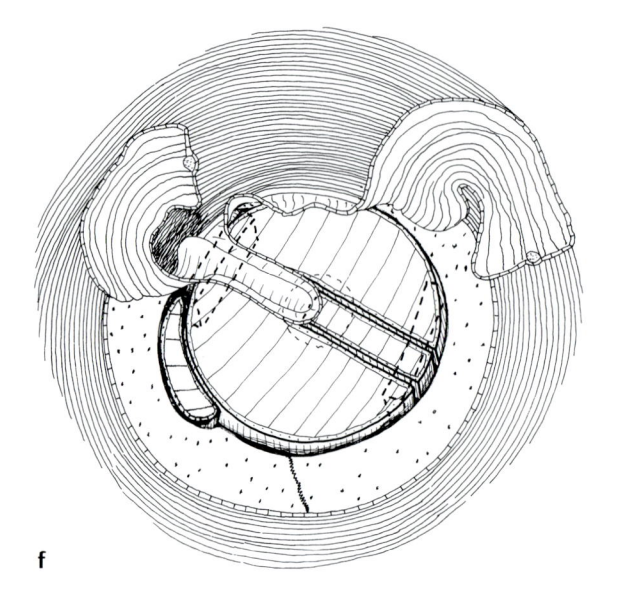

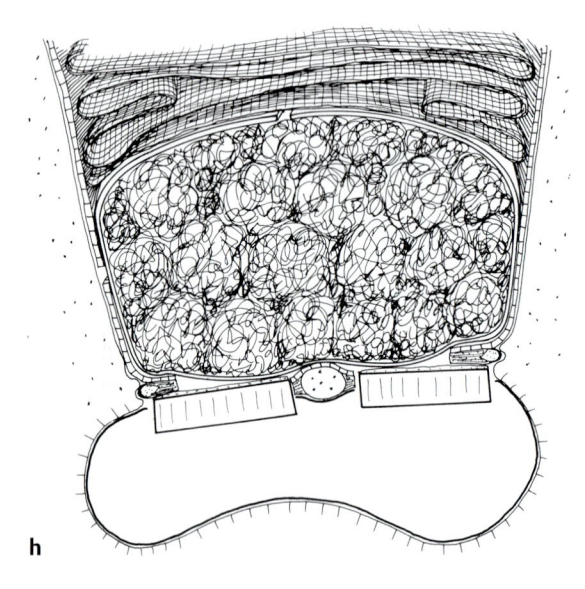

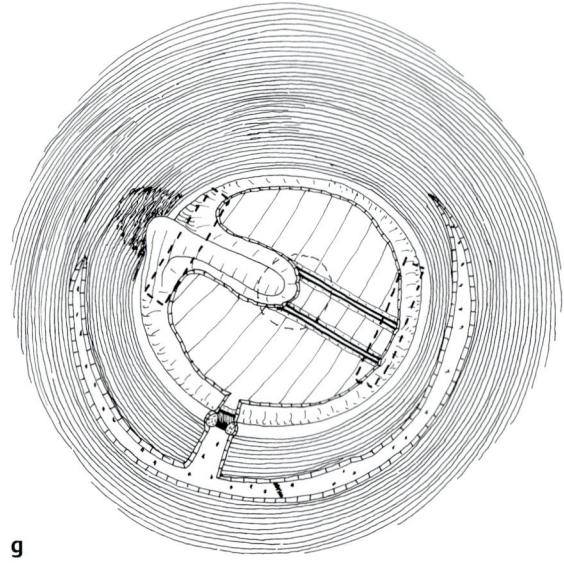

Fig. 6.2f–h

f A small palisade is placed between the umbo and the inferior support cartilage. A superoposterior defect of the scutum is covered with a small palisade. A Gelfoam ball supports the upper end of the malleus palisade; support of the palisade with a Gelfoam ball is easy and effective.

g The tympanomeatal flaps are replaced, together with the fibrous annulus and remnants of the eardrum.

h Side view of underlay tympanoplasty type 1 with broad cartilage palisades at the level of the umbo, and packing of the ear canal. Two broad palisades are positioned at the level of the bony annulus. Several strips of blue silicone foil cover the eardrum and the ear canal skin. After placing several pieces of Gelfoam, the foils are turned inward. The lateral end of the ear canal is closed by gauze moistened with hydrocortisone–oxytetracycline ointment.

annulus and supported by the interposed incus (**Fig. 6.4b**). After replacement of the tympanomeatal flaps (**Fig. 6.4c**), the connection between the shaped and reduced interposed autogenous incus and the broad palisades is good (**Fig. 6.4d**).

Similar solid interposition prostheses can be made and shaped from cortical bone, tragal cartilage, and homogenous incus.

Retracted and Adherent Malleus Handle in a Total Perforation with Defective Incus

The pathogenesis of such a condition is as follows: Chronic or recurrent secretory otitis media and long-lasting tubal dysfunction cause diffuse atrophy and retraction of the entire pars tensa, including resorption of the long process of the incus and adhesion of the umbo to the promontory. Because of severe purulent acute otitis media, the thin and atrophic pars tensa becomes necrotic and may disappear, resulting in a total perforation.

In the endaural approach, the edges of the perforation are cleaned and the two tympanomeatal flaps with the anterior fibrous annulus are elevated. The defective incus is removed. Using a curved incudostapedial knife, the adhesions between the umbo and the promontory are cut and the eardrum remnant is separated from the promontory. Under the inferior half of the bony annulus three small pieces of cartilage are placed to support the inferior semilunar palisade (**Fig. 6.5a**). The eardrum remnants connected to the umbo and to the retracted malleus handle are elevated as a malleus flap. Then the malleus handle is elevated to its normal position (**Fig. 6.5b**). The autogenous incus is shaped to become more flat and is placed onto the stapes head and under the malleus handle (Bernal-Sprekelsen, personal communication 2006). The large semi-

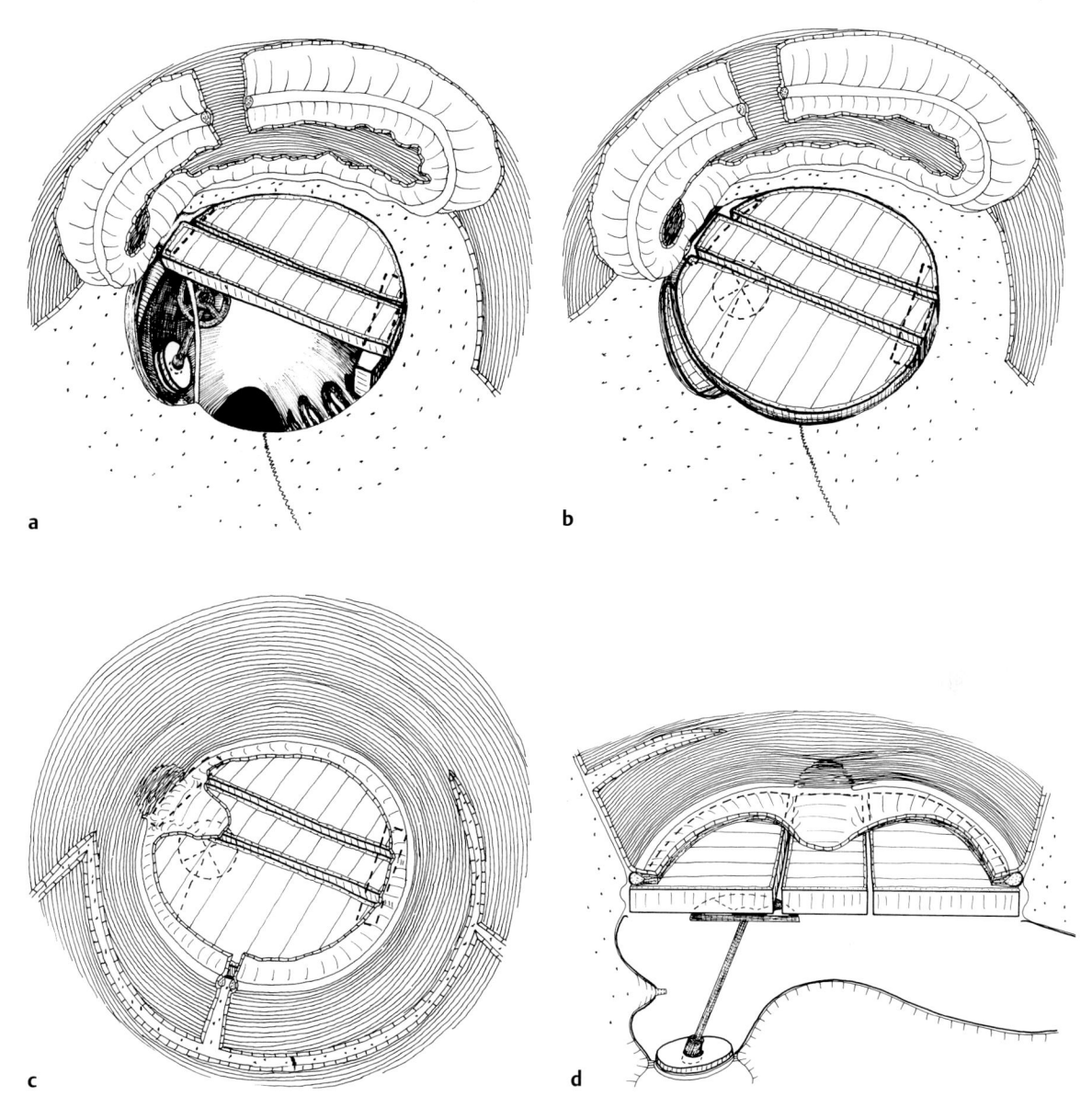

Fig. 6.3a–d Reconstruction of a total perforation without ossicles using broad cartilage palisades and titanium TORP prosthesis.

a The edges of the perforation are cleaned of epithelium. In endaural approach and swing-door technique, an inferior and a superior tympanomeatal flap are elevated together with the fibrous annulus, exposing the bony annulus. The epithelium around the attic region is elevated. The footplate is cleaned and a Hüttenbrink cartilage guide is placed onto the footplate (Hüttenbrink et al. 2004). A Kurz titanium TORP prosthesis is placed through the hole of the guide onto the footplate. Onto the eminence of the tensor tympani muscle a small cartilage palisade is placed, similar to the architrave. In the hypotympanum a 3 mm × 2 mm piece of cartilage is placed to support the inferior ends of the palisades. The anterior semilunar palisade is placed onto the architrave and onto the cartilage in the hypotympanum. The second palisade replaces the malleus, it is supported by the cartilage and the head of the TORP prosthesis.

b The third palisade covers the posterior half of the tympanic cavity. It is placed and adapted to the head of the TORP prosthesis and the chorda tympani as well as the palisade on the tensor tympani and partly on the facial nerve. The bony defect after drilling of the posterosuperior scutum is covered with a small palisade.

c The tympanomeatal flaps with the eardrum remnant are replaced.

d Side view with some perspective at the level of the footplate of an underlay cartilage tympanoplasty type 3 with broad palisades. The Kurz titanium TORP prosthesis has contact with two palisades, which are placed at the level of the bony annulus.

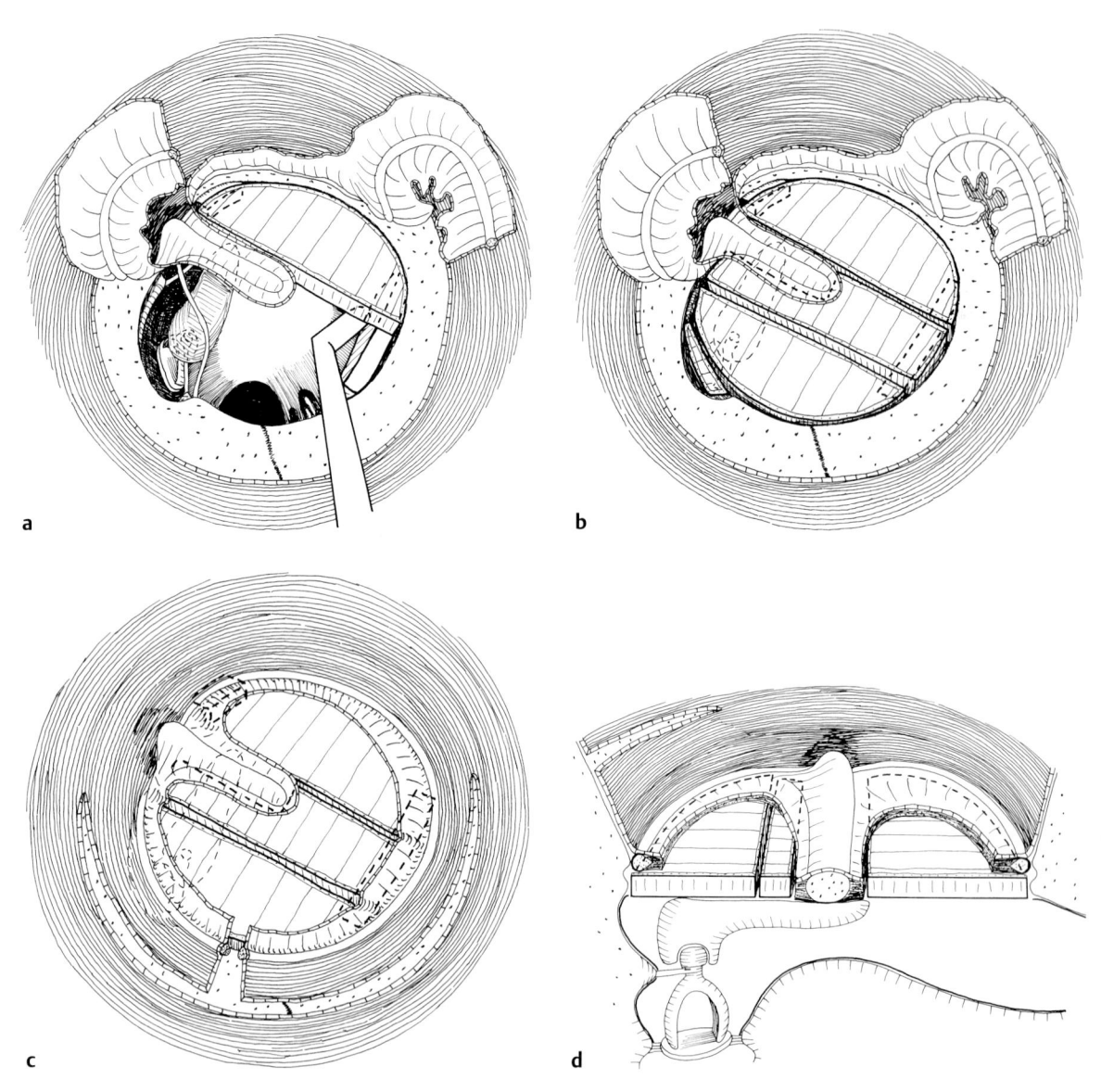

Fig. 6.4a–d Cartilage underlay tympanoplasty type 2 with broad palisades and interposition of autogenous incus in total perforation and missing long process of the incus.

a   The edges of the perforation are cleaned of epithelium and the undersurface of the eardrum is scarified. The incus is removed and shaped; a hole is drilled for the stapes. The incus body is reduced and flattened, allowing placement of the broad palisade. The short process of the incus is flattened and placed under the malleus handle. The anterior palisade is placed close to the bony annulus and is supported by a piece of cartilage placed into the hypotympanum. Superiorly, an architrave-like piece of cartilage supports the superior end of the cartilage.

b   The second palisade is adapted to the malleus handle and has a good contact with the incus. The large posterior semilunar palisade is supported by the incus and inferiorly by the cartilage in the hypotympanum.

c   Tympanomeatal flaps and the eardrum remnants are replaced.

d   Side view with some perspective of cartilage broad palisade tympanoplasty type 2 with incus interposition. The incus is reduced and flattened to accommodate the broad palisade, allowing good contact with the eardrum.

lunar palisade is placed under the umbo, preventing new retraction of the malleus handle. The anterosuperior palisade is supported by the tip of the short process of the interposed incus (**Fig. 6.5c**). The posterosuperior palisade is placed onto the flattened interposed incus body (**Fig. 6.5 d**). After replacement of the tympanomeatal flaps and of the malleus flap, the elevated epithelium from the promontory partly covers all three palisades (**Fig. 6.5e**).

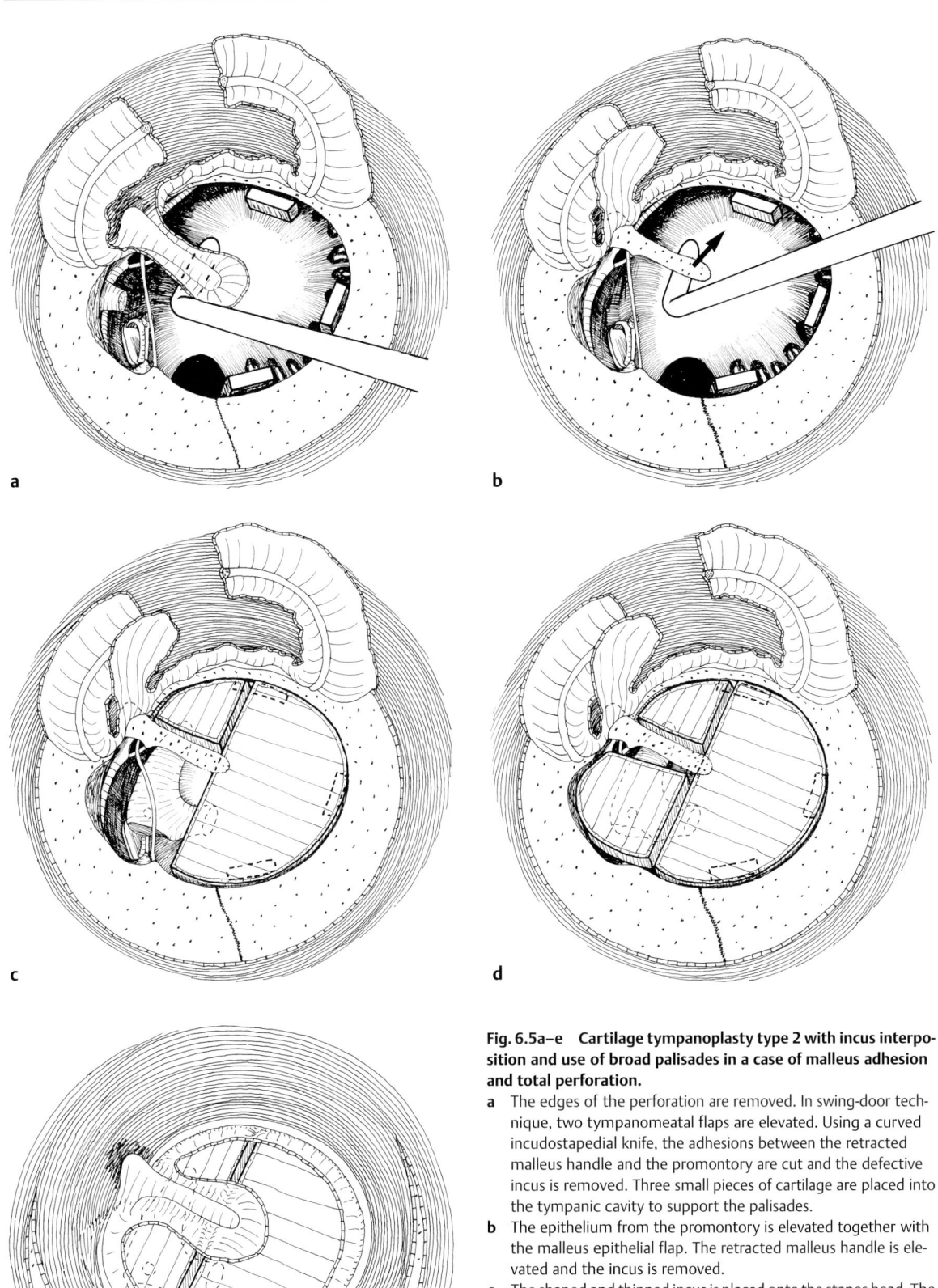

Fig. 6.5a–e Cartilage tympanoplasty type 2 with incus interposition and use of broad palisades in a case of malleus adhesion and total perforation.

a The edges of the perforation are removed. In swing-door technique, two tympanomeatal flaps are elevated. Using a curved incudostapedial knife, the adhesions between the retracted malleus handle and the promontory are cut and the defective incus is removed. Three small pieces of cartilage are placed into the tympanic cavity to support the palisades.
b The epithelium from the promontory is elevated together with the malleus epithelial flap. The retracted malleus handle is elevated and the incus is removed.
c The shaped and thinned incus is placed onto the stapes head. The large inferior palisade is placed onto the three "cartilage supports" but under the umbo to prevent retraction. The anterosuperior palisade is also supported.
d The posterosuperior palisade rests on the incus.
e The malleus flap with the epithelium removed from the promontory is replaced onto the palisades.

Broad Palisades and Various Tympanomastoidectomies

The approach of the Bernal-Sprekelsen group to cholesteatoma is retrograde drilling, following the cholesteatoma toward the attic and the antrum and further to the mastoid process (Bernal-Sprekelsen et al. 2003).

After starting in retroauricular or endaural approach, from the ear canal and the scutum, the drilling is continuing to the attic and to the antrum and—depending on the size of the cholesteatoma—possibly to eventual canal wall down mastoidectomy. The extension of cholesteatoma is thus the selection criterion for either a canal wall down procedure, or a canal wall up procedure.

In canal wall up procedure the ear canal defect, after an atticotomy and a small atticoantrotomy, may be closed with broad cartilage palisades and/or other cartilage grafts, remaining a preserved ear canal.

In canal wall down procedures, open cavities are obliterated partially or totally with cartilage from the cavum conchae. Cartilage cut into smaller pieces is used to fill up the anterior epitympanum and antrum and to cover the horizontal semicircular canal. The use of small pieces of cartilage to fill up the cavity or its various pockets is intended to occupy the space and indirectly to prevent retractions. If a large cartilage plate is used, potential retraction may occur at its edges, especially if the plate is not perfectly accommodated to the walls of the cavity or not supported by other cartilage pieces.

Accordingly, a wide entrance to the cavity has to be ensured by a meatoplasty with excision of the conchal cartilage, for use in obliteration of the cavity.

Closure of an Atticotomy with Broad Cartilage Palisades

Atticotomy is a common procedure in attic cholesteatoma, allowing extension of surgery to the antrum and mastoid process. Various canal wall up and canal wall down mastoidectomy methods have been described and are used (see Tos 1995, pp. 36–38). Some atticotomy and atticoantrotomy methods closed with cartilage-perichondrium composite islands grafts will be shown in Chapters 14 to 17. Here only an example is shown of how an attic defect can be closed by broad cartilage palisades.

After removal of the attic cholesteatoma in endaural approach, the atticotomy is prepared to accommodate the broad palisades: A groove is drilled along the defect of the ear canal wall. Anteriorly and posteriorly the bone is smoothened and partly removed to facilitate placement of the anterior and the posterior palisades. The cog (a bony spur in the anterior attic wall; see MMES_2 Figs. 85–87) is fashioned to support the anterior palisade (**Fig. 6.6a**). The anterior palisade is placed on the cog, which makes a safe entrance to the eustachian tube (**Fig. 6.6b**). The contact to the malleus head is established, and the contact to the anterior half of the eardrum is very good as well. The posterior palisade (**Fig. 6.6c**) has good contact with the posterior part of the ossicular chain and does not need any support.

I recommend covering the entire attic region with the fascia (**Fig. 6.6d**). The epithelialization is then safer and faster (**Fig. 6.6e**).

Results in Tympanoplasty with Broad Cartilage Palisades

Bernal-Sprekelsen et al. (2003) report on 362 consecutive ears operated on during a 6-years period from October 1992 to October 1998 for previously nonoperated cholesteatoma with cartilage tympanoplasty and ossiculoplasty. One hundred and seventy-seven tympanoplasties were tympanomastoidectomies with radical canal wall down procedures (CWD), and 185 were conservative tympanomastoidectomies with canal wall up procedures (CWU).

Anatomical Results

For the 362 operated ears with a mean follow-up of 54 months (36–106 months) after cholesteatoma surgery, results were very good:
- **Reperforations:** 6 (1.7%); all were closed again with cartilage.
- **Retraction pockets:** 9 (2.5%); mainly because the cartilage supports the anterior epitympanum and the part of the eardrum that was not reconstructed with the cartilage.
- **Recurrent cholesteatomas:** 8 (2.2%).
- **Extrusion of a TORP prosthesis:** 1 (0.28%).
- **Residual cholesteatoma** was not found.

Functional Results

Results were measured using a four-frequency pure-tone average air–bone gap (PTA-ABG).
- At 54 months follow-up, the overall preoperative and postoperative PTA-ABGs were 34.4 dB and 18.1 dB, respectively.
- For the PORP group, preoperative and postoperative PTA-ABGs were 28.3 dB and 16.8 dB, respectively. For the
- TORP group, preoperative and postoperative PTA-ABGs were 40.5 dB and 19.4 dB, respectively

No significant differences between postoperative results with the TORP and with the PORP were found:
- **TORP with CWU group:** postoperative PTA-ABG was 18.1 dB.

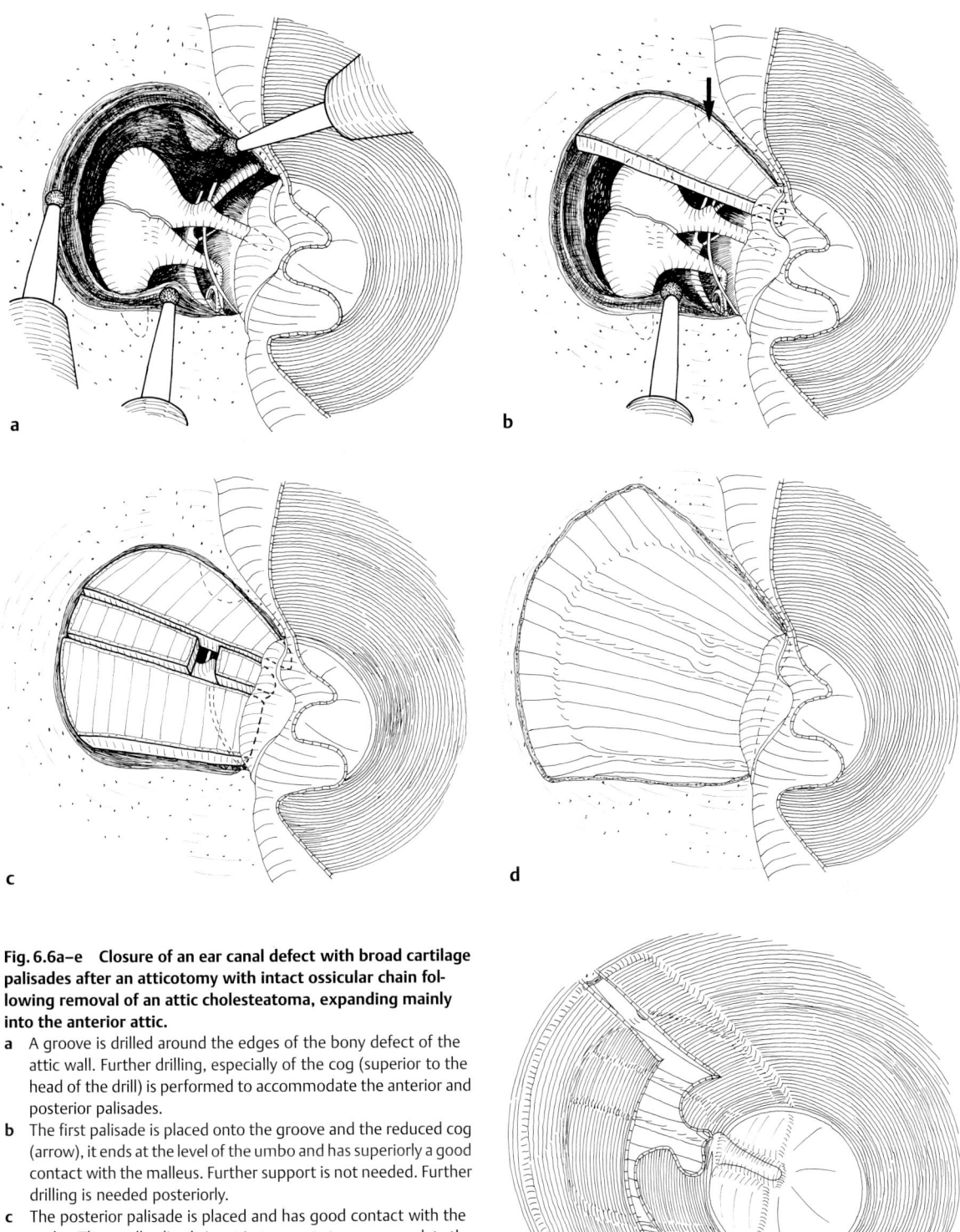

Fig. 6.6a–e Closure of an ear canal defect with broad cartilage palisades after an atticotomy with intact ossicular chain following removal of an attic cholesteatoma, expanding mainly into the anterior attic.

a   A groove is drilled around the edges of the bony defect of the attic wall. Further drilling, especially of the cog (superior to the head of the drill) is performed to accommodate the anterior and posterior palisades.

b   The first palisade is placed onto the groove and the reduced cog (arrow), it ends at the level of the umbo and has superiorly a good contact with the malleus. Further support is not needed. Further drilling is needed posteriorly.

c   The posterior palisade is placed and has good contact with the umbo. The small palisade is cut in two parts to accommodate the short process of the malleus.

d   The ear canal is covered with the fascia ending under the eardrum

e   The superior tympanomeatal flaps and ear canal skin flaps are replaced.

Table 6.1 Overall functional results in 362 ears at mean 54 months follow-up (Bernal-Sprekelsen et al. 2003)

Postoperative air–bone gap	No. of ears	Percentage	Cumulative percentage
0–10 dB	108	29.8	29.8
11–20 db	117	32.3	62.1
21–30 dB	81	22.4	84.1
>30 dB	56	15.5	100.0
Total	362	00.0	100.0

- **TORP with CWD group:** postoperative PTA-ABG was 20.7 dB.
- **PORP with CWU group:** postoperative PTA-ABG was 15.4 dB.
- **PORP with CWD group:** postoperative PTA-ABG was 18.8 dB.

In 56 ears, the autologous incus could be interposed as a PORP or as TORP columella. In 306 ears, the Ceravital or the Ionos prosthesis was used as a PORP between the head of the stapes and the cartilage palisade, or as a TORP columella between the footplate and the cartilage palisade.

Postoperative Air–Bone Gap at Mean Follow-up (54 months) after Surgery
Table 6.1 shows an air–bone gap within 20 dB in 62.1 % of 362 ears, which is good in relation to severity of the series with cholesteatoma and defective ossicular chain.

Comparison of ABG Closure in CWU and CWD in Combination with PORP and TORP Ossiculoplasty
Average ABG improved at all frequencies, but the improvement of ABG was significantly better in CWU procedures than in CWD procedures for frequencies 0.5 kHz and 1 kHz.

In a separate study, 30 months after cartilage tympanoplasty type 3 with broad palisades and titanium TORP prosthesis, Menéndez-Colino and Bernal-Sprekelsen (2002) found an ABG closure in the range 0–10 dB in 43 % of ears. The results were better with a titanium TORP prosthesis with a weight of 4 mg than with the Ionos cement prosthesis with a weight of about 60 mg. The good results with titanium prostheses are presumably due to the light weight of the titanium TORP prosthesis (Menéndez-Colino et al. 2004).

Postoperative Complications
Anacusis appeared in two ears; in one of them because of a footplate fracture during removal of tympanosclerosis. In five other ears, some sensorineural hearing loss occurred.

Author's Comments and Recommendations

The Longest Follow-up Period

The study of Bernal-Sprekelsen et al. (2003) is the only study on broad cartilage palisades. This study also has the longest mean follow-up period (54 months) among all studies on cartilage palisade tympanoplasty. This is astonishing if we consider that cartilage palisade tympanoplasty began 40 years ago (Heermann and Heermann 1967; Heermann et al. 1970; Heermann 1977; 1978; 1991, 1992).

Our study on cartilage palisade tympanoplasty after surgery for sinus and tensa retraction cholesteatoma in children has a somewhat shorter follow-up period of 34 months (Andersen et al. 2002, 2004). However, 10-year results of this study have recently been published (see Chapter 4, page 84).

Evaluation of Hearing Results in Tympanoplasty Type 1 with Broad Cartilage Palisades Is Needed

The ears with intact ossicular chain are not included in the evaluation of Bernal-Sprekelsen et al. (2003). Knowledge of the efficiency of broad palisades with intact ossicular chain is very important and desirable to establish the extent of hearing improvement caused by palisades alone. In our series of cholesteatoma in children treated with small cartilage palisades, the postoperative hearing was best in the group with tympanoplasty type 1 and intact ossicular chain (Andersen et al. 2002, 2004). In the cartilage strip method, excellent hearing results were found in 30 ears with tympanoplasty type 1, with closure of the air–bone gap to within 0–10 dB in 63 % of the ears (Neumann et al. 2002).

It will be important to see whether the postoperative hearing is best in ears with intact ossicular chain and the perforation closed with broad cartilage palisades.

Support of Broad Palisades by Small Pieces of Cartilage

Heermann used to place a palisade-like short piece of cartilage onto the eminence of the tensor tympani muscle—an architrave—to support the most anterior palisade. This anterior palisade was placed under the bony annulus, and was often supported by a piece of cartilage placed in the anterior hypotympanum. Bernal-Sprekelsen used the support used by Heermann and added support at other places as well, especially in the posterior hypotympanum. Such placement of pieces of cartilage can be done before or after placement of the palisades, and apparently the cartilage pieces in the tympanic cavity did not cause any sequelae. The Gelfoam placed into the tympanic cavity will disappear and also will not cause any sequelae.

References

Andersen J, Cayé-Thomasen P, Tos M. Cartilage palisade tympanoplasty in sinus and tensa retraction cholesteatoma. Otol Neurotol 2002;23:825–831.

Andersen J, Cayé-Thomasen P, Tos M. A comparison of cartilage palisades and fascia in tympanoplasty after surgery for sinus or tensa retraction cholesteatoma in children. Otol Neurotol 2004;25:856–863.

Bernal-Sprekelsen M, Tomás Barberán M. Indicationes, tecnica y resultados anatomicos de la tympanoplastica con cartilago en empalizada. [Indications, techniques and anatomic results of the tympanoplasty using palisade cartilage] Acta Otorrinolaringol Esp 1997;48:279–286.

Bernal-Sprekelsen M, Tomás Barberán M, Romaguera Lliso MD. Resultados funktionales preliminaries de la timpanoplastica con cartilao en empalizada. [Preliminary functional results of tympanoplasty with palisade cartilage] Acta Otorrinolaringol Esp 1997;48:341–346.

Bernal-Sprekelsen M, Romaguera Lliso MD, Sanz Gonzalo JJ. Cartilage palisades in type 3 tympanoplasty: anatomic and functional long-term results. Otol Neurotol 2003;24:38–42.

Heermann J. Entwicklung von der Haut-zur Faszien-und zur Knorpeltympanoplastik (Epitympanon-Antrum-Mastoidplastik). Laryngol Rhinol Otol (Stuttg) 1977;56:267–270.

Heermann J. Auricular cartilage palisade tympano-epitympano-antrum- and mastoid- plasty. Clin Otolaryngol 1978;3:443–446.

Heermann J. Thirty years autograft tragal and conchal cartilage perichondrium palisade tympanum, epitympanum, antrum and mastoid plasties: 13 000 cases. In: Charachon R Garcia-Ibanez E. eds. Long Term Results and Indications in Otology and Otoneurology. Amsterdam: Kugler Publications; 1991:159–164.

Heermann J. Autograft tragal and conchal palisade cartilage and perichondrium in tympanomastoid reconstruction. Ear Nose Throat J 1992;71:344–349.

Heermann J, Heermann H. Sieben Jahre Faszien – Knorpel- Dachschindel –Tympanoplastik und Antrum-Mastoidplastik. Z Laryngol Rhinol Otol 1967;46:370–382.

Heermann J, Heermann H, Kopfstein E. Fascia and cartilage palisade tympanoplasty. Nine years' experience. Arch Otolaryngol 1970; 91:228–241.

Hüttenbrink KB, Zahnert T, Beutner D, Hofmann G. The cartilage guide: a solution for anchoring a columella prosthesis on footplate. Laryngorhinootologie 2004;83:450–456.

Menéndez-Colino LM, Bernal-Sprekelsen M. Reconstriccion timpano-osicular. Resultados funcionales de timpanoplastia con cartilago en empalizada y protesis de titanio. Estudo piloto. [Tympanic-ossicular reconstruction. Functional results using cartilage palisades and titanium prostheses] Acta Otorrinolaringol Esp 2002;53:718–724.

Menéndez-Colino LM, Bernal-Sprekelsen M, Alobid I, Traserra-Coderch J. Preliminary functional results of tympanoplasty with titanium prostheses. Otolaryngol Head Neck Surg 2004;131: 747–749.

Neumann A, Hennig A, Schultz-Coulon HJ. Morphologische und funktionelle Ergebnisse der Knorpelpalisadentympanoplastik. HNO 2002;50:935–939.

Tos M. Manual of Middle Ear Surgery. Vol. 2. Mastoid Surgery and Reconstructive Procedures. New York, Stuttgart: Thieme; 1995: 36–38.

7 Cartilage Strips in Underlay Tympanoplasty Techniques

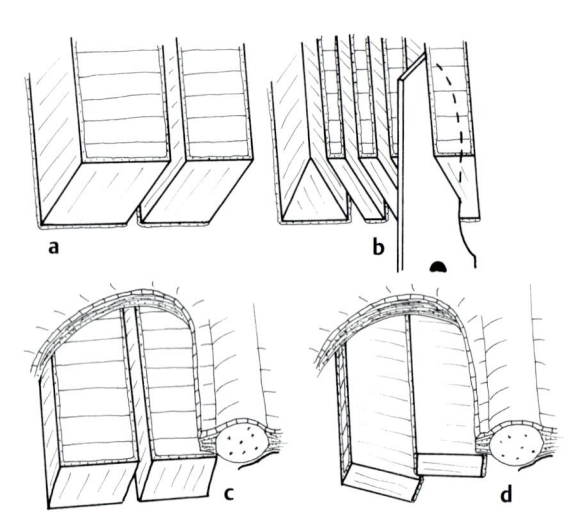

Fig. 7.1a–d Characteristics of palisades and strips.
a Palisades are cut perpendicularly to the piece of cartilage as a full-thickness graft covered completely by the perichondrium.
b Strips are cut obliquely, the thickness is one-half or one-third of the thickness of the palisades and the strips of perichondrium are small.
c The palisades are placed close to each other, but still with a small distance between successive palisades.
d The strips are placed in the manner of roof tiles.

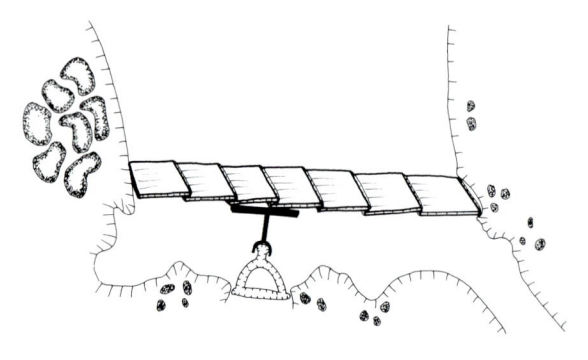

Fig. 7.2 Redrawing of the schematic side view of the cartilage strips method published by Neumann et al. (2003) The seven cartilage strips, cover the total perforation and the head of the titanium PORP prosthesis. They are placed like roof tiles and are extremely thin.

Definition

Neumann published a paper entitled "Cartilage palisade tympanoplasty of Heermann" (Neumann 1999), but the drawings were different from the usual palisades of Heermann (Heermann and Heermann 1967; Heermann et al. 1970). They looked like thin strips, with small belts of perichondrium.

Here the cartilage strip method is separated from the cartilage palisade methods because of the following substantial differences:

1. **Cutting, thickness, and shape:** Cartilage palisades are cut from a piece of cartilage in rectangular 0.5–2 mm wide belts, through the full thickness of tragal or conchal cartilage (**Fig. 7.1a**). The cartilage strips (as I term them) can be cut in an oblique manner, resulting in strips of half thickness, or even one-third thickness of tragal or conchal cartilage (**Fig. 7.1b**).
2. **Covering with perichondrium:** Cartilage palisades are totally covered on the ear canal side by the perichondrium (**Fig. 7.1a**). Because the cartilage strips are considerably smaller than the palisades, the strips of perichondrium are also small and may be on both sides (**Fig. 7.1b**).
3. **Position of palisades and strips:** Palisades are placed close to each other, with a small gap (**Fig. 7.1c**). The positioning of strips is like the laying of tiles on a roof (**Fig. 7.1 d**). The edge of one strip is placed onto (or under) the edge of the previous strip (Neumann 1999).

Comparison of the schematic drawing of the thickness, shape and the position of the strips in the side view (Neumann et al. 2002, 2003), using extremely thin strips (**Fig. 7.2**), with the side view of cartilage palisades (see **Figs. 4. 11b, 4.18 f**), are the strongest arguments for separation of the cartilage strip methods and the cartilage palisade methods. Even with the thicker strips (**Fig. 7.3**), the difference between these two methods is evident.

Palisade methods are criticized for the distances between the palisades, allowing growth of the epithelium during the period of epithelialization of the new eardrum. Later, retraction of the epithelium between the palisades, caused by negative pressure may occur. In addition, perforations may appear if there is a large distance between two palisades. Because the edges of a strip are covered by the preceding strip in a tile-like manner, the method of cartilage strips can obviate such retractions or perforations. This constitutes a very important difference between the two methods.

The cartilage strip method is novel and has been used mainly by Neumann and his co-workers, but recently Kazikdas et al. (2007) have published results of the cartilage strip technique, comparing it with the technique using fascia.

Harvesting and Shaping of the Cartilage Strips

Harvesting of the cartilage is easy and is similar to the harvesting of cartilage used for palisades. Because the strips are thinner than the palisades, a smaller tragal or conchal cartilage piece is needed than for the thicker palisades.

The cartilage can be harvested from the tragus, concha, cymba, triangular fossa, or scapha (see Chapter 3). For closure of a total perforation, a 10 mm × 8 mm piece of tragal cartilage (see **Fig. 3.21**) or conchal cartilage (see **Figs. 3.25, 3.33**) is needed.

In endaural approach, the tragal cartilage can also be harvested through the intercartilaginous incision of Heermann (see **Fig. 3.23**).

Kazikdas et al. (2007) harvests the cartilage graft from the cymba.

Cutting and Shaping of the Cartilage Strips

The harvested piece of cartilage is covered with perichondrium on both sides. The perichondrium is removed from the convex side—which is the anterior side of the tragal cartilage and the posterior side of the conchal cartilage. The removed perichondrium has several applications (see Chapter 4).

Small strips are 0.9–1.0 mm wide, which is the thickness of conchal or tragal cartilage. With a perpendicular cut through the tragal cartilage, a thick strip (0.4–0.6 mm), or a thin (0.2–0.3 mm) strip can be made. The perichondrium is attached on one side only and will measure between 0.2 and 0.6 mm, depending on the thickness of the strips (**Fig. 7.4a**).

Small strips cut from a concave piece of concha or cymba cartilage are usually thin (**Fig. 7.4b**).

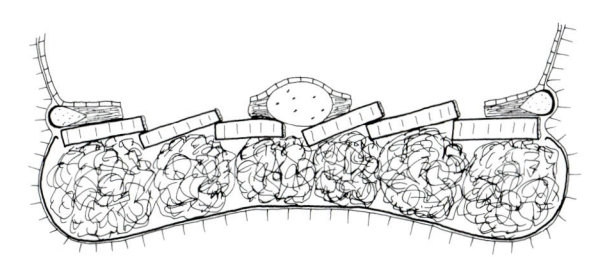

Fig. 7.3 Underlay technique with cartilage strips. Side view of the reconstructed eardrum with one-third to one-half thickness cartilage strips at the level of the umbo in a case of total perforation. The anterior strip is placed at the level of the anterior annulus and is supported by Gelfoam balls. The next strips are placed onto the previous strips like tiles on a roof.

Wide strips are 1.1–3.0 mm wide; they are thin because they are cut in an oblique manner. The perichondrium belt is small, measuring 0.2–0.3 mm (**Fig. 7.4c**). The wide and thin strips adapt better to each other (**Fig. 7.5**) than do thick strips (see **Fig. 7.3**).

Thinning the Edges of the Strips

To achieve better adaptation of the edges of the strips and to avoid edges on the eardrum, which may disturb epithelialization of the eardrum, I propose thinning of some edges of the strips (**Fig. 7.6a–c**).

Eardrums reconstructed using edge-free strips appear better, with less prominent or lower edges, and have faster epithelialization (**Fig. 7.7**).

More Perichondrium on the Cartilage Strips

In Chapter 4, I argued for cartilage palisades covered with perichondrium on both sides, and more likely advantages than disadvantages were noted.

In the cartilage strip method the lack of perichondrium is evident: In a thin, wide cartilage strip, only a strip of 2 mm is present. By cutting the tragal or conchal cartilage, covered on both sides with perichondrium, two strips of perichondrium will be attached on two edges of each strip (**Fig. 7.8**), with a 100% increase in the perichondrium covering.

When cutting the edges of strips with perichondrium, small flaps of preserved perichondrium are created. These flaps become connected to the neighboring strips (**Fig. 7.9**)

7 Cartilage Strips in Underlay Tympanoplasty Techniques

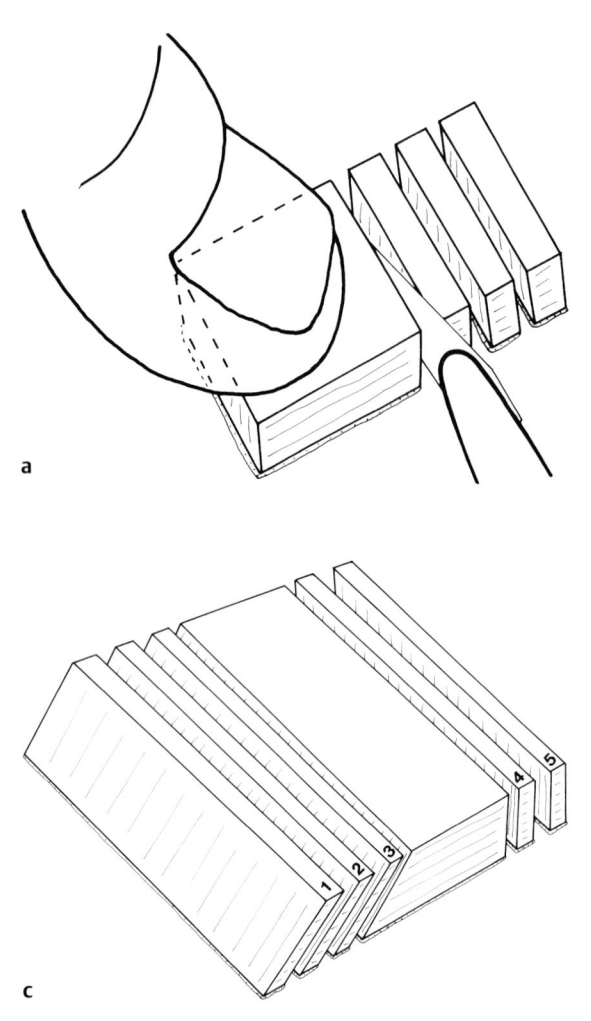

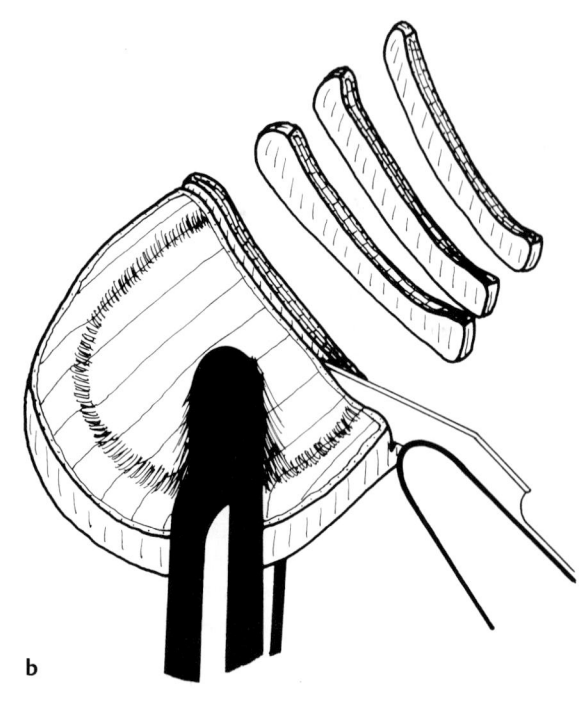

Fig. 7.4a–c Cutting and shaping of the cartilage strips.
a Perpendicular cuts of the tragal cartilage result in small strips with various thickness. The perichondrium is on one end only and measures 0.2–0.6 mm.
b Cutting cartilage strips from a slightly concave piece of concha cartilage with perichondrium on the concave side. The strips are thin and small.
c Comparison of cutting broad or the small cartilage strips. Strips cut in an oblique manner are broad (1, 2, 3), strips cut in the perpendicular manner are small (cuts 4 and 5).

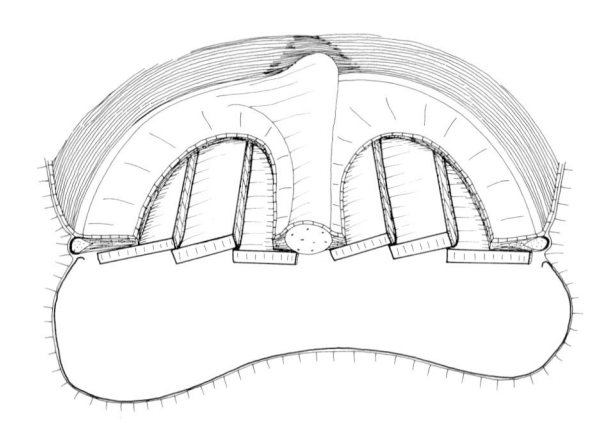

Fig. 7.5 Side view with some perspective of the superior half of the eardrum in a total perforation closed with underlay grafting with cartilage strips. The edge of the perforation and the border of the eardrum are cleaned of keratinized epithelium. The epithelium on the outer aspect of the malleus handle is left in place. The anterior strip is placed under the anterior border of the perforation. Subsequent strips are positioned on the edge of the preceding strip, slightly overlapping each other like roof tiles.

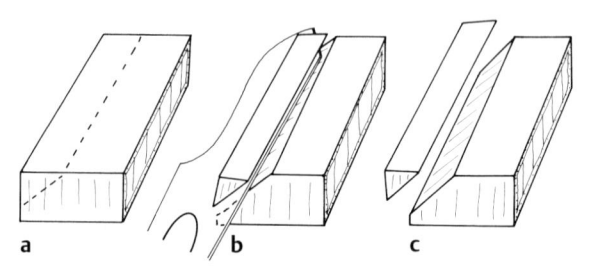

Fig. 7.6a–c Cutting the edges of thick cartilage strips.
a Normal thick strip.
b Using a scalpel with a No. 15 blade, the edge of the strip is cut off.
c The edge has been cut off and the edge of the neighboring cartilage strip can be placed on the lower edge.

Indications for Cartilage Strips in Underlay Techniques

Indications for underlay tympanoplasty with cartilage strips are the same as for cartilage palisade tympanoplasty:
- Posterosuperior retractions and perforations
- Atelectasis and adhesive otitis media
- Total and subtotal retractions and perforations
- Ears with poor tubal function; ears with negative preoperative Valsalva maneuver
- Ears with thick and moist middle ear mucosa
- Recurrent surgery
- Reconstruction of previous radical cavities without ossicles

If the results turn out be better and more stable in the long-term than can be achieved with fascia or perichondrium, the indications for surgery can be widened to cases with sequelae of chronic otitis media with good tubal function.

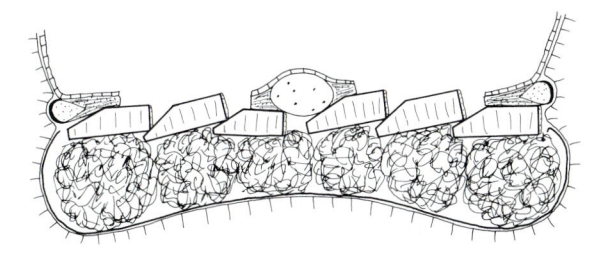

Fig. 7.7 Side view of a reconstructed eardrum, using thick strips with edges removed. The cartilage strips are placed onto the cut and chamfered edge of the previous strip, resulting in a thinner and smoother eardrum without sharp edges.

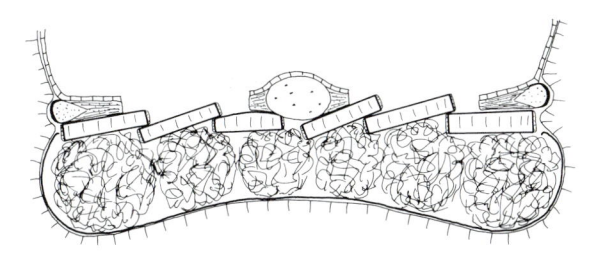

Fig. 7.8 Side view of a reconstructed eardrum using strips with perichondrium on both edges.

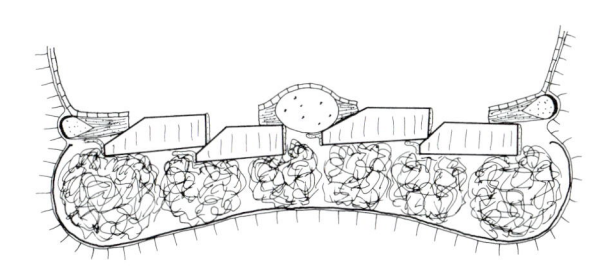

Fig. 7.9 Side view of a reconstructed eardrum using thick strips with perichondrium on both edges and with chamfered edges. The small flaps of perichondrium at the cut edges are turned onto the neighboring strip.

Surgical Techniques

All three approaches—transcanal, endaural, and retroauricular—can be used depending on the pathology and the surgeon's philosophy, otosurgical school of thought and personal preference. The techniques differ when dealing with various perforations and various ossiculoplasties.

Posterior Perforation

Posterior perforation and the posterior pathologies will most often be treated in underlay swing-door technique. To be able to see any remnants of a retraction and observe the condition of the ossicles, the posterior tympanomeatal flap has to be elevated.

Underlay Cartilage Strip Technique in Tympanoplasty Type 1

First, the edges of the perforation are cleaned and the undersurface of the eardrum scarified; then two tympanomeatal flaps are elevated. Some bone from the scutum is removed by drilling (**Fig. 7.10a**). The first strip is placed along the malleus handle and onto Gelfoam balls in the tympanic cavity. The subsequent strips are placed onto the edges of the preceding strips (**Fig. 7.10b**). Inferiorly, Gelfoam supports the strips; superiorly, they are lying on the chorda tympani. The cartilage strips are relatively light and after replacement of the tympanomeatal flaps they will adhere to the replaced and scarified eardrum remnant (**Fig. 7.10c**). Additional support of Gelfoam is not needed. Placement of Gelfoam on the ear canal side for 3 weeks will further stabilize the strips.

Underlay Cartilage Strip Technique in Tympanoplasty Type 3

A titanium columella is placed onto the footplate. The head of the columella is stabilized by the chorda tympani. The first strip is placed along the malleus handle and onto the head of the columella (**Fig. 7.11a**). The edges of the following strips are placed onto the preceding strips (**Fig. 7.11b**) and the tympanomeatal flap with the eardrum remnant is replaced (**Fig. 7.11c**).

7 Cartilage Strips in Underlay Tympanoplasty Techniques

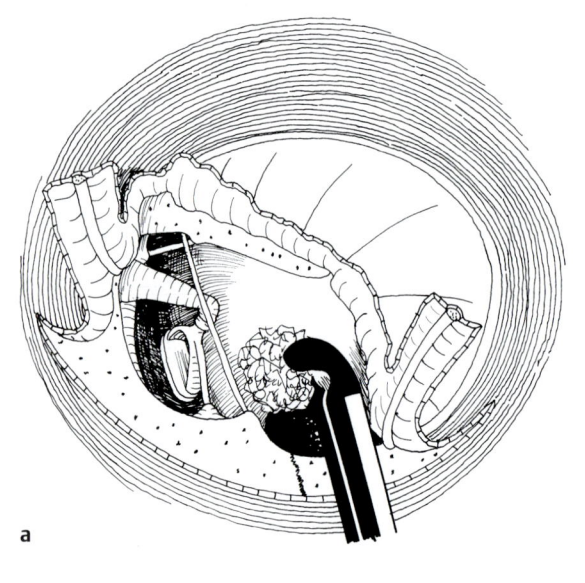

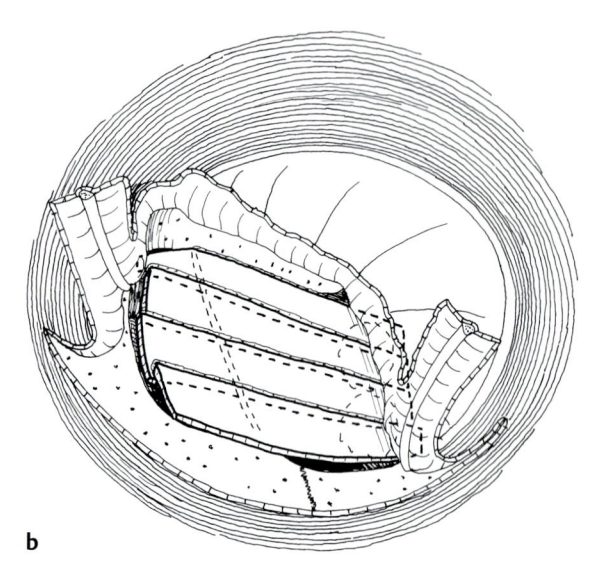

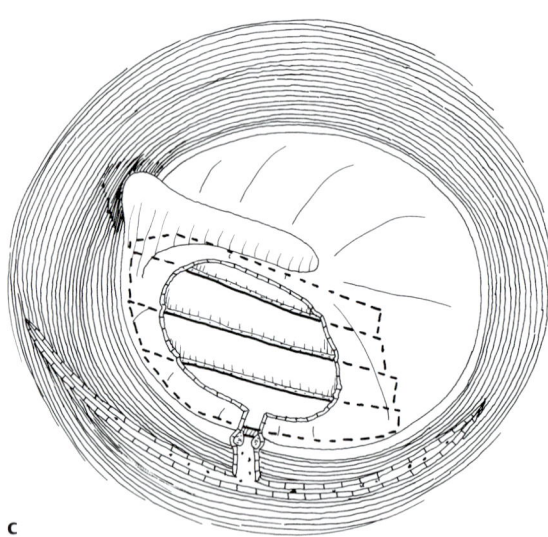

Fig. 7.10a–c Underlay cartilage strips in posterior perforation with intact ossicular chain.

a The edges of the perforation are removed, and the mucosa of the eardrum remnant is scarified. In swing-door technique, two tympanomeatal flaps are elevated. Gelfoam balls are placed into the tympanic cavity.

b The anterior strip is placed along the malleus handle and onto the chorda tympani. The following strips are placed onto the edges of the previous strips. The inferior ends of the strips are supported with Gelfoam balls, the superior ends are resting on the chorda tympani.

c After replacement of the tympanomeatal flaps and the eardrum remnants, the strips will adhere to the scarified undersurface of the eardrum remnant.

Inferior Perforation

Underlay Cartilage Strip Technique without Tympanomeatal Flap

This technique can easily be performed with underlay placement of the cartilage strips. The inferior half of the tympanic cavity is filled with Gelfoam balls and the anterior strip is placed under the anterior eardrum remnant (**Fig. 7.12a**). The edge of each of the next strips is placed onto the its neighboring strip (**Fig. 7.12b**).

Underlay Cartilage Strip Technique with Large Tympanomeatal Flap

This technique provides a good view of the tympanic cavity. To achieve this, the edges of the perforation have first to be cleaned and the undersurface of the eardrum scarified. This is best done before elevation of the eardrum. The inferior half of the tympanic cavity is filled with Gelfoam balls to support the cartilage strips. The first strip is placed at the level of the anterior bony annulus. The edges of the remaining strips are placed onto the previously placed strips (**Fig. 7.13a**). The scarified eardrum will adhere to the strips after replacement of the tympanomeatal flap (**Fig. 7.13b**).

Total Perforation

Total and subtotal perforation, especially as a result of removal of a total retraction, adhesive otitis, or tensa retraction cholesteatoma, will often be reconstructed with the underlay cartilage tympanoplasty, using either palisades (see Chapter 4), strips, or total cartilage–perichondrium composite island graft (see Chapter 17). The most

Surgical Techniques   119

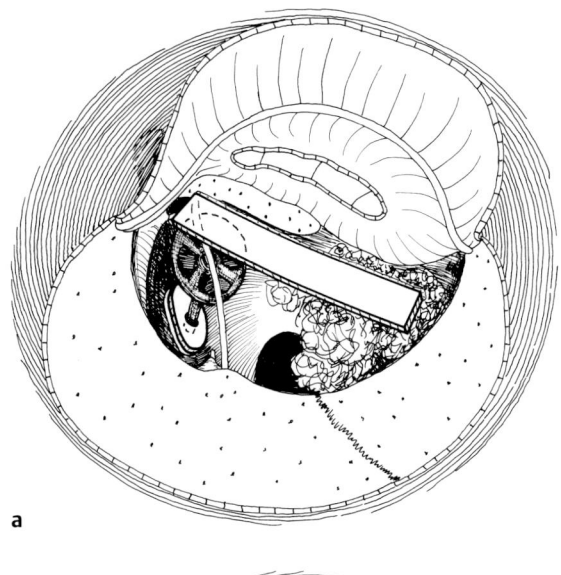

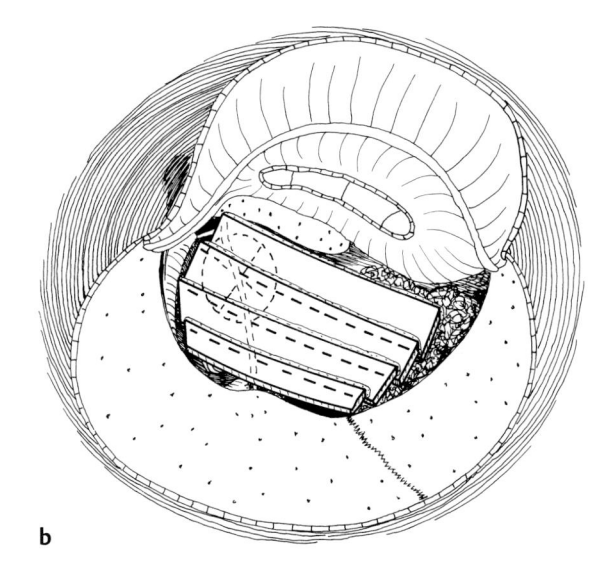

Fig. 7.11a–c Cartilage strip tympanoplasty of type 3 in posterior perforation and missing stapes crura.

a The edges of the perforation are cleaned and the undersurface of the eardrum remnant is scarified. A large tympanomeatal flap is elevated. A 0.2 mm thick Hüttenbrink cartilage guide with a 0.8 mm round hole is placed onto the footplate (Hüttenbrink et al. 2004). The foot of the titanium Kurz columella is placed through the 0.8 mm hole onto the footplate. The head of the columella is stabilized by the chorda. The first strip is placed along the malleus handle and onto the head of the columella.

b The second and the third strips are placed onto the head of the columella as well. The edge of each strip is placed onto the neighboring strip. The fourth strip is placed onto the chorda and is further supported with Gelfoam.

c The tympanomeatal flap with the eardrum remnant is replaced.

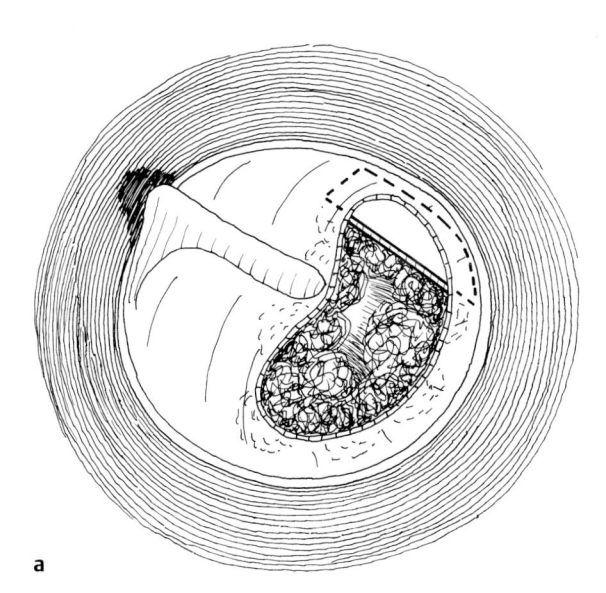

Fig. 7.12a, b Cartilage strip technique in inferior perforation without tympanomeatal flap.

a The edges of the perforation are removed and the undersurface of the eardrum is scarified. The lower part of the tympanic cavity is filled with Gelfoam balls. The first strip is placed under the anterior edge of the perforation.

b The subsequent strips are placed onto the edges of the preceding strips; the short strip on the umbo is laid similarly.

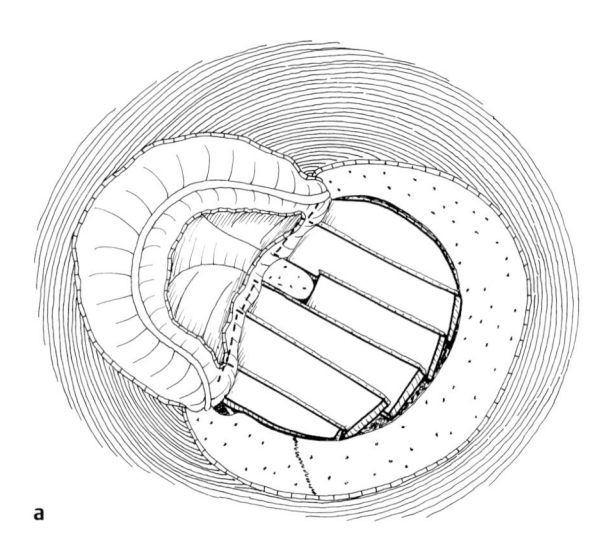

Fig. 7.13a, b Cartilage strip tympanoplasty in inferior perforation with elevation of a tympanomeatal flap.
a The tympanomeatal flap is elevated, the cavity is filled with Gelfoam balls, and the anterior strip is placed. The subsequent strips are placed on the preceding strips. The short umbo strip is placed in contact with the denuded umbo.
b The tympanomeatal flap with the eardrum remnant is replaced.

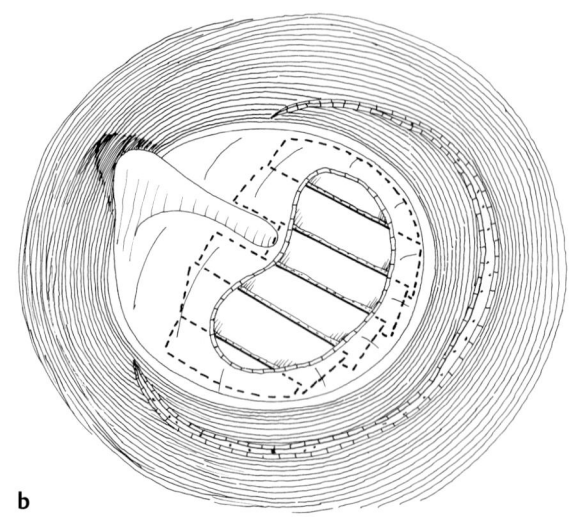

common underlay techniques start with the raising of a large tympanomeatal flap or with the swing-door technique raising two flaps.

Underlay Cartilage Strip Technique in Tympanoplasty Type 1 with the Elevation of a Large Tympanomeatal Flap

The tympanic cavity is filled with Gelfoam balls (**Fig. 7.14a**) The first strip is placed at the level of the bony annulus and is adapted to the curve of the bony annulus. The following strips are placed with their edges on the edges of the preceding strips (**Fig. 7.14b**). After replacement of the tympanomeatal flap and the eardrum remnant (**Fig. 7.14c**), and after solid packing of the ear canal for 3 weeks, conditions for complete epithelialization are good.

Underlay Cartilage Strip Technique in Tympanoplasty Type 2 with Interposition of a Shaped Autogenous Incus

A large tympanomeatal flap is elevated. Gelfoam is placed in the tympanic cavity. The incus is removed and shaped; in particular the lateral aspect of the incus is flattened to accommodate the cartilage strips, and it is placed onto the stapes head. The anterior strip is shaped in relation to the bony annulus (**Fig. 7.15a**). The edge of the next strip is placed onto the edge of the preceding strip. The strips also lie on the short process of the incus. The short malleus strip is placed under the umbo. The posterior strips are placed onto the flattened incus (**Fig. 7.15b**). The replaced scarified eardrum remnant adheres to the strips (**Fig. 7.15c**).

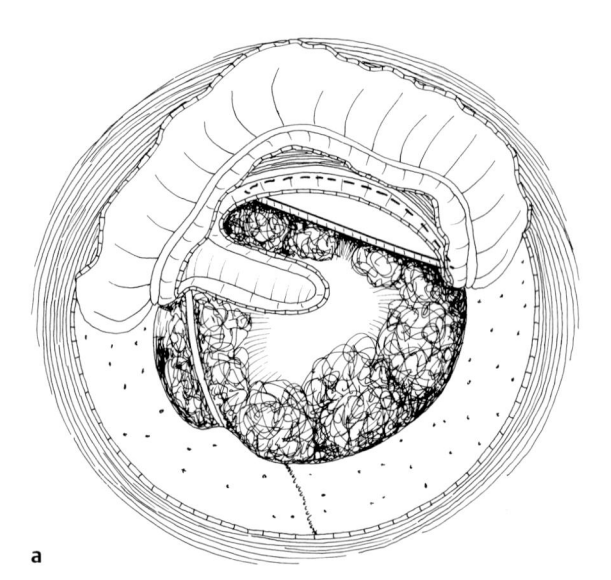

Fig. 7.14a–c Cartilage strip tympanoplasty type 1 in total perforation with intact ossicular chain.
a The edges of the perforation are removed, the undersurface of the ear drum is scarified, and the tympanic cavity is filled with Gelfoam. The anterior strip is placed close to the bony annulus.

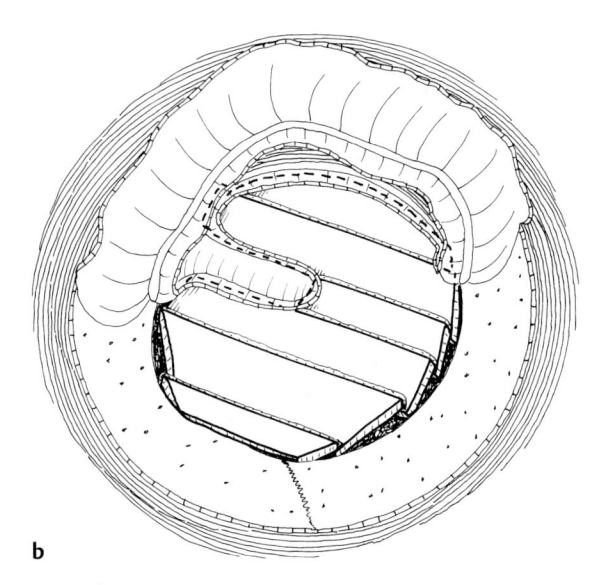

Fig. 7.14b, c
b The edge of the next palisade is placed onto the anterior palisade; the other palisades are placed on the edges of the neighboring palisades.

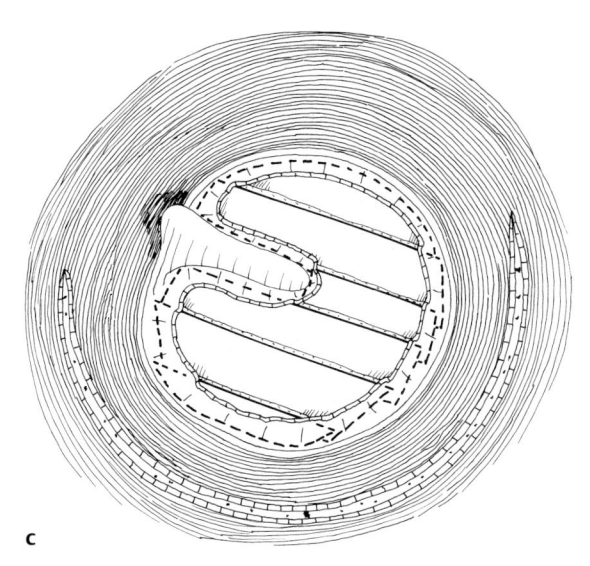

c The tympanomeatal flap with the eardrum remnant is replaced.

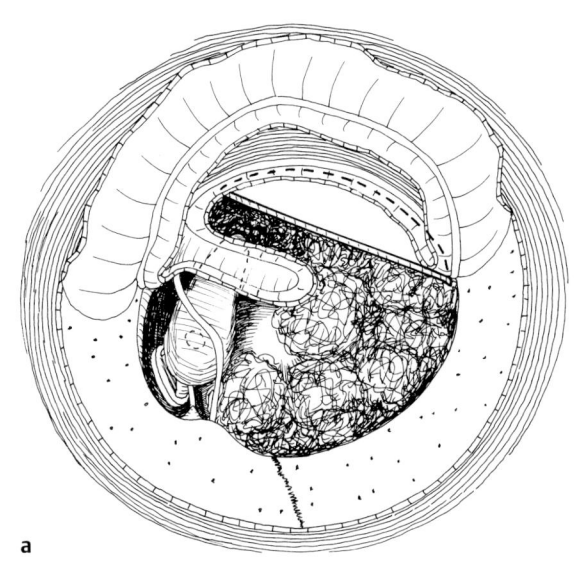

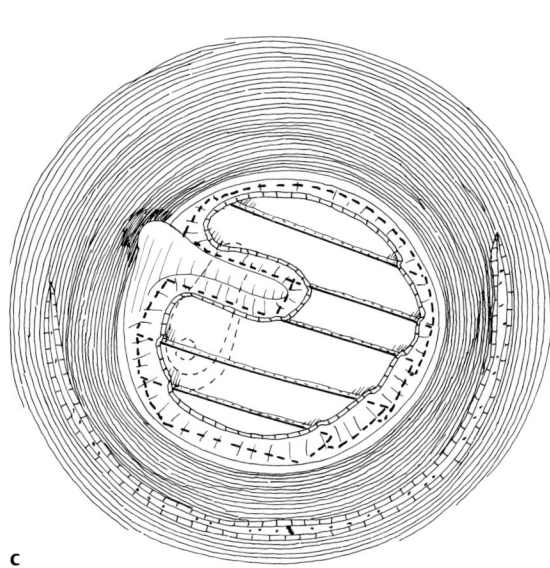

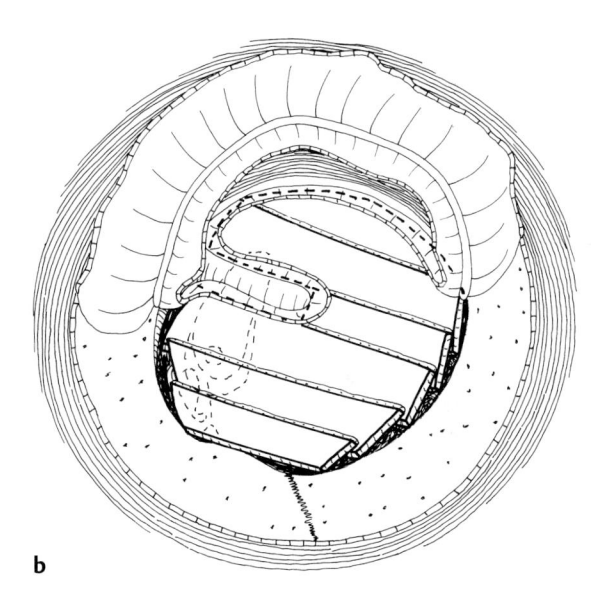

Fig. 7.15a–c Cartilage strip tympanoplasty type 2 with incus interposition in a total perforation and missing long process of the incus.
a The defective incus is removed, shaped, flattened, and placed onto the stapes head. The thinned short process is placed under the malleus handle. The cavity is filled with Gelfoam and the first palisade is placed under the anterior remnant of the eardrum.
b Subsequent strips are placed onto the edges of the previous palisades.
c The tympanomeatal flap with the eardrum remnant is replaced.

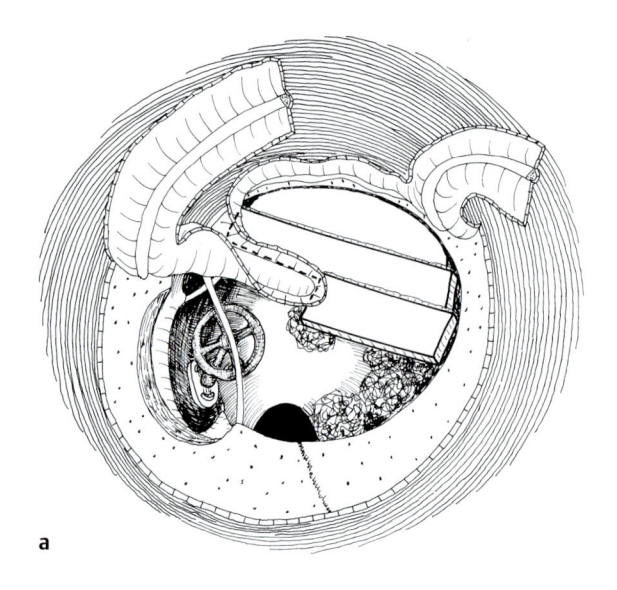

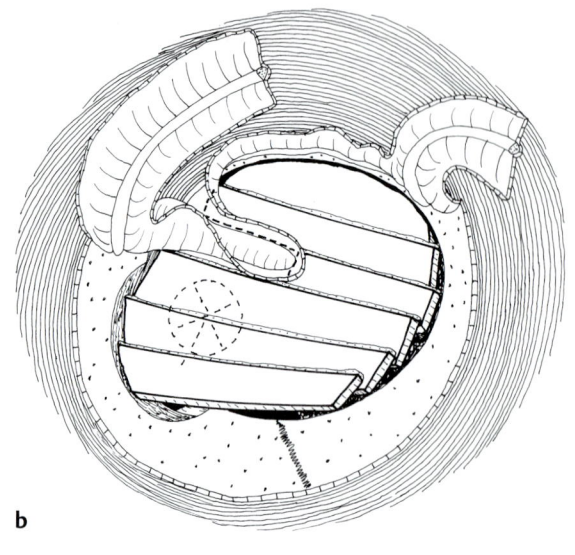

Fig. 7.16a–c Cartilage underlay strip tympanoplasty type 3 in total perforation and missing stapes.
a The edges of the perforation have been removed, and the undersurface of the eardrum has been scarified. Two tympanomeatal flaps are elevated in a swing-door technique. The tympanic cavity is filled with Gelfoam. The missing stapes is replaced with the Kurz TORP columella, placed onto the footplate. The anterior strip is placed under the anterior border of the eardrum, close to the bony annulus. The next two strips are placed with their edges on the neighboring palisades.
b The posterior strips are placed onto the head of the columella like roof tiles.
c The tympanomeatal flaps with the eardrum remnant are replaced.

Underlay Cartilage Strip Technique in Tympanoplasty Type 3 with Placement of a Kurz Titanium Columella between the Footplate and the Eardrum

In a swing-door technique, two tympanomeatal flaps are elevated, providing good visualization of the anterior part of the tympanic cavity. After the usual work on the eardrum remnant and placement of Gelfoam in the tympanic cavity, the titanium columella is placed onto the footplate. The anterior and posterior strips are placed like roof tiles (**Fig. 7.16a, b**). The posterior strips are positioned on the head of the prosthesis. The replaced tympanomeatal flaps further stabilize the strips (**Fig. 7.16c**).

Tunnelplasty

To keep the first anterior strip in a lateral position, small cubes of cartilage are placed in the anterior attic, mostly onto the eminence of the eustachian tube, and the hypotympanum (**Fig. 7.17**). This is done especially in cases with open anterior attic and missing malleus, or after canal wall down mastoidectomy. Neumann fairly often performed tunnelplasty to support middle ear aeration by keeping open the tympanic ostium of the eustachian tube (Neumann 1999; Neumann et al. 2002, 2003).

Reconstruction of the Eardrum and the Attic Wall with Cartilage Strips

In cases of total perforation and attic wall defect or posterosuperior scutum defect, Neumann (1999) begins by first placing cartilage strips in inferosuperior direction to cover the total perforation (**Fig. 7.18a**) and then 3–4 strips to cover, in an oblique anteroposterior direction, the attic defect and the superior ends of the posterior strips (**Fig. 7.18b, c**). This excellent principle of Neumann, with double covering of bony defects of the superior and posterosuperior attic defects, can be extended to larger bony defects.

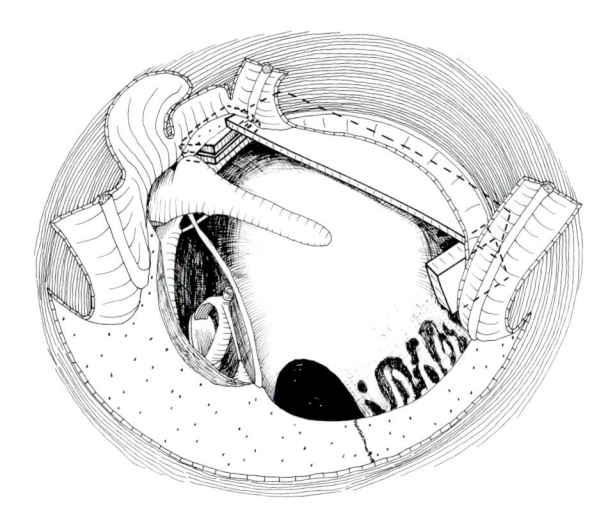

Fig. 7.17 A tunnelplasty with a cartilage strip. Two small pieces of cartilage are placed onto the eminence of tensor tympani muscle. The anterior strip is placed under the eardrum remnant supported by the small piece of cartilage placed vertically in the hypotympanum, under the inferior end of the strip.

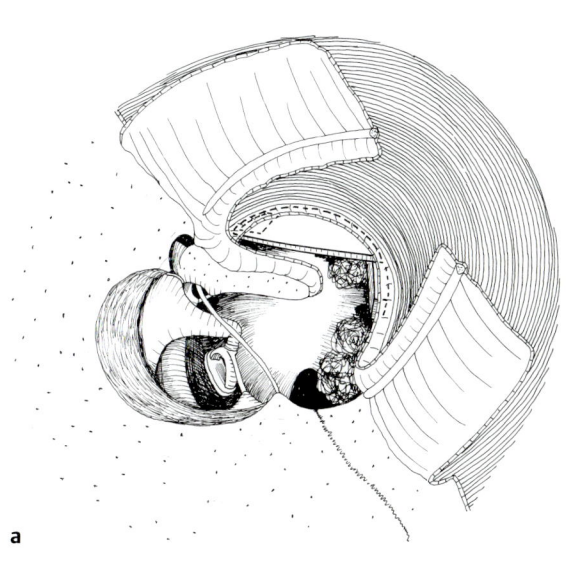

Fig. 7.18a–c Reconstruction of bony defects in the attic with cartilage strips.
a   In retroauricular approach, atticotomy and tunnelplasty are performed. The edges of the total perforation are cleaned, the undersurface of the eardrum remnant is scarified, and the tympanic cavity is filled with Gelfoam balls.
b   The total perforation is covered with anterior cartilage strips as usual. The long posterior strips continue up to the drilling of the attic and are solidly supported by the bone, closing the attic defect.
c   Three cartilage strips are placed in an oblique anteroposterior direction and will be totally covered by the two large tympanomeatal flaps.

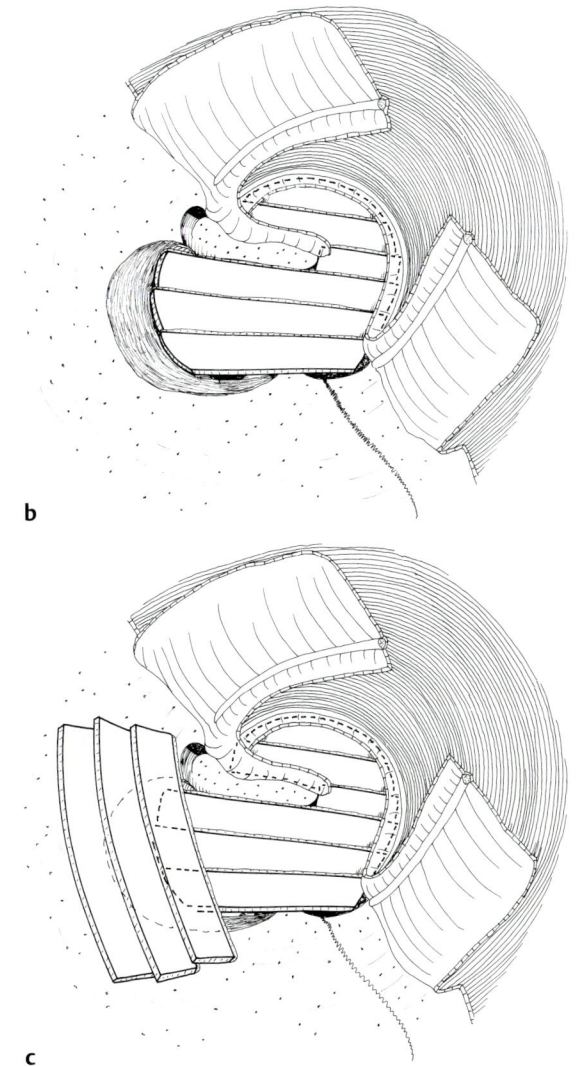

Covering the Cartilage Strips with Perichondrium

As indicated previously, the presence of more perichondrium on the cartilage strips will be advantageous. Kazikdas et al. (2007) in fact modified the underlay cartilage strip method by using the perichondrium at the end of surgery to cover the strips. The perichondrium can be placed as on-lay graft or as partly on-lay, partly underlay graft (as used by Ferekidis et al. [2003] in his modification of the cartilage palisade technique [see **Figs. 4.18a–h, 4.19d, 4.20c, 4.21**]) or as an underlay graft (as used by Dubreuil [personal communication 2006] in his modification of cartilage palisade technique [see **Fig. 4.23e, f**]).

Kazikdas et al. (2007) did not make clear whether the perichondrium is placed as an underlay or on-lay graft, but this is of little importance. What is important is the improved possibility of adhesion of the small strips with the corresponding perichondrium to the laterally placed perichondrium, which will be epithelialized and vascularized.

Table 7.1 Pre- and postoperative air–bone gap (mean of 0.5, 1, 2, and 4 kHz) in 84 ears, 1–3 years after cartilage strip underlay technique

Air–bone gap (dB)	No. of ears	
	Preoperative	Postoperative
0–10	2	25
11–30	48	50
31–50	34	9

Table 7.2 Pre- and postoperative air–bone gap (mean of 0.5, 1, 2, and 4 kHz) in 30 ears with intact ossicular chain and tympanoplasty type 1, 1–3 years after surgery

Air–bone gap (dB)	No. of ears	
	Preoperative	Postoperative
0–10	1	19
11–30	20	10
31–50	9	1

Table 7.3 Pre- and postoperative air–bone gap (mean of 0.5, 1, 2, and 4 kHz) in 31 ears with tympanoplasty type 2 with interposition of a PORP prosthesis (22 ears) or with a cartilage anulus–stapes plate (CASP) (9 ears)

Air–bone gap (dB)	No. of ears			
	Preoperative		Postoperative	
	PORP	CASP	PORP	CASP
0–10	0	0	0	2
11–30	13	5	14	7
31–50	9	4	8	0

Results of Surgery

Neumann et al. (2002) published results of 84 ears operated by the cartilage strip method at the Hospital of Neuss during the 2-year period from October 1997 to October 1999.

Indications for Surgery
Surgery was performed for the following indications: cholesteatoma in 28 ears, adhesive otitis in 22 ears, dry subtotal perforation in 17 ears, chronic mesotympanic otitis in 12 ears, and second-look operation in 5 ears.

Ossicular Chain, Ossiculoplasty and Tympanoplasty Type
In 30 ears the ossicular chain was intact and tympanoplasty type 1 was performed. In 22 ears the incus was defective but the stapes was intact and a tympanoplasty type 2 was performed with interposition of the titanium PORP prosthesis between the stapes head and the eardrum with the malleus handle. In 9 ears with intact stapes an annulus–stapes–plate method (see **Fig. 1.8c**) of Heermann was used (Heermann et al. 1970).

In 23 ears the stapes was absent; tympanoplasty type 3 was performed and the titanium TORP prosthesis was placed onto the footplate.

Postoperative Evaluation
The first evaluation was performed 1–3 years after the surgery (mean 21 months).

Anatomical results at the Evaluation
The cartilage strips were visible in all ears and were not fused into a cartilage plate. In 2 ears (2.4%) a recurrent perforation was found. No extrusion of the titanium prosthesis was found.

Hearing Results
The air–bone gap was better 1–3 years after surgery (**Table 7.1**) in the entire series of 84 ears.

From 30 ears with intact ossicular chain and tympanoplasty type 1 the postoperative air–bone gap was within 10 dB in 19 ears (63%) (**Table 7.2**). This is in fact the most important message in relation to effectiveness of the underlay cartilage strip technique. However, a more detailed analysis of hearing, by splitting the 11–30 dB group into an 11–20 dB and a 21–30 dB group will allow a better comparison with the PORP group and TORP group as well as with the annulus–stapes-plate group.

In 31 ears the stapes was present; a tympanoplasty type 2, with interposition of a PORP prosthesis between stapes head and the eardrum was performed in 22 ears and a Heermann annulus–stapes-plate in 9 ears (**Table 7.3**).

The results with PORP prosthesis were surprisingly poor. Not one ear had the air–bone gap improved to a better level than 10 dB. Among the 9 patients with the annulus–stapes plate, 2 ears (22%) had the air–bone gap improved within 10 dB. In comparison with tympano-

Table 7.4 Pre-and postoperative air–bone gap (mean of 0.5, 1, 2, and 4 kHz) in 23 ears with tympanoplasty type 3, using titanium TORP prosthesis, placed onto the footplate

Air–bone gap (dB)	No. of ears	
	Preoperative	Postoperative
0–10	1	4
11–30	10	19
31–50	12	0

Table 7.5 Mean preoperative and postoperative PTA-ABG in 34 ears inserted a TORP and in 27 ears inserted a PORP during cartilage strip tympanoplasty

PTA-ABG (dB)	No. of ears			
	Preoperative		Postoperative	
	TORP	PORP	TORP	PORP
0–10	1	0	9	2
11–30	15	15	24	17
31–50	18	12	1	8

plasty type 1 with 63 % air–bone gap closure within 10 dB, the achievement with PORP prosthesis was poor.

The results of 23 ears with tympanoplasty type 3 and TORP prosthesis were satisfactory (**Table 7.4**) in relation to the severity of the series. Air–bone gap closure within 10 dB was achieved in 4 ears (17 %).

In a second evaluation of 61 ears by Neumann et al. (2003), 27 ears with tympanoplasty type 2 (titanium PORP) and 34 ears with tympanoplasty type 3 (titanium TORP) were included. The mean follow-up time was 38 months, range 375–1265 days (Neumann et al. 2003). Here only ears with cartilage strip tympanoplasty and titanium prosthesis of the Tübingen type of Kurz were studied and compared.

The anatomical results were the same as previously, with no graft failures and no retractions.

The hearing results were evaluated as pure tone average minus air–bone gap average (PTA-ABG) for frequencies 0.5, 1, 2, and 4 kHz and the difference in hearing between the PORP series and the TORP series was compared (**Table 7.5**). The hearing results were surprisingly poor in the PORP series compared with the TORP series and ears with intact ossicular chain.

Comparison of Results of Underlay Cartilage Strip Technique with Fascia Grafting

Kazikdas et al. (2007) presented a comparison between results with fascia on 28 ears, and with underlay cartilage strips on 23 ears operated during a 6-year period from 2000 to 2006. Both groups can be classified in the group of sequelae of chronic otitis media without cholesteatoma.

Pathology and Indications
In both groups the perforations were subtotal, and the ossicular chain was intact. The ears were dry with normal middle ear mucosa at least one month before operation.

Observation Period
The mean follow-up period was 18.7 months, range 7–33 months.

Anatomical Results
Graft take was achieved in 22 ears (95.7 %) with cartilage strip technique, and in the fascia group in 21 ears (75 %). The difference did not reach but was close to the level of statistical significance ($p = 0.059$). The only small perforation in the cartilage group was presumably caused by dislocation of the strips.

Hearing Results
Pure-tone average (PTA): *Cartilage group:* preoperative 31.4 ± 10.7 dB; postoperative 22.4 ± 12.0 dB. *Fascia group:* preoperative 42.2 ± 14.6 dB; postoperative 29.7 ± 17.0 dB. The differences are not statistically significant, but there is a tendency to better hearing in the cartilage group.

Air–bone gap (ABG) and speech reception threshold (SRT): Differences were not statistically significant but there was a tendency to smaller air–bone gap in the cartilage group.

Conclusion on Results of the Underlay Cartilage Strip Technique

The anatomical results are apparently the same as, or even better than, with fascia.

The hearing results are based on two existing reports on series with intact ossicular chain (Neumann et al. 2002, 2003). Hearing was good and definitively not poorer than that achieved with fascia (Kazikdas et al. 2007). The use of light cartilage strips seems not to produce any deterioration in postoperative hearing.

More clinical research is needed in relation to the poorer results with PORP than with TORP prostheses.

Author's Comments and Recommendations

It is my hope that separation of the cartilage palisade method from the cartilage strips method will be broadly accepted, allowing the possibility of comparison of the long-term results between the two methods.

By oblique cutting of the cartilage graft, the strips may be made thin. With rectangular cutting, thick strips can be made. The hearing of reconstructed eardrums with thin strips can be directly compared with the hearing of eardrums reconstructed using thick strips. Thus the influence of the thickness of the reconstructed eardrum on hearing can be directly investigated in terms of the cartilage strip method. Such a study cannot be performed for the palisade method.

Placement of the strips like roof tiles allows some support from the adjacent strips. In this way reconstructed eardrum appears solid after completed epithelialization.

Because the strips are lighter than the palisades, support by Gelfoam is presumed to be sufficient, in addition to the tendency of the strips to adhere to the undersurface of the eardrum. Support of the cartilage strips by placement of pieces of cartilage in the hypotympanum and/or in the epitympanum may be used in a few difficult cases.

If further clinical studies show results at least as good as or better than results achieved with fascia or perichondrium, the cartilage strips method will become a commonly used and popular method in the closure of dry perforations in cases with sequelae of chronic otitis media.

References

Ferekidis EA, Nikolopoulos TP, Kandiloros DC, . Chondrotympanoplasty: a modified technique of cartilage graft tympanoplasty. Med Sci Monit 2003;9:73–78.

Heermann J, Heermann H. Sieben Jahre Faszien – Knorpel- Dachschindel –Tympanoplastik und Antrum-Mastoidplastik. Z Laryngol Rhinol Otol 1967;46:370–382.

Heermann J, Heermann H, Kopstein E. Fascia and cartilage palisade tympanoplasty. Nine years' experience. Arch Otolaryngol 1970;91:228–243.

Hüttenbrink K-B, Zahnert T, Beutner D, Hofmann G. The cartilage guide: a solution for anchoring a columella prostheses on the footplate. Laryngorhinootologie 2004;83:450–456.

Kazikdas KC, Onal K, Boyraz I, Karabulut E. Palisade cartilage tympanoplasty for management of subtotal perforations: a comparison with the temporalis fascia technique. Eur Arch Otorhinolaryngol 2007;264:985–989.

Neumann A. Die "Knorpelpalisadentympanoplastik" nach Heermann. HNO 1999;47:1074–1088.

Neumann A, Hennig A, Schultz-Coulon H-J. Morphologische und funktionelle Ergebnisse der Knorpelpalisadentympanoplastik. HNO 2002;50:935–939.

Neumann A, Schultz-Coulon H-J, Jahnke K. Type 3 tympanoplasty applying the palisade cartilage technique: a study of 61 cases. Otol Neurotol 2003;24:33–37.

8   Cartilage Strips in On-lay Tympanoplasty Techniques

Definition

There are no publications in the literature dealing with on-lay technique with cartilage strips. On-lay technique with cartilage strips involves reconstruction of the eardrum by placement of thin cartilage strips in the manner of roof tiles onto the denuded eardrum remnant. I have used this technique several times in closure of various types and various sizes of eardrum perforations.

The arguments for separation of the on-lay cartilage strip method from the other cartilage methods are the same as described in Chapter 7:
1. The strips differ from the palisades in thickness, shape, and cutting.
2. The covering of the strips with the perichondrium is much more sparse than that of the palisades, which are totally covered on one side.
3. The strips are positioned like roof tiles; the palisades are placed close to each other but still with some small distance between them.

The on-lay technique requires removal or elevation of the epithelium around the perforation. Such methods are delicate and demanding but they represent the minimally invasive surgery, without raising the tympanomeatal flap with the fibrous annulus. Failure of on-lay myringoplasty is nearly always caused by the surgeon, most often because of insufficient deepithelialization of the eardrum remnant and insufficient covering of the denuded area of the eardrum.

Harvesting and Shaping of the Cartilage Strips

Harvesting and shaping the cartilage is the same as for underlay techniques described in Chapter 7. For on-lay technique, slightly shorter strips are needed than for underlay technique. Thin strips are preferred for on-lay technique, in particular in small anterior and inferior perforations, requiring oblique cutting (see **Fig. 7.4c**). I recommend harvesting the cartilage graft covered with the perichondrium on both sides. Using oblique cutting of the graft (**Fig. 8.1**), strips 0.3 mm thick and 1.5–2 mm wide strips can be cut with the perichondrium attached on both edges.

Using perpendicular cutting of the tragus or concha grafts with perichondrium on both sides, strips 0.3–0.5 mm thick and 0.9 mm wide are cut. To cover the anterior and a small inferior perforation, 0.3 mm thick strips can be used. To cover a large inferior perforation, subtotal or total perforations 0.4–0.5 mm thick strips or even thicker strips may be needed. In such cases the edges of

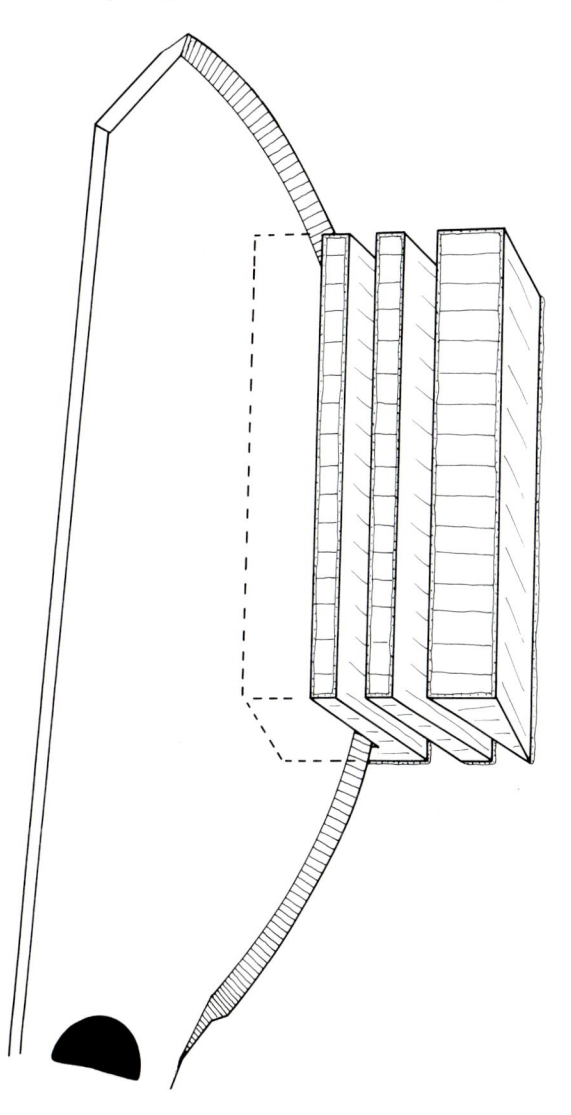

Fig. 8.1 Oblique cutting of the tragal cartilage, covered on both sides with the perichondrium, resulting in thin and thick cartilage strips. The cutting is done with a 23-blade scalpel.

the cartilage strips may be chamfered (see **Fig. 7.6a–c**) to obtain a smoother and thinner eardrum, without edges (see **Fig. 7.7**).

Indications for Surgery

Indications for use of cartilage strips instead of fascia or perichondrium are the same as for palisades, that is, in cases where a postoperative retraction is to be expected: recurrent tympanoplasty, retractions, atelectasis, adhesive otitis, cholesteatoma, ears with poor tubal function, and negative preoperative Valsalva maneuver.

If future clinical research shows that thin cartilage strips provide good and stable hearing, or even better hearing results than with fascia or perichondrium, the indications may become wider and include all perforations.

The On-lay Cartilage Strip Techniques

Anterior Perforation

In anterior perforation the on-lay technique is the most logical closure. Several different methods of elevation of epithelial flaps or removal of epithelium around the perforation may be used; here only two of the most often used methods are illustraded. On-lay methods are also described Chapters 5, 11, 12, 23 and 24, and partly in Chapters 18, 25, and 26.

Partial Elevation of Small Epithelial Flaps

After a small anterior circumferential incision, two ear canal skin flaps and a superior malleus flap are elevated. The remaining epithelium around the perforation is removed (**Fig. 8.2a**). Two thin cartilage strips, with the perichondrium on both ends are placed like roof tiles onto the denuded lamina propria (**Fig. 8.2b, c**) The epithelial flaps are replaced in such a way that parts of the cartilage strips are covered with the epithelium (**Fig. 8.2 d**).

In another method, described in Chapter 5, all epithelium around the perforation is elevated as flaps (see **Fig. 5.5b–d**). The replaced flaps can cover a substantial part of the cartilage palisades or strips (see **Fig. 5.5e**).

The Anterior Swing-Door Incision with Elevation of a Superior and an Inferior Skin Flap, Together with the Surrounding Epithelium

The eardrum epithelium is carefully elevated, including the epithelium from the malleus handle (**Fig. 8.3a, b**). After placement of two cartilage strips, to cover the perforation (**Fig. 8.3c**) the epithelium and the skin flap are replaced, covering large parts of the cartilage strips (**Fig. 8.3 d**).

A technique with elevation of a large anterior tympanomeatal flap, together with the epithelium surrounding the anterior perforation is used in Chapter 5 and is illustrated in **Fig. 5.7a–d**.

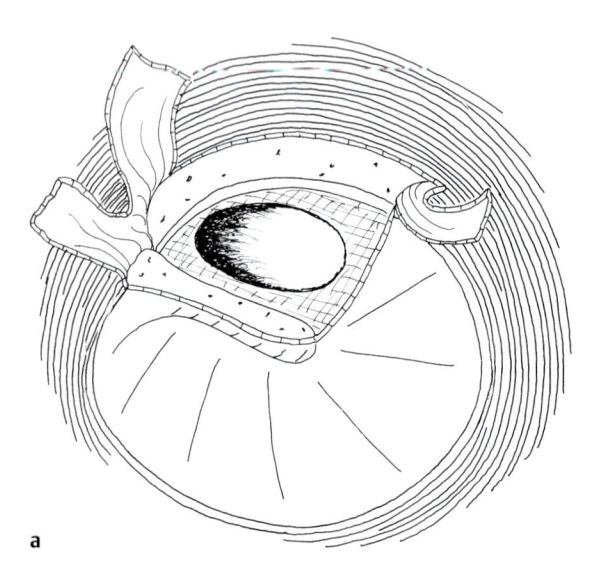

a

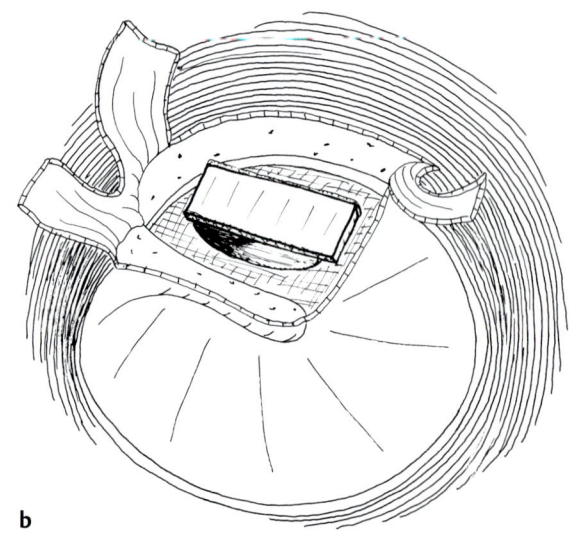

b

Fig. 8.2a–d Closure of an anterior perforation with thin cartilage strips using the method of elevation of two ear canal skin flaps and malleus flap.
a The margins of the perforation are cleaned of epithelium. After an anterior circumferential incision, inferior and superior flaps are elevated together with the epithelium. The superior malleus flap is also elevated. The perforation is ready for placement of the cartilage strips.
b The first strip is placed onto the anterior perforation.

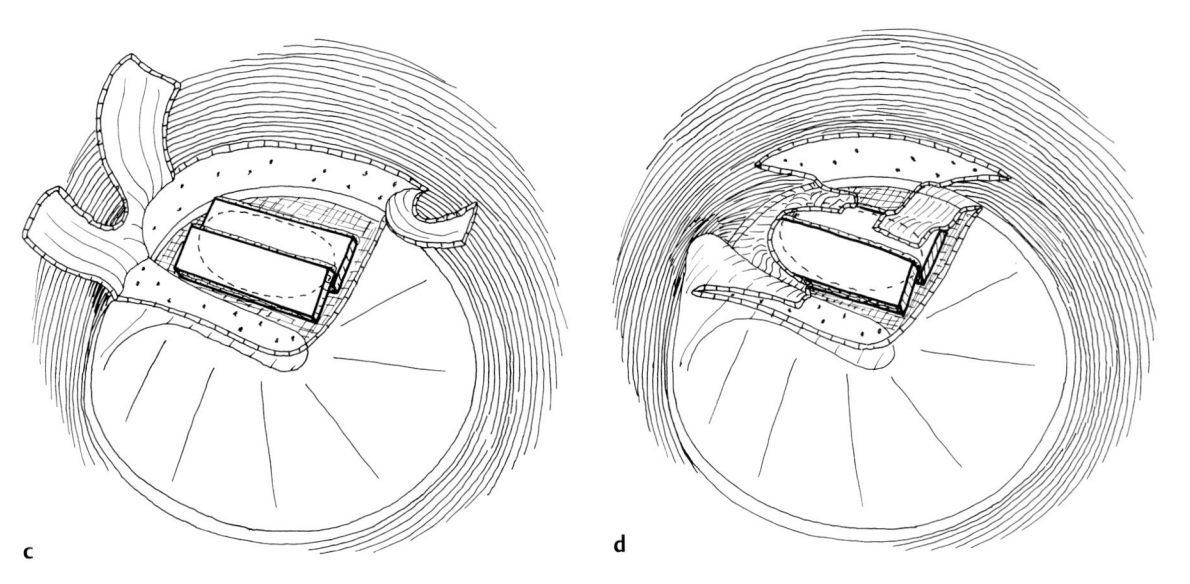

Fig. 8.2c, d
c The second strip is placed slightly overlapping the first strip. The perforation is closed.
d The skin flaps are replaced, partly covering the cartilage strips.

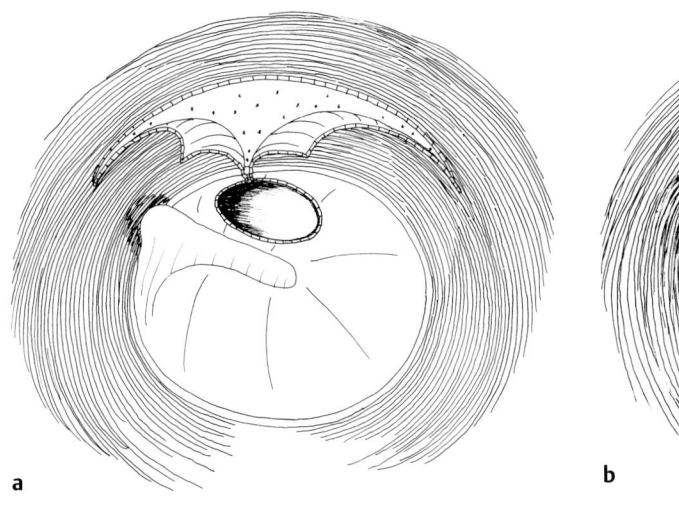

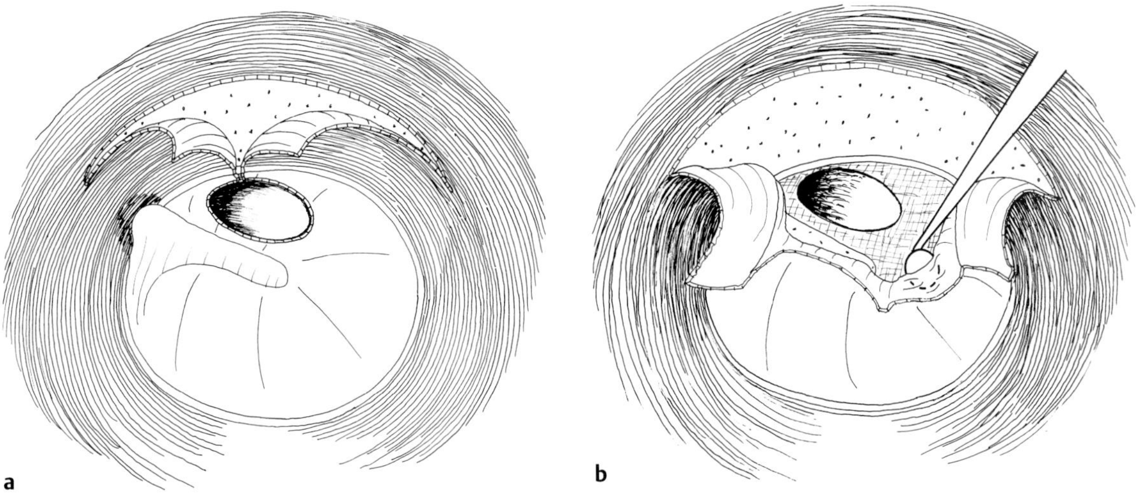

Fig. 8.3a–d The anterior swing-door incision with elevation of two skin flaps together with the epithelium surrounding the anterior perforation.
a A circumferential incision and a vertical incision at the 3-o'clock position are performed.
b Using mainly a round knife, the epithelium is carefully separated from the lamina propria. It is usually possible to preserve the intact epithelium.
c The first cartilage strip is placed onto the edges of the perforation. The second strip is partly placed onto the first.

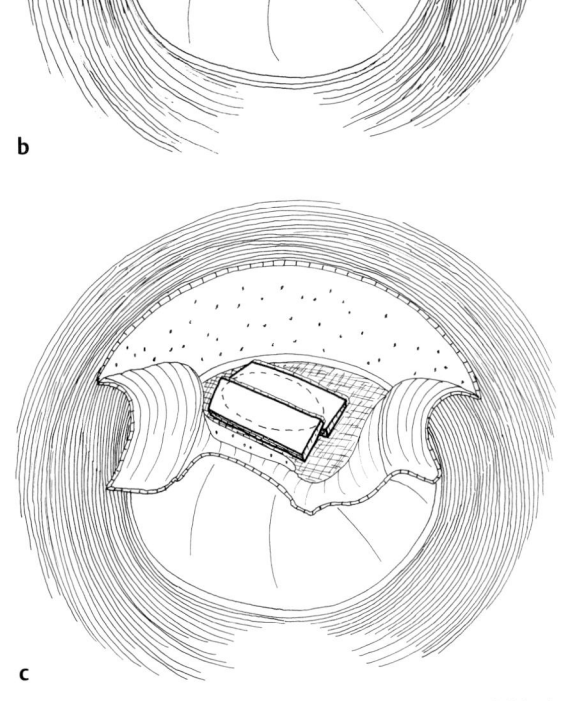

Fig. 8.3d ▷

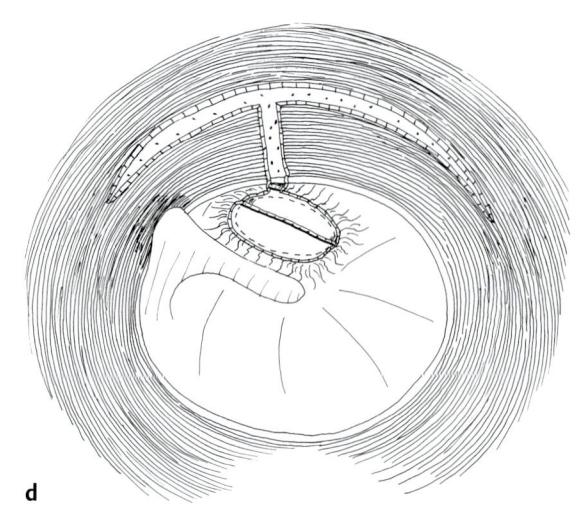

Fig. 8.3d The skin flaps are replaced, with all the epithelium.

Inferior Perforation

Inferior perforation is suitable for on-lay cartilage strip tympanoplasty and several methods of elevation or removal of the epithelium surrounding the perforation are used.

Elevation of Superior Epithelial Flaps

Along the inferior annulus the ear canal skin with the epithelium from the eardrum remnant is removed. Along the superior edge of the perforation the epithelium of the eardrum is elevated (**Fig. 8.4a**). The cartilage strips are placed like roof tiles; first the anterior strip is placed, then the next is placed onto the edge of the previous strip (**Fig. 8.4b**) and the superior flaps are replaced (**Fig. 8.4c**).

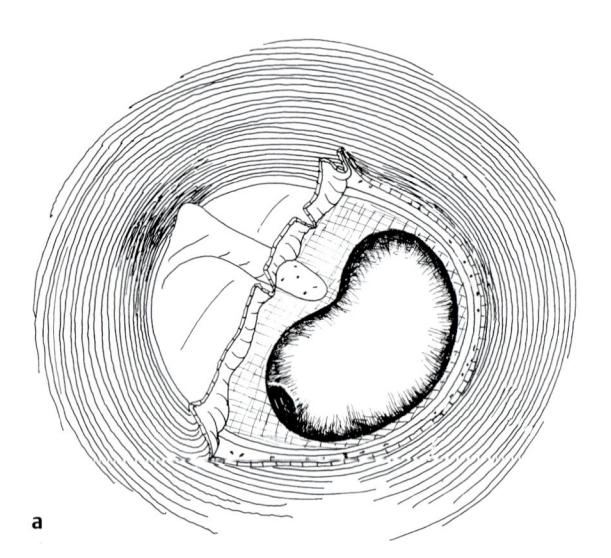

Fig. 8.4a–c Closure of a large inferior perforation with elevation of superior epithelial flaps and on-lay cartilage strip technique.
a Superiorly, the epithelial flaps are elevated. Inferiorly, after a circumferential incision, the epithelium is removed. The entire annulus and the inferior edge of the perforation are cleaned of epithelium.
b The first strip is placed onto the anterior edge of the perforation. The following strips overlapping each other slightly, like roof tiles.
c The superior flaps are replaced.

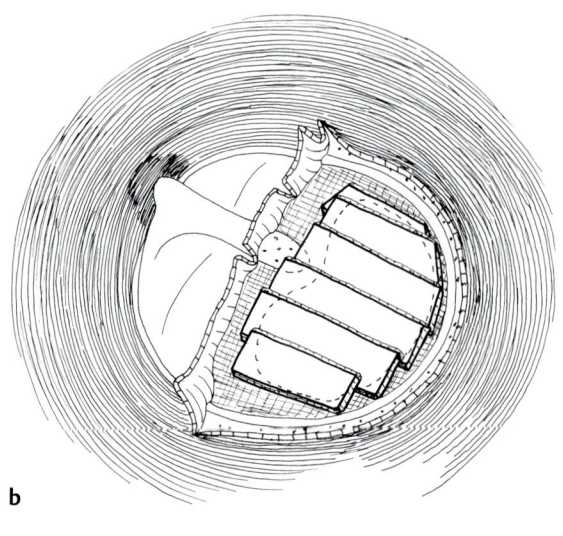

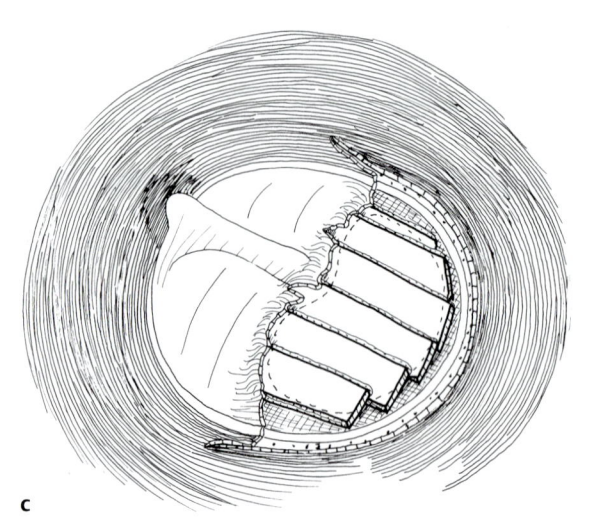

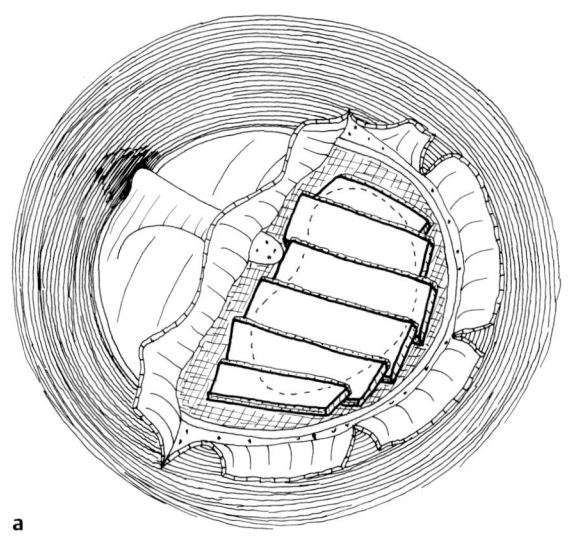

Fig. 8.5a, b Elevation of epithelium along the edges of the inferior perforation.
a First the superior epithelium is elevated, then the epithelium along the inferior border of the perforation is elevated. Thin cartilage strips with the perichondrium on both edges are placed like roof tiles onto the denuded lamina propria.
b The epithelial flaps are replaced and cover the ends of the strips.

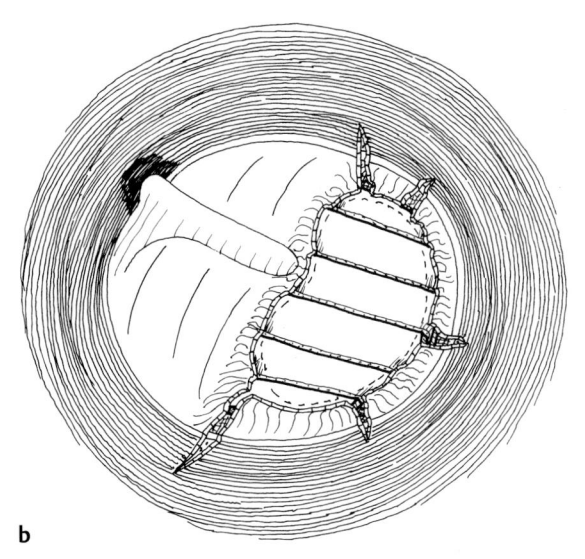

Elevation of Epithelial Flaps along the Edges of the Inferior Perforation

Superior epithelial flaps are elevated using an incudostapedial knife. Epithelium along the inferior edge of the perforation is elevated piece by piece (**Fig. 8.5a**) along the inferior fibrous annulus. The perforation is covered with six thin cartilage strips, with perichondrium on both edges and positioned like roof tiles. After replacement of all epithelial flaps (**Fig. 8.5b**) closure is solid and epithelialization rapid.

Elevation of a Large Inferior Tympanomeatal Skin Flap together with the Surrounding Eardrum Epithelium

It is often easy to elevate epithelium from the fibrous annulus and the eardrum remnant (**Fig. 8.6a**). Five cartilage strips are placed like roof tiles onto the denuded lamina propria (**Fig. 8.6b**). The epithelial flaps are replaced (**Fig. 8.6c**). Rapid epithelialization is expected because the superior and inferior ends of the cartilage strips are covered with epithelial flaps.

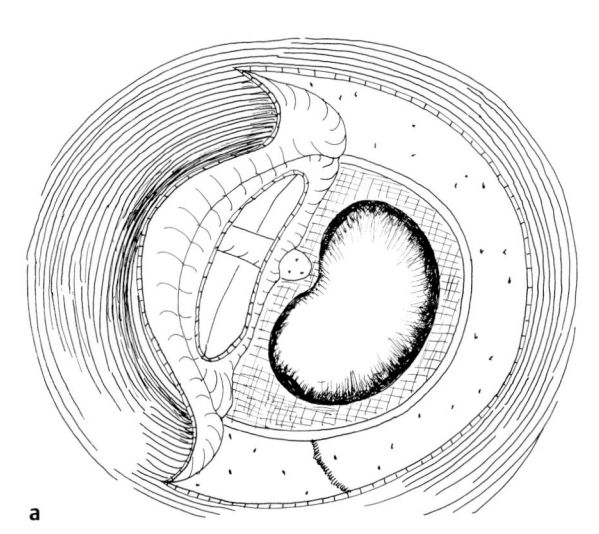

Fig. 8.6a–c Elevation of a large tympanomeatal skin flap with the eardrum epithelium surrounding a large inferior perforation.
a The borders of the perforation are cleaned. A circumferential incision is made from the 9-o'clock to the 3-o'clock position. The skin flap and the surrounding epithelium are elevated.
b Five cartilage strips cover the perforation.

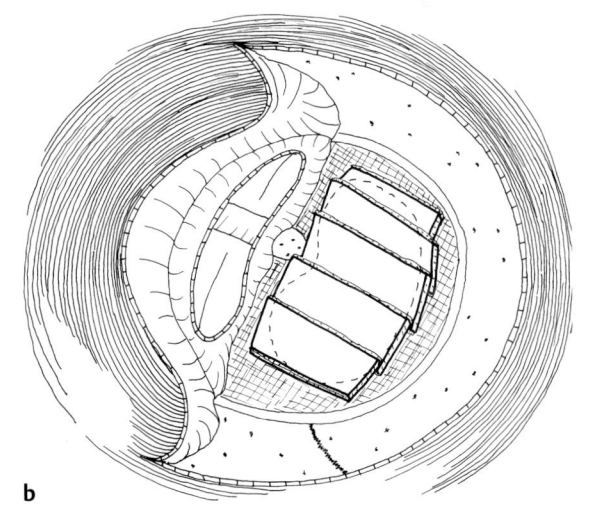

Fig. 8.6c ▷

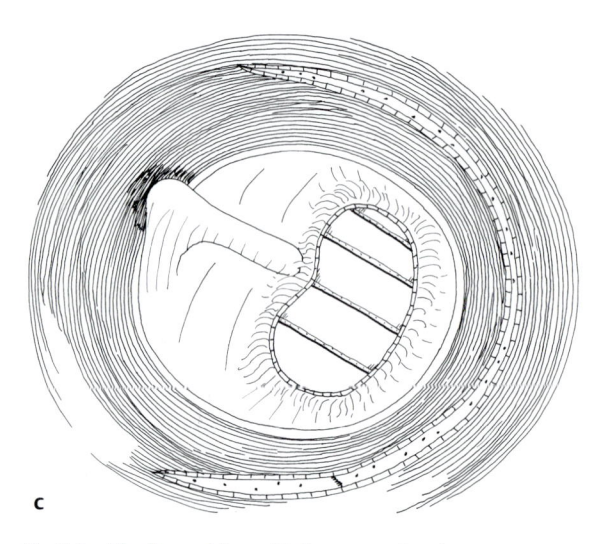

Fig. 8.6c The flap and the epithelium are replaced.

Total Perforation

The thickness of the strips can be changed in relation to the pathology of the middle ear mucosa and tubal function. With normal mucosa and normal tubal function, 0.3 mm thick and up to 3 mm wide strips should be sufficient. In case of severe pathology, such as retractions, adhesive otitis media, recurrent surgery, poor tubal function, or thick or moist middle ear mucosa, thicker cartilage strips, such as 0.4–0.5 mm, can be used.

Three methods of elevation of the skin and epithelium flaps around the perforation for on-lay techniques will be illustrated. All three methods are suitable in total perforation, subtotal perforation, and inferior perforation:
1. Technique with outward elevation of the eardrum epithelium and the skin flaps (**Fig. 8.7a**).
2. On-lay technique with elevation of three superior epithelial flaps and removal of the epithelium around the inferior border of the perforation (**Fig. 8.8a**).
3. On-lay technique with elevation of a large tympanomeatal flap together with the epithelium of the eardrum around the perforation (**Fig. 8.9a**).

Outward Elevation of the Eardrum Epithelium and the Skin Flaps

This method is a combination of my method (Tos 1980) of elevation of the three superior skin flaps, exposing the superior part of the tympanic cavity, and elevation of three epithelium–skin flaps along the inferior fibrous annulus (**Fig. 8.7a, b**). The entire denuded lamina propria and the fibrous annulus are exposed and seven thin cartilage strips are placed onto the denuded lamina propria. The strips are covered along both edges by the perichondrium and are placed like roof tiles; the second strip is placed on the edge of the first strip and the edges of the subsequent strips are placed onto the edges of the previous strips. After replacement of the epithelium flaps (**Fig. 8.7c, d**) the superior and inferior ends of the cartilage strips are covered with the epithelium, allowing rapid epithelialization.

On-lay Technique with Elevation of Three Superior Epithelial Flaps

The three epithelial flaps are elevated and an inferior belt of the ear canal skin with the attached epithelium from the eardrum is removed (**Fig. 8.8a**). Six relatively thick cartilage strips are placed like roof tiles (**Fig. 8.8b**). After replacement of the superior flaps, the epithelialization may take some time because of the lack of epithelium along the inferior annulus (**Fig. 8.8c**). Preservation of the epithelium as shown in **Fig. 8.7c** may be a better solution.

On-lay Technique with Elevation of a Large Tympanomeatal Flap

After a circumferential incision between the 10-o'clock and 2-o'clock positions, a large skin flap is elevated together with the attached eardrum epithelium (**Fig. 8.9a**). Five thin cartilage strips are placed like roof tiles (**Fig. 8.9b**). The edge of the second strip is placed onto the edge of the anterior (first) strip and so on. After replacement of the tympanomeatal flap, the epithelium will cover the superior and the inferior ends of the strips (**Fig. 8.9c**).

On-lay Cartilage Strips in Ossiculoplasty

On-lay Cartilage Strip Tympanoplasty Type 3 with a Columella

Cartilage strips are thinner than palisades and can more easily be placed onto the head of a titanium TORP columella in a case with total perforation and missing stapes. In relation to ossiculoplasty, the on-lay technique with placement of the cartilage strips onto the lamina propria allows more space for the head of the columella than in underlay technique where the cartilage strips are placed under the lamina propria.

After elevation of a large tympanomeatal flap with the surrounding eardrum epithelium, a Hüttenbrink cartilage guide is placed onto the footplate (Hüttenbrink et al. 2004). Through the 0.8 mm hole of the guide the foot of the Kurz titanium columella is placed and stabilized by the chorda tympani (**Fig. 8.10a**). The three anterior cartilage strips are placed like roof tiles onto the lamina propria. The edge of the short strip is placed onto the edge of the previous strip, providing good support for this short strip. The posterior strips are again placed like roof tiles onto the lamina propria and onto the head of the titanium prosthesis (**Fig. 8.10b**). After replacement of the tympanomeatal flap with the epithelial flaps, the covering of the ends of the strips is good (**Fig. 8.10c**).

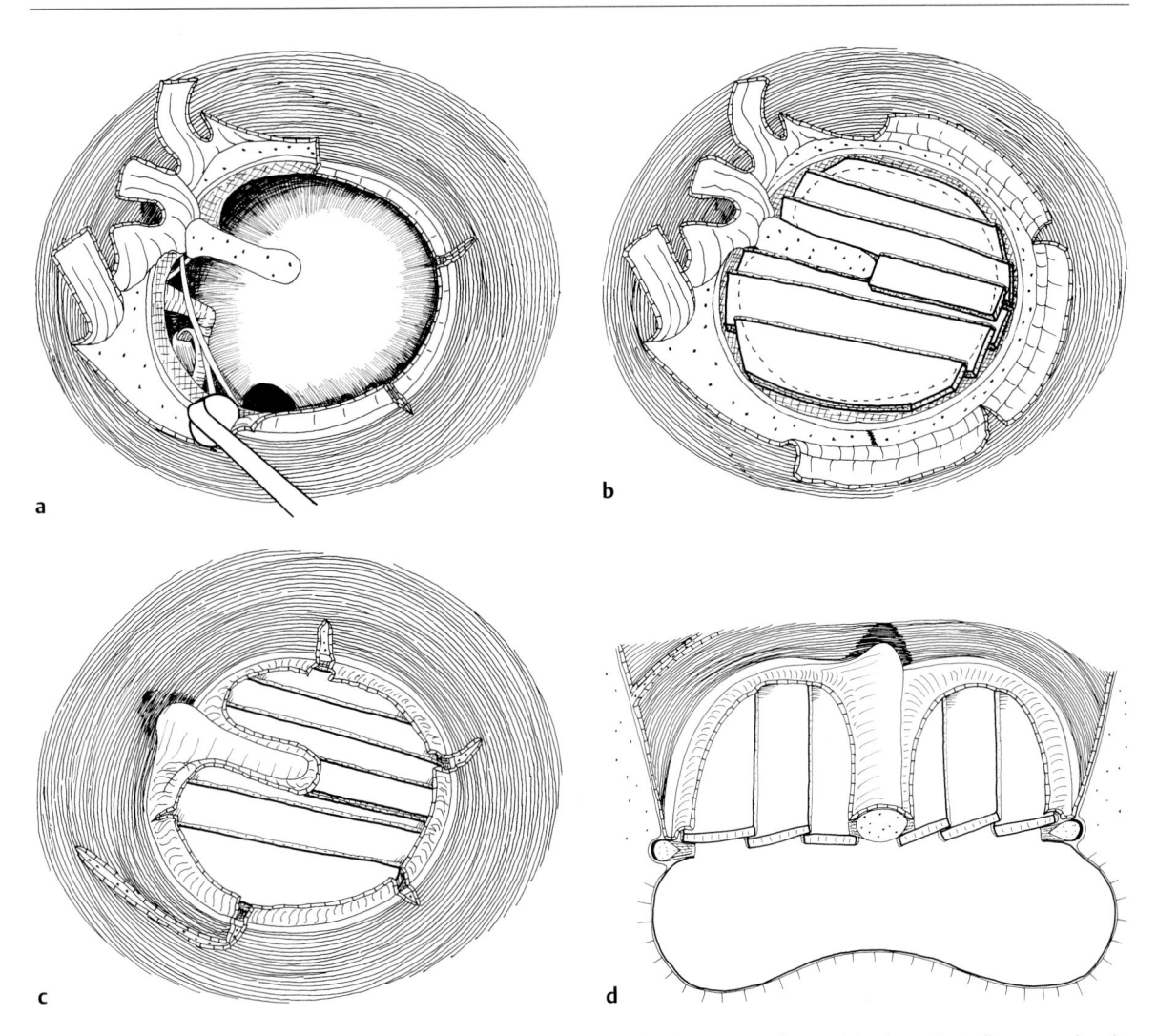

Fig. 8.7a–d Outward elevation of the eardrum epithelium and skin flaps in total perforation.

a Three superior skin and epithelium flaps are elevated. Two small vertical incisions are made at the 5-o'clock and 7-o'clock positions.
b The epithelium from the eardrum remnant, with the attached ear canal skin, is elevated outward as three flaps. Seven thin cartilage strips with the perichondrium on both edges are placed on each other like roof tiles.
c The three superior flaps and the three inferior flaps are replaced.
d Side view with some perspective at the level of the umbo of the on-lay cartilage strip closure of a total perforation. The anterior strip is placed onto the anterior lamina propria. The edges of the following strips are placed onto the edges of the previous strips, in the manner of roof tiles.

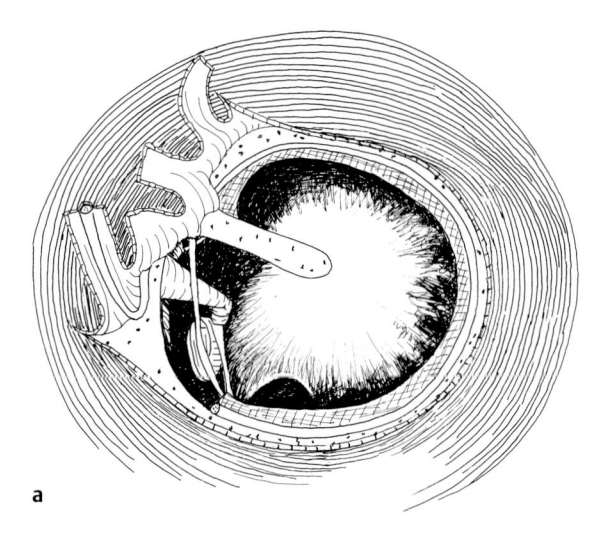

8 Cartilage Strips in On-lay Tympanoplasty Techniques

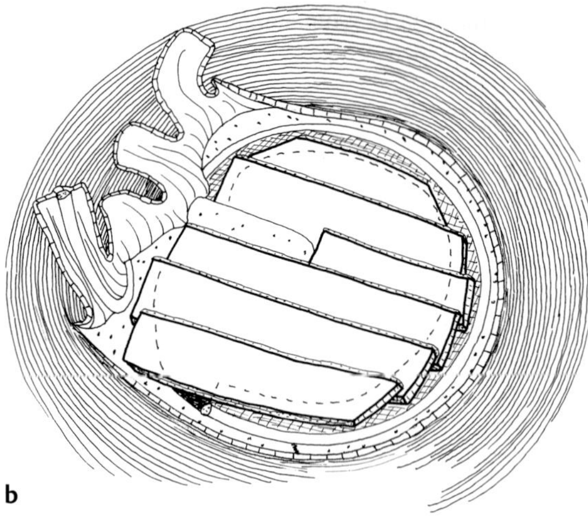

Fig. 8.8 a–c On-lay technique with elevation of three superior skin flaps with the eardrum epithelium in total perforation to be closed with on-lay cartilage strips.
- **a** The epithelium is removed from the edges of the perforation and the three superior skin flaps and the eardrum epithelium are elevated. Along the inferior border of the perforation a strip of the epithelium and ear canal skin is removed. The posterosuperior fibrous annulus is elevated, allowing a good view of the sinus tympani.
- **b** The five long strips and a short strip are placed onto the edges of the perforation. The short strip extends from the umbo to the annulus. The posterosuperior part of the annulus is elevated to achieve a better view of the tympanic sinuses. In this region the posterior cartilage strip is positioned as an underlay graft.
- **c** The flaps are replaced.

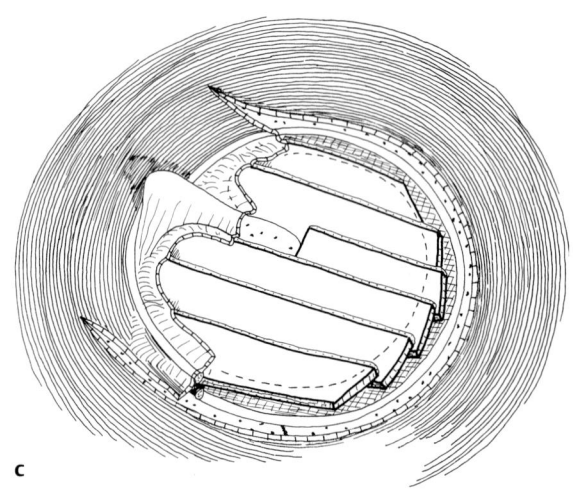

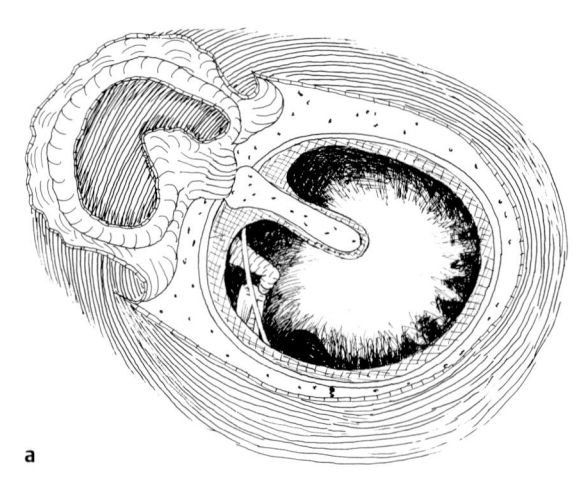

Fig. 8.9 a–c Elevation of a large tympanomeatal flap in a total perforation to be covered with on-lay cartilage strips.
- **a** A large circumferential incision with elevation of a skin flap is completed.
- **b** Cartilage strips are placed onto the annulus and positioned slightly overlapping each other like roof tiles.

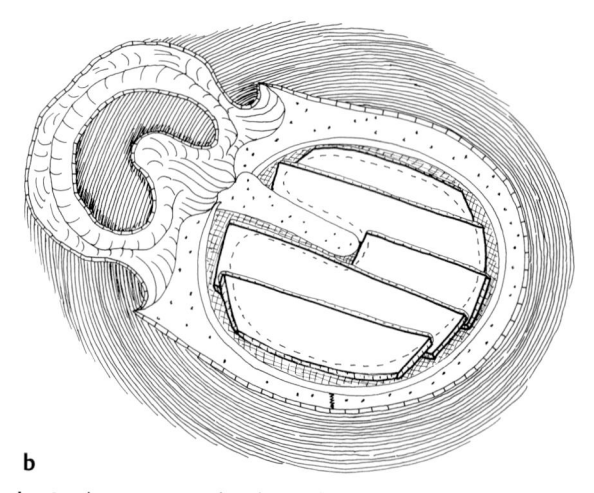

On-lay Cartilage Strip Tympanoplasty Type 2 with Interposition of the Incus

Several methods of interpositions can be used in cases of total perforation and missing long process of the incus; these are described in MMES_1, Figs. 689–976). If possible I prefer to use a shaped autogenous incus.

The three superior skin and epithelial flaps are elevated. Along the inferior annulus three small vertical incisions are performed (**Fig. 8.11a**) to facilitate outward elevation of the eardrum epithelium and the adjacent skin (**Fig. 8.11b**). The incus is removed and shaped, with slight flattening of the body, and a groove is made for the head of the stapes. The incus body is placed onto the head of the stapes, its short process under the malleus handle. The anterior cartilage strips are placed onto the lamina propria in the manner roof tiles. The short strip is placed onto the edge of the neighboring strip and also has contact with the malleus handle. The posterior palisades are placed like roof tiles onto the lamina propria and the incus body (**Fig. 8.11c**). After replacement of the epithelium and the

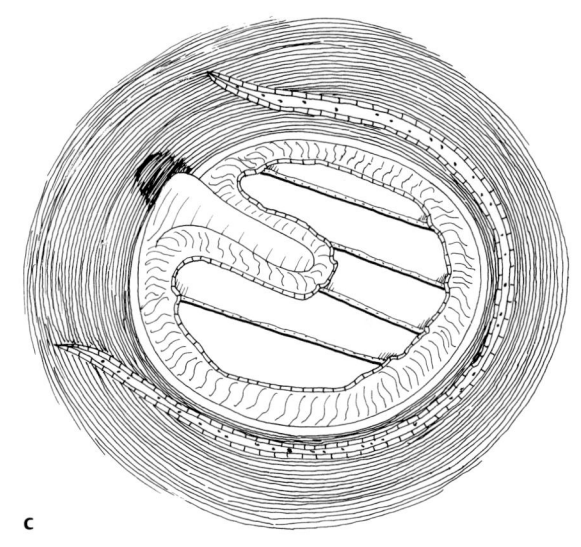

Fig. 8.9c
c The flaps are replaced and the epithelium covers the superior and inferior ends of the strips.

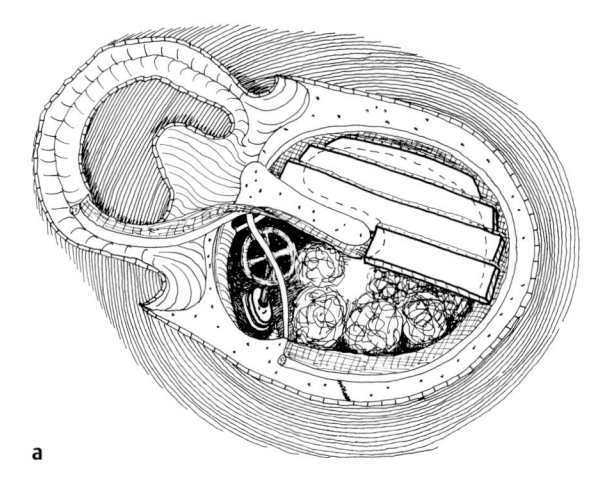

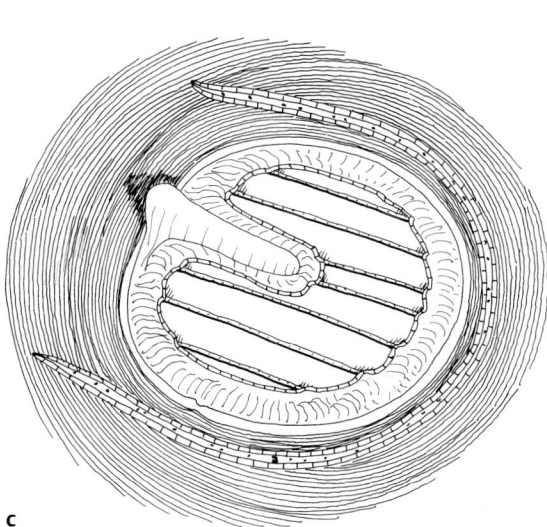

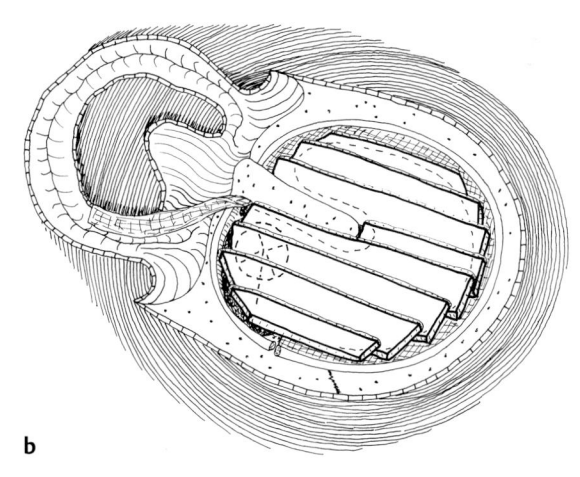

Fig. 8.10a–c On-lay cartilage strip tympanoplasty type 3 with a titanium columella in a case with total perforation and missing stapes.
a A large tympanomeatal skin flap with eardrum epithelium is elevated. A Hüttenbrink cartilage guide is placed onto he footplate. The Kurz titanium columella is placed through the hole of the guide onto the footplate. The head is stabilized by the chorda tympani and Gelfoam. The four anterior cartilage strips are placed like roof tiles onto the denuded lamina propria of the anterior half of the tympanic cavity.
b The posterior cartilage strips are placed like roof tiles onto the head of the columella and onto the denuded lamina propria.
c The tympanomeatal flaps and the epithelial flaps are replaced, covering the inferior and superior ends of the cartilage strips.

Fig. 8.11a–e On-lay cartilage strip tympanoplasty type 2 with interposition of a shaped autogenous incus between the stapes head and the malleus handle in a case with total perforation and missing long process of the incus.

a Three superior skin flaps are elevated. Three small vertical incisions of the eardrum epithelium and skin are made along the inferior annulus. The incus is removed.

b The shaped incus with a groove for the stapes head and with slightly flattened body to accommodate the cartilage strips is interposed in the classic manner. The anterior thin cartilage strips with the perichondrium on both edges are placed like roof tiles onto the denuded lamina propria.

c The posterior cartilage strips are placed like roof tiles onto the incus body and the lamina propria.

d The epithelial flaps and the skin flaps are replaced, covering the superior and inferior ends of the strips.

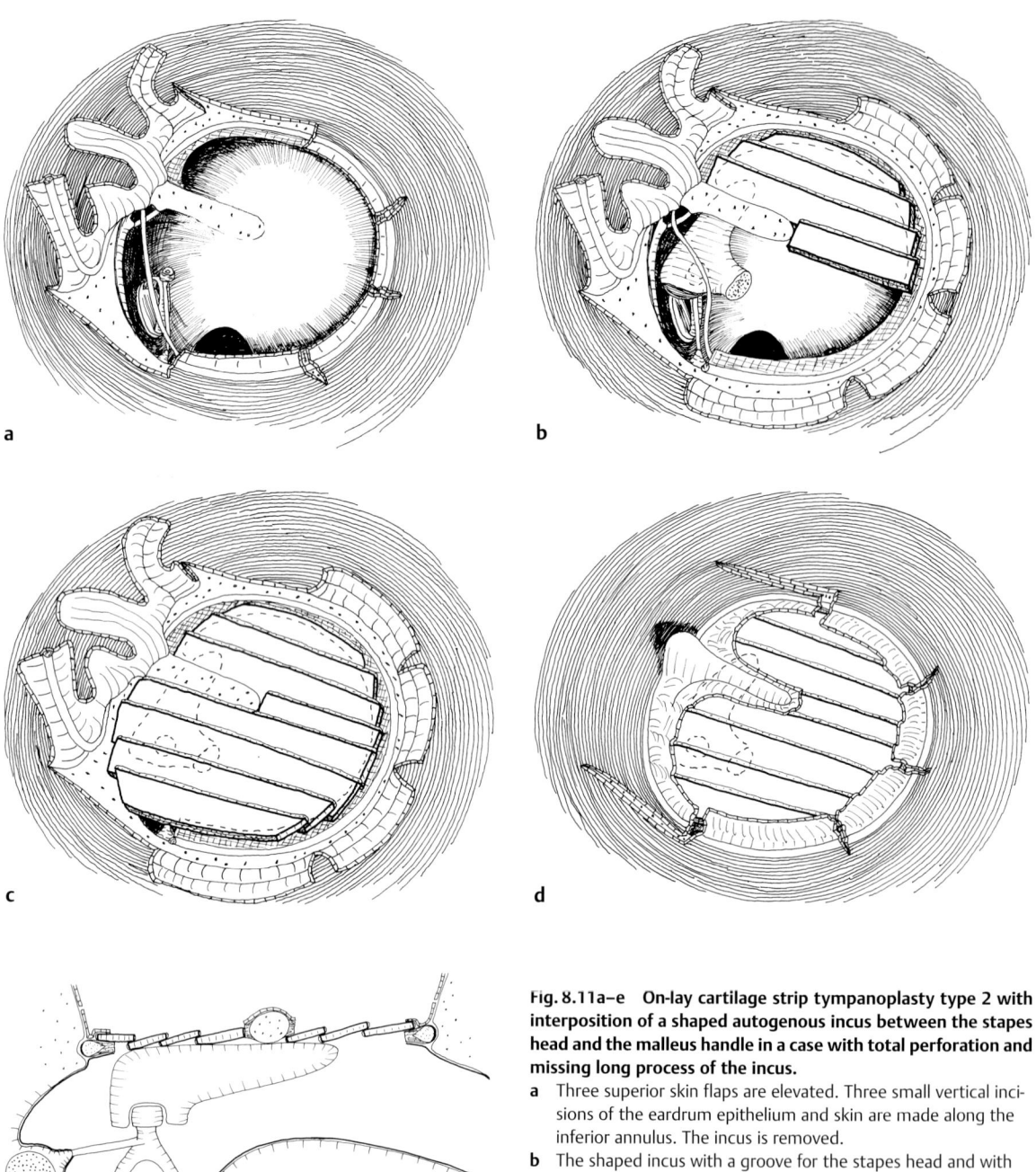

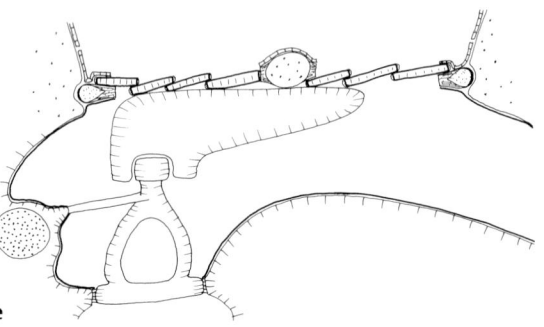

e Side view of on-lay cartilage strip tympanoplasty type 2 with interposition of a shaped incus between the head of the stapes and the malleus handle. There is a good connection between the strips and the incus. The placement of the cartilage strips like roof tiles is apparent. Both edges of the strips are covered by small belts of perichondrium.

skin flaps, the ends of the strips are covered with the epithelium (**Fig. 8.11 d, e**).

Results of Surgery

There are no publications on the results of on-lay methods. I have performed about 30 tympanoplasties using on-lay cartilage strips in closure of anterior, inferior, and total perforations. Two to three months after surgery, all perforations were closed and the postoperative hearing was not poorer than expected. However, there was no systematic follow-up study of these patients.

Author's Comments and Recommendations

On-lay technique is suitable for cartilage strips in closing of anterior, inferior, and total perforations, mainly because the strips do not need any support. There is no need for an architrave or for placement of any other piece of cartilage in the hypotympanum. In contrast to fascia and perichondrium, cartilage strips placed on the denuded lamina propria will be able to resist the eventual pressure from the ear canal, and the under-pressure from the middle ear. The cartilage strips will remain on the edges of the perforation and will not move into the tympanic cavity.

In my opinion, thin cartilage strips placed as on-lay grafts provide the best possibility of achieving hearing results as good as or even better than those obtained with fascia or perichondrium. This assertion can easily be proved or disproved.

The anatomical results are definitely better with cartilage palisades or cartilage strips than tympanoplasties with fascia or perichondrium. All publications showing results indicate that the numbers of reperforations, retractions, and reoperations are higher after tympanoplasty with perichondrium or fascia than with palisades or strips.

Need for Clinical Research

It is to be hoped that many clinical studies on on-lay cartilage strip tympanoplasty will be undertaken in the future; for example:
- Comparison of results in the on-lay cartilage strip method with those using fascia or perichondrium in similar pathologies.
- Comparison of results using on-lay cartilage strips with those using underlay cartilage strips in similar pathologies.
- Comparison of results using on-lay cartilage strips with those using on-lay cartilage palisade technique or underlay cartilage palisade technique.
- Comparison of results in closure of the total perforation using on-lay cartilage strip technique with results of closure of the total perforation with a total cartilage–perichondrium composite graft.

References

Hüttenbrink K-B, Zahnert T, Beutner D, Hofmann G. The cartilage guide: a solution for anchoring a columella prostheses on the footplate. Laryngorhinootologie 2004;83:450–456.

Tos M. Stability of myringoplasty based on late results. ORL J Otorhinolaryngol Relat Spec 1980;42:171–81.

9 The Dornhoffer Cartilage Mosaic Tympanoplasty

Definition

In 2000, Dornhoffer presented a new technique which here I will call "Dornhoffer cartilage mosaic tympanoplasty." Dornhoffer called it "palisade technique," but he clearly noted that his technique "differs from the palisade technique of Heermann: instead of placing rectangular strips of cartilage in the side to side manner, an attempt is made to use one major full-thickness piece of cartilage, in a semilunar shape, which is placed directly under and against the malleus handle, or on the top of the prosthesis" (Dornhoffer 2003, 2006).

The cartilage is cut into several pieces that are subsequently assembled together like the pieces of a jigsaw puzzle to reconstruct the tympanic membrane (**Fig. 9.1**). The shapes and sizes of the cartilage pieces may vary greatly (**Fig. 9.2**), depending on the size and shape of the perforation and on the ossiculoplasty method as well as on the ossiculoplasty material. For example, an interposed incus in a type 2 tympanoplasty and a cartilage piece of full thickness may occupy too much space in the posterosuperior part of the tympanic cavity.

The Heermann cartilage palisade method is defined as reconstruction of the eardrum with relatively long, 0.5–3 mm wide, full-thickness cartilage strips covered on one side with perichondrium, placed side by side and close to each other. Usually they are placed in the inferosuperior direction. The order of placement of the palisades is rather strictly stipulated, starting with the most anterior palisade.

In contrast to the palisade technique, the cartilage mosaic technique is more "liberal": the pieces are of various shapes and various sizes, cut to cover a particular defect, either as one or two large pieces or several small pieces. The mosaic method is a new, innovative and creative technique, and is worthy of a separate description and separate evaluation of the primary and late results, rather than being treated as a modification of the palisade technique (Tos 2008).

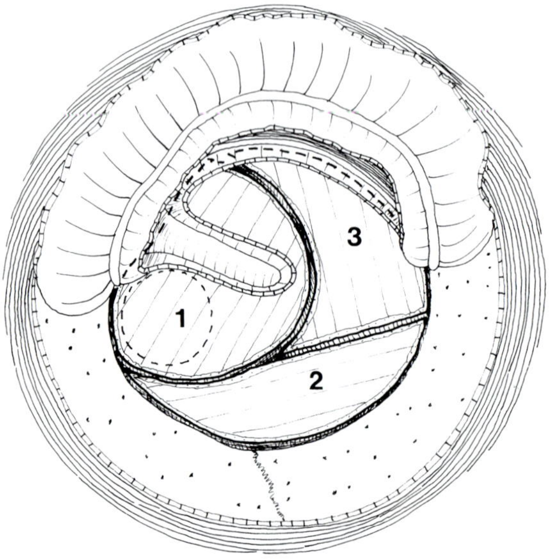

Harvesting and Trimming of the Cartilage

In the transcanal and the endaural approaches, Dornhoffer (1997) uses tragal cartilage (see **Figs. 3.21, 3.23a–c**). In the retroauricular approach, the cymba cartilage (see **Fig. 3.27**) or the concha cartilage (see **Figs. 3.26, 3.27**) is used. The cymba cartilage is slightly thinner (1.0 mm), and more curved than the concha cartilage, which additionally is irregular in certain areas. Because of the curvature, the cymba cartilage is less suitable for the total tensa cartilage–perichondrium composite island graft (Dornhoffer 1999, 2000), but it is very suitable for the cartilage mosaic tympanoplasty (Dornhoffer 2003). The tragus cartilage is also suitable for the mosaic tympanoplasty.

After harvesting of the tragus or the cymba graft, the perichondrium is removed from the convex side. This convex side is turned toward the tympanic cavity. On the concave side, the cartilage is covered by the perichondrium (**Fig. 9.2**).

Fig. 9.1 Example of the Dornhoffer cartilage mosaic tympanoplasty. A total perforation with missing stapes is reconstructed with a TORP and three pieces of full-thickness cartilage, covered on the ear canal side with the perichondrium. First a large oval piece is placed under the malleus handle, covering the head of the TORP prosthesis. The second cartilage piece covers the posteroinferior part, and the third piece covers the anteroinferior part of the tympanic cavity (Dornhoffer 2006).

Indications for Cartilage Mosaic Tympanoplasty

Indications are the same as for cartilage palisade tympanoplasty or for cartilage-perichondrium composite grafts. The following conditions may benefit from the Dornhoffer cartilage mosaic tympanoplasty:
- Posterior, inferior, subtotal, or total perforations with poor tubal function and/or with negative preoperative Valsalva maneuver
- Recurrent perforations
- Retractions or atelectasis
- Adhesive otitis
- Cholesteatoma
- Perforations with thick, moist middle ear mucosa
- Reconstruction of the eardrum in old cavities

Surgical Techniques of Cartilage Mosaic Tympanoplasty

The mosaic tympanoplasty is suitable for closure of a posterior perforation, a large inferior perforation, a subtotal or a total perforation.

In contrast to the palisade technique of Heermann, in which the first palisade is the most anterior palisade (see Chapters 4 and 5), in the mosaic technique the reconstruction of the eardrum can start at any place in the tympanic cavity. Dornhoffer (2003, 2006) always supports the cartilage pieces with Gelfoam balls.

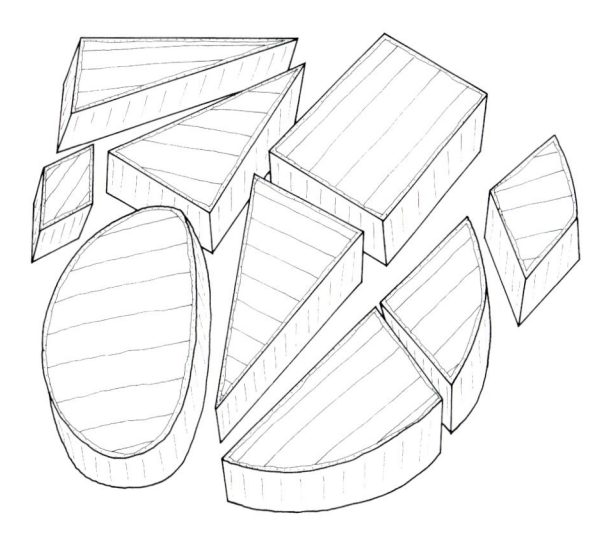

Fig. 9.2 Several pieces of full-thickness for the cartilage mosaic tympanoplasty, covered with the perichondrium, cut from a large tragus or cymba graft.

Posterior Perforation

Tympanoplasty Type 1

A swing-door incision is made, allowing elevation of a superior and an inferior tympanomeatal flap (**Fig. 9.3a**). The first superior cartilage piece is placed under the malleus handle, as superiorly as possible. It rests on the chorda tympani. The second piece is placed under the umbo and is supported by Gelfoam. After replacement of the two flaps (**Fig. 9.3b**), rapid epithelialization of the perichondrium will take place.

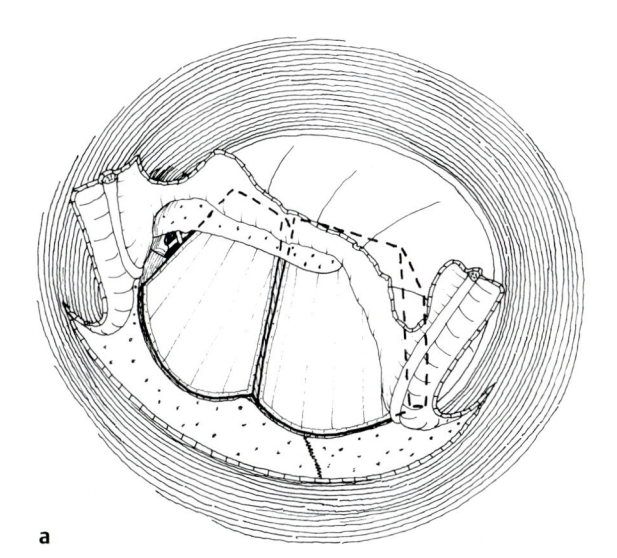

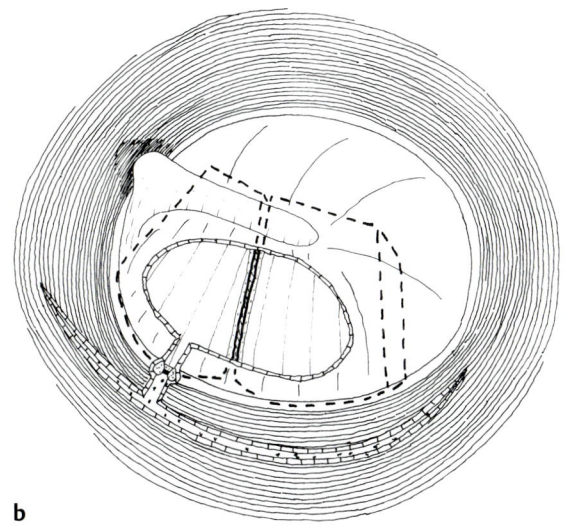

Fig. 9.3a, b Closure of the posterior perforation with intact ossicular chain, using cartilage mosaic tympanoplasty.
a After cleaning of the edges of the perforation, scarification of the undersurface of the eardrum, and the making of swing-door incisions, two tympanomeatal flaps are elevated. The undersurface of the malleus handle is also scarified and Gelfoam balls are placed under the malleus region. The first piece of cartilage is placed under the malleus handle. The second piece is placed inferior to the first piece. Both pieces are supported by Gelfoam.
b The tympanomeatal flaps are replaced, covering most of the cartilage.

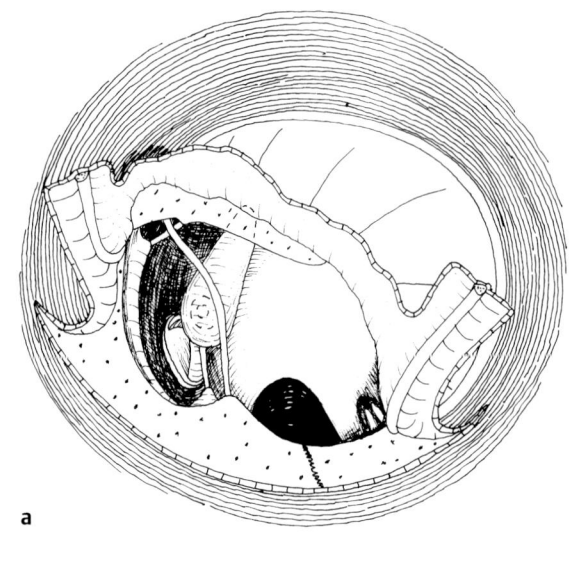

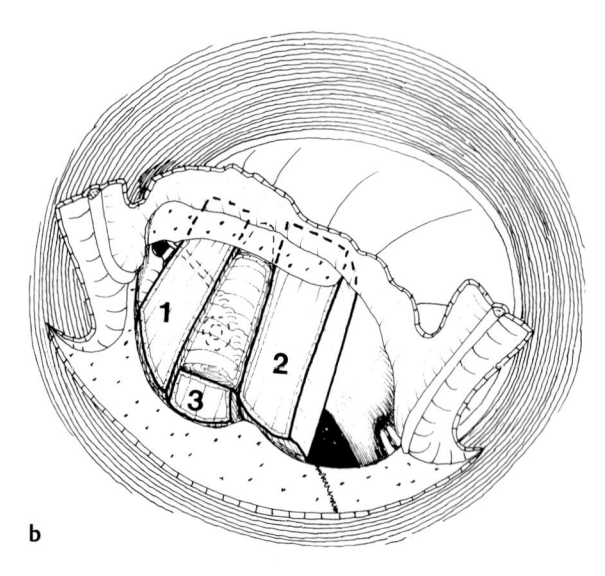

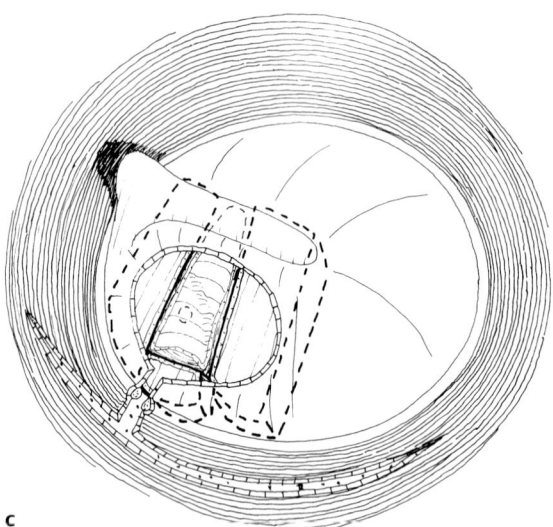

Fig. 9.4a–c Closure of a posterior perforation after tympanoplasty type 2 with interposition of the autogenous incus, using the Dornhoffer cartilage mosaic tympanoplasty.
a After the posterior swing-door incision is made, two tympanomeatal flaps are elevated. The defective incus is removed and shaped. A groove is made on the remnant of the long process and the body is flattened to accommodate the cartilage pieces.
b The first cartilage piece is placed superior to the incus body and is supported by the chorda tympani. The second cartilage piece is placed inferior to the incus and also under the malleus handle. A small third piece is placed posterior to the incus body, which is covered by a free perichondrium flap.
c The tympanomeatal flaps are replaced.

Tympanoplasty Type 2

When the long process of the incus is missing and the malleus handle is present, a tympanoplasty type 2 will be performed using an autogenous incus. The incus should be slightly flattened to allow covering with the cartilage pieces placed close to the incus (**Fig. 9.4a**). The first cartilage piece covers the area superior to the incus body and ends under the malleus handle. The second piece is placed inferior to the interposed incus, also ending under the malleus handle. Thus, the incus body and the short process of the incus are not covered with cartilage (**Fig. 9.4b**), but early epithelialization is to be expected after replacement of the tympanomeatal flaps (**Fig. 9.4c**).

Tympanoplasty Type 3

After removal of the epithelium from the edges of the perforation and after scarification of the undersurface of the eardrum remnant, a large tympanomeatal flap is elevated, exposing the footplate (**Fig. 9.5a**). The cartilage guide (Hüttenbrink et al. 2004) is placed onto the footplate and the titanium columella is placed through the hole of the guide onto the footplate (**Fig. 9.5a**). The head of the prosthesis is stabilized by the chorda tympani. The first cartilage piece covers the superior half of the head of the columella, the second piece covers the inferior part (**Fig. 9.5b,c**).

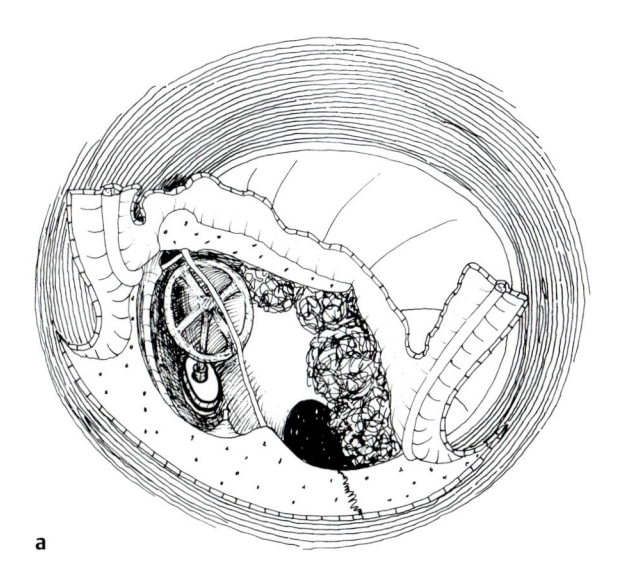

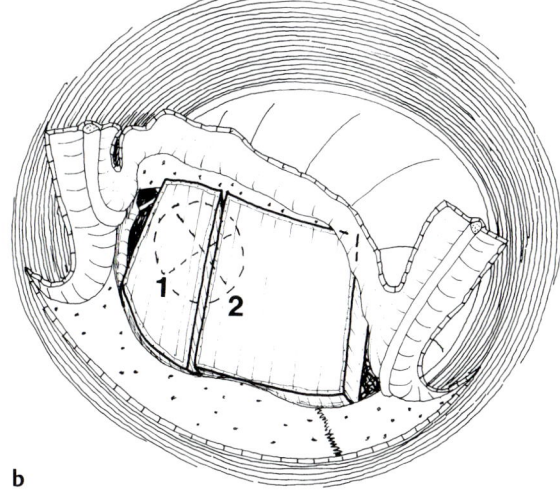

Fig. 9.5a–c Cartilage mosaic tympanoplasty type 3 in a posterior perforation, using a Kurz titanium columella.
a The edges of the perforation are cleaned, the undersurface of the eardrum is scarified, and two tympanomeatal flaps are elevated. The columella is placed onto the footplate through a hole made in the cartilage guide.
b The first cartilage piece is placed onto the upper half of the head of the columella at the level of the malleus handle. The second piece is placed onto the inferior part of the head of the columella, also at the level of the malleus handle.
c The epithelium flaps and the tympanomeatal flaps are replaced.

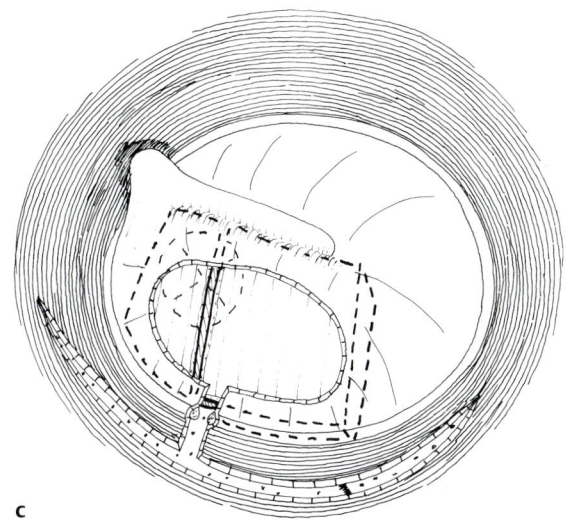

Inferior Perforation

A large inferior perforation can easily be closed by cartilage mosaic tympanoplasty. After cleaning of the edges of the perforation and scarification of the undersurface of the eardrum remnant, a large tympanomeatal flap is elevated. The inferior half of the tympanic cavity is filled with Gelfoam balls. The first cartilage piece is placed into the anterosuperior part of the tympanic cavity, at the level of the bony annulus and under the malleus handle (**Fig. 9.6a**). The second, semilunar cartilage piece is placed along the inferior bony annulus, and the third piece into the posterosuperior quadrant. After replacement of the tympanomeatal flaps (**Fig. 9.6b**), rapid epithelialization begins.

The side view at the level of the umbo region shows the two cartilage pieces covered with perichondrium lying medially under the umbo and laterally under the lamina propria, making the eardrum slightly concave (**Fig. 9.6c**).

The cartilage pieces cut from cymba cartilage are intrinsically slightly concave.

Subtotal Perforation

In a subtotal perforation, three pieces of full-thickness cartilage with the perichondrium may close the perforation satisfactorily. The pieces on both sides of the malleus handle (**Fig. 9.7a**) and a semicircular piece along the inferior bony annulus can firmly close the perforation. Gelfoam balls in the tympanic cavity support the cartilage pieces, and the adhesion of the perichondrium to the undersurface of the eardrum remnant may be quite effective after replacement of the tympanomeatal flaps (**Fig. 9.7b**). Small, thin slices of cartilage or pieces of perichondrium can be placed into any gaps between two or more pieces.

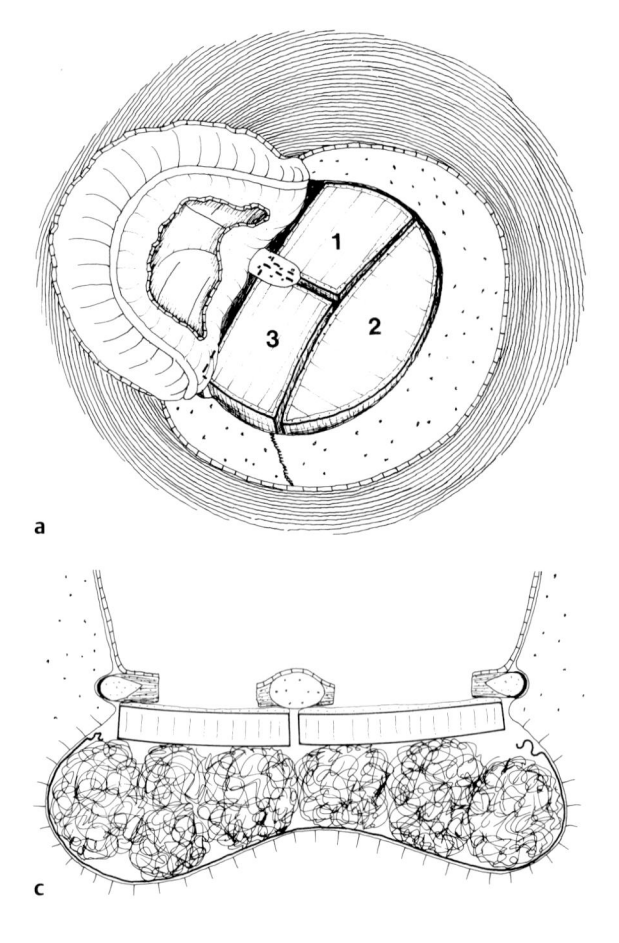

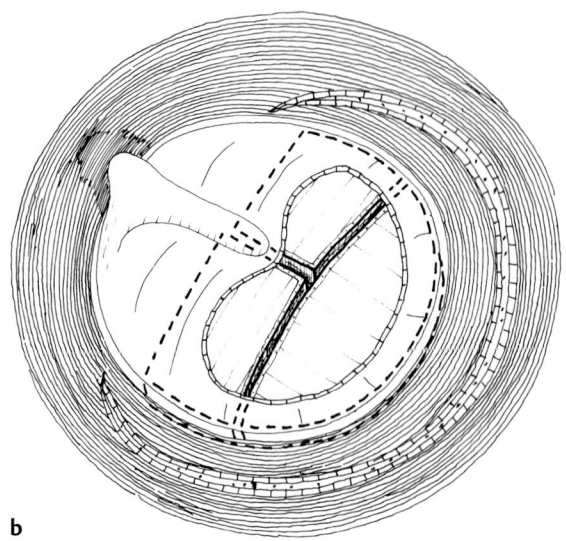

Fig. 9.6a–c Closure of a large inferior perforation using a cartilage mosaic tympanoplasty.
a The edges of the perforation are cleaned and the undersurface of the eardrum is scarified. A large tympanomeatal flap is elevated. The tympanic cavity is filled with Gelfoam balls. The first piece is placed into the anterior part of the tympanic cavity. The second, semilunar, piece is placed along the inferior bony annulus. The third piece covers the posterior part of the tympanic cavity.
b The tympanomeatal flap is replaced.
c Side-view of the cartilage mosaic tympanoplasty at the level of the umbo. The two pieces are positioned medially under the umbo and laterally under the eardrum remnants, making the eardrum slightly concave. The pieces are supported by Gelfoam balls.

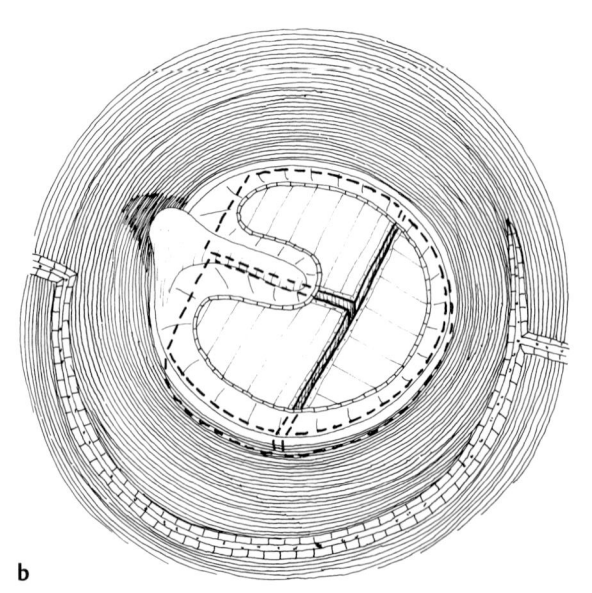

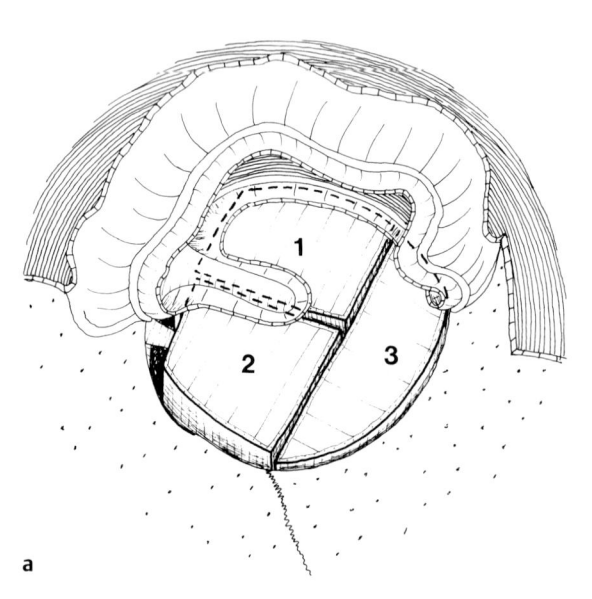

Fig. 9.7a, b Cartilage mosaic tympanoplasty closing a subtotal perforation.
a After cleaning the edges of the perforation and scarifying the undersurface of the eardrum remnant, a large tympanomeatal flap is elevated in retroauricular approach. The tympanic cavity is filled with Gelfoam balls. The first piece is placed in the anterosuperior part of the tympanic cavity at the level of the bony annulus and under the malleus handle. The second piece is placed in the posteroinferior part of the tympanic cavity, and along the inferior bony annulus a semilunar third piece is placed.
b The tympanomeatal flap and the posterior ear canal skin are replaced.

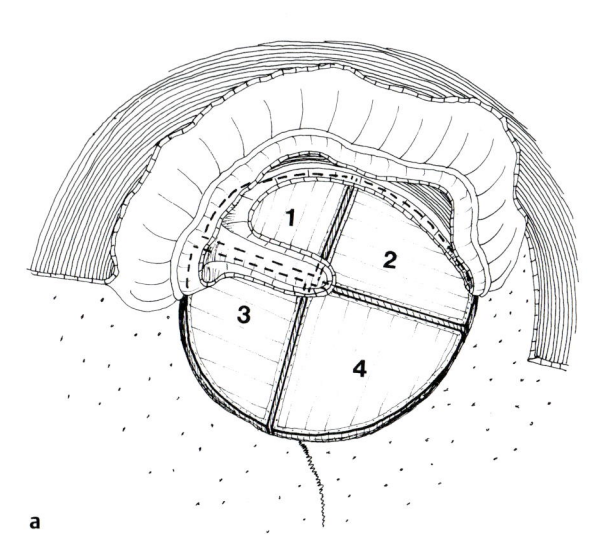

Fig. 9.8a, b Cartilage mosaic tympanoplasty in closure of a total perforation with intact ossicular chain.
a After cleaning the edges of the perforation and scarifying the undersurface of the malleus handle and eardrum remnant, the tympanic cavity is filled with Gelfoam balls, except around the stapes region. The first piece is placed into the anterosuperior quadrant, the second into the anteroinferior quadrant, the third under the posterosuperior quadrant, supported by the chorda tympani. The fourth piece is placed in the posteroinferior quadrant. All four pieces have some contact with the malleus handle and the umbo.
b The tympanomeatal flap is replaced.

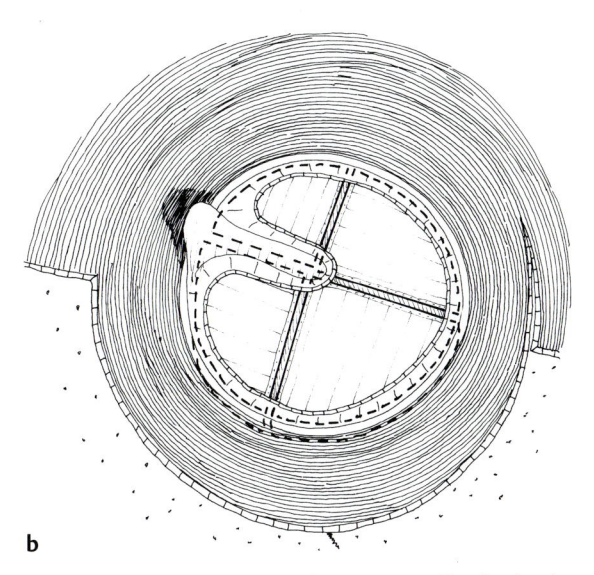

Total Perforation

Closure of a total perforation is the most common indication for the cartilage mosaic tympanoplasty (Dornhoffer 2003, 2006). Total retraction or atelectasis, adhesive otitis, and tensa retraction cholesteatoma will at the end of the surgery have a total tensa perforation, which can be closed with Dornhoffer mosaic tympanoplasty.

Tympanoplasty Type 1

In a case of intact ossicular chain, the cartilage pieces may be of different sizes and shapes and the placement of the pieces may start at any place. In the actual reconstruction (**Fig. 9.8a**) the first piece covers the anterosuperior quadrant, the second piece the anteroinferior quadrant, the third piece the posterosuperior quadrant, and the fourth piece the posteroinferior quadrant. The pieces are supported with Gelfoam balls. After replacement of the tympanomeatal flap (**Fig. 9.8b**), the epithelialization of the eardrum can begin.

Tympanoplasty Type 2

In case of defective long process of the incus with intact stapes and malleus handle, a titanium prosthesis or another PORP prosthesis can be used. When using the autogenous incus, a groove is made on the remnant of the long process to be placed onto the head of the stapes. The short process of the incus is flattened to the same level as the cartilage pieces. The tympanic cavity is filled with Gelfoam balls. The first cartilage piece covers the anterosuperior quadrant; it has some contact with the interposed short process of the incus (**Fig. 9.9a**). The second piece is placed superior to the interposed incus and under the malleus handle. It is supported by the chorda tympani. The large third piece covers the inferoposterior part of the tympanic cavity; its anterior edge is placed under the malleus handle. The fourth piece covers the anteroinferior quadrant and has some contact with the umbo. A small piece of cartilage is placed behind the interposed incus. After replacement of the tympanomeatal flap (**Fig. 9.9b, c**) the conditions are good for rapid epithelialization.

Tympanoplasty Type 3

In tympanoplasty type 3, without stapes crura, various columellae can be shaped and used, such as autogenous incus or cortical bone, or columellae made of various biocompatible materials (see MMES_1, pp. 348–382) and of metals, in particular the titanium columella. Columellae with a large and flat head are most suitable for the mosaic cartilage tympanoplasty.

An example of the Kurz titanium columella is illustrated in **Fig. 9.10a**). The foot of the prosthesis is placed through the hole of the cartilage guide and onto the footplate. The head of the columella is stabilized by the chorda tympani. The first piece is placed in the anterosuperior part of the tympanic cavity. The second piece is placed onto the head of the columella (**Fig. 9.10b**) and the next three pieces cover the inferior half of the tympanic cavity (**Fig. 9.10c, d**).

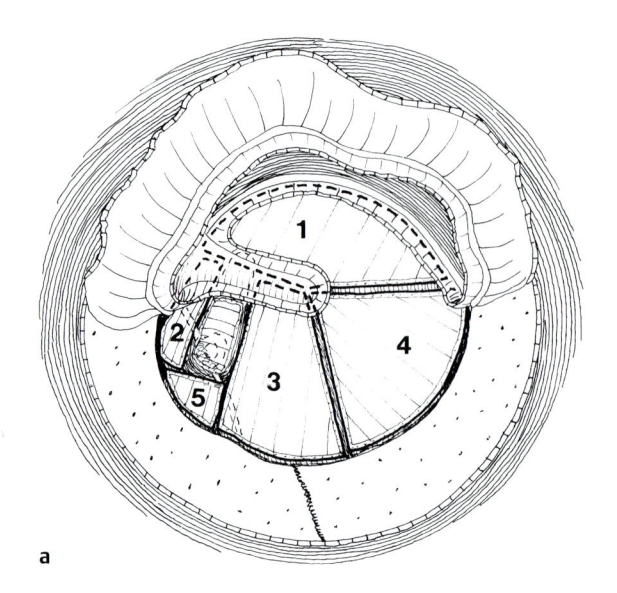

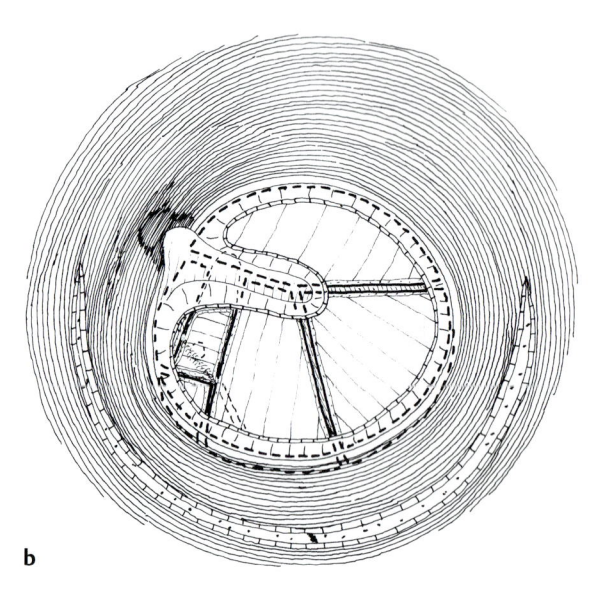

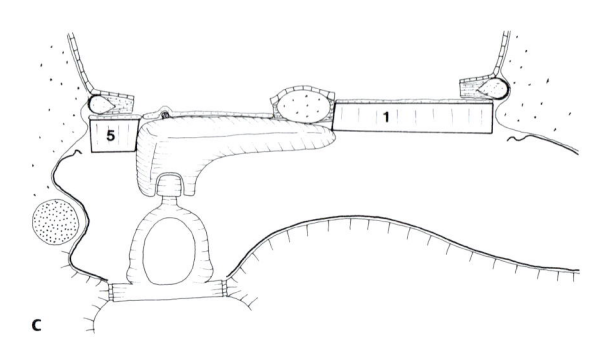

Fig. 9.9a–c Cartilage mosaic tympanoplasty in closure of a total perforation with interposition of the incus.

a The tympanomeatal flap is elevated after scarification of the undersurface of the eardrum remnant. The shaped incus is placed onto the head of the stapes and under the malleus handle. The first piece is placed onto the anterosuperior area, having some contact with the interposed short process of the incus. The small second piece is placed posterior to the interposed incus. The third piece is placed under the malleus handle covering the posterior part of the tympanic cavity. The fourth piece is placed along the inferior bony annulus with some contact with the distal edge of the umbo. A small fifth piece is placed posterior to the incus. A free perichondrium flap covers the interposed incus. All four main pieces have good contact with the bony annulus and some contact with the umbo.

b The tympanomeatal flap is replaced.

c Side view of cartilage mosaic tympanoplasty type 2 with incus interposition, at the level of the stapes. The shaped and flattened incus body, with a groove, is placed onto the stapes head. The short process of the incus touches the anterosuperior cartilage piece (1). The posterosuperior piece (5) is touching the flattened incus body, which is covered by a small free perichondrium flap.

Results of Surgery

Dornhoffer (2003) published extensive documentation on the results of 1000 patients treated with cartilage tympanoplasty. These results are summarized in Chapter 17, but the results achieved with pars tensa cartilage-perichondrium composite island grafts and cartilage mosaic tympanoplasty are not described separately for each method.

No results on cartilage mosaic tympanoplasty have been published elsewhere. Dornhoffer is presumably the only surgeon with a large series of the cartilage mosaic tympanoplasty cases and cases with total pars tensa composite graft. Hopefully, the results of these two methods will be evaluated separately, compared, and published.

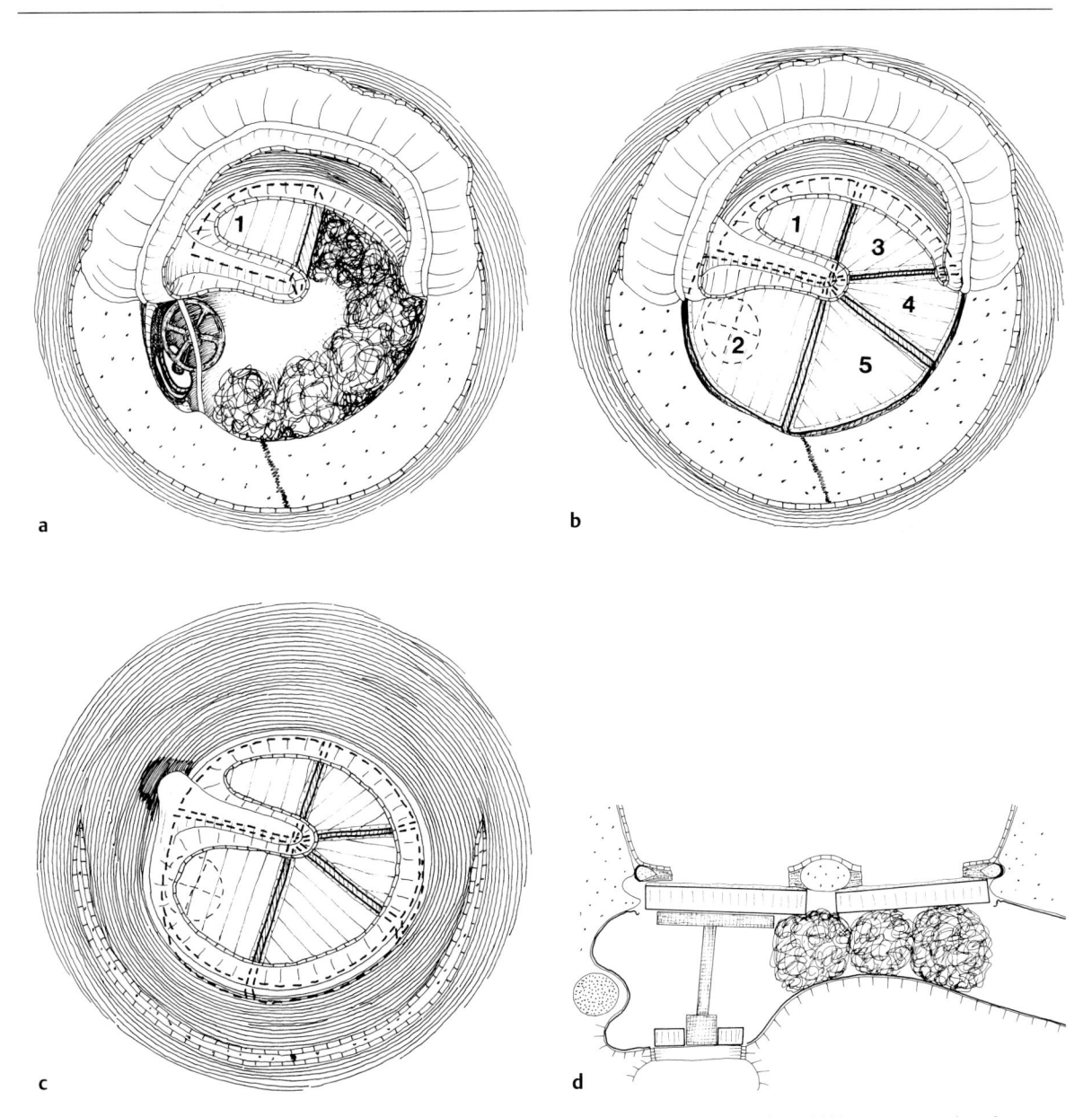

Fig. 9.10 a–d Cartilage mosaic tympanoplasty type 3, closing a total perforation and covering a titanium columella.

a After cleaning the edges of the perforation and scarifying the undersurface of the eardrum remnant, a large tympanomeatal flap is elevated. A cartilage guide is placed onto the footplate and a Kurz titanium columella is placed through the hole of the guide onto the footplate. The posterior edge of the first piece is placed under the anterior edge of the malleus handle and covers the anterosuperior quadrant of the tympanic cavity, which is filled with Gelfoam balls.

b The second piece is placed onto the head of the columella and just under the posterior edge (or at the level) of the malleus handle. The third, fourth, and fifth pieces cover the inferior part of the tympanic cavity.

c The tympanomeatal flap is replaced.

d Side view at the level of the footplate, of the cartilage mosaic tympanoplasty type 3 with a titanium columella and with closure of a total perforation. The foot of the columella is placed through the hole of the cartilage guide onto the footplate. The head of the prosthesis is covered with a cartilage piece, which has contact with the malleus handle. The columella is rather short. The anterior piece also has contact with the malleus handle. Gelfoam balls support the cartilage piece.

Author's Comments and Recommendations

It is important that this mosaic cartilage tympanoplasty technique remains distinct from the classic Heermann cartilage palisade technique described in Chapters 4, 5, and 6, and from the cartilage strips method of Neumann (1999), described in Chapters 7 and 8. The differences in reconstruction of the eardrum are large. Moreover, the reconstruction of the eardrum is much more liberal than with palisades or strips, which always start with the anterior palisade/strip. In mosaic tympanoplasty, the first pieces of cartilage, of various shapes and sizes, can be placed in any quadrant of the eardrum.

In Chapters 10 and 11, the techniques of thin foils (0.2–0.3 mm) and thin plates (0.4–0.5 mm) without perichondrium are described. Construction of the eardrum with foils and thin plates also differs from the mosaic cartilage tympanoplasty in three important respects:

1. Although the placement of the foils or the thin plates is of the mosaic fashion, the thin foils are overlapped or underlapped with each other, which means, that two foils can be placed on each other in the same region, making two or even three layers of cartilage. This is not the case in the Dornhoffer mosaic cartilage tympanoplasty.
2. In mosaic cartilage tympanoplasty the cartilage is used as full-thickness piece; foils are 0.2–0.3 mm thick and thin plates are 0.4–0.5 mm thick.
3. The full-thickness cartilage is covered with the perichondrium on the concave (ear canal) side; foils or thin plates are not covered with perichondrium.

In Chapters 12 and 13 the techniques with thick (0.5–1.0 mm) cartilage plates, without perichondrium are described and illustrated. These techniques also differ from the Dornhoffer mosaic cartilage technique: the cartilage plates do not have the perichondrium attached and are placed under a fascia graft or a separate perichondrium graft.

In 95 patients with recurrent perforation after a previous tympanoplasty with temporalis fascia, revision surgery of the Dornhoffer group was performed (Boone et al. 2004). At the revision tympanoplasty, 42% of the patients were under the age of 18 years. Twenty-one percent of 95 patients were actively draining at the recurrent surgery. The reconstruction of the eardrum was either with Dornhoffer total cartilage–perichondrium composite island graft (see Chapter 17) or with Dornhoffer underlay cartilage mosaic. Primary closure of the perforation was successful in 95%. Preoperatively, the average PTA-ABG at four frequencies (500, 1000, 2000, 3000 Hz) was 24 ± 13.8 dB, and was 12.2 ± 7.3 dB after the operation. Again, the results of the two different methods were not evaluated separately.

References

Boone RT, Gardner EK, Dornhoffer JL. Success of cartilage grafting in revision tympanoplasty without mastoidectomy. Otol Neurotol 2004;25:678–681.

Dornhoffer JL. Hearing results with cartilage tympanoplasty. Laryngoscope 1997;107:1094–1099.

Dornhoffer JL. Surgical modification of the difficult mastoid cavity. Otolaryngol Head Neck Surg 1999;120:361–367.

Dornhoffer JL. Surgical management of the atelectatic ear. Am J Otol 2000;21:315–321.

Dornhoffer JL. Cartilage tympanoplasty: Indications, techniques, and outcomes in a 1000 patient series. Laryngoscope 2003;113(11):1844–1856.

Dornhoffer JL. Cartilage tympanoplasty. Otolaryngol Clin North Am 2006;39:1161–1176.

Hüttenbrink K-B, Zahnert T, Beutner D, Hofmann G. The cartilage guide: a solution for anchoring a columella prostheses on the footplate. Laryngorhinootologie 2004;83:450–456.

Neumann A. Die "Knorpelpalisadentympanoplastik" nach Heermann. HNO 1999;47:1074–1088.

Tos M. Cartilage tympanoplasty methods. Proposal of a classification. Otolaryngol Head Neck Surg 2008;139(6):747–758.

10 Underlay Tympanoplasty with Cartilage Foils and Thin Plates

In this chapter two areas need to be distinguished: (1) Underlay tympanoplasty using cartilage foils cut with the Kurz precision cartilage knife; (2) Underlay tympanoplasty with thin cartilage plates (0.1–0.5 mm) cut with a scalpel, resulting in varying thickness of individual plates.

Definition

Cartilage foils are thin slices of cartilage without perichondrium, with a thickness of 0.2–0.3 mm. Thin cartilage plates may have a thickness of 0.4 mm. The foils and thin plates are usually cut with the Kurz precision cartilage knife. They may be of various shapes and various sizes, depending on the graft harvested. Some are elongated similar to strips; some have a size of a quarter or a half of the eardrum; the largest may cover the entire total perforation (**Fig. 10.1a–e**).

Cartilage foils were introduced and applied in Dresden by Hüttenbrink (personal communication, 2001) and his co-workers (Mürbe et al. 2002). Experimentally, the Dresden group has shown that in case of poor tubal function an overlapping positioning of thin cartilage foils—like the leaves of tulip blossom—provides a good stabilization of the reconstructed eardrum (Mürbe et al. 2002). The thickness of the normal eardrum is 0.1 mm, thus the eardrum reconstructed with 0.2–0.3 mm thick foils will still be thicker than the normal eardrum but will have acoustic qualities like those of a normal eardrum. The placement of the foils is similar to that of dried fascia grafts. They can be placed as underlay or as on-lay grafts (Morra, personal communication and video, 2006). In this chapter, the underlay placement of cartilage foils will be described.

Thin cartilage plates (lamellae, when elongated) may be applied in a similar way to foils, i.e., with overlap. Mayeleh, Helshiki, Portmann and Negrevergne from three different Portmann Institutes have published results of a new cartilage mosaic method, placing thin cartilage plates similarly to the placement of cartilage foils (Abou Mayaleh et al. 2005). The thickness of these plates is less than 0.5 mm.

Thick cartilage plates, such as half-thickness plates of 0.5 mm, three-quarter-thickness plates of 0.6–0.8 mm, and full-thickness plates of 0.9 and 1.0 mm, are also not covered with perichondrium. They are applied similarly to composite grafts, but they are not covered and are not suspended by the perichondrium flaps, which represents a considerable difference from composite island grafts. The methods with thick cartilage plates are described and illustrated in Chapters 12 and 13.

It is difficult to determine the exact thickness of the cartilage plate, especially if the thickness differs within the plate. However, no progress can be made without an attempt to follow a classification of the many cartilage grafts. There must be a difference in hearing between the eardrum reconstructed with 0.2 mm thick foils and one reconstructed with 0.7 mm thick plates. On the other side, the resistance against the negative middle ear pressure may be smaller in the eardrum reconstructed with 0.2 mm thick foils than with 0.7 mm thick cartilage plates.

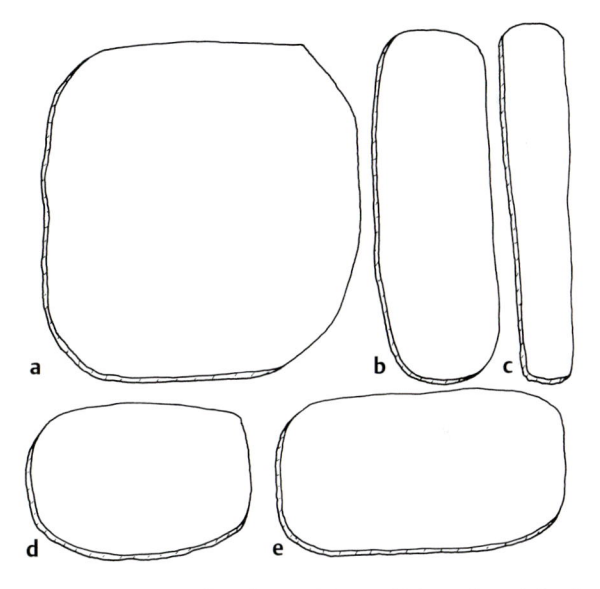

Fig. 10.1a–e Examples of some 0.2 mm thick cartilage foils of various sizes, cut with the Kurz Precision Cartilage Knife.
a   Maximal size to be placed into the recess.
b, c Two lamella-like foils (small and long).
d, e Foils of the size for one and for two eardrum quadrants.

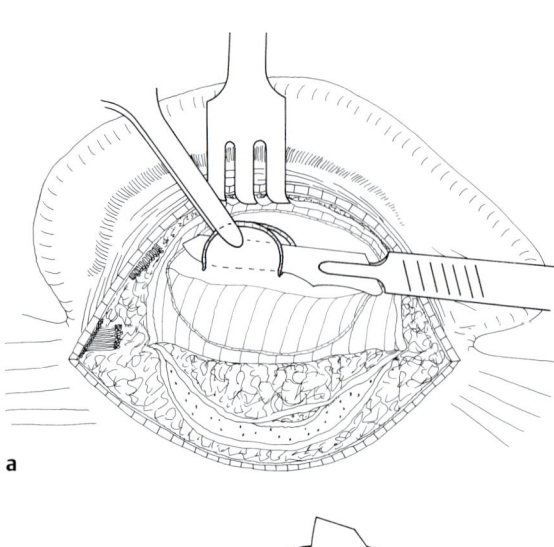

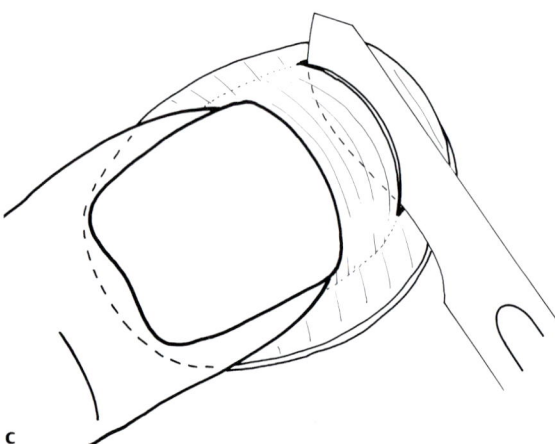

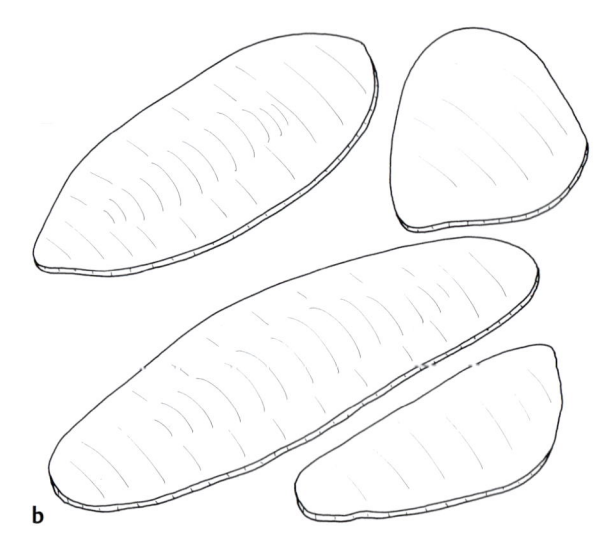

Fig. 10.2a–c Harvesting, cutting, and shaping of the thin cartilage plates, foils, and lamellae for cartilage mosaic tympanoplasty.
a In Portmann's posterosuperior incision, a large area of the conchal eminence is exposed. An incision of the subcutaneous tissue and the conchal perichondrium is made superiorly, exposing a large area of the convex conchal cartilage. Several tangential cuts are made with the scalpel, to harvest about 8–10 pieces of cartilage. A piece of perichondrium is removed as well. The remaining perichondrium and subcutaneous tissue are replaced.
b Cartilage plates of various thicknesses (lamellae when elongated) harvested by tangential cutting of the exposed conchal cartilage. Usually they are thinnest peripherally and thickest in the center.
c Tangential cutting of a cartilage plate, to make it thinner in the center.

Harvesting and Elaboration of Cartilage Foils and Thin Plates

The harvesting of cartilage to be used for foils and thin plates is easy, because no large grafts and no perichondrium flaps are needed. An incision 2 mm medial to the dome of the tragus is recommended (see **Fig. 3.21**) for cosmetic reasons. If the endaural approach with intercartilaginous incision is used, the tragus cartilage is harvested through the intercartilaginous incision (see **Fig. 3.23a–c**). Conchal cartilage can be used as well, especially in cases with retroauricular approach (see **Figs. 3.26–3.28**).

A 5 mm × 5 mm to 9 mm × 9 mm tragus graft or concha graft is adequate for elaboration of foils, because three foils can be cut with the Kurz precision cartilage knife or other knives.

In the 1970s (Overbosch 1971) and in the 1980s (Yamamoto et al. 1984) homogenous cartilage from the nasal septum was used. Foils and thin plates of 0.1, 0.2, 0.3, and 0.4 mm thickness were cut using a dermatome. The plates were covered with fascia.

Portmann's Tangential Cutting of Conchal Thin Plates and Lamellae

In Portmann's posterosuperior incision (MMES_1, Figs. 123–131) the skin and the subcutaneous tissue are elevated, exposing the eminence of the concha. A flap of the subcutis and the perichondrium is elevated and turned backward, exposing a large area of the cartilage (**Fig. 10.2a**). Using an 11- or 15-blade scalpel, several tangential cuts of the conchal cartilage are made and several thin pieces of cartilage are cut. The maximum thickness is less than 0.5 mm. Toward the periphery of the graft the thickness of the plate decreases to 0.2 mm (**Fig. 10.2b**). These thin plates are used for mosaic cartilage tympanoplasty. If the cartilage plates are too thick in some places, they can be thinned by tangential cutting (**Fig. 10.2c**). A 0.5 mm thick cartilage plate can easily be thinned using the Kurz precision cartilage knife.

Indications for Surgery

The thickness of the foil is 0.2–0.3 mm—twice that of the normal eardrum. Closure of a simple dry perforation may give the same good acoustic result as closure with fascia or perichondrium, and the same or better anatomical result. Thus, indications may be as wide as they are for the use of fascia or the perichondrium.

On the basis of excellent anatomical and functional results, Abou Mayaleh et al. (2005) have widened the indication for cartilage mosaic tympanoplasty to all types of perforations and all types of tympanoplasty, especially the recurrent perforations, and perforations evolving on an inflammatory context and/or dysfunction of the eustachian tube. The authors recommend especially that anterior and inferior perforations be treated with the cartilage mosaic tympanoplasty, regardless of the ossicular chain status.

Underlay Techniques with Foils and Thin Plates

In underlay techniques the edge of the perforation has to be removed and cleaned of epithelium. The undersurface of the eardrum remnant has to be scarified and denuded, facilitating adherence of the foil to the eardrum remnant. The tympanomeatal flap, with the eardrum remnant, has to be elevated and the foils are placed and adapted to the undersurface of the eardrum. Adaptation of large foils may be difficult, so several small foils may be placed to cover a total perforation (see **Fig. 2.8**). One foil is placed under the previous foil—an "underlapping" arrangement. One foil is placed onto the previous foil—an overlapping. Both overlapping and underlapping can be employed in the same ear.

Examples of underlay techniques with foils and thin plates will be presented for posterior, inferior, and total perforations. An example using thin plates in Portmann mosaic technique is also presented.

Posterior Perforation

Posterior perforation is suitable for repair by cartilage foil technique. First the edge of the perforation is removed and cleaned, then the undersurface of the eardrum is scarified (**Fig. 10.3a**). After elevation of the tympanomeatal flap, Gelfoam balls are placed into the inferior part of the tympanic cavity, to support the two thin and light foils. The first is placed along the malleus handle, the second covers the most posterior part of the tympanic cavity and overlaps the first foil (**Fig. 10.3b**). Both are superiorly supported by the chorda tympani. After replacement of the tympanomeatal flap (**Fig. 10.3c**), rapid and complete epithelialization will take place.

Inferior Perforation

After the usual cleaning of the perforation and scarification of the under surface of the eardrum remnant, a large inferior tympanomeatal flap is elevated. Gelfoam is placed into the hypotympanum and around the umbo to support the foils (**Fig. 10.4a**). The first foil covers the anterior half, the second covers the posterior half of the tympanic cavity and overlaps the first foil. The third foil overlaps the second foil. After replacement of the tympanomeatal flap (**Fig. 10.4b**), conditions are good for epithelialization of the cartilage foils.

Total Perforation

Total perforation may be just a sequela of a non-cholesteatomatous chronic otitis media or the result of removal of a total retraction, of adhesive otitis media, or of tensa retraction cholesteatoma. The tubal function may be either abnormal or normal. In more severe pathology, the thickness of the foils can be increased to 0.3 mm and the extent of overlapping or underlapping can be increased, resulting in a thicker reconstructed eardrum.

All approaches can be used in cartilage foil technique; here the retroauricular approach is used and a large tympanomeatal flap is elevated, the edges of the perforation are cleaned, and the undersurface of the eardrum remnant is scarified. The first, the anterosuperior, foil is supported with Gelfoam (**Fig. 10.5a**). The large posterior foil is supported superiorly by the chorda tympani, inferiorly by Gelfoam. The third foil overlaps both other foils (**Fig. 10.5b**).

Tympanoplasty Type 2 with Incus Interposition

In the case of missing long process of the incus, the interposition of the autogenous incus is the best and in the long term the most stable ossiculoplasty method (**Fig. 10.6a**). The incus can be interposed and shaped in various ways (MMES_1, Figs 716–764). Usually a groove is made on the incus body to accommodate the stapes head. The end of the short process of the incus is usually visible on the anterior side of the malleus handle, allowing placement of the anterior foil onto the end of the short process. The second foil covers the body of the interposed incus. The lateral side of the incus body should be flattened to provide optimal contact to the foil. The third foil covers the inferoposterior quadrant and overlaps both foils. After replacement of the two tympanomeatal flaps with the denuded eardrum remnants, the foils are supposed primarily to stick to and later to adhere and grow to the eardrum remnants (**Fig. 10.6b**). Our knowledge of the processes taking place in the sticking together ("gluing") and active adherence between large areas of the "naked" foil and the scarified edge of the eardrum is scanty.

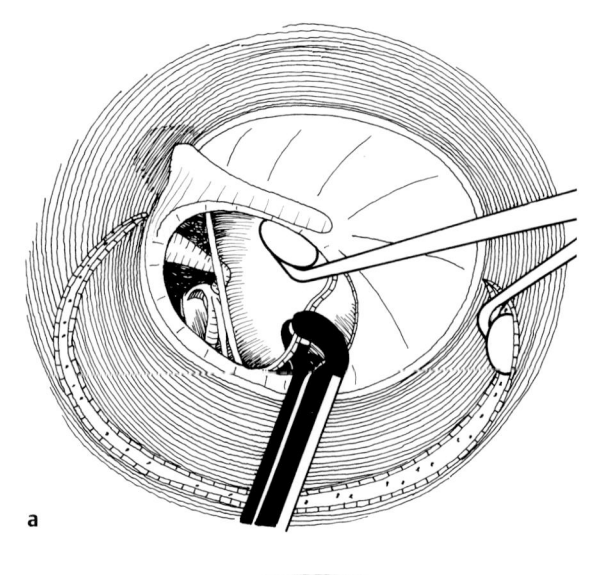

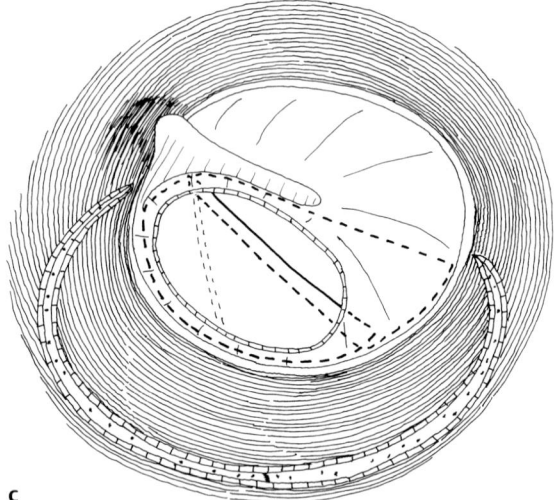

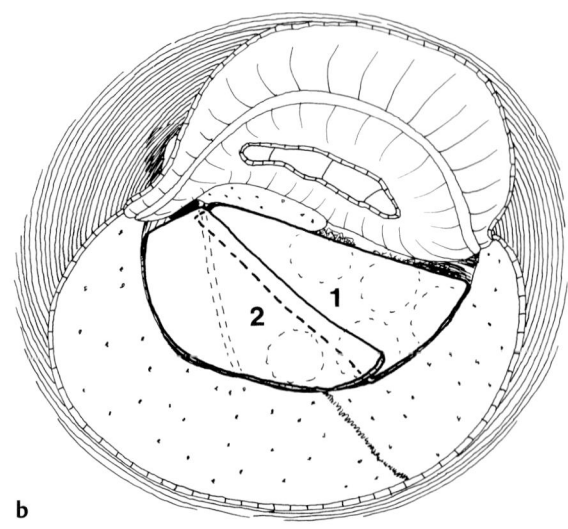

10 Underlay Tympanoplasty with Cartilage Foils and Thin Plates

Fig. 10.3a–c Underlay technique with cartilage foils to close a posterior perforation.

a The undersurface of the eardrum is scarified and the epithelium around the edge of the perforation is removed. A posterior circumferential skin incision is made.

b The tympanomeatal flap is elevated. After scarification of the posterior aspect of the malleus handle, a large foil is placed along the malleus handle (1), supported superiorly by the chorda tympani, inferiorly by Gelfoam balls. The second large foil (2) is placed overlapping the first foil and is additionally supported by the chorda tympani.

c The tympanomeatal flap is replaced and the foils will attach to the eardrum remnant by surface tension.

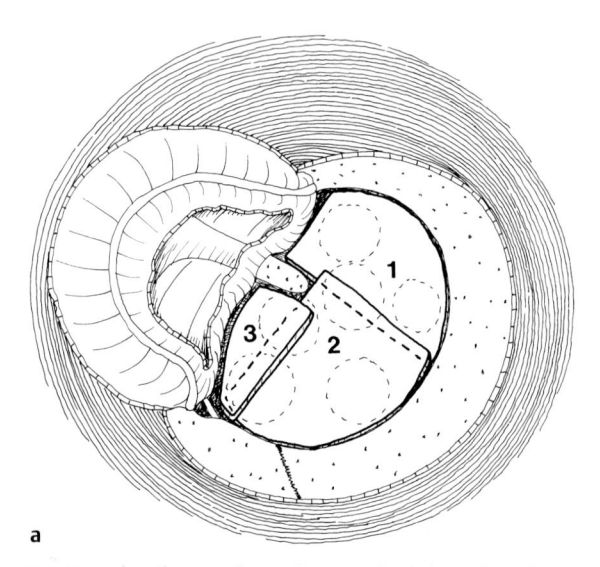

Fig. 10.4a, b Closure of an inferior perforation with underlay placement of cartilage foils.

a A large inferior circumferential incision is made, and the tympanomeatal flap is elevated. Some Gelfoam balls are placed into the hypotympanum and under the umbo to support the foils. The first foil is placed in the anterior hypotympanum, the second in the posterior hypotympanum, slightly overlapping the first foil. The small third foil overlaps the second foil.

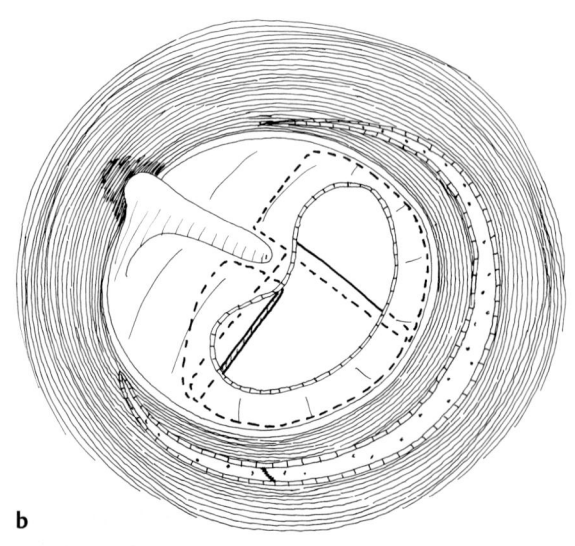

b The tympanomeatal flap is replaced.

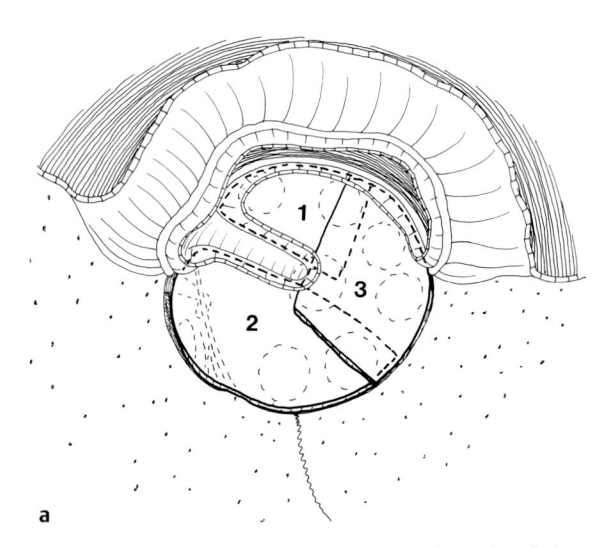

Fig. 10.5a, b Closure of a total perforation with cartilage foils in a retroauricular approach.
a A large tympanomeatal flap is elevated and Gelfoam balls are placed into the anterior and inferior parts of the tympanic cavity. The first foil covers the anterosuperior quadrant, the large second foil covers the posterior half, and the third foil covers the inferior part of the tympanic cavity, overlapping the first and the second foil.
b The tympanomeatal flap is replaced.

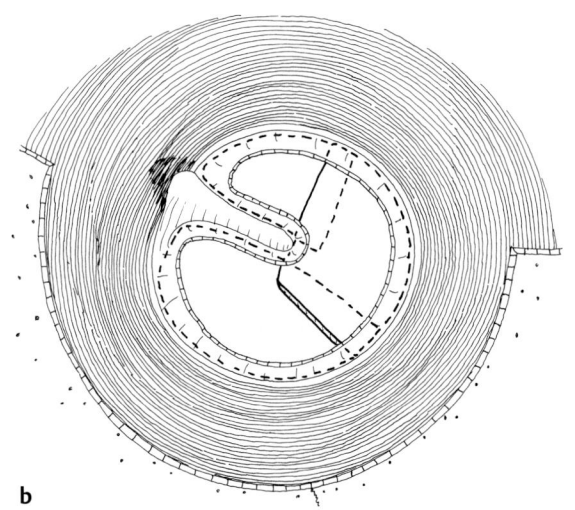

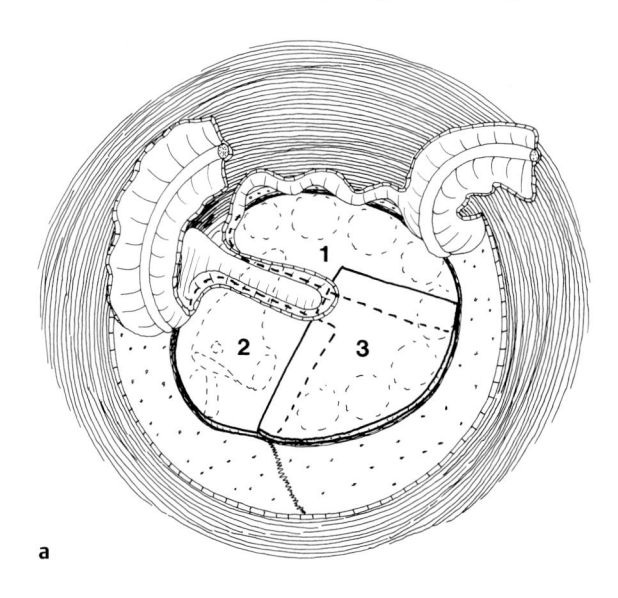

Fig. 10.6a, b Tympanoplasty type 2 with interposition of autogenous incus and closure of a total perforation with underlay-placed cartilage foils.
a With a swing-door incision two tympanomeatal flaps are elevated. The incus body with a groove is placed onto the stapes head; the short process of the incus is under the malleus handle. The large first foil covers the anterior half of the tympanic cavity and is supported by the short process of the incus and the Gelfoam balls. The second foil covers the interposed incus body. The third foil overlaps both foils.
b The tympanomeatal flaps are replaced.

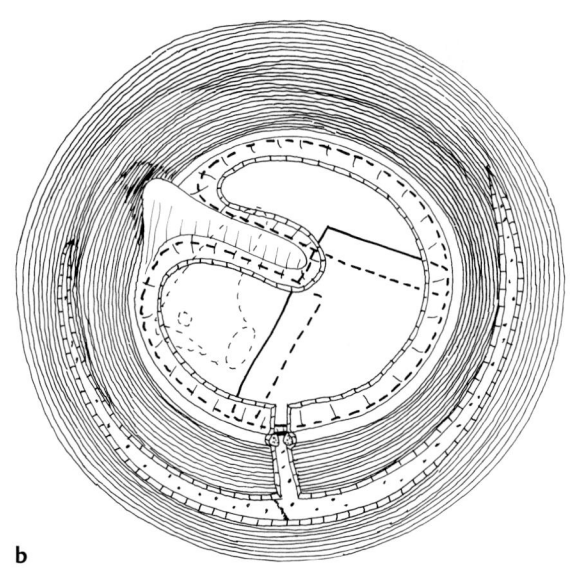

Tympanoplasty Type 3 with Kurz Titanium Columella (TORP)

In the case of missing stapes and total perforation, the tympanomeatal flap is elevated and a cartilage guide is placed onto the footplate. Through the hole of the guide, a titanium TORP prosthesis is placed onto the footplate (**Fig. 10.7a**) The head of the TORP is stabilized by the chorda tympani. The first foil covers the anterosuperior quadrant of the eardrum, the second covers most of the inferior tympanum and overlies the first foil. The third foil covers the posterior part of the tympanic cavity; it overlies the second foil and underlies the fourth foil, being placed onto the head of the prosthesis (**Fig. 10.7b**). A fifth foil also covers the head of the prosthesis: altogether, two foils with a total thickness of 0.4–0.5 mm cartilage are placed onto the prosthesis (**Fig. 10.7c**).

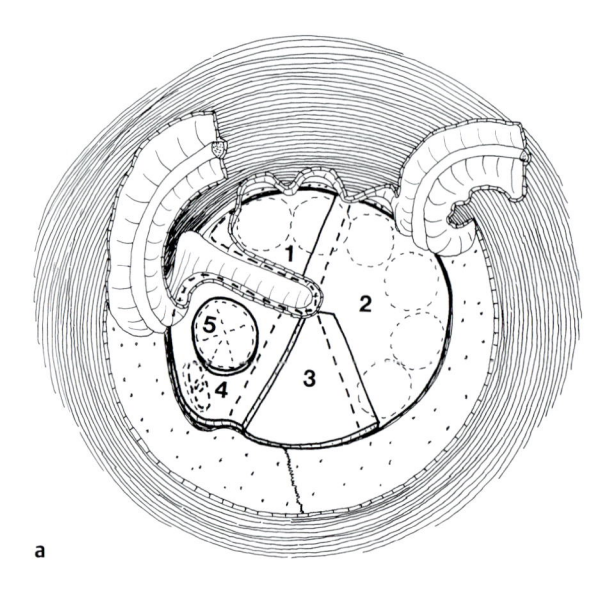

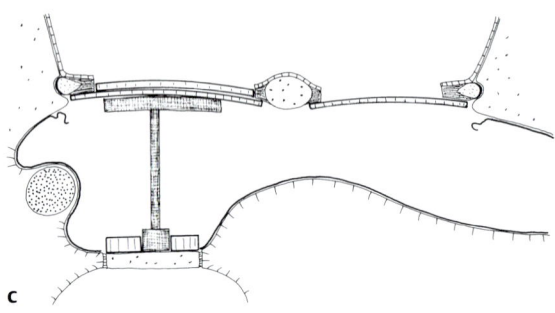

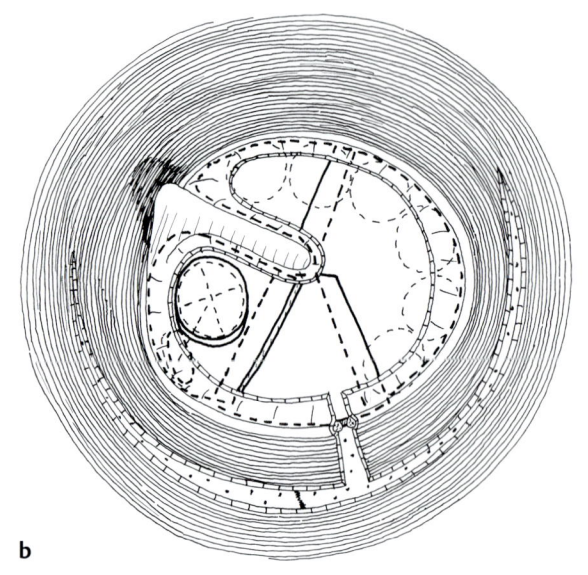

Fig. 10.7a–c Tympanoplasty type 3 with a TORP titanium prosthesis in a case of total perforation and missing stapes, closed with cartilage foils.
a After removal of the edge of the perforation and scarification of the undersurface of the eardrum, two tympanomeatal flaps are elevated. A cartilage guide and the foot of the prosthesis are placed onto the footplate. Gelfoam balls are placed into the anterior and inferior parts of the tympanic cavity. The four cartilage foils are placed into the anterior, inferior, and posterior parts of the tympanic cavity. A fifth foil covers the head of the prosthesis.
b The tympanomeatal flaps are replaced.
c Side view of reconstructed eardrum with two cartilage foils onto the TORP prosthesis. The cartilage guide is placed onto the footplate and the shaft of the prosthesis is placed onto the footplate. The anterior tympanum is covered with one foil only.

The Portmann Mosaic Underlay Cartilage Tympanoplasty with Foils or Thin Plates

In the retroauricular approach of Portmann (MMES_1, Figs 123–131), a posterosuperior incision 2–3 mm behind the retroauricular fold and a periosteal incision around the entrance of the bony ear canal are made. The postauricular skin is elevated, exposing the conchal cartilage for harvesting (see **Fig. 10.2a–c**).

The edges of the total perforation are cleaned. In the retroauricular approach, a large tympanomeatal flap is elevated and the undersurface of the eardrum remnant is scarified. The first and second foils or plates, both can be used, cover the anterior quadrants, with overlapping (**Fig. 10.8a**) The third foil or plate partly overlaps the second foil or plate. The fourth overlaps the third. The fifth foil or plate, resembling a small lamella, overlaps all the other four beneath the umbo. After replacement of the tympanomeatal flap (**Fig. 10.8b**) the foils and plates are covered with perichondrium or fascia, gluing all together with tissue fluid. Gelfoam is not used as support. The different foils or plates are overlapping each other; or are held in place only by surface tension. The perichondrium, placed as an on-lay graft, stabilizes the plates or foils.

It is the covering with perichondrium as an on-lay perichondrium graft that makes this method a modification of the underlay technique.

Results after Surgery with Cartilage Foils or Thin Plates Covered with Perichondrium

The Portmann group presented anatomical and functional results in 94 patients 3.5 years (range 3–7 years) after cartilage mosaic tympanoplasty (Abou Mayaleh et al. 2005). Nine patients were operated on both ears, making a total of 103 ears. The age distribution was 3–10 years, 19.4%; 10–20 years, 26.2%; 20–50 years, 40.8%; and 40–75 years 13.5%. The causes of the perforation were cholestea-

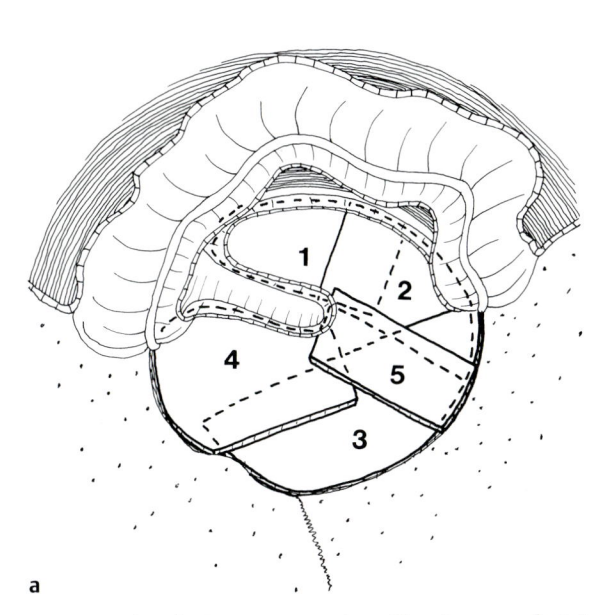

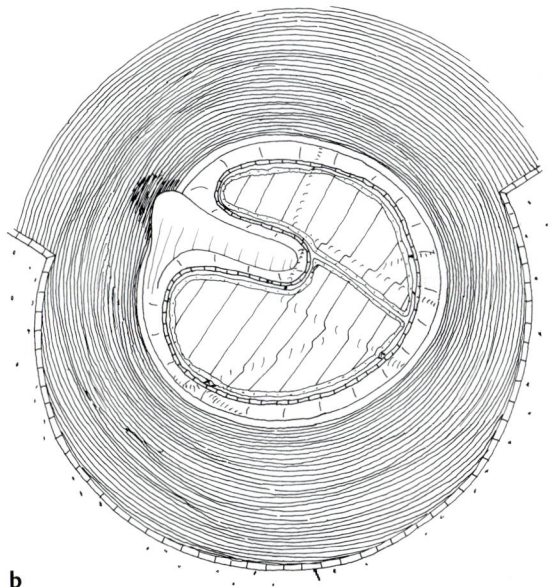

Fig. 10.8a, b The Portmann mosaic cartilage tympanoplasty in a total perforation.
a A large tympanomeatal flap is elevated and then the first thin plate or foil is placed as an underlay graft to cover the anterosuperior quadrant. The second thin plate or foil covers the anteroinferior quadrant and overlaps the first. The third covers the inferoposterior quadrant and partly overlaps the second. The fourth covers the posterosuperior quadrant and overlaps the third foil or plate. The fifth is placed inferior to the umbo, partly overlapping the other four.
b The tympanomeatal flap is replaced. The perichondrium covers the foils or plates as an on-lay graft.

toma 54.4%; non-cholesteatomatous chronic otitis media 20.4%; sequelae to secretory otitis with tubal dysfunction 17.5%; traumatic perforation 4.8%; severe tympanosclerosis 2.9%.

Anatomical Results
Perforations were closed in 93.2% of 103 ears. Retraction was found in one ear. The total rate of success was 92.2%. The position of the cartilage plates was satisfactory in 98% of the ears and the tympanic cavity was aerated in 97% of the ears.

Functional Results
Pre- and postoperative hearing was evaluated as the mean of 500 Hz, 1000 Hz, 2000 Hz and 4000 Hz.

The mean preoperative air–bone gap was 26.5 dB and the mean postoperative gap was 14.6 dB. The mean air–bone gap gain was 12.5 dB (range 0–40 dB).

In three, originally small, perforations the mean hearing gain was 7.4 dB; in 29 perforations with original size of one-quarter of the eardrum the mean hearing gain was 14.5 dB; in 41 ears with perforation one-half the size of the eardrum the mean gain was 17 dB; but in 23 perforations with original size of three-quarters of the eardrum the mean gain was only 6.2 dB. Similarly, in 7 subtotal perforations the mean gain was only 5.5 dB.

Generally, the anatomical and the functional results were good 3–7.5 years after surgery.

In 2006, B. Morra from Turin reported as a personal communication and in a video, the results of 383 patients operated in the period between 2000 and 2004, using underlay cartilage foils for the reconstruction of the eardrum. Of these patients, 191 had a cholesteatoma, 108 had a recurrent perforation, 70 had atalectasis, and 12 pediatric chronic otitis. At minimum 1 year after surgery, 4.2% of patients had a recurrent perforation, and 1.5% had a recurrent cholesteatoma. The overall preoperative average PTA-ABG (in the four frequencies 0.5–3 kH) was 29.2 dB +/−12.3 dB, and the postoperative PTA-ABC was 16.3 +/−9.9 db ($p > 0.05$). The anatomic and functional results were good.

No results from other surgeons have been published.

Author's Comments and Recommendations

The cartilage foil methods are very flexible and the thickness of the new eardrum can be doubled or tripled during the surgery by placing one, two or even three foils on each other. Because of the overlapping or underlapping of the foils, the irregularity of the eardrum constructed with foils is small in contrast to the irregularity produced with palisades.

Technically, the underlay foil technique and the on-lay foil techniques appear easy. The low weight of the foils makes it easier for the foils to 'glue' and then actively adhere to the undersurface of the scarified eardrum remnant. I still place some Gelfoam into the tympanic cavity to support the foils, but Abou Mayaleh et al. (2005) did not use Gelfoam or any other support and they did not observe dislocation of the foils into the tympanic cavity.

The on-lay placement of the foils onto the denuded lamina propria can be done precisely and the edges of the foils can be covered by the elevated eardrum epithelium, promoting rapid epithelialization of the foils.

The method using foils is to me the most interesting cartilage method, because during surgery the surgeon can make the eardrum thicker or thinner and thereby influence hearing.

However, we do not yet know how thick an eardrum reconstructed with cartilage foils should be to achieve optimal hearing. I am convinced that clinical studies of the postoperative hearing after reconstruction of the eardrum with 0.2 mm, 0.3 mm or 0.4 mm thick foils will be able to demonstrate the optimal thickness of the reconstructed eardrum.

The postoperative hearing after reconstruction of the eardrum with foils should be compared with results from series of patients with eardrums reconstructed using full-thickness cartilage–perichondrium composite grafts, cartilage palisades, or other cartilage tympanoplasty methods.

References

Abou Mayaleh H, Heshiki R, Portmann D, Negrevergne M. Tympanoplastie de renforcement en mosaïque de cartilage (differences avec la technique en palisade). [Reinforcing tympanoplasty with cartilage mosaic (differences from the palisade technique)] Rev Laryngol Otol Rhinol (Bord) 2005;126:181–189.

Mürbe D, Zahnert T, Bornitz M, Hüttenbrink K-B. Acoustic properties of different cartilage reconstruction techniques of the tympanic membrane. Laryngoscope 2002;112:1769–1776.

Overbosch HC. Homograft myringoplasty with micro-sliced septal cartilage. Pract Otorhinolaryngol (Basel) 1971;33:356–357.

Yamamoto E, Iwanaga M, Morinaka S. Use of micro-sliced homograft cartilage plates in tympanoplasty. Acta Otolaryngol Suppl 1984; 419:123–129.

11 On-lay Tympanoplasty with Cartilage Foils and Thin Plates

Definition

Thin cartilage foils with a thickness of 0.2 or 0.3 mm (see **Fig. 2.8**), or thin cartilage plates, with a thickness of 0.4 mm, are placed as on-lay grafts onto the denuded lamina propria (see **Fig. 2.9**). There is no difference between the cartilage foils used as on-lay grafts and those used in underlay tympanoplasty (Hüttenbrink, personal communication, 2001; Mürbe et al. 2002). The on-lay method with cartilage foils has not yet been published in the literature.

Inspired by Wullstein (1959, 1960), since the early 1960s I have performed on-lay tympanoplasty with fascia or with perichondrium in anterior, inferior, subtotal, and total perforations (Tos 1969,1972a, b, c) with satisfactory results. As a proponent of on-lay tympanoplasty, I sporadically performed about 15 on-lay tympanoplasties using cartilage foils in the period 2001–2005. The drawings for on-lay tympanoplasty are based on my long experience with the on-lay fascia tympanoplasty and these 15 on-lay tympanoplasties with cartilage foils.

Harvesting and Elaboration of Cartilage Foils and Thin Plates

There are no major differences in harvesting and elaboration of the cartilage foils between on-lay tympanoplasty and underlay tympanoplasty, as described in Chapter 10.

Full-thickness tragus or conchal cartilage pieces of 4 mm × 4 mm for small or of 8 mm × 8 mm for total perforation are harvested. The perichondrium is removed on both sides. With the Kurz Precise Cartilage Knife (see Chapter 3), three 0–2 mm thick foils can be cut.

The shape and the size of the foils needed for on-lay tympanoplasty is determined after elevation or removal of the epithelium surrounding the edge of the perforation. Usually the on-lay graft has to cover a 0.5 mm wide edge of the denuded lamina propria. Thus, 1 mm is added to the posteroanterior diameter and to the superioinferior diameter of the perforation to achieve the appropriate size and shape of the cartilage foil. A rectangular, 4 mm long hook is suitable for measurement of the perforation and the cartilage foil. As in underlay tympanoplasty, the perforation in on-lay tympanoplasty can be covered with two minor foils, overlapping each other.

Thin cartilage plates, cut with the scalpel from the concha as shown by Abou Mayaleh et al. (2005) (see **Fig. 10.2**) can also be used in on-lay technique.

Indications for On-lay Tympanoplasty with Cartilage Foils and Thin Plates

As for underlay tympanoplasty with foils and thin plates, the indications for on-lay tympanoplasty with cartilage foils and thin plates are wide because closure of the perforation with one or two foils may give the same acoustic results as with fascia or perichondrium. The anatomical results may even be better with cartilage foils than with fascia or perichondrium. Resistance against retraction may be stronger with the eardrum reconstructed with cartilage foils than with the eardrum reconstructed with fascia or perichondrium.

On-lay Techniques with Foils and Thin Plates

In the on-lay techniques the epithelium around the perforation has to be either elevated from the lamina propria as small epithelial flaps or removed; it can be elevated in some places, in other places it has to be removed. The most elegant and minimally invasive on-lay surgery is based on elevation of the epithelium all the way around the perforation, placing the foils onto the denuded lamina propria, and replacing the elevated epithelial flaps onto the thin cartilage foil. The cartilage foils can easily be placed exactly onto the denuded eardrum remnant (see **Fig. 2.9**). The foils can be cut exactly in relation to the size of the perforation and their overlapping is easily done. Furthermore, no support of the foils is needed.

As in tympanoplasty with fascia, in anterior, inferior, subtotal, and total perforations I prefer transcanal on-lay techniques, mainly because such methods are minimally invasive and need no support. Cartilage foils seem to be a good material for on-lay closure of any perforation, regardless of the size of the perforation.

Anterior Perforation

The anterior perforation is the best-suited perforation for the on-lay technique. The tympanoplasty can most often be performed through a transcanal approach with the ear speculum or through an endaural approach. Moreover, the on-lay technique is minimally invasive and a tympanotomy is often not necessary.

Several **methods of elevation of the epithelium** are described and used in this book:
1. The anterior swing-door technique, with elevation of two skin flaps, together with all other epithelial flaps (see **Figs. 5.5a–e, 8.3a–d**).
2. Technique with partial removal of the epithelium (**Figs. 5.6a–d, 8.2a–d**).
3. Technique with elevation of a large anterior skin flap (**Fig. 5.7a–d**).

The **methods of removal of the epithelium around the perforation** are also suitable for the on-lay placement of the foils (see MMES_1, Figs. 431–435).

The **methods with partial removal of the epithelium combined with the elevation of the epithelial flaps** can be used as well (see MMES_1, Figs. 447–452). The fastest epithelializaton of the foils occurs when all the epithelium is preserved and can cover the edges of the foils (see MMES_1, Figs. 455–570).

In this chapter only the technique with anterior elevation of two skin flaps together with the elevation of all other epithelial flaps will be illustrated, in connection with the on-lay placement of the foils (**Fig. 11.1a**). A trimmed foil is placed onto the denuded edges of the lamina propria. The skin flaps are pulled from the ear canal onto the cartilage foil, and the other flaps are replaced, partly covering the edges of the foil (**Fig. 11.1b**). A moist, flattened disk of Gelfoam covers the anterior half of the tympanic membrane.

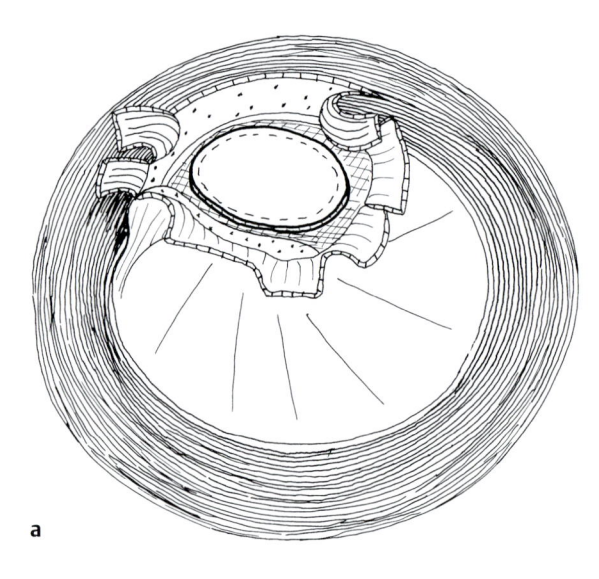

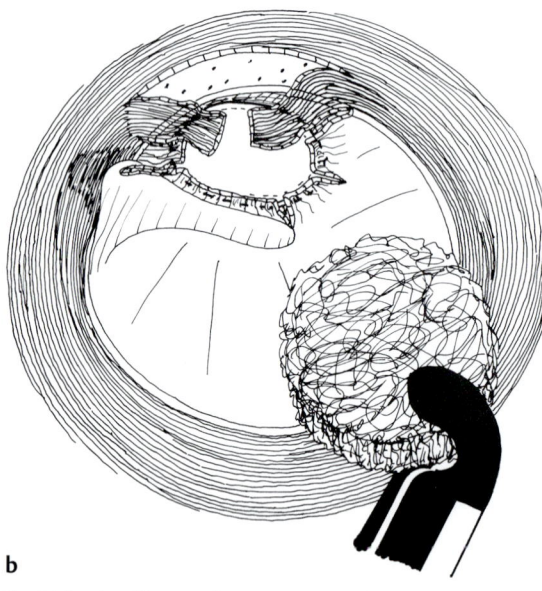

Fig. 11.1a, b Closure of an anterior perforation by placing a trimmed cartilage foil as on-lay graft onto the denuded lamina propria.
a With a small anterior swing-door incision and a radial incision at the 2-o'clock position, two skin flaps and several epithelial flaps around the perforation are elevated. The cartilage foil is shaped and placed onto the denuded lamina propria.
b The epithelial flaps are replaced, covering the edges of the foil. The two skin flaps are pulled over the edge of the foil. The anterior part of the eardrum is covered with a flat disk of moistened Gelfoam. The Gelfoam fixes the cartilage foil and the epithelial flaps.

Inferior Perforation

Inferior perforation is also very suitable for on-lay techniques with use of cartilage foils. Several **methods of elevation of the epithelium** surrounding the inferior perforation have been illustrated previously:
1. Partial elevation of the superior epithelium flaps and removal of the remaining epithelium along the inferior border of the perforation (see **Figs. 5.9b–f, 8.5a, b**).
2. Elevation of a large tympanomeatal flap together with the surrounding epithelium (see **Figs. 5.10a, b, 5.11a, b, 8.6b, c**).
3. Outward elevation of the surrounding epithelium and the ear canal skin (see **Figs. 5.12a–c, 5.13a, b**).

The three methods described are suitable for closure of an inferior perforation with foils placed as on-lay grafts.

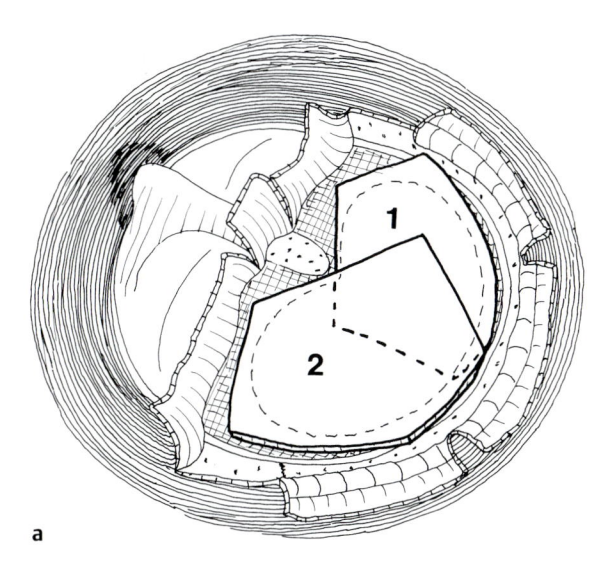

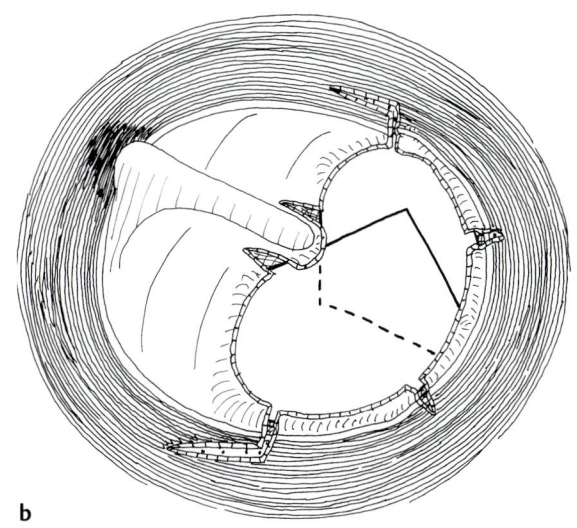

Fig. 11.2a, b Closure of an inferior perforation with on-lay cartilage foils after elevation of epithelial flaps.
a Four small radial incisions of the eardrum epithelium are performed. Using a round knife or an incudostapedial knife, epithelium is elevated from the superior border of the perforation and from the umbo region. Then elevation is continued around the inferior border, creating three flaps with the eardrum epithelium and ear canal skin. First an anterior foil and then a posterior foil are placed onto the denuded lamina propria. The posterior foil overlaps the anterior foil.
b The small epithelial flaps are replaced, covering the edges of the foils.

The **methods of removal of the epithelium** around the perforation can also be used in on-lay tympanoplasty with cartilage foils (see MMES_1, Figs. 436–439). Also the **methods of part removal and part elevation of the epithelium** (see MMES_1, Figs. 471–476) can often be used with cartilage foils.

Here the method of outward elevation of the epithelium and the skin is described (**Fig. 11.2a**). First, the superior flaps are elevated. Four small radial incisions are made at the 5-o'clock and 7-o'clock positions and three epithelial flaps along the inferior border of the perforation are elevated. The first cartilage foil is placed onto the denuded lamina propria, covering the anterior part of the perforation. The posterior part of the perforation is closed by the second foil, which overlaps the first foil. After replacement of the epithelial flaps, the edges of the foils are covered with the epithelium, allowing rapid epithelialization (**Fig. 11.2b**).

Total Perforation

For total perforations, several **methods of elevation of the epithelial flaps** can be used in on-lay technique with cartilage foils:
1. On-lay technique with elevation of three superior epithelial flaps and removal of the skin and epithelium around the inferior part of the perforation (see **Fig. 5.14a**).
2. On-lay technique with elevation of a large tympanomeatal flap, together with the epithelial flaps (see **Figs. 5.16a–c, 5.17a, b**).
3. Elevation of three superior flaps and elevation of four inferior epithelial flaps (see **Figs. 8.7a–c, 8.11a–d, 11.3a–c**).

The third method attempts to preserve all epithelium in a minimally invasive manner and will be used to illustrate the on-lay foil technique. It represents a combination of my technique of elevation of three superior flaps (Tos 1980) with elevation of the inferior flaps (Calcaterra 1972).

First, the three superior flaps are elevated (**Fig. 11.3a**); then the three inferior radial incisions of the epithelium are made and four inferior epithelial flaps are elevated outward. Because all foils meet each other at the umbo region, a Gelfoam ball is placed here to support the foils around the umbo. First the anterosuperior foil and then the anteroinferior foil are placed, overlapping the first foil (**Fig. 11.3b**). The third foil overlaps the second foil and the fourth foil overlaps the third foil. A fifth, lamella-like foil is placed between the umbo and the inferior part of the fibrous annulus. After replacement of the epithelial flaps (**Fig. 11.3c**), the reconstruction of the new eardrum should appear quite solid. Where there is some doubt, with fear of a later retraction, further small foils can be placed onto the suspect regions.

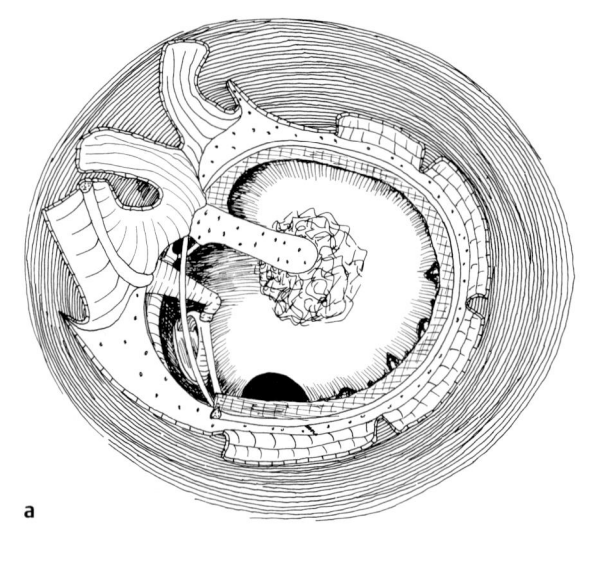

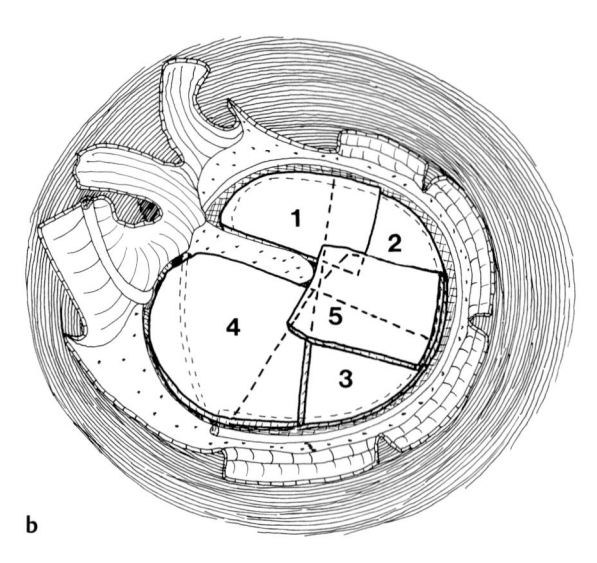

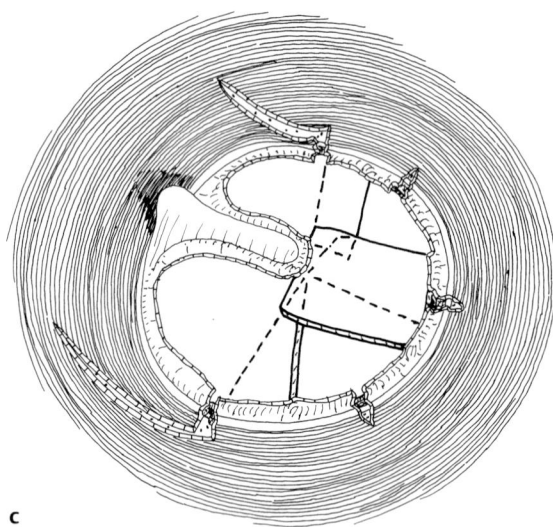

Fig. 11.3a–c A combination of elevation of three superior and three or four inferior epithelial flaps and the on-lay closure of the total perforation with cartilage foils.

a Superoposterior and superoanterior circumferential ear canal skin incisions and five small radial incisions of the eardrum epithelium along the border of the perforation are performed. Using a round knife or an incudostapedial knife, the epithelial flaps and the skin flaps are elevated all the way around the total perforation; the lamina propria and the edge of the perforation are cleaned of epithelium. The fibrous annulus and a small belt of the ear canal bone are exposed. A Gelfoam ball is placed under the umbo. The posterosuperior fibrous annulus is elevated as well, to improve the view to the footplate.
b The first foil is placed onto the denuded anterior lamina propria and onto the lamina propria along the anterior edge of the malleus handle. The second foil overlaps the first foil, the third foil overlaps the second foil, the fourth foil overlaps the third foil. Finally a broad lamella is placed as the fifth foil to cover the region inferior to the umbo.
c The tympanomeatal flaps are replaced.

Tympanoplasty Type 2 with Interposition of the Incus and Covering the Total Perforation with Cartilage Foils

A large tympanomeatal flap with the eardrum epithelium is elevated. The lamina propria and the edge of the perforation are carefully cleaned of any remnants there may be of the squamous epithelium. The defective incus is removed and shaped, to be placed onto the head of the stapes. A groove for the head of the stapes head is made on the incus and the head is flattened to accommodate the foils (**Fig. 11.4a**). The first foil covers the anterior half of the tympanic cavity. The second foil covers the inferoposterior part of the cavity and overlaps the anterior foil. The third foil covers the superoposterior part of the cavity and the interposed incus (**Fig. 11.4b**). The tympanomeatal flap is replaced, covering the edges of the foils and the malleus handle (**Fig. 11.4c**).

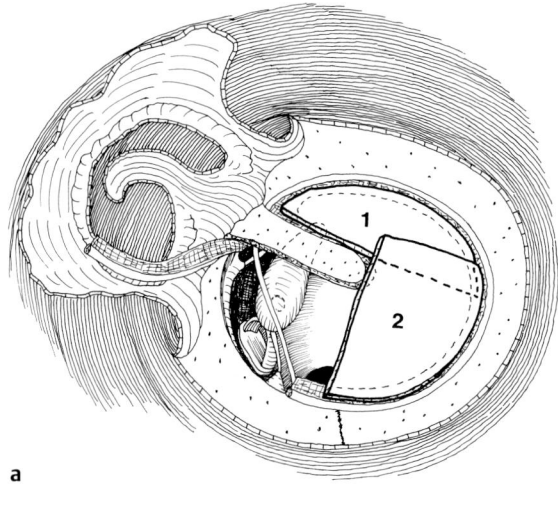

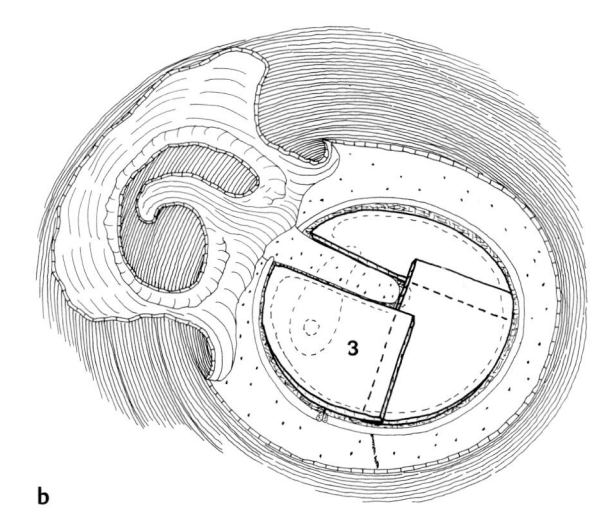

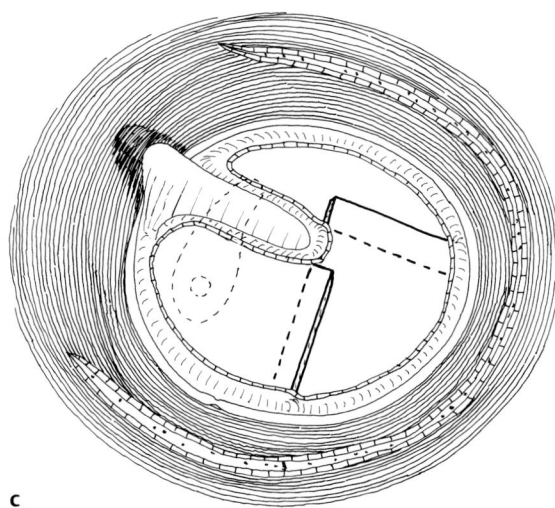

Fig. 11.4a–c Cartilage tympanoplasty type 2 with interposition of the shaped incus between stapes and the malleus handle and closure of the total perforation with foils.

a A large tympanomeatal flap with epithelial flaps is elevated and the lamina propria is cleaned of epithelium. The autogenous incus is shaped, with a groove to be placed onto the head of the stapes. The first foil covers the anterior half of the tympanic cavity. The second foil covers the inferoposterior quadrant and overlaps the first foil.
b The third foil is placed onto the shaped and flattened incus body and the denuded lamina propria. It overlaps the second foil.
c The tympanomeatal flap and the epithelial flaps are replaced.

Tympanoplasty Type 3 with the Shaped Autogenous Incus as a TORP Columella and Closure of the Total Perforation Using Cartilage Foils

The three superior tympanomeatal and the three inferior epithelial flaps are elevated outward, exposing the lamina propria and the fibrous annulus (**Fig. 11.5a**). For missing stapes, the defective long process of the incus is removed and shaped as a TORP columella. The short process of the incus is placed onto the footplate, the remnant of the long process is shaped and placed under the malleus handle (**Fig. 11.5a**). The foils are placed onto the cleaned lamina propria: the large anterior foil is placed first, then the inferior foil, partly overlapping the anterior foil, followed by the posterior foil, covering the incus and overlapping the inferior foil. On the superior and inferior sides of the incus two small foils (5) are placed to reinforce the superior foil and make it thicker (**Fig. 11.5a**). The tympanomeatal flaps and the epithelial flaps are replaced, covering the edges of the foils (**Fig. 11.5b, c**).

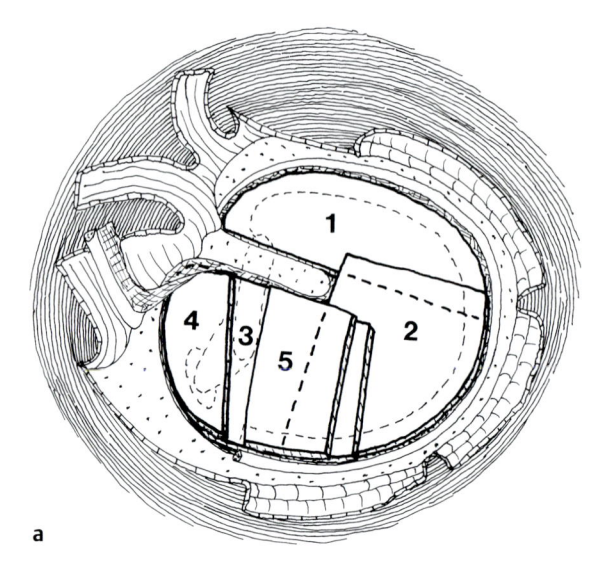

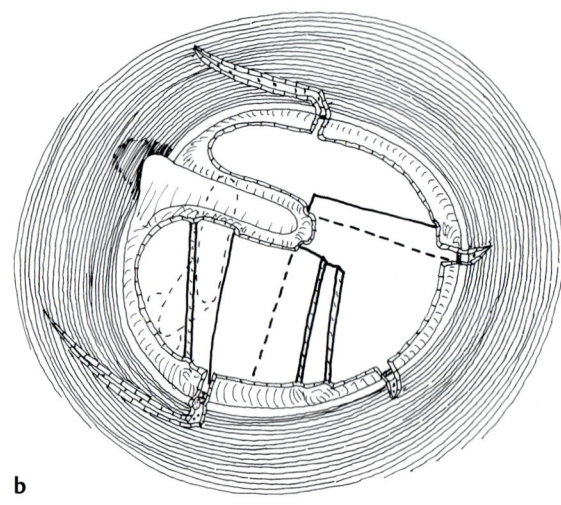

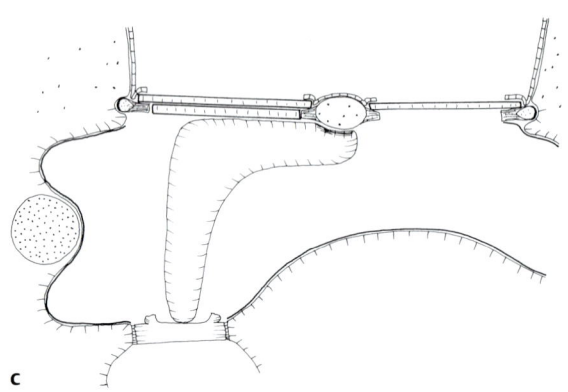

Fig. 11.5a–c Cartilage tympanoplasty type 3 with autogenous incus as a TORP columella and a total perforation covered with on-lay cartilage foils.

a Three superior tympanomeatal flaps and three inferior epithelial flaps are elevated outwards. First, the defective incus is removed and shaped. The shaped short process of the incus is placed onto the footplate, the shaped incus body under the malleus handle. A large anterior foil is placed first, onto the denuded lamina propria. The second foil covers the inferoposterior quadrant and overlaps the first foil. The third foil covers the interposed incus and overlaps the second foil. Two additional foils are placed onto the third foil: one superior to the incus and one inferior to the incus.
b The tympanomeatal flaps and the epithelial flaps are replaced.
c Side view at the level of the footplate of cartilage tympanoplasty type 3 with an autogenous incus as a columella and closure of a total perforation with on-lay cartilage foils. The anterior foil lies on the denuded lamina propria. The posterior foil lies on the flattened incus. Another foil is placed onto the posterior foil and onto the denuded posterior lamina propria, thickening the posterior part of the eardrum in on-lay tympanoplasty.

Results after On-lay Tympanoplasty with Cartilage Foils

No results of surgery after on-lay tympanoplasty with cartilage foil have been published. Primary results were good in 15 patients, 3 months after on-lay tympanoplasty with cartilage foils that I performed. The perforations were closed in all ears and the hearing was good. The epithelialization of the cartilage was rapid and complete.

Author's Comments and Recommendations

The on-lay placement of the foils onto the denuded lamina propria can be done precisely and the edges of the foils can be covered by the elevated eardrum epithelium, promoting rapid epithelialization of the foils.

The cartilage foil method is, in my opinion, the most interesting and promising cartilage method, because during surgery the surgeon can make the eardrum thicker or thinner and can thereby influence the hearing.

However, we do not yet know how thick an eardrum reconstructed with cartilage foils should be to achieve optimal hearing. I am convinced that clinical studies of the postoperative hearing after reconstruction of the eardrum with 0.2 mm, 0.3 mm or 0.4 mm thick foils will be able to demonstrate the optimal thickness of the reconstructed eardrum.

The postoperative hearing after reconstruction of the eardrum with foils should be compared with results from series of patients with eardrums reconstructed using full-thickness cartilage–perichondrium composite island grafts, cartilage palisades, or other cartilage tympanoplasty methods.

The great advantage of cartilage foils is their easy placement, either onto the denuded lamina propria or under the eardrum.

References

Calcaterra TC. The window shade technique of tympanic membrane grafting. Laryngoscope 1972;82:45–49.

Abou Mayaleh H, Heshiki R, Portmann D, Négrevergne M. Tympanoplastie de renforcement en mosaique de cartilage (differences avec la technique en palisade). Rev Laryngol Otol Rhinol (Bord) 2005;126:181–189.

Mürbe D, Zahnert T, Bornitz M, Hüttenbrink K-B. Acoustic properties of different cartilage reconstruction techniques of the tympanic membrane. Laryngoscope 2002;112:1769–1776.

Tos M. Tympanoplastik ved kronisk suppurativ otitis media. Ugeskr Laeger 1969;131:1385–1392.

Tos M. Tympanoplasty in chronic adhesive otitis media. Acta Otolaryngol 1972a;73:53–60.

Tos M. Assessment of the results of tympanoplasty. J Laryngol Otol 1972b;86:487–500.

Tos M. Results of tympanoplasty with modified radical mastoidectomy. Acta Otolaryngol 1972c;74:61–65.

Tos M. Stability of myringoplasty based on late results. ORL J Otorhinolaryngol Relat Spec 1980;42:171–181.

Wullstein H. Fundamentals and tasks of plastic surgery in operation for restoration of hearing. J Laryngol Otol 1959;73:515–525.

Wullstein HL. Operationen zur Verbesserung des Gehöres. Stuttgart: Thieme; 1960:291–307..

12 On-lay Tympanoplasty with Thick Cartilage Plates

Definitions

Cartilage plates do not have attached perichondrium and are used as reinforcement of the eardrum, either of the entire eardrum or of parts of it. At the end of the procedure the cartilage plates will usually be covered with fascia, or with free perichondrium. The cartilage plates are not suspended by the perichondrium flaps, as are the cartilage–perichondrium composite island grafts, which is the most important characteristic of cartilage plates.

Cartilage plates can be used in on-lay tympanoplasty as described in this chapter, or in underlay tympanoplasty as described in Chapter 13. In on-lay cartilage tympanoplasty the cartilage plate is placed onto the eardrum remnant (Jansen 1963; Weichselbaumer 1968; Kleinsasser and Glanschneider 1969; Kleinfeldt et al. 1975).

After the palisade technique, on-lay cartilage plate tympanoplasty is the oldest cartilage tympanoplasty method, started by Klaus Jansen in the early 1960s.

Harvesting and Elaboration of the Cartilage Plates

Usually autogenous concha or tragus cartilage is used to elaborate the cartilage plates, as a full-thickness graft, as a three-quarter-thickness graft, or as a half-thickness graft. Autogenous septum cartilage was harvested and first used by Salen (1964) in myringoplasty, as described in Chapter 1. Jansen (1963) used allogenous nasal septum cartilage, later autogenous cartilage, and even perichondrium that was separately harvested from the nasal septum.

There are no differences between the harvesting and elaboration of autogenous cartilage plates used for on-lay cartilage tympanoplasty and those for underlay tympanoplasty; the details of elaboration and thinning are described in Chapter 13.

Homogenous Cartilage

In the 1960s and 1970s, homogenous cartilage from the nasal septum or from the outer ear was often used in middle ear surgery (Jansen 1963, 1968, Smyth and Kerr 1967, 1970, Overbosch 1971, Raivio and Siirala, 1973, Yamamoto et al. 1985). Most often, the septum cartilage was micro-sliced to 0.1, 0.2, 0.3 and 0.4 mm thick foils or plates. The surgical methods were similar to the methods using autogenous grafts. Homogenous cartilage is no longer used.

The surgical techniques used with autogenous cartilage foils and thin plates have been shown in Chapters 10 and 11.

Homogenous Eardrum Implantation

The implantation of the homogenous eardrum also began in the 1960s (Marquet 1966, 1968; Brandow 1969; Betow 1975, 1982). Because of fear of infection, especially with HIV and with the hepatitis virus, the use of homografts was abandoned worldwide in the 1990s, except in Belgium. In that country, surgery with homogenous cartilage and homogenous eardrum continues, and there have been no reports of viral transmission and infection (Decat et al. 1997).

In some countries, cartilage can be donated from persons screened for diseases contraindicated to transplantation after specific guidelines. The harvested cartilage is sterilized with gamma irradiation (Schulte et al. 1998).

On-lay Techniques with Thick Cartilage Plates

Although homogenous cartilage cannot be used today, the surgical techniques in which homogenous cartilage plates were used previously can still be employed, though now with autogenous cartilage plates.

On-lay tympanoplasty has been popular since the 1960s and 1970s, especially when using cartilage plates covered with a fascia graft or a free perichondrium graft.

The goal of using cartilage plates is to reinforce the eardrum and stabilize and protect the various columellae or interposed ossicles, i.e., the various TORP and PORP prostheses.

The Jansen Cartilage Plate On-lay Tympanoplasty

Jansen (1963) was the first to start using homogenous cartilage plates, taken from the septum. He used an on-lay technique, which at that time was a popular method, either in tympanoplasty alone or together with his "intact canal wall mastoidectomy." Jansen used the transcanal approach through the ear canal speculum, starting with small radial skin incisions around the annulus, and with elevation of large posterior and small anterior skin flaps, exposing a belt of the bony ear canal, the fibrous annulus, and the cleaned lamina propria of the eardrum remnant (**Fig. 12.1a**). After removal of the bone along the postero-superior scutum, the tympanic sinuses are visible. A half-thickness cartilage plate without perichondrium, but with a cut-out for the malleus handle, is placed onto the umbo and onto the denuded eardrum remnant (**Fig. 12.1b**). A round fascia graft covers the malleus handle, the cartilage plate, the fibrous annulus, and the ear canal bone (**Fig. 12.1c**). After replacement of the skin flaps rapid epithelialization will take place (**Fig. 12.1 d, e**).

Tympanoplasty Type 2 or Type 3 and Cartilage Plates

In cholesteatoma, Jansen (1963) performed intact canal wall mastoidectomy and tympanoplasty. In the case of intact stapes and missing long process of the incus, Jansen made a hole through the posterosuperior part of the cartilage plate and connected a cartilage prosthesis between the head of the stapes and the perichondrium, or the fascia covering the cartilage plate. Today I replace the cartilage prosthesis with a shaped bony prosthesis, either a shaped incus remnant or the cortical bone (**Fig. 12.2a**).

When the stapes is missing, a long cartilage columella between the footplate and the perichondrium is today replaced with a columella made from an incus or from a piece of the cortical bone (**Fig. 12.2b**). The relatively thin and long cartilage columella will certainly become soft, with poor sound transmission as a result.

The Titanium Columella and Cartilage Plates

Instead of cartilage or cortical bone, nowadays a titanium columella will most often be placed between the footplate and the cartilage plate (**Fig. 12.3a, b**). There is no need to create a hole in the cartilage plate. The fascia or the perichondrium covers the entire cartilage plate and the upper part of the malleus handle, allowing rapid epithelialization.

The head of a titanium PORP prosthesis can be placed under the cartilage plate, without making a hole in the cartilage plate, as shown in **Figs. 4.9b, c, 4.10–4.12, 4.13a, 4.14a**.

"Cartilage Boards" On-lay Technique

Weichselbaumer (1968) placed a full-thickness cartilage plate, roughly pear-shaped, onto the denuded lamina propria of the eardrum remnant, to close a large perforation (**Fig. 12.4a**). The superior end, with a small groove, is placed onto the head of the stapes. The method is termed "cartilage boards" (*Knorpelbretter*).

I propose total closure of the perforation, especially in the posterosuperior region, either by enlarging the upper part of the cartilage plate or by adding three small pieces of cartilage. After covering the cartilage with fascia (**Fig. 12.4b**) and replacement of the skin flaps, the closure seems to be solid (**Fig. 12.4c**).

In the case of a low stapes, a 1.5 mm × 1.5 mm cartilage plate with a groove is placed onto the stapes head. The cartilage plate is thereby further elevated to the level of the eardrum.

Cartilage Plates in Stabilization of the Columella

Kleinsasser and Glanschneider (1969), used half-thickness cartilage plates, harvested from the tragal cartilage through intercartilaginous incision (**Fig. 17.5a–c**). The cartilage plates are placed as on-lay grafts, onto the denuded lamina propria, and covered by a fascia graft. In tympanoplasties after canal wall down mastoidectomies (**Fig. 12.5a–d**) the superior edge of the plate is supported by small balls of fibrous tissue placed onto the eminence of the facial nerve and the eminence of the tensor tympani muscle. The footplate and the cartilage plate are connected with columellae (**Fig. 12.5a, b**), the stapes is connected with the cartilage plate by a bony prosthesis (**Fig. 12.5c, d**).

These days the footplate will be connected with the cartilage plate by a shaped columella made of cortical bone, or the shaped incus (**Fig. 12.6a–c**), or by a titanium TORP columella. Between the stapes and the cartilage plate a PORP titanium prosthesis or a shaped incus may be used (**Fig. 12.6d**).

Full-Thickness Cartilage Plate

Kleinfeldt et al. (1975) used a full-thickness concha cartilage plate, without perichondrium. The size of the plate is slightly larger than the size of the perforation. The cartilage plate was **often pressed thinner** in the Cottle cartilage press. Additionally, the cartilage plate is thinned along the edge of the graft with a scalpel (**Fig. 12.7**). The cartilage plate is covered with fascia. The surgical on-lay technique is similar to the Jansen technique.

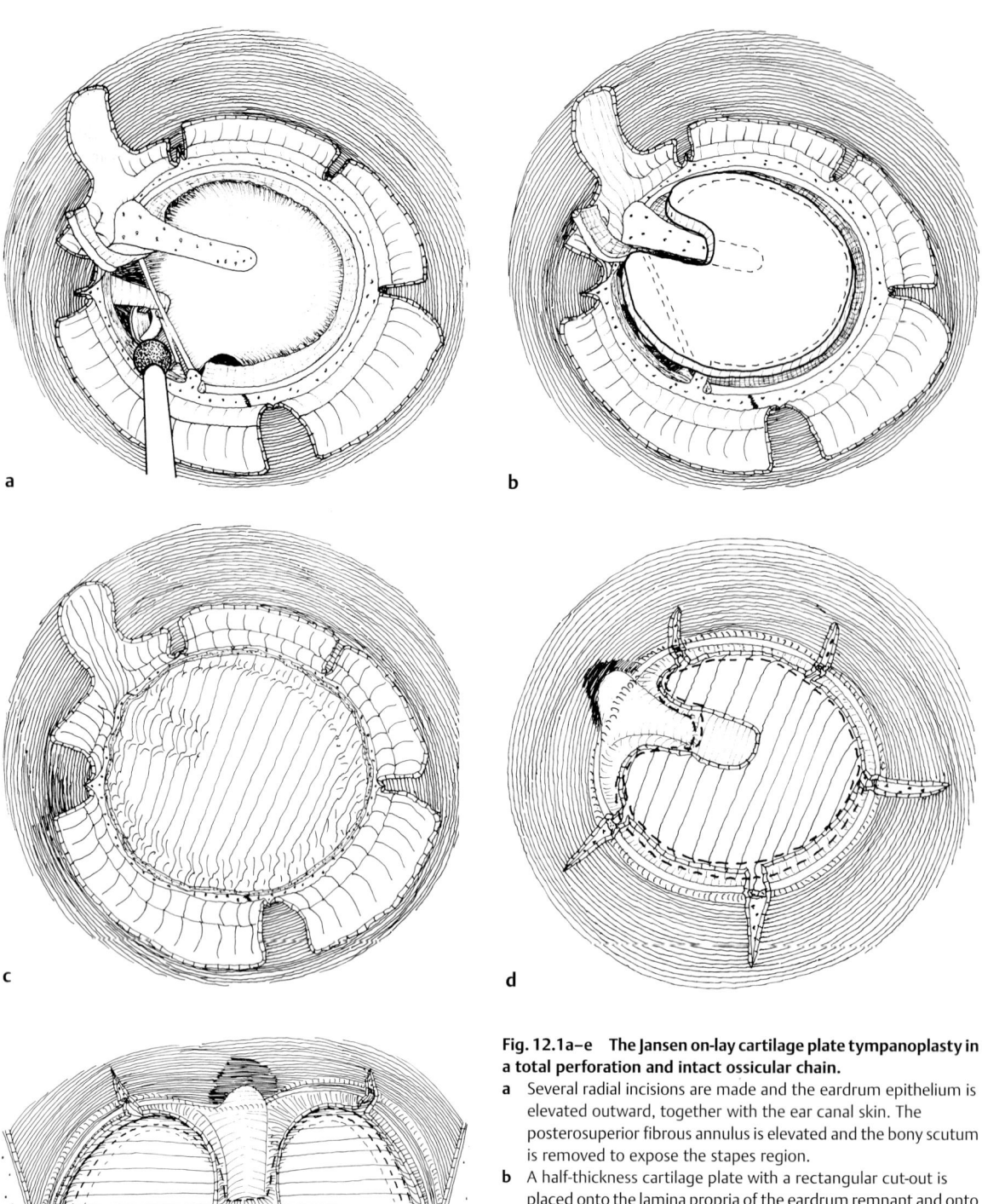

12 On-lay Tympanoplasty with Thick Cartilage Plates

Fig. 12.1a–e The Jansen on-lay cartilage plate tympanoplasty in a total perforation and intact ossicular chain.

a Several radial incisions are made and the eardrum epithelium is elevated outward, together with the ear canal skin. The posterosuperior fibrous annulus is elevated and the bony scutum is removed to expose the stapes region.

b A half-thickness cartilage plate with a rectangular cut-out is placed onto the lamina propria of the eardrum remnant and onto the inferior part of the malleus handle and the umbo.

c The fascia covers the cartilage plate, the superior half of the malleus handle, the fibrous annulus and the ear canal bone.

d The tympanomeatal flaps are replaced along with the malleus flap.

e Side view, with some perspective, of the on-lay closure of a total perforation with a cartilage plate and fascia at the level of the umbo. The cartilage plate lies on the umbo and the denuded lamina propria of the eardrum. The fascia covers the cartilage plate, the lamina propria, the fibrous annulus, and the ear canal bone.

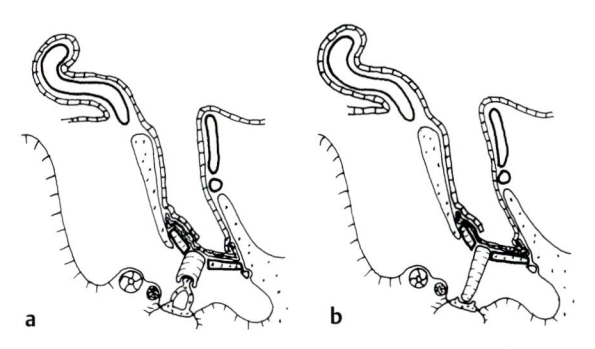

Fig. 12.2a, b The intact canal wall mastoidectomy and tympanoplasty.
a Type 2 tympanoplasty, with interposition of a shaped incus between the head of the stapes and the fascia, covering the cartilage plate. A hole is made on the cartilage plate.
b Type 3 tympanoplasty with a columella of shaped incus, placed between the footplate and the undersurface of the fascia. The columella penetrates the hole in the cartilage disk.

Results of Surgery with Cartilage Plates

Results of the Early On-lay Techniques

Among the 100 tympanoplasties using the technique described, Jansen (1963) found only two discharging ears 3 weeks after surgery. Jansen claims that the sound conduction is restored, but no audiological data are presented. The sound vibration is transmitted from the new eardrum via the cartilage columella, but it is now well known that cartilage in a long columella becomes soft, with poor transmission.

Weichselbaumer (1968) claims that the hearing gain is satisfactory with his methods and that it often covers the entire frequency range. However, no audiological pre- and postoperative data are presented.

Kleinsasser and Glanschneider (1969) presented good documentation of audiological data and good results with their methods of cartilage plates. The postoperative hearing was better with the bony columella than with the cartilage columella. Results were best after placement of a bony prosthesis between the stapes head and the cartilage plate.

At follow-up 2 years after 100 tympanoplasties with total and subtotal perforations, Kleinfeldt et al. (1975) obtained an anatomical success rate of 98%, with intact eardrum. Among 84 ears with intact ossicular chain and tympanoplasty type 1, the postoperative hearing was normal (0–10 dB) in 66 ears, improved in 15 ears, and unchanged in 3 ears. Among 16 ears with tympanoplasty type 3, or with adhesive otitis, the results were poor, with unchanged preoperative hearing in 14 ears.

Kleinfeldt et al. conclude that the sound transmission of a pressed, full-thickness cartilage plate placed as on-lay graft may provide excellent functional results in cases with intact ossicular chain.

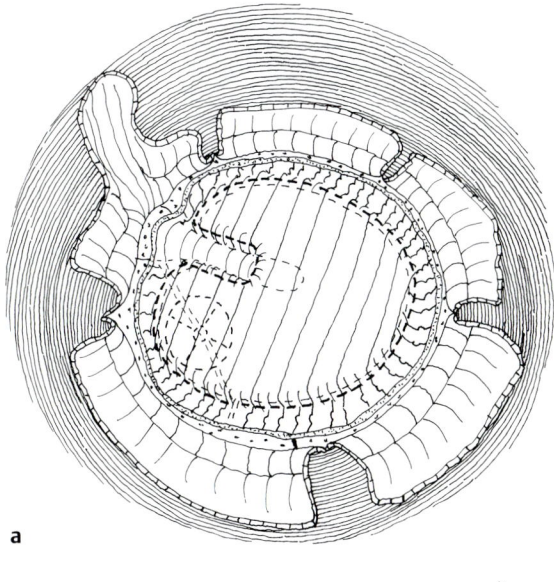

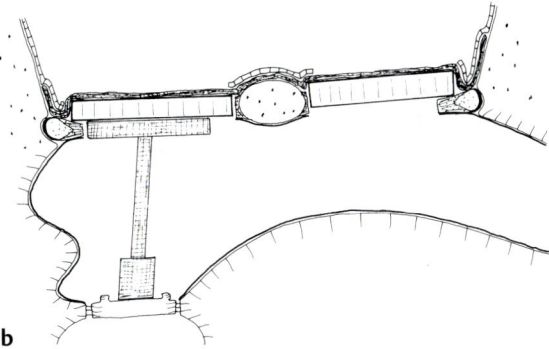

Fig. 12.3a, b Placement of a Kurz titanium columella between the footplate and the cartilage plate in an on-lay tympanoplasty type 3.
a The skin flaps are elevated together with the epithelium of the eardrum remnant. A titanium columella is placed onto the footplate and a half-thickness cartilage plate with a rectangular cut-out is placed onto the denuded lamina propria of the eardrum and partly onto the umbo. The fascia covers the cartilage and the denuded bone. Finally, the skin flaps will be replaced.
b Side view at the level of the footplate of the on-lay tympanoplasty type 3 with a cartilage plate, covered with a fascia graft. The head of the Kurz titanium columella has good contact with the undersurface of the cartilage plate, which is placed onto the lamina propria of the eardrum remnant and onto the umbo.

Author's Comments and Recommendations

The comments are based on on-lay and underlay tympanoplasty methods (Chapter 13) with thick cartilage plates.

The definition of cartilage plates is not strict and cannot be strict. The most important and constant characteristic of the cartilage plate is the lack of a perichondrium flap, while the thickness, placement and covering of the cartilage plates may have several variations.

Fig. 12.4a–c The "cartilage boards" technique in a total perforation with missing malleus handle and long process of the incus.
a Several small vertical skin incisions are performed, all the way around the fibrous annulus. The epithelium of the eardrum remnant and the adjacent ear canal skin is elevated. The superoposterior fibrous annulus is elevated and the bone of the scutum is removed to expose the stapes region. The remnant of the malleus is cleaned. A large, half-thickness, autogenous, concha cartilage plate, shaped to the form of a pear, is placed onto the denuded eardrum remnant. The upper, smaller end of the plate, with a groove, is placed onto the stapes head. My recommendation is to place three small palisades around the upper border of the plate.
b The cartilage plate and the denuded ear canal wall are covered with the fascia graft.
c The skin flaps are replaced.

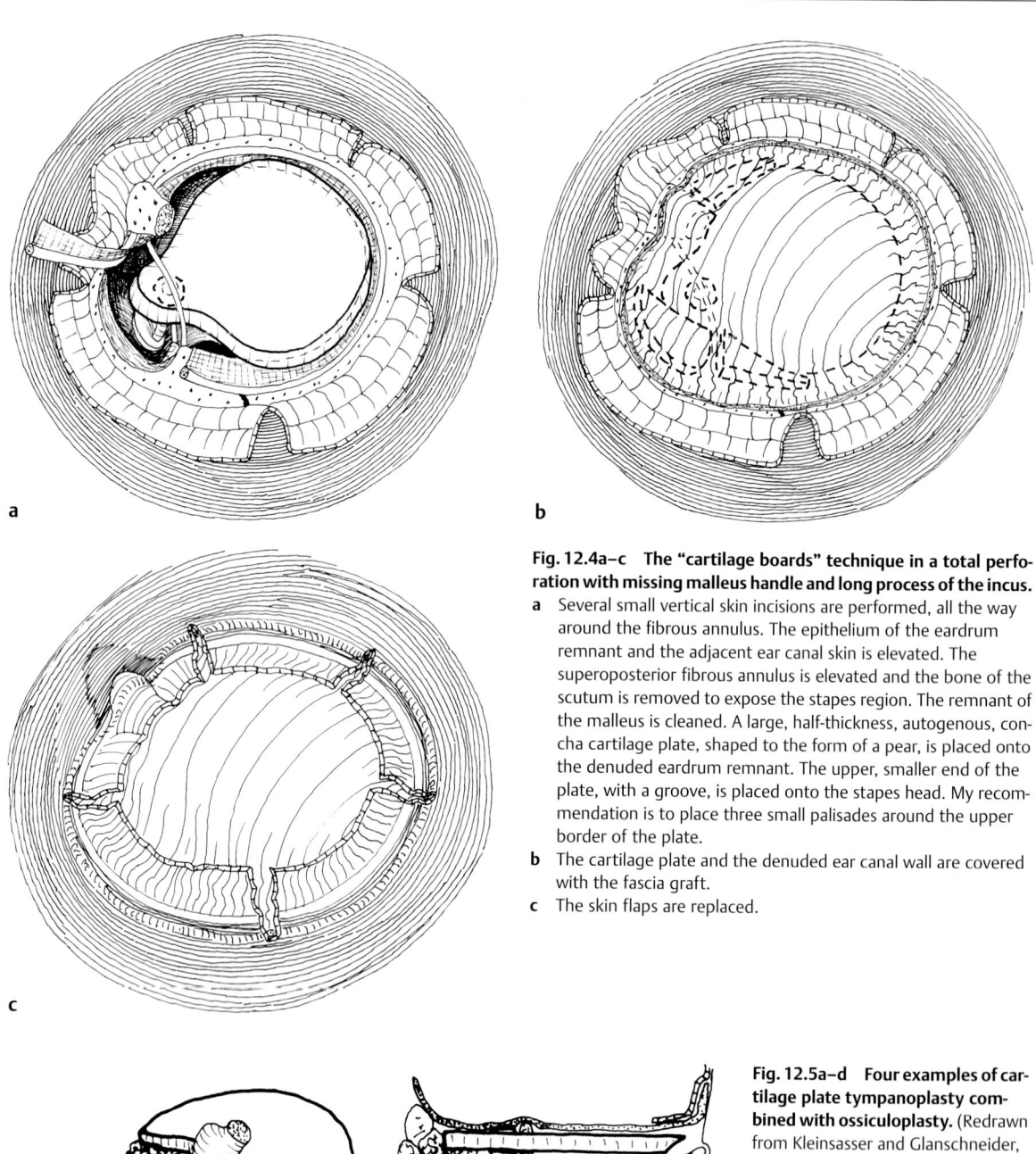

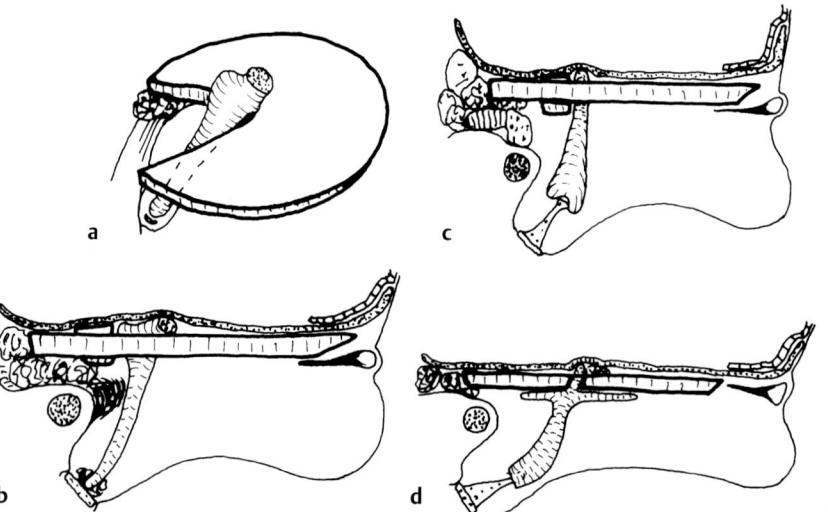

Fig. 12.5a–d Four examples of cartilage plate tympanoplasty combined with ossiculoplasty. (Redrawn from Kleinsasser and Glanschneider, 1969.) In all four examples, full-thickness cartilage plates are used; they are covered with fascia. The inferior end of the plate is placed onto the eardrum remnant. The superior end is in the attic supported by the fibrous tissue.
a Through a cut-out in the cartilage plate, the malleus handle is placed as a columella The cartilage plate and the neck of the malleus will be covered by the fascia.
b The columella is a shaped malleus, protruding through the cartilage plate and contacting the fascia.
c, d Prostheses formed from the shaped incus connect the stapes with the cartilage plate and are stabilized by the holes made through the cartilage plate.

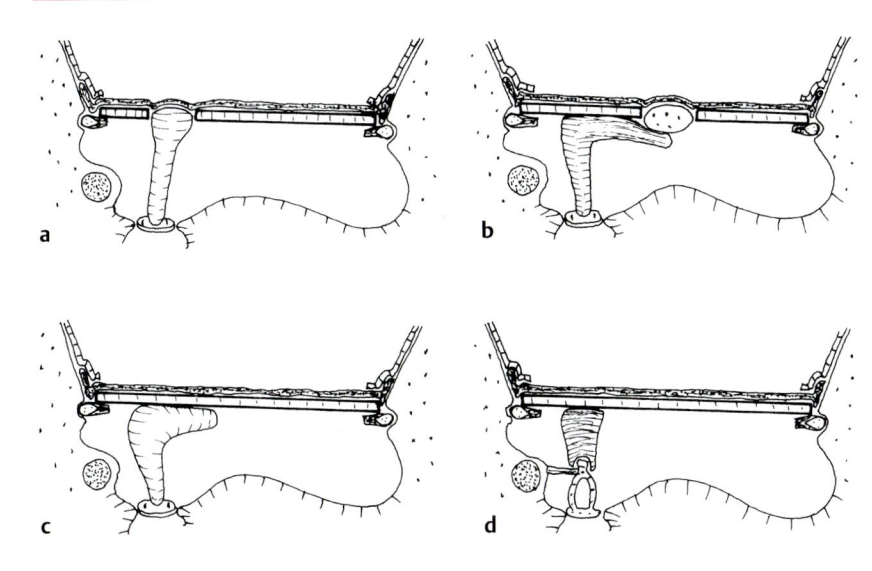

Fig. 12.6a–d Four alternative examples of ossiculoplasty combined with half thickness cartilage plates. In all four examples the half-thickness cartilage plates are placed onto the eardrum and are covered with fascia.
a Through a cut-out in the cartilage plate a shaped malleus handle is placed as a columella.
b, c The L-shaped columella made of cortical bone (**b**) and the incus columella (**c**) are placed between the footplate and the cartilage plate.
d A prosthesis made of cortical bone connects the stapes head with the cartilage plate.

The **thickness** of the plate ranges from full thickness (1.1 mm) (Kleinfeldt et al. 1975; Puls 2003) to 0.4 mm (Martin et al. 2004). Both extremes have produced good hearing results.

Placement of the cartilage plate is also of great interest: Some surgeons use on-lay technique and place the cartilage plate onto the denuded lamina propria. Others use underlay technique and place the cartilage plate in various ways: under the anterior bony annulus and onto the posterior ear canal wall (Martin et al. 2004). Often the plates are simply placed under the scarified eardrum remnant, either without support or with support from Gelfoam.

Covering of cartilage plates also varies. The plates are often covered with fascia, occasionally with loosened perichondrium, or with areolar tissue (Aidonis et al. 2005). Only rarely is there no covering of the cartilage plates (Puls 2003).

The **fate of the cartilage** covered with the perichondrium or without covering is discussed in Chapter 27. Although there is controversy about the outcome of several experiments, the perichondrium does improve the nutrition of the cartilage, and grafts implanted with perichondrium show less degenerative change and less fibrosis than grafts without perichondrium. On the other hand, fibrosis of the cartilage graft presumably does not lead to major anatomical or functional consequences, as observed on cartilage columellae and cartilage struts.

There is a need for clinical studies on late results of surgery with various cartilage grafts. Histological studies of implanted grafts collected at recurrent surgery will improve our knowledge of fate of the cartilage.

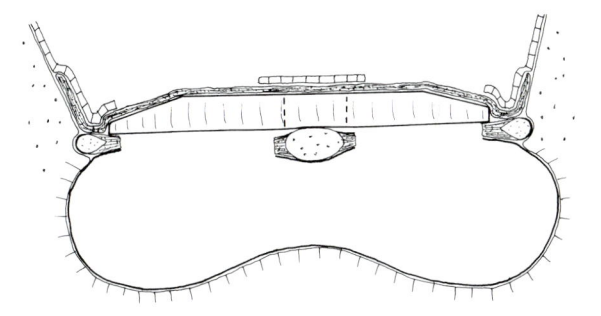

Fig. 12.7 Side view of the full-thickness cartilage plate tympanoplasty at the level of the umbo, as used by Kleinfeldt et al. (1975). The edge of the cartilage plate is thinned to accommodate its positioning onto the lamina propria of the eardrum. The cartilage plate is placed onto the umbo and onto the denuded lamina propria of the eardrum remnant.

Effect of the Thickness of The Cartilage Disk on Hearing

As shown in most of the chapters, the thickness of the graft may vary from 0.2 mm to the full thickness of the tragus cartilage of 1.0 mm or of the concha cartilage of 1.1 mm. The thicker and more rigid the cartilage graft is, the more stable and resistant is the reconstructed eardrum against fluctuation of the air pressure in the tympanic cavity. A thick and rigid cartilage graft is stable, but it has poorer sound transmission than a thin cartilage graft. Thus, the best cartilage graft is an optimal compromise between two demands: good sound transmission and anatomical stability of the reconstructed eardrum.

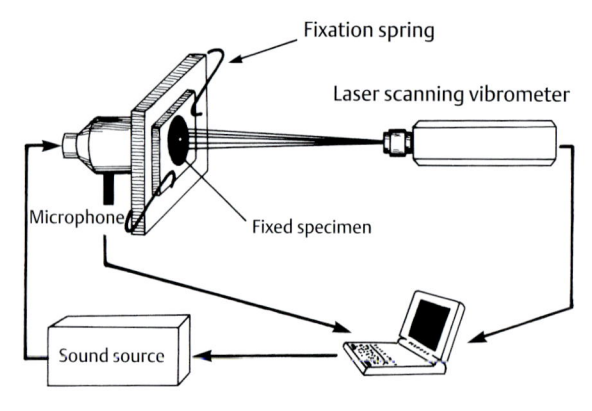

Fig. 12.8 The Dresden experimental external auditory canal–tympanic membrane model for measurements of vibration amplitudes of various cartilage grafts. A sound source transmits sound through a plastic tube to the cartilage graft, which is clamped between two aluminum plates with a central hole for the graft to be evaluated. A microphone registers the sound in the tube (representing the ear canal). The scanning laser Doppler micrometer registers the vibration of 133 equidistant predefined points. (Redrawn from Mürbe et al. 2002.)

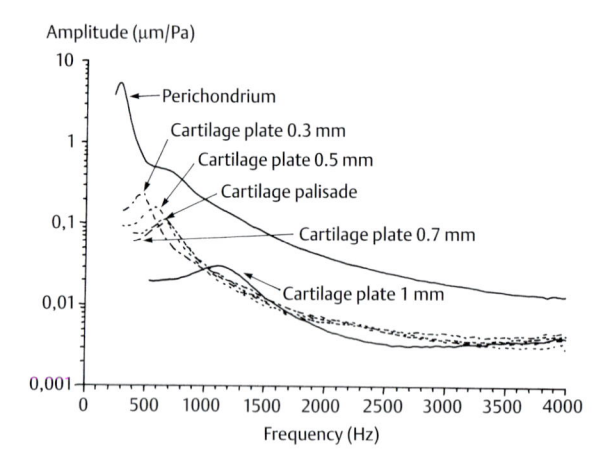

Fig. 12.9 Frequency response function for cartilage plates of various thicknesses of palisades and perichondrium. Curves represent the average of all amplitude spectra of the measured points; displacement amplitude is given in micrometers per pascal. (Redrawn after Mürbe et al. 2002.)

Experimental Investigation of the Use of Cartilage in Tympanic Membrane Reconstruction

An excellent experimental research program, inspired by Hüttenbrink, on biomechanical aspects of middle ear reconstruction, especially on acoustic and mechanic properties of different materials and grafts, has been carried out during the last 15 years in Dresden, Germany (Hüttenbrink 2004; Zahnert et al. 1997, 1999, 2000; Mürbe et al. 2002).

A new method of introducing sound onto the eardrum and a new way of measuring its vibration have enabled the testing of the acoustic properties of various grafts.

Methods

Sound with **white noise pressure levels of 70–90 dB** is transmitted through a plastic tube (length 2 cm, inner diameter 8 mm) representing the ear canal onto a fresh human tympanic membrane, fascia, perichondrium, or various cartilage grafts (**Fig. 12.8**). The eardrum and other grafts (of 10 mm × 10 mm) were clamped between two aluminum plates (60 mm × 60 mm × 6 mm and 30 mm × 30 mm × 6 mm respectively), with a central hole (8 mm in diameter) for evaluation of the graft. The vibrational amplitudes due to the noise were measured by laser Doppler vibrometry (Zahnert et al. 1997).

Sound Pressure Response

Perichondrium
Studies have shown that the perichondrium and the temporalis fascia have similar amplitude–frequency responses for dynamic excitation to the normal tympanic membrane. The frequency response function of the perichondrium (**Fig. 12.9**) has a peak in the amplitude at low frequencies (highest peak at 300 Hz), which is typical for soft membranes. Temporalis fascia has similar amplitude–frequency curves to the perichondrium, with the peak at 350 Hz. The tympanic membrane has a much smoother frequency curve with a resonance peak at 400 Hz, but the amplitude–frequency curves of the perichondrium, fascia, and the eardrum do not differ greatly from each other (Zahnert et al. 2000, Fig. 5).

Cartilage Plates
Cartilage plates with an area of 10 mm × 10 mm and thicknesses of 0.3 mm, 0.5 mm, 0.7 mm, and 1.0 mm respectively were examined. Ten plates in each thickness group were cut with the Kurz Precise Cartilage Knife (**Fig. 3.36**) and tested for sound pressure response and static pressure loading. The amplitude–frequency curves of the four thickness are shown in **Fig. 12.9**. The vibrational amplitudes are highest for the 0.3 mm thick plate, with a peak at 550 Hz. The vibrational amplitudes for the half-thickness plate (0.5 mm) are considerably higher than those of the full-thickness plate (1.0 mm). Considering both the stability and the vibratility, Zahnert et al. (2000) concluded that half-thickness cartilage plates are the best for reconstruction of the eardrum. However, Atef et al. (2007) found no differences in postoperative hearing between full-thickness and half-thickness grafts.

Cartilage Palisades

Full-thickness cartilage plate was cut into 2 mm wide parallel palisades that were placed edge to edge. Vibration maxima occur between the palisades, leading to reduced transmission characteristics, which are nevertheless similar to those of the tympanic membrane. The vibrational amplitudes are slightly lower than those of the half-thickness plate (**Fig. 12.9**) and cartilage island grafts (**Fig. 12.10**), but our own studies showed that 3 years after surgery for cholesteatoma better hearing results were obtained with cartilage palisades than with fascia (Uzun et al. 2003, 2004; Tos et al. 2005).

Cartilage Composite Island Grafts

Small (4 mm diameter) and a large (7 mm) full-thickness cartilage island grafts were also investigated. The sound-induced vibrational amplitudes were large for the small and the large cartilage island grafts (**Fig. 12.10**). The amplitudes of cartilage islands were larger than those of palisades and plates.

Conclusions of the Experimental Studies

The sound transmission properties of the reconstructed eardrum are strongly influenced by the reconstruction techniques as well as the material characteristics. The choice of surgical technique should take into account requirements based on mechanical stability and the acoustic transfer characteristics of the transplant.

Clinical Research on the Thickness of Cartilage Grafts

To date, apparently only one paper directly addresses the effect of the thickness of the cartilage disk in tympanoplasty.

Atef et al. (2007) performed a prospective clinical study on two randomly allocated groups of patients with central perforations and intact ossicular chain. In the first group, cartilage–perichondrium composite full-thickness island grafts were used; in the other group, half-thickness composite underlay grafts were used. Inclusion criteria were dry central perforation and an air–bone gap not exceeding an average of 25 dB for the frequencies 500, 1000, 2000, and 4000 Hz.

In the first group, 30 patients were treated **with full-thickness graft**, with one recurrent perforation. In the second group, **half- thickness grafts** were used in 32 patients, with one recurrent perforation. The sites of the perforations in the first group were: 2 anterior, 6 posterior, 20 subtotal. In the second they were: 1 anterior, 9 posterior, and 19 subtotal perforations.

The mean preoperative PTA-ABG in the first group was 21.3 ± 3.72 dB, and in the second group was 22.07 ± 2.62 dB. The average postoperative PTA-ABG 8–9 months after surgery was 10.44 ± 2.21 dB in the first group, and 10.28 ± 1.65 dB in the second group.

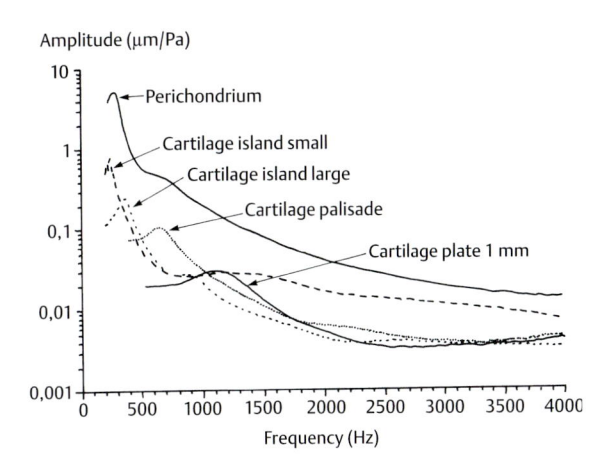

Fig. 12.10 Frequency response function for the small and large cartilage–perichondrium composite island grafts compared with perichondrium, cartilage palisades, and thick plates. Curves represent the average of all amplitude spectra of the measured points; displacement amplitude is given in micrometers per pascal. (Redrawn after Mürbe et al. 2002.)

The **anatomical** results were good, with a failure of 3% in both groups. The postoperative hearing was the same in both groups. The authors recommend the use of full-thickness island grafts and emphasize that "this study contradicts the work of Zahnert et al. (2000)." More such studies are needed.

Problems with Curling

In a prospective comparison of the results in the group of patients with full-thickness cartilage grafts and the group with half-thickness grafts, Atef et al. (2007) mentioned that "after slicing the cartilage to half of its thickness, the graft curls on itself, which sometimes makes underlay grafting of the tympanic membrane very difficult." Unfortunately, the authors did not specify how often the curling appeared, whether the curling prevented placement of the graft, or whether the curling caused poor anatomical results. One might expect that the curling could cause inadequate attachment of the composite graft to the undersurface of the eardrum remnant, and a subsequent re-perforation, but both groups had only one perforation each.

During the last four years of writing this book, I have desperately searched for some literature on curling of the cartilage, but I have found nothing that could be used. On thinning a full-thickness island graft, with the perichondrium on one side, to a half-thickness graft, one might expect that the perichondrium would contract and cause the edge of the thinned cartilage to curl. The edge and the peripheral part of a cartilage disk become elevated in relation to the undersurface.

The curling problem may explain why the cartilage plates are first cleaned of the perichondrium on both sides and then, at the end of the surgery, the cartilage plate is covered with the fascia or the free perichondrium.

To prevent such curling, I propose in Chapter 23 four incisions of the perichondrium—the "anti-curling incisions" (see **Figs. 23.3b, 23.4b, c, 23.6b, c, 23.7b, c, 23.9b, c, 23.10b, 23.11b, c**). The peripheral belt of perichondrium is too small to elevate the edge of the cartilage disk. Nevertheless, a systematic study is needed to validate the anti-curling incisions. In contrast, the creation of the butterfly graft by Eavey (1998) actually exploits the curling of the round cartilage. The edge of a round cartilage graft, covered on both sides by the perichondrium, is incised midway and parallel to the two outlaying sheets of the perichondrium (see **Figs. 25.2–25.5, 25.10a, b**) resulting in curling of both edges of the graft.

Optimal Graft Thickness for Different Sizes of the Perforation

Lee et al. (2007) experimentally studied the optimal graft thickness in relation to the size of the perforation. Three different sizes of perforation were made, representing 15%, 55%, and 85% of the eardrum. A cartilage plate was used to repair the eardrum perforation and then the new eardrum–cartilage coupled complex was loaded into a three-dimensional biomechanical model for analysis. The amplitude–frequency responses for different cartilage thickness were compared with those for a natural eardrum. The results show that, first, in cases with 85% perforation the amplitude–frequency responses were most similar to those of the natural eardrum at lower frequencies. The authors concluded that the optimal thicknesses of the graft are 0.1–0.2 mm for medium and large perforations. For small perforations, a cartilage of less than 1.0 mm is a good compromise between mechanical stability and low acoustic transfer loss.

References

Aidonis I, Robertson TC, Sismanis A. Cartilage shield tympanoplasty: a reliable technique. Otol Neurotol 2005;26:838–841.

Atef A, Talaat N, Fahti A, Mosleh M, Safwat S. Effect of the thickness of the cartilage disk on the hearing results after perichondrium–cartilage island flap tympanoplasty. ORL J Otorhinolaryngol Relat Spec 2007;69:207–211.

Betow C. Reconstruction of the middle ear and the posterior osseous wall of the auditory canal with homograft (reconstruction of old radical cavities). Trans Am Acad Ophthalmol Otolaryngol 1975; 80:573–576.

Betow C. 20 years of experience with homografts in ear surgery. J Laryngol Otol Suppl 1982;5:1–28.

Brandow EC. Homograft tympanic membrane transplant in myringoplasty. Trans Am Acad Ophthalmol Otolaryngol 1969;73: 825–835.

Decat M, Polet MA, Gersdorff M. Use of costal cartilage in middle ear surgery. Acta Otorhinolaryngol Belg 1997;51:17–21.

Eavey RD. Inlay tympanoplasty: cartilage butterfly technique. Laryngoscope 1998;108:657–661.

Hüttenbrink K-B. Biomechanical aspects of middle ear reconstruction. In: Jahnke K, ed. Middle Ear Surgery. Stuttgart, New York: Thieme; 2004:1–51..

Jansen C. Cartilage tympanoplasty. Laryngoscope 1963;73: 1288–1302.

Jansen C. The combined approach for tympanoplasty. J Laryngol Otol 1968;82:779–793.

Kleinfeldt D, Vick U, Lübcke P-F. Zur Verwendung von autologem Ohrmuschelknorpel zur Doppeltransplantatplastik des Trommelfelles. HNO 1975;23:13–15.

Kleinsasser O, Glanschneider D. Knorpelplätchen zur Befestigung von Columellen und zum Überbrückung grosser Trommelfelldefekte bei der Tympanoplastik. Z Laryngol Rhinol Otol 1969;48: 590–599.

Lee C-F, Chen J-H, Chou Y-F, Hsu L-P. Optimal graft thickness for different sizes of tympanic membrane perforation in cartilage tympanoplasty: a finite element analysis. Laryngoscope 2007;117:725–730.

Marquet J. Reconstructive microsurgery of the eardrum by means of a tympanic membrane homograft: preliminary report. Acta Otolaryngol 1966;62:459–464.

Marquet J. Myringoplasty by eardrum transplantation. Laryngoscope 1968;78:1329–1336.

Martin C, Thimoshenko AP, Martin C, Bertholon P, Prades JM. Malleus removal and total cartilage reinforcement in intact canal wall tympanoplasty for cholesteatoma. Ann Otol Rhinol Laryngol 2004;113:421–425.

Mürbe D, Zahnert T, Bornitz M, Hüttenbrink K-B. Acoustic properties of different cartilage reconstruction techniques of the tympanic membrane. Laryngoscope 2002;112:1769–1776.

Overbosch HC. Homograft myringoplasty with micro-sliced septal cartilage. Pract Otorhinolaryngol (Basel) 1971;33:356–357.

Puls T. Tympanoplasty using conchal cartilage graft. Acta Otorhinolaryngol Belg 2003;57:187–191.

Raivio M, Siirala U. Conserved homoplastic cartilage in tympanoplasty. Acta Otolaryngol 1973;75:282–283.

Salen B. Myringoplasty using septum cartilage. Acta Otolaryngol Suppl 1964;188(Suppl. 188):82–93.

Schulte DL, Driscoll CL, McDonald TJ, Facer GW, Beatty CW. Irradiated rib cartilage graft for reconstruction of the tympanic membrane: preliminary results. Am J Otol 1998;19:141–144.

Smyth GDL, Kerr AG. Homologous grafts for ossicular reconstruction in tympanoplasty. Laryngoscope 1967;77:330–336.

Smyth GDL, Kerr AG. Cartilage homografts-experimental and clinical aspects. Acta Otorhinolaryngol Belg 1970;24:53–59.

Tos M, Uzun C, Cayé-Thomasen P. Andersen J. Tympanometry after tympanoplasty with cartilage palisades or fascia after surgery for tensa cholesteatoma in children. In: Lim DJ, Bluestone CD, Casselbrant M, eds. Hamilton, Ontario :BC Decker, Inc.; 2005:321–322.

Uzun C, Cayé-Thomasen P, Andersen J, Tos M. A tympanometric comparison of tympanoplasty with cartilage palisades or fascia after surgery for tensa cholesteatoma in children. Laryngoscope 2003;113:1751–1757.

Uzun C, Cayé-Thomasen P, Andersen J, Tos M. Eustachian tube function in tympanoplasty with cartilage palisades or fascia after cholesteatoma surgery. Otol Neurotol 2004;25:864–872.

Weichselbaumer W. Über Lappenunterfütterung und Columellaeffekte bei Tympanoplastikken. Z Laryngol Rhinol Otol 1968;33: 508–513.

Yamamoto E, Iwanaga M, Morinaka S. Use of micro-sliced homograft cartilage plates in tympanoplasty. Acta Otolaryngol Suppl 1985;419:123–129.

Zahnert T, Bornitz M, Hüttenbrink KB. Acustische und mechanische Eigenschaften von Trommelfelltransplantaten. Laryngorhinootologie 1997;76:717–723.

Zahnert T, Schmidt R, Vogel U, Hüttenbrink KB. Experiments and finite element calculations on the acoustic transfer characteristics of gold and titanium middle ear prosthesis. Eur Arch Otorhinolaryngol 1999;256:53.

Zahnert T, Hüttenbrink KB, Mürbe D, Bornitz M. Experimental investigations of the use of cartilage in tympanic membrane reconstruction. Am J Otol 2000;21:322–328.

13 Underlay Tympanoplasty with Thick Cartilage Plates

Definitions

In this method the cartilage plates, of thickness 0.5–1.1 mm but usually without attached perichondrium, are placed as a reinforcement of the eardrum, either under the entire eardrum or under a part of the eardrum. Often the cartilage plates are covered either with the fascia or free perichondrium, or with areolar tissue from the temporal region.

In underlay tympanoplasty technique the cartilage plates are supposed to adhere to the undersurface of the eardrum, or to the fascia or to the free perichondrium. Sometimes the plates are supported by Gelfoam placed into the tympanic cavity. The cartilage plates are sometimes supported by the chorda tympani, long process of the incus, or the stapes head. Often the thinned edge of the cartilage plate is placed onto the bony annulus as an underlay graft (Martin 1979, Martin et al. 2004).

Harvesting and Elaboration of the Autogenous Cartilage Plates

Nowadays only autogenous cartilage from the tragus or the concha are used. A 10 mm × 10 mm piece with the perichondrium attached on one or on both sides is harvested. Perichondrium is removed from both sides and the plate can be cut to the desired thickness in various ways: (1) The cartilage plate may be held with two fingers and sliced to the desired thickness with the scalpel (see **Fig. 3.34a**), or with a razor blade. (2) The cartilage plate is held firmly against a wooden tongue blade and split with a safety razor blade (see **Fig. 3.34b**). (3) The cartilage is held with a surgical forceps and split with a scalpel (see **Fig. 3.34c**). (4) Using Hildmann cartilage slicing clamp (see **Fig. 3.35**) cartilage can be safely sliced with a scalpel or a safety razor blade. (5) The safest thinning is performed using Kurz Precise Cartilage Knife (see **Fig. 3.36**). The removed perichondrium can later be separately placed onto the cartilage, but under the eardrum remnant.

The Underlay Tympanoplasty Techniques with Thick Cartilage Plates

The cartilage plate of thickness of 0.5–1.1 mm is placed under the eardrum remnant and under the fibrous annulus. It is covered either with the fascia (Martin 1979) or with the areolar tissue harvested from the outer side of the temporalis fascia (Aidonis et al. 2005), or the cartilage plate may not be covered at all (Puls 2003).

Cartilage Plate Covered with Fascia

Reinforcement of the eardrum with a half-thickness cartilage plate has been used in France for many years (Martin et al. 1973; Martin 1979; Martin et al. 2004). The cartilage plates are without perichondrium and the peripheral part of the plate is thinner than the central part.

In an excellent study of cholesteatoma surgery with staged intact canal wall mastoidectomy and posterior atticotympanotomy, Martin et al. (2004) distinguished between partial and total reinforcement. In the method of **partial reinforcement** of the tympanic membrane, the incus and malleus head are removed, but the malleus handle is preserved. The cholesteatoma was removed and the removed or resorbed bony ear canal wall was reconstructed. The partial reinforcement of the tympanic membrane was done with fragments of the cartilage plates and covered with the fascia or with the perichondrium.

In **total reinforcement** of the tympanic membrane, first proposed by Roulleau and Martin (1998), the entire malleus is removed and a large cartilage plate, 0.4 mm thick, covers the entire tympanic cavity

The anterior edge of the plate is placed under the bony annulus (**Fig. 13.1a, b**), the posterior part is placed onto the posterior ear canal bone. The cartilage plate is covered with a large piece of fascia, placed anteriorly under the fibrous annulus.

In the **second-stage** procedure, an ossiculoplasty was performed in both groups. The head of the prosthesis is flattened and placed under the cartilage plate, with the largest contact area possible (**Fig. 13.1b**)

Cartilage Plate Covered with Areolar Tissue—a Cartilage Shield Tympanoplasty?

Aidonis, Robertson, and Sismanis (2005) from Virginia University, Richmond, used the postauricular approach and harvested cartilage from the concha. Perichondrium is removed from both sides of the cartilage graft. Areolar tissue overlaying the temporalis fascia is harvested to cover the cartilage plate, instead of the fascia. The vascular strip is elevated out of the ear canal. After cleaning of the edges of the perforation, and scarification of the undersurface of the eardrum, a radial skin incision is made (**Fig. 13.2a**). Two tympanomeatal flaps and the malleus flap are elevated. Gelfoam placed into the tympanic cavity supports the cartilage disk (**Fig. 13.2b**). The cartilage disk, with a cut-out wedge, is placed medial to the malleus handle (**Fig. 13.2c**) and covered with the areolar tissue (**Fig. 13.2d**). After replacement of the skin flaps (**Fig. 13.2e**), the reconstruction is firm (**Fig. 13.2f**) and epithelialization will be rapid. The authors called their method cartilage shield tympanoplasty.

Recently, Kyrodimos, Sismanis, and Santos (2007) from the same hospital published results of the same method as described in the previous paper. The method was called Type 3 cartilage "shield" tympanoplasty. In retroauricular approach, the areolar tissue that overlies the temporalis fascia is harvested. The round piece of cartilage is removed and **the perichondrium removed on both sides.** A wedge is cut out for the malleus handle. The edges of the perforation are denuded; two tympanomeatal flaps and the malleus flap are elevated; the intact and mobile stapes is inspected; and the tympanic cavity is filled with wet Gelfoam balls. The round full-thickness cartilage disk, slightly larger than the eardrum, is placed onto the stapes head, which in this book is called tympanoplasty type 2 (myringostapediopexy). The areolar tissue covers the cartilage and the tympanomeatal flaps are replaced (see **Fig. 13.2a–f** for a case with intact ossicular chain).

Cartilage Shield Tympanoplasty of Moore

Moore (2002) harvested a large piece of triangular fossa, removed the perichondrium on one side, and shaped it as a large total graft to be placed onto the bony groove drilled onto the anterior bony annulus. He also called this graft cartilage shield graft. The graft may be shaped with excision of a V-shaped notch to accommodate the malleus handle or excision of a U-shaped notch to accommodate an interposed incus.

In case of a missing malleus, Moore removed the entire eardrum remnant and placed a large cartilage shield plate onto the bony annulus.

The drilling of the anterior and inferior bony annulus is shown in Chapter 17 (see **Figs. 17.12a–h**, **17.13a–c**). In Chapters 18 and 19, but especially in Chapter 20, the drilling of the anterior and inferior bony annulus takes place in

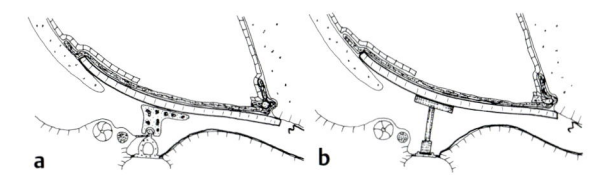

Fig. 13.1a, b Side view of the total reinforcement with underlay placement of the cartilage plate in canal wall up mastoidectomy and tympanoplasty. In the first stage the malleus is removed and a large cartilage plate is placed posteriorly onto the ear canal wall, anteriorly under the bony annulus. Fascia covers the cartilage plate and is placed onto the ear canal bone, but under the anterior fibrous annulus. In the second stage 18 months later, a hydroxyapatite PORP is interposed between the stapes head and the cartilage plate (**a**), or a columella between the footplate and the cartilage plate (**b**).

procedures described in these chapters (see **Figs. 20.14a–e**, **20.15b–h**, **20.16a–f**). A large cartilage shield plate can be safely placed onto the bony annulus. For reconstruction of the middle ear, Moore used either total shield graft or notched shield graft in case of incus interposition. When the cartilage graft was inserted, it was placed so that the concave side with its perichondrium was lateral and the convex surface without perichondrium was medial. Posteriorly and posteriorly-superiorly the cartilage graft was approximated to the new contours of the external auditory canal.

Tympanoplasty with Cartilage Plates Only

In all methods described in this chapter, the cartilage plates were covered either with the fascia or the perichondrium, or with the areolar tissue, but Puls (2003) did not cover the cartilage plates at all. Puls uses full-thickness concha cartilage without perichondrium.

After refreshing the edges of the perforation, two tympanomeatal flaps are elevated (**Fig. 13.3a**). A full-thickness cartilage plate is tailored to be slightly larger than the perforation. It is placed close to the malleus handle, onto the chorda tympani, and is supported inferiorly by Gelfoam (**Fig. 13.3b**). After replacement of the skin flaps there should be no problem with epithelialization (**Fig. 13.3c**).

In total and subtotal perforation a V-shaped notch is cut out to fit the handle of the malleus, similar to **Fig. 13.2c**. Ossiculoplasty is performed with a Plastipore PORP or TORP, placed under the cartilage plate.

Tympanoplasty with Crushed Autogenous Cartilage Plate

It has been reported that after nasal surgery cartilage will warp in time (Gibson and Davis 1958) and large cartilage plates may twist in the middle ear in later years (Heermann et al. 1970). Although there are no reports of warping or twisting of the cartilage plates placed in into the tym-

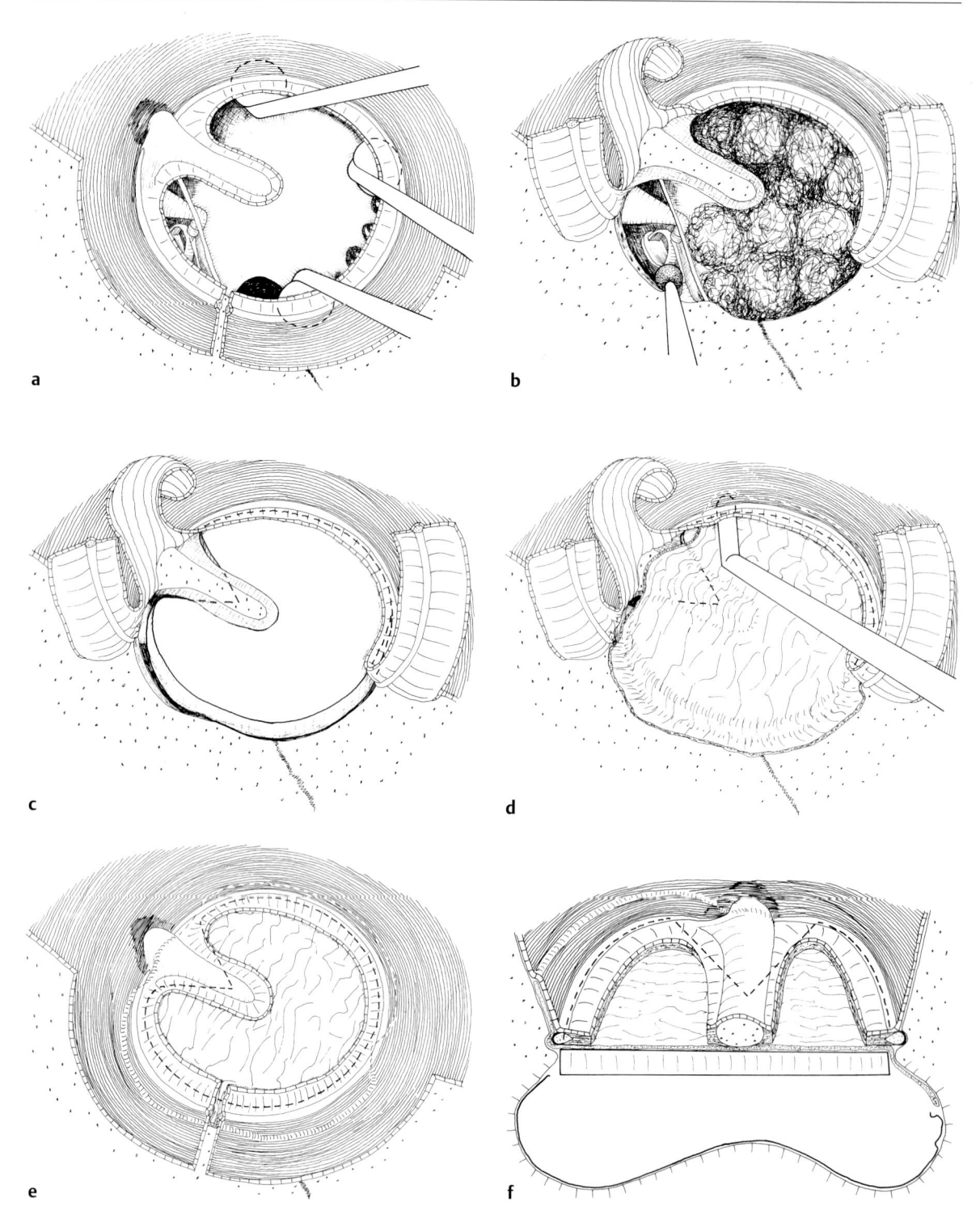

Fig. 13.2a–f Underlay placement of the cartilage plate in a total perforation and intact ossicular chain.

- **a** The edges of the perforation are cleaned, the undersurface of the eardrum is scarified, and a vertical skin incision is made.
- **b** The two tympanomeatal flaps and the malleus flap are elevated. The posterosuperior bony annulus is removed, exposing the tympanic sinuses. The tympanic cavity is filled with Gelfoam.
- **c** The full-thickness cartilage plate with a cut-out wedge is placed medial to the malleus handle, and under the anterior eardrum remnant.
- **d** Areolar tissue covers the cartilage disk and the malleus handle, and posteriorly may cover an area of the ear canal bone. Anteriorly, the areolar tissue is pushed under the eardrum remnant.
- **e** The tympanomeatal flaps and the malleus flap are replaced.
- **f** Side view with some perspective at the level of the umbo. The cartilage plate is placed under the umbo and is covered with the areolar tissue.

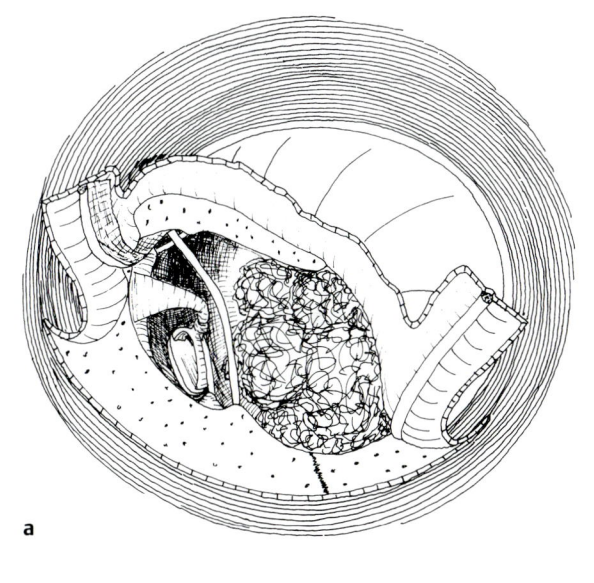

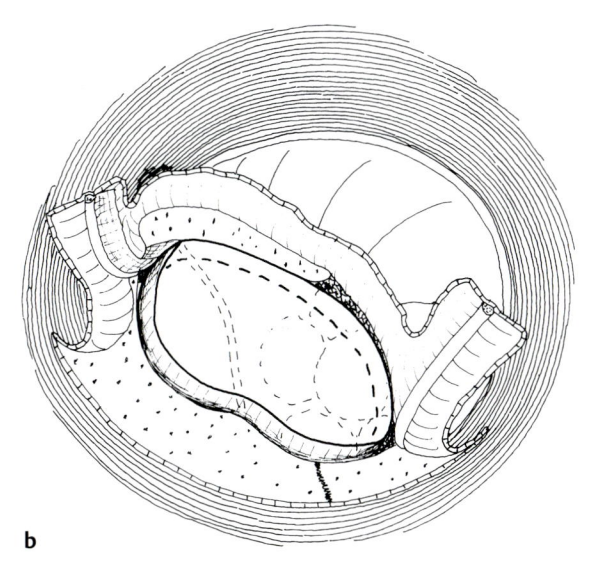

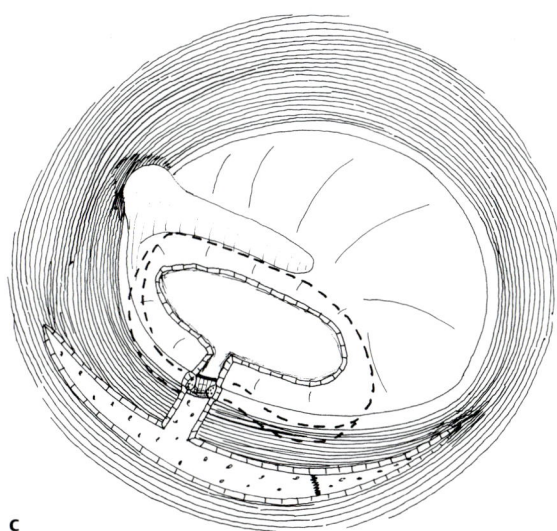

Fig. 13.3a–c An example of closure of a posterior perforation with a full-thickness cartilage plate without covering of the plate.
a After cleaning of the edge of the posterior perforation and scarification of the undersurface of the eardrum, two tympanomeatal flaps are elevated. Gelfoam balls will support the cartilage plate.
b The cartilage plate without the perichondrium, tailored to fit exactly to the perforation is supported superiorly by the chorda and inferiorly by the Gelfoam balls..
c The two tympanomeatal flaps are replaced and pulled in the posterior direction to reduce the epithelial defect.

panic cavity, Park (1995) believes that crushing of the cartilage plate prevents warping and twisting.

Using a specially designed translucent plastic crusher, Park (1995) crushed 5 mm × 5 mm pieces of autogenous concha, tragus, and septum cartilage (**Fig. 13.4**). A remarkable reduction of the thickness and expansion of the area of the cartilage was achieved. The author recommends that crushed cartilage plates be used in tympanoplasty and has used crushed cartilage in 16 cases for reconstruction of the bony defect of the attic. In 24 cases the eardrum was reinforced with crushed cartilage in the same underlay technique as with noncrushed cartilage plates. None of the crushed pieces of cartilage showed twisting or bending, although the follow-up time was apparently not very long.

Crushing induces multiple, irregular fracture lines on the cartilage that have no directional preponderance. Thus, the stress forces on both sides are relieved and a post-grafting contraction in any particular direction is prevented (Park 1995).

Late results after tympanoplasty with crushed cartilage plates are needed as there are no other reports on this very interesting issue.

Tympanoplasty with Irradiated Homogenous Rib Cartilage Plates

Rib cartilage is taken from human donors who meet the Mayo Clinic's guidelines for autopsy tissue donation (Schulte et al. 1998). The rib cartilage is harvested, packaged in three special envelopes, and gamma irradiated.

In surgery, the cartilage plates are cut with a scalpel (**Fig. 13.5**). The plate is shaped in relation to the size of the perforation and placed as an underlay graft. The cartilage plate is covered with the fascia and the tympanomeatal

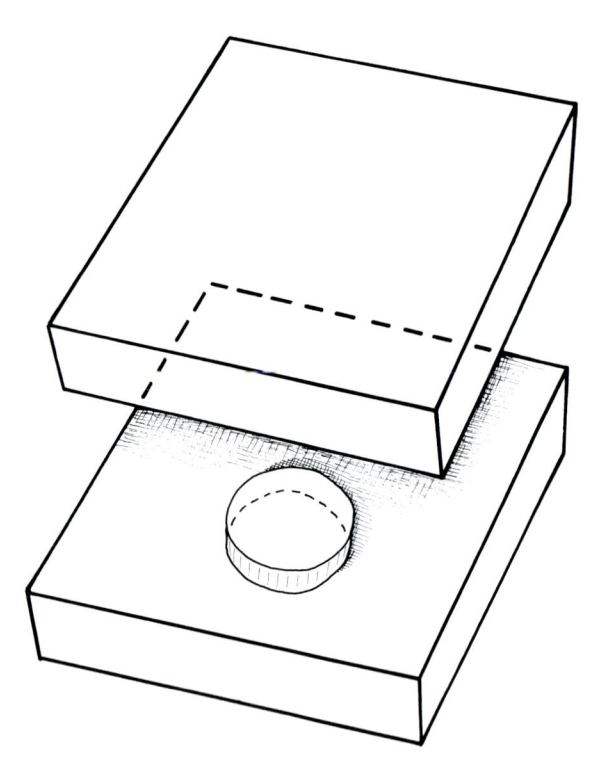

Fig. 13.4 Schematic illustration of cartilage crushing using the translucent plastic crusher of Moon Suh Park (Park 1995). The cartilage is placed onto the lower plate; it is covered by the upper plate, which will crush the cartilage. The crushing of the cartilage can be observed through the upper plate. The pieces of cartilage are crushed gently until they begin to crack grossly.

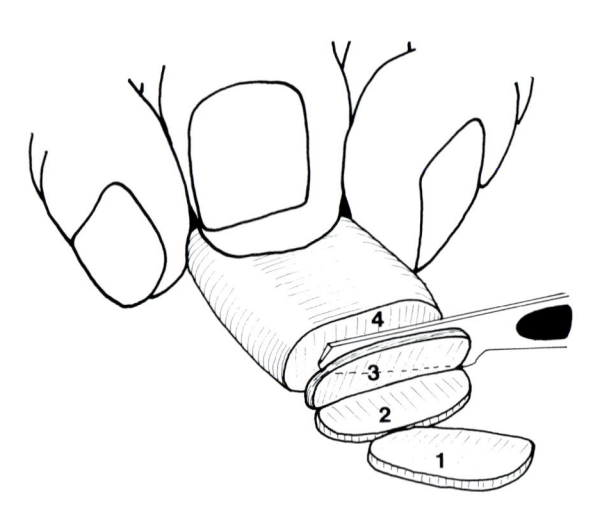

Fig. 13.5 Irradiated homologous rib cartilage being cut into plates with a scalpel.

flaps are replaced. The surgical underlay technique is similar to the other underlay techniques using cartilage plates.

Reinforcement of the Tympanic Membrane with Cartilage Plates after Removal of Congenital Cholesteatoma

In a large series of 117 children operated on for congenital cholesteatoma (Lazard et al. 2007), the patients were divided in two groups. In the first group, with 12 children, suffering from limited cholesteatoma not involving the ossicular chain, the cholesteatomas were entirely and easily removed in one stage, without sign of recurrence.

In the second group, with 105 children, a second-look operation was performed systematically. Within this group, at the first operation on 69 children (65.7%), a full-thickness cartilage reinforcement of the tympanic membrane and reconstruction of the attic wall was carried out, whereas in 9 children (8.6%) a partially destroyed wall was not repaired. At the second-look operation, residual cholesteatoma was found in 41% of cases, and postoperative retraction pockets in 15% of cases. The sites of the retractions were mainly the posterosuperior part of the eardrum and the attic recess. Retraction pockets occurred despite cartilage reinforcement of the tympanic membrane in 56.3% cases, but retraction pockets were located outside of the zone of the initial reinforcement/reconstruction, confirming the protective role of cartilage grafts with respect to the retraction process (Lazard et al. 2007).

Results of Surgery with Cartilage Plates

Results of Recent Underlay Techniques

The two series of Martin et al. (2004)—with intact canal wall mastoidectomy and tympanoplasty in the first stage and tympanotomy with an eventual ossiculoplasty in the second stage—are very impressive, with 416 cholesteatomas operated on.

Hearing results of the **first** series, of 240 ears with cholesteatoma (71.7% attic, 16.7% sinus, and 10.0% tensa retraction cholesteatoma after Tos's classification [Tos 1983; Tos and Lau 1989]), treated with **partial reinforcement** without removal of the malleus handle, were the same as in the **second** series of 176 cholesteatomas (79% attic, 9.1% sinus, and in 12.0% tensa retraction cholesteatoma), with **total reinforcement** and removal of the entire malleus.

In the **first** series, the mean preoperative air–bone gap at frequencies 0.5, 1, 2, and 3 kHz was 22.9 ± 12.7 dB. The mean postoperative air–bone gap was 13.8 ± 10.7 dB.

In the **second** group the mean preoperative hearing was 21.9 ± 10.2 dB. The mean postoperative hearing gain was 11.9 ± 8.8 dB.

Mean closure of the air–bone gap was 9.2 ± 13.8 dB in the **first** series and 10.2 ± 11.2 dB in the **second** series.

Statistically there were no differences in hearing results between the two series.

No extrusion of the prosthesis was found in either group of the patients.

Reinforcement of the whole tympanic membrane with a conchal or tragal cartilage graft results in a significantly reduced rate of recurrent cholesteatoma, which decreased from 26.9% in the first group to 8.5% in the second group. Martin has used cartilage plates as underlay grafts for many years and did not report twisting and warping.

Aidonis et al. (2005), in their series of 61 patients, found a take rate of 98.4%. The average pre- and postoperative pure-tone air–bone gaps were 34.4 ± 14.1 dB and 24.0 ± 13.7 dB, respectively ($p < 0.005$). Thus, cartilage shield tympanoplasty, **covering the cartilage with areolar tissue**, is a reliable method with good results.

Out of 114 patients who had cartilage tympanoplasty with areolar tissue (Kyrodimos et al. 2007), 52 patients had defects of the ossicular chain, but intact and mobile stapes, covered with cartilage plate (a myringostapediopexy in tympanoplasty type 2, where the cartilage disk is placed onto the stapes head). The primary procedure included 29 patients, revision surgery 23 patients. The overall preoperative average PTA-ABG was 31.35 ± 12.7 dB; the postoperative PTA-ABG (at mean follow-up of 24 months, range 12–36 months) was 20.3 ± 10.43 dB ($p < 0.0001$).

Graft take was successful in all patients. There was no postoperative graft lateralization or retraction.

The same group from Virginia University in Richmond (Sismanis et al. 2008) has performed revision surgery with the same surgical technique—cartilage shield tympanoplasty. Over 9 years (January 1998–December 2006), 43 patients with total perforation underwent 46 procedures (**Fig. 13.2a–f**). At the latest mean follow-up of 22 months (range 6–110 months) the anatomical results were excellent, with graft take of 93.5%. The mean preoperative ABG was 33.6 ± 13.2 dB; the postoperative ABG was 25.7 ± 11.3 dB. The overall mean improvement of mean ABG was 11.22 dB ($p < 0.0001$). Taking into consideration that this was revision surgery, the results were good and stable.

Among 83 patients operated from 1995 to 1999, at 2-years follow-up Moore (2002) obtained an integrity of the eardrum of 100%, as measured by tympanometry.
- *Hearing:* 51% of the patients were in the poor category at 5 kHz, compared with 14% postoperatively.
- At 1 kHz, 52% of patients had poor audiological status preoperatively, compared with 16% postoperatively.
- At 2 kHz, 18% of patients had poor hearing > 30 dB, compared with 25% postoperatively. The improvement of hearing was statistically significant ($p < 0001$) at all four frequencies.
- 98% of patients had a 30 dB or less conductive hearing loss at 2 kHz at least 2 years after ossiculoplasty. These were all revision tympanoplasty cases.

Puls (2003), in 91 ears, **without covering the cartilage** plate with fascia in tympanoplasty type 1, achieved an air–bone gap closure within 20 dB in 88%, and in 72% of 43 tympanoplasties type 2 with intact stapes and interposition of a prosthesis and in 45.5% of the 17 cases in tympanoplasty type 3 with a columella.

With crushed cartilage plate, among 53 cases, Park (1995) achieved an air–bone closure within 20 dB in 40% of ears, and a re-perforation in 8 ears (15%).

In grafting with **irradiated rib cartilage** (Schulte et al. 1998), among 36 cases the average speech reception threshold improved from 35.6 dB to 30.5 dB. The average air–bone gap improved from 13.3 dB to 12.6 dB.

Author's Comments and Proposals

Classification of Cartilage Shield Tympanoplasty

Cartilage tympanoplasty has previously not had a classification of the various methods. During the last 5 years of the writing of this book, 23 different cartilage tympanoplasty methods have been collected and a classification has been elaborated as described in Chapter 2 and published in *Otolaryngology – Head and Neck Surgery*, as an invited article (Tos 2008). The 23 methods were divided into six groups:
- Group A: Cartilage tympanoplasty with palisades, strips, and slices (Chapters 4–9)
- Group B: Cartilage tympanoplasty with foils, thin plates, and thick plates (Chapters 10–13)
- Group C: Cartilage tympanoplasty with cartilage-perichondrium composite island grafts (Chapters 14–17)
- Group D: Cartilage tympanoplasty with **special total** pars tensa cartilage–perichondrium composite island grafts (Chapters 18–20)
- Group E: Cartilage tympanoplasty with small cartilage–perichondrium islands grafts for anterior, inferior and subtotal perforations (Chapters 21–24)
- Group F: Special cartilage tympanoplasty methods, such as inlay butterfly tympanoplasty and composite chondroepithelial clip tympanoplasty: the triple "C" technique (Chapters 25 and 26)

The **cartilage shield T-tube tympanoplasty** is described in Chapter 20. It is defined as a total pars tensa cartilage–perichondrium composite island graft with a large perichondrium flap surrounding the full-thickness cartilage disk, which is covered with perichondrium on the ear canal side and has an **implanted T-tube**.

The cartilage shield tympanoplasties of Aidonis et al. (2005), Kyrodimos et al. (2007), and Sismanis et al. (2008) use a full-thickness cartilage disk, without perichondrium covering and without a peripheral perichondrium flap. Thus the disk is a thick cartilage plate and belongs to the topic of this chapter.

The term "cartilage shield" can be used for the majority of cartilage disks thicker than 0.2 mm, because they are able to protect (or shield) against retraction.

Moore (2002) called his cartilage tympanoplasty either a total shield cartilage tympanoplasty or a notched shield cartilage tympanoplasty.

If the term "cartilage shield" is used for a support for placement of the areolar tissue, then several other methods, in which the cartilage is covered with fascia or with the perichondrium, could also be called cartilage shield tympanoplasty, which would diminish the value of the classification; the term "underlay cartilage tympanoplasty with thick cartilage" should rather be used.

References

Aidonis I, Robertson TC, Sismanis A. Cartilage shield tympanoplasty: a reliable technique. Otol Neurotol 2005;26:838–841.

Gibson T, Davis WB. The distortion of autogenous cartilage grafts: its cause and prevention. Br J Plast Surg 1958;10:257–274.

Heermann J, Heermann H, Kopfstein E. Fascia and cartilage palisade tympanoplasty. Nine years' experience. Arch Otolaryngol 1970;91:228–241.

Kyrodimos E, Sismanis A, Santos D. Type 3 cartilage "shield" tympanoplasty: an effective procedure for hearing improvement. Otolaryngol Head Neck Surg 2007;136:982–985.

Lazard DS, Gilles R, Denoyelle F, Chauvin P. Congenital cholesteatoma: risk factors for residual disease and retraction pockets—a report on 117 cases. Laryngoscope 2007;117:634–637.

Martin H. La chirurgie de renforcement du tympan. J Fr Otorhinolaryngol Audiophonol Chir Maxillofac 1979;28:195–196.

Martin H, Cajgfinger H, Gignoux B, De la Oudot J. chirurgie de renforcement du tympan [Surgical reinforcement of the tympanum] [Article in French. Ann Otolaryngol Chir Cervicofac 1973;90:119–122.

Martin C, Thimoshenko AP, MartinC, Bertholon P, Prades JM. Malleus removal and total cartilage reinforcement in intact canal wall tympaoplasty for cholesteatoma. Ann Otol Rhinol Laryngol 2004;113:421–425.

Moore GF. Revision tympanoplasty utilizing fossa triangularis cartilage. Laryngoscope 2002;112:1543–1554.

Park MS. Tympanoplasty using autologous crushed cartilage. Rev Laryngol Otol Rhinol (Bord) 1995;116:365–368.

Puls T. Tympanoplasty using conchal cartilage graft. Acta Otorhinolaryngol Belg 2003;57:187–191.

Roulleau P, Martin C. Traitement chirurgical. In: Les Monographies du CCA Wagram. Poches de retraction et etats pre-cholesteatomateux. Paris: CCA Wagram, 1998;26:41–61..

Schulte DL, Driscoll CL, McDonald TJ, Facer GW, Beatty CW. Irradiated rib cartilage graft for reconstruction of the tympanic membrane: preliminary results. Am J Otol 1998;19:141–144.

Sismanis A, Dodson K, Kyrodimos E. Cartilage "shield" grafts in revision tympanoplasty. Otol Neurotol 2008;29(3):330–333.

Tos M. Treatment of cholesteatoma in children. A long-term study of results. Am J Otol 1983;4:189–197.

Tos M, Lau T. Recurrence and the condition of the cavity after surgery for cholesteatoma using various techniques. In: Tos M, Thomsen J, Peitersen E, eds. Cholesteatoma and Mastoid Surgery. Amsterdam: Kugler & Ghedini; 1989;863–869..

Tos M. Cartilage tympanoplasty methods. Proposal of a classification. Otolaryngol Head Neck Surg 2008;139(6):747–758.

14 Superior (or Attic) Cartilage–Perichondrium Composite Island Graft Tympanoplasty

Definition

A superior, or attic, cartilage–perichondrium composite island graft is generally defined as a round, semicircular, or other shaped cartilage plate with attached perichondrium on one side (**Fig. 14.1a–e**). The perichondrium flaps surround the cartilage. The lateral flap is the largest and is placed onto the lateral wall of the ear canal. The medial flap is the shortest and it is placed medially onto the short process of the malleus and under the superior part of the eardrum. There may be some perichondrium on the inferior or the superior side of the cartilage. Milewski (1991) recommends perichondrium flaps as large as possible around the cartilage island.

The shape and the size of the cartilage plate depend on the size and shape of the defect of the bone in the attic region. The cartilage plate covers the bony defect like a cork, and the surrounding perichondrial flaps, placed onto the bone, prevent the cartilage plate from dislocating deeper into the attic or/and the antrum.

In the tympanic cartilage–perichondrium composite island grafts, the cartilage faces the tympanic cavity. This prevents formation of adhesions between the graft and the middle ear mucosa. For the superior cartilage island graft it is apparently not important whether the cartilage faces toward the attic or toward the ear canal. Moreover, there are various constructions and shapes of the island flaps and various placements of the graft. The origin and size of the attic defects as well as the basic disease may also have significant influence on the shape and size of the graft and the outcome of surgery.

Some authors cover the cartilage island graft with the fascia (Adkins and Osguthorpe 1984).

Indications for Surgery

Cartilage offers the advantage of being readily available in sufficient quantities. In the endaural approach the tragus cartilage, and in the retroauricular approach the concha cartilage can be harvested without other separate incisions. Cartilage is well tolerated in the attic region and it is easy to cut to the proper shape and size. It is therefore the most commonly used graft to repair any attic defect.

The indications for surgery can be divided into three major groups:

1. Resorption of the bone of the scutum in **attic retractions** after chronic secretory otitis media. The characteristic of attic retractions is that they are very common and manifest themselves with various degrees of severity. Most retractions are small and completely harmless and will remain harmless during the entire life of the individual. Some will progress and become deeper, and some may have clear signs of bone resorption of the scutum, resulting in a larger access to the retraction and improved self-cleaning of the retraction. Some few retractions will have recurrent problems with self-cleaning and will eventually be candidates for surgery. A few retractions will develop a condition of **attic precholesteatoma** with accumulation of debris and crust formation within the retraction. Inflammation takes place behind such a crust, leading to proliferation of keratinized squamous epithelium and formation of microcholesteatomas and resulting in a growth of attic cholesteatoma and bone resorption (Tos 1981; Sudhoff and Tos 2000, 2001).

In our epidemiological studies of three cohorts of Danish children, followed from birth to the age of 16 years by tympanometry and otomicroscopy, at least one episode of secretory otitis media was found in 80% of otherwise healthy children (Tos and Poulsen 1978; Tos et al. 1978, 1979, 1982a, b; Tos 1983; Tos et al. 1984). A relatively high percentage of these children developed pathological changes of the pars tensa (Tos and Poulsen 1979;Tos et al. 1984; Tos et al. 1990a; Stangerup et al. 1994) or attic retractions, or both (Tos et al. 1982a, b; Stangerup et al. 1994).

In our classification of attic retractions into four grades (**Fig. 14.2**), bone resorption of the scutum occurred in types 3 and 4 (Tos and Poulsen 1980). The conclusion of our long-term epidemiological studies on secretory otitis and its sequelae, particularly on the eardrum of the attic retraction, is that secretory otitis is an extremely common disease and is the cause of pathological changes of the pars tensa and/or the pars flaccida (attic retractions). Most of the attic retractions are harmless and will remain so throughout life. A few will progress and very few will have problems with self-cleaning of the retraction and subsequent accumulation of debris. If conservative treatment is not effective then surgery may be considered. Surgery

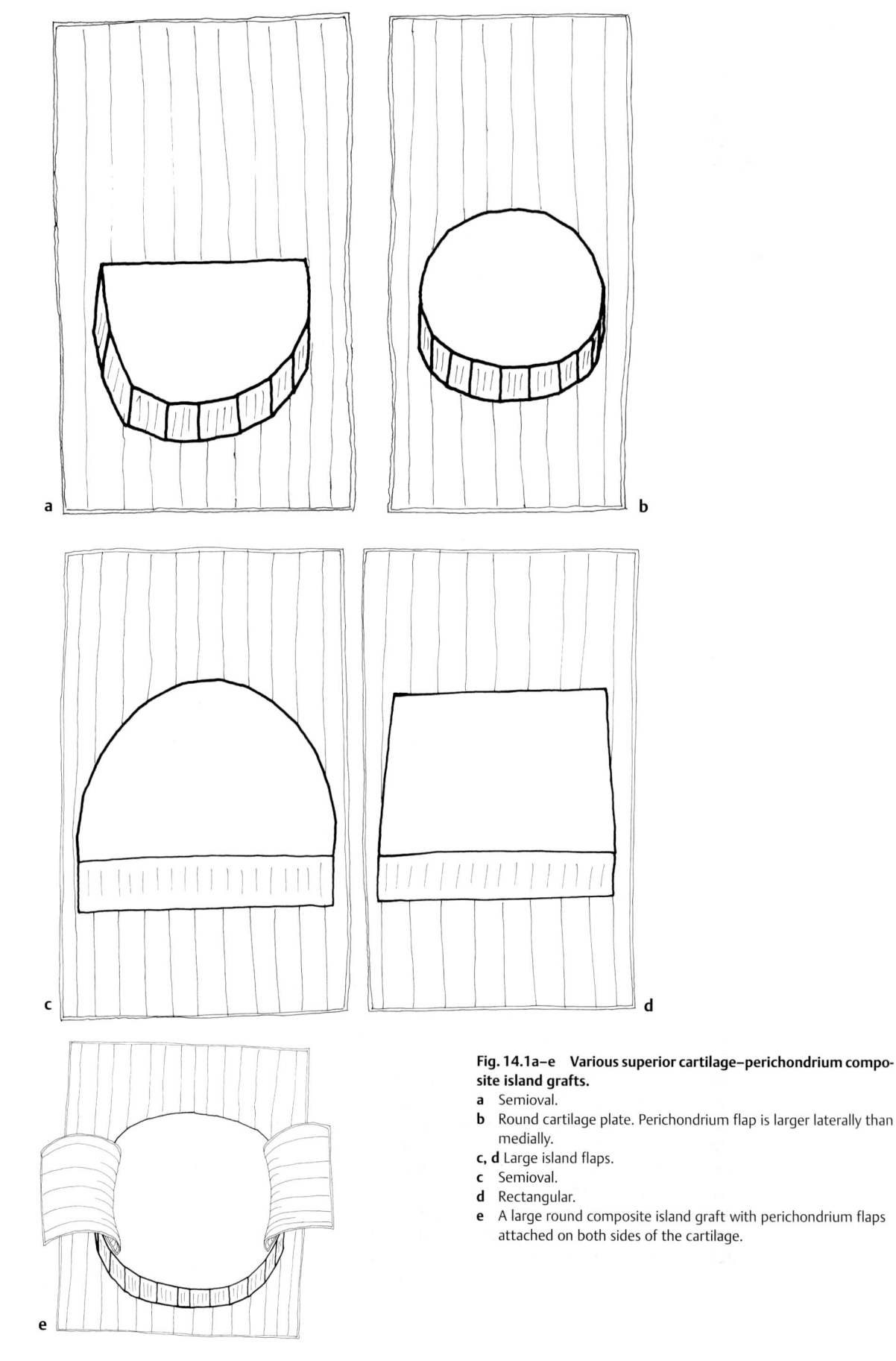

Fig. 14.1a–e Various superior cartilage–perichondrium composite island grafts.
a Semioval.
b Round cartilage plate. Perichondrium flap is larger laterally than medially.
c, d Large island flaps.
c Semioval.
d Rectangular.
e A large round composite island graft with perichondrium flaps attached on both sides of the cartilage.

can be an enlargement of the entrance to the retraction or a total removal of the retraction and reconstruction of the bony defect of the scutum with an attic cartilage island graft.
2. Bone resorption of the scutum in **attic cholesteatoma**. Sometimes, especially in children, bone resorption of the scutum may be sparse, even in a very invasive and aggressive cholesteatoma (Tos 1981).
3. **Surgical defects of the scutum** caused by previous operations with removal of the attic wall and current operations such as atticotomy, atticoantrotomy, and types of canal wall up mastoidectomy.

Surgical Methods for Closure of Bony Defects of the Scutum

McCleve Technique

The first surgeon to use the attic island graft was McCleve (1969). He placed the perichondrium toward the attic and the cartilage toward the ear canal (**Fig. 14.3**). A perichondrium flap elevated from the concave side of the cartilage is turned medially and placed under the eardrum. McCleve included the dome of the tragus cartilage in the island graft and, after elevating the perichondrium of the concave side (**Fig. 14.4a**), placed the dome end of the graft medially, and turned the perichondrium attached to the dome under the eardrum.

In a situation with reconstruction of the scutum after atticoantrotomy without the ossicles, the cartilage island graft is placed with the dome end under the eardrum. The perichondrium faces the antrum and continues laterally onto the ear canal wall and medially under the eardrum (**Fig. 14.4b**).

Later, McCleve (1985) added a modification of the attic island graft for cases without ossicles, and in particular for cases without the malleus. The cartilage faces the antrum; the perichondrium faces the ear canal, but it continues under the eardrum (**Fig. 14.4c**).

Fleury Technique

Fleury et al. (1974) used cartilage with perichondrium on both sides, creating two medial and two lateral perichondrium flaps (**Fig. 14.5**). The graft is placed onto the border of the defect in the ear canal wall with the lateral inner perichondrium flap covering the inner side and the outer perichondrium flap covering the outer side of the ear canal wall (**Fig. 14.6**). Medially, both the medial perichondrium flaps are placed on the neck and the short process of the malleus.

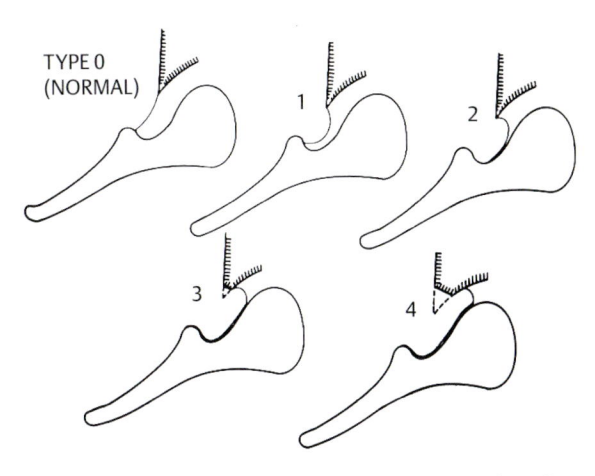

Fig. 14.2 Classification of attic retractions (Tos and Poulsen 1980).
Type 1: The retraction of the Schrapnell membrane is not touching the neck of the malleus.
Type 2: The Schrapnell membrane is touching the neck of the malleus; in half of cases it is permanently adherent to the neck and in the other half it is not.
Type 3: The Schrapnell membrane is retracted and adherent to the neck and head of the malleus and there is slight resorption of the bone of the scutum, i. e., the entrance to the retraction is enlarged.
Type 4: The bone resorption of the scutum is extensive and the access to the retraction is enlarged. The epithelial membrane is adherent to the malleus head and incus body.

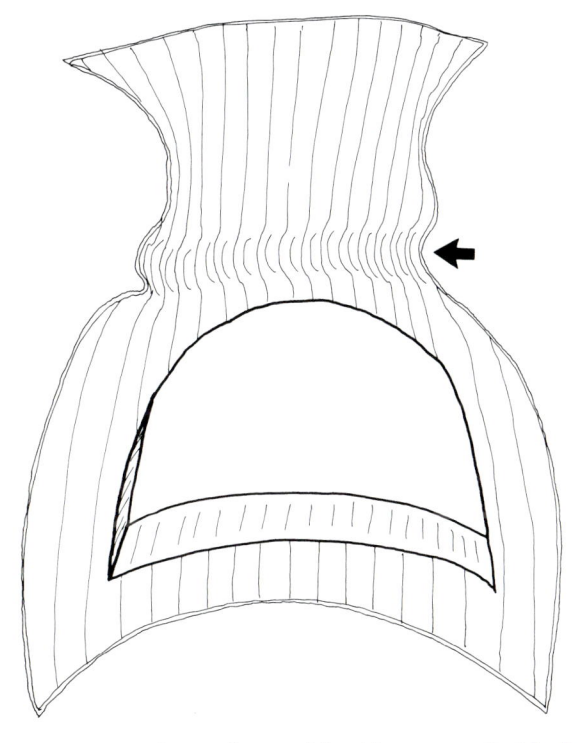

Fig. 14.3 Superior cartilage–perichondrium composite island graft applied by McCleve (1969). A special perichondrium flap is elevated from the concave side of the tragal cartilage, but it is still attached to the dome (arrow). This flap is placed under the eardrum and the shaped cartilage plate is placed into the bony defect of the attic.

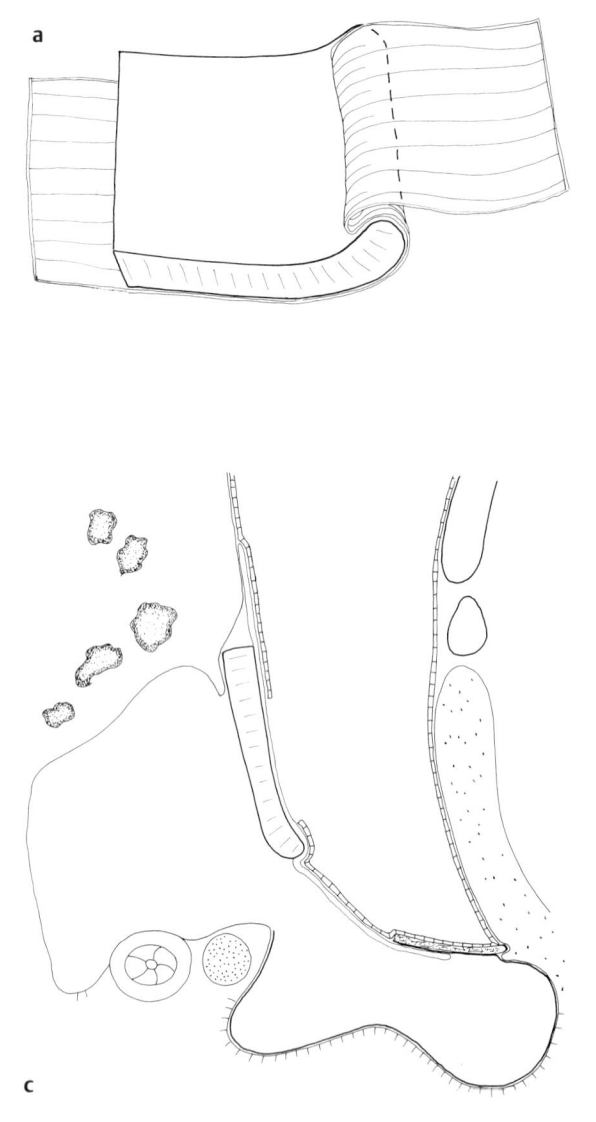

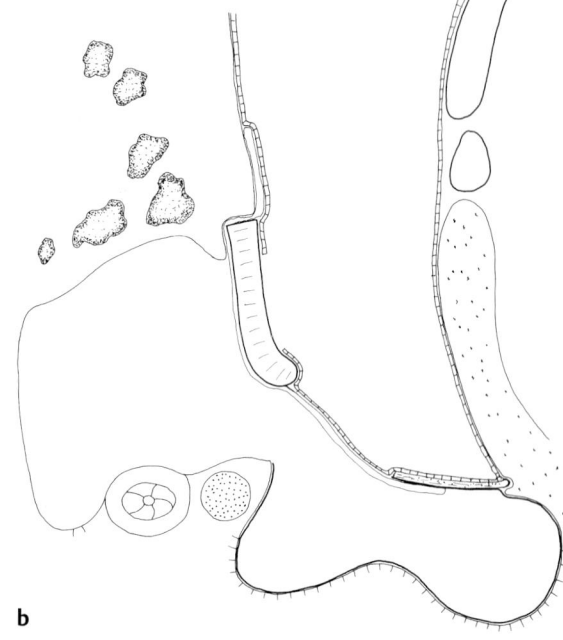

Fig. 14.4a–c

a **Superior cartilage–perichondrium composite island graft as used by McCleve.** A large piece of the tragal cartilage with the dome is harvested. From the concave (posterior) side of the tragal cartilage the perichondrium is elevated up to the edge of the dome and this part will be placed under the eardrum. The perichondrium of the other side is placed on the lateral wall of the ear canal and turned to the attic.

b **McCleve superior cartilage island graft in a case of reconstruction of the scutum after atticoantrotomy and a missing malleus.** The perichondrium faces the antrum, but is placed onto the ear canal wall and under the eardrum. The dome of the tragus cartilage is placed medially.

c **The McCleve cartilage island graft in a similar situation as shown in the previous drawing, but with the perichondrium facing the ear canal.** The perichondrium placed under the eardrum is elevated from the opposite site of the cartilage.

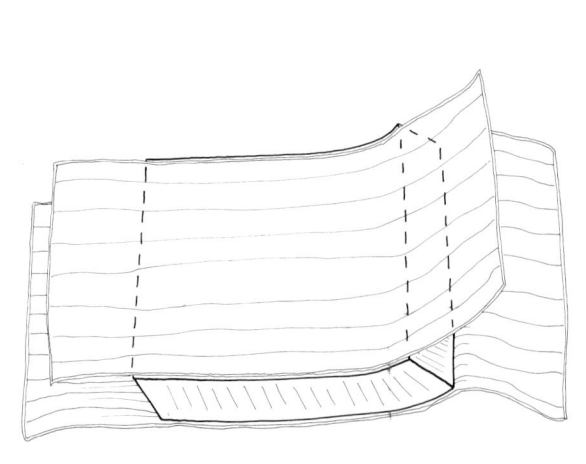

Fig. 14.5 Fleury superior composite cartilage island graft with perichondrium on both sides and with two lateral and two medial perichondrium flaps.

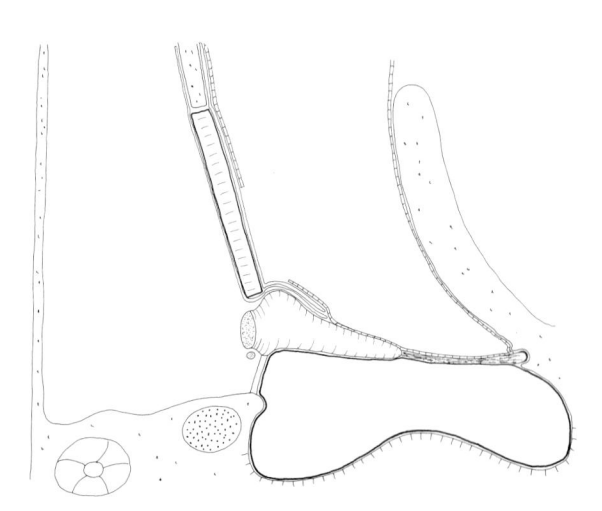

Fig. 14.6 Scutumplasty with Fleury's superior cartilage–perichondrium composite island grafts. The cartilage is placed onto the defective ear canal wall and is supported laterally by two perichondrium flaps, placed on both sides of the ear canal wall. Medially, both perichondrium flaps are placed onto the short process of the malleus.

Adkins Technique

In this technique the dome end of the tragus cartilage is harvested and is shaped appropriately to the size of the scutum defect (Adkins and Osguthorpe 1984; Adkins 1990). The perichondrium is then elevated from the concave side of the tragus up to the dome but is left in continuity over the dome and with the perichondrium on the other side (see **Figs. 14.7, 14.8**).

After completion of the atticotomy, a groove is drilled along the borders of the bony defect with a diamond drill (**Fig. 14.9a**). The cartilage is placed onto the groove and the lateral perichondrium flap is adjusted onto the lateral ear canal wall (**Fig. 14.9b**). The medial flap is placed under the superior part of the eardrum. A large piece of fascia is placed as a bag onto the cartilage–perichondrium island graft (**Fig. 14.9c**) and folded out over the ear canal wall (**Fig. 14.9d**). After replacement of the ear canal skin flaps and the medial epithelium flaps (**Fig. 14.9e**) this reconstruction of the attic defect with two grafts seems to be quite firm (**Fig. 14.9f**).

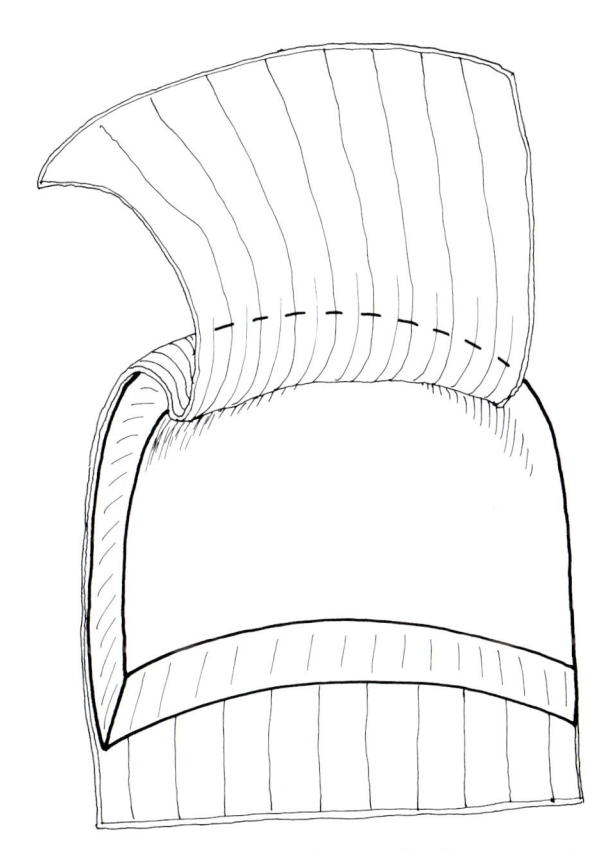

Fig. 14.7 Adkins superior cartilage–perichondrium composite island graft. The perichondrium is elevated up to the dome. This part will support the lateral part of the graft and cover the ear canal wall. The small medial perichondrium grafts is placed onto the short process of the malleus and under the superior part of the eardrum.

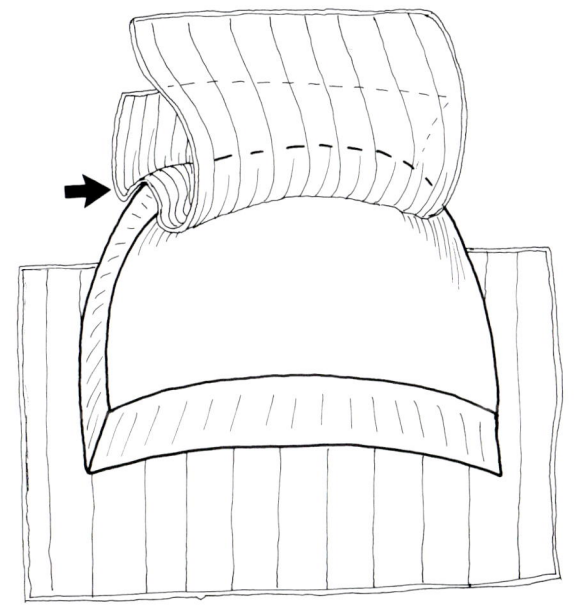

Fig. 14.8 Adkins superior cartilage–perichondrium composite island graft surrounded by four perichondrium flaps: lateral flap; medial flap; inferior flap; superior flap. The lateral flap is connected to the opposite perichondrium by the dome perichondrium (arrow).

Fig. 14.9a–f Closure of a large defect of the bony ear canal wall after atticotomy and removal of an attic cholesteatoma with the technique of Adkins.

a Atticotomy is performed and completed and attic cholesteatoma removed. A groove is drilled all the way along the border of the bony defect.
b The cartilage is placed onto the bone and adapted to the groove. The lateral perichondrium flap is adapted to the posterior bony wall of the ear canal. The medial perichondrium flap is placed onto the short process of the malleus and the superior part of the bony annulus covering the superior part of the tympanic cavity.
c A fascia bag containing two or three Gelfoam balls is placed onto the cartilage.
d The fascia is spread over the ear canal wall and the perichondrium and is placed under the eardrum remnant and under the ear canal skin.
e The eardrum, the epithelial flaps, and ear canal skin are replaced.

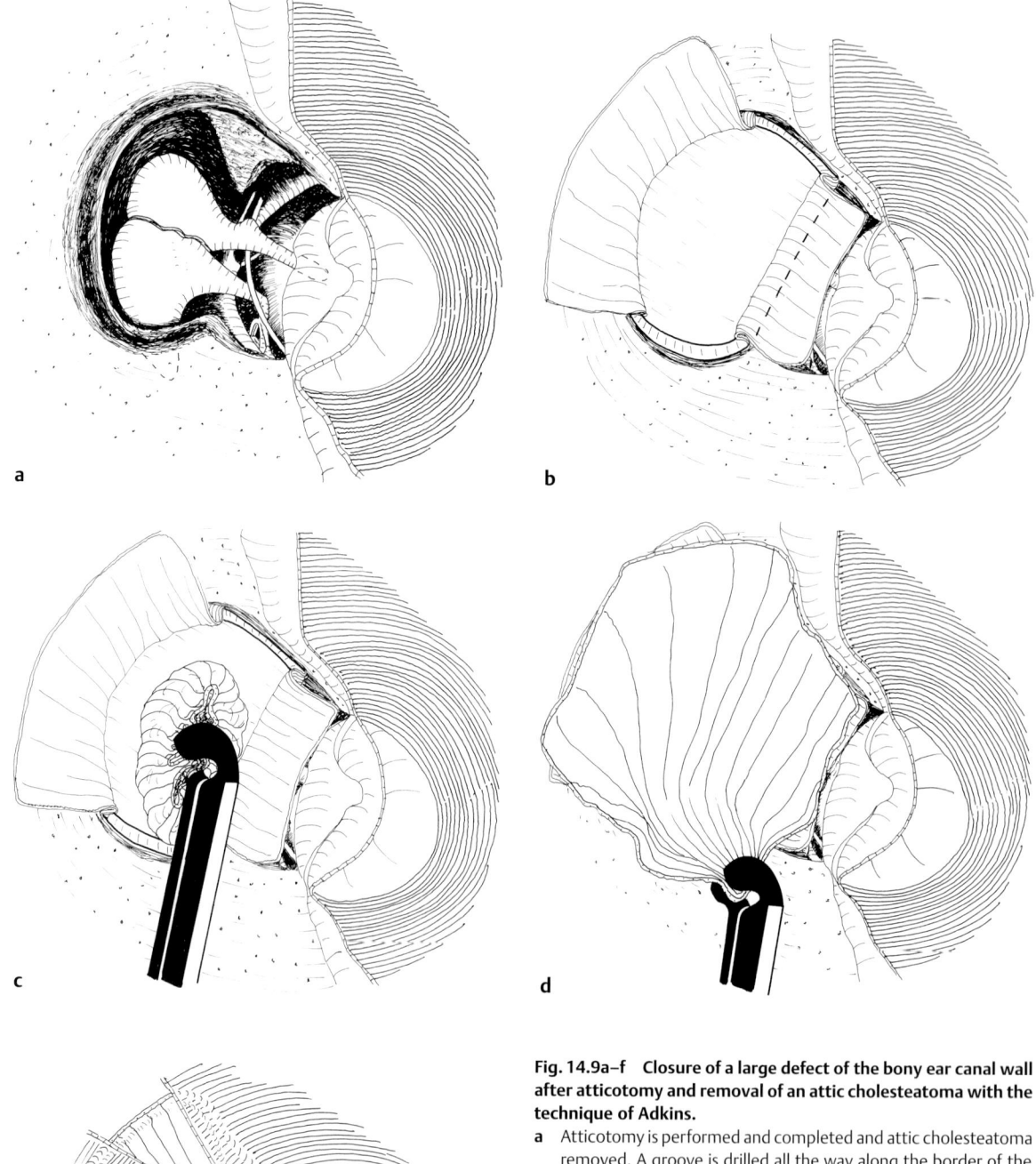

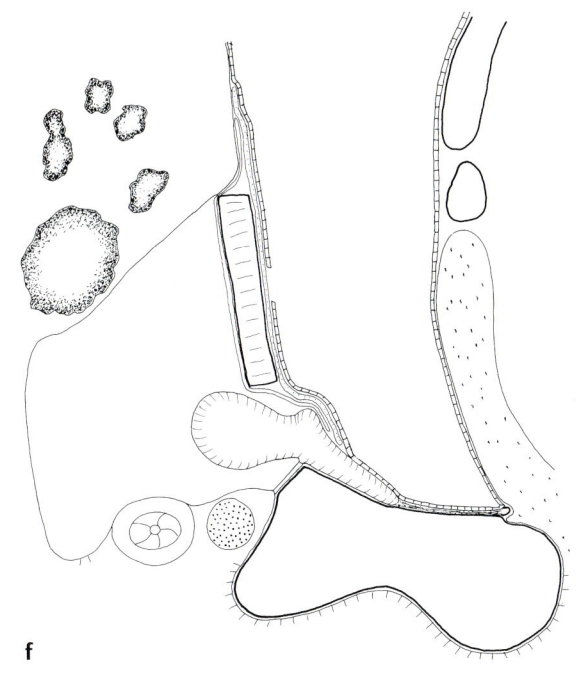

Fig. 14.9f

f Side view of the Adkins technique of closure of the bony defect after atticotomy with superior cartilage–perichondrium composite island graft and fascia. The cartilage is placed in a groove with the lateral perichondrium flap stabilizing the cartilage. The medial perichondrium flap, together with the fascia, closes the tympanic cavity.

Black Technique

For scutumplasty after a canal wall up mastoidectomy, Black (1992) used a combination of hydroxyapatite plate, bone paste, and thinned cartilage–perichondrium island graft. After a completed canal wall up mastoidectomy and the total removal of squamous epithelium, a groove is drilled into the root of the zygoma and a hydroxyapatite plate is fitted, to cover the bony defect of the attic from the mastoid side. The size of the plate depends on the size of the defect of the attic and the anatomical situation in the anterior attic (**Fig. 14.10a**). Onto this plate is placed a bone paste (**Fig. 14.10b**). The bone paste thus fills out all the bony defect of the ear canal wall. The defect and the bone paste including the surrounding ear canal wall are covered with the slightly thinned cartilage island graft (**Fig. 14.10c**). The lateral and medial perichondrium flaps cover the ear canal wall and medially also the superior tympanic cavity as an underlay graft (**Fig. 14.10 d**).

If the hydroxyapatite plate was not stable, Black placed a 4 mm × 14 mm and 0.5 mm thick piece of Silastic doubled over at the level of the hydroxyapatite plate. This acts as a spring and is intended to hold the hydroxyapatite plate in place during the critical first three months (**Fig. 14.10e**).

Honda Scutumplasty

Honda (1992) applied concha cartilage as free graft because its slightly concave shape fits best in the scutum defect. First a groove is drilled along the edges of the bony defect (**Fig. 14.11a**). Then fascia is placed onto the groove and fixed with fibrin glue (**Fig. 14.11b**). Onto the fascia and onto the groove a shaped piece of concha cartilage is placed and fixed with fibrin glue (**Fig. 14.11c**). The skin flaps are replaced and cover most of the cartilage free graft (**Fig. 14.11 d**).

Quinn Technique

More recently, Koury and co-workers (2005) published an interesting scutumplasty, which they used on 16 patients with cholesteatoma after a combined-approach tympanoplasty. All patients were operated by S. J. Quinn.

Employing a retroauricular approach, two pieces of cartilage are harvested, each covered on one side with perichondrium. One piece is adapted to the size and the shape of the scutum defect and will be placed into the bony defect of the attic wall. The medial end of the cartilage free graft lies at the level of the neck of the malleus (**Fig. 14.12**). On the attic side the cartilage is covered with fascia that continues laterally on the back side of the thin ear canal wall. The second piece of conchal cartilage is placed in the attic, perpendicular to the cartilage graft filling the attic defect, to act as a buttress. This cartilage can be further stabilized on the deep aspect by the use of fascia strips.

On the ear canal side the cartilage is covered with perichondrium without any additional flaps around the cartilage (**Fig. 14.12**). Another fascia graft is placed onto the perichondrium. This fascia continues as an on-lay graft onto the malleus handle and superior part of the eardrum. Laterally the fascia covers part of the ear canal wall.

In this method the cartilage is not an island graft. It is covered with the perichondrium, but it does not have perichondrium flaps. The cartilage is a free graft. The interesting aspect of this technique is the covering of both sides of the cartilage graft with the fascia.

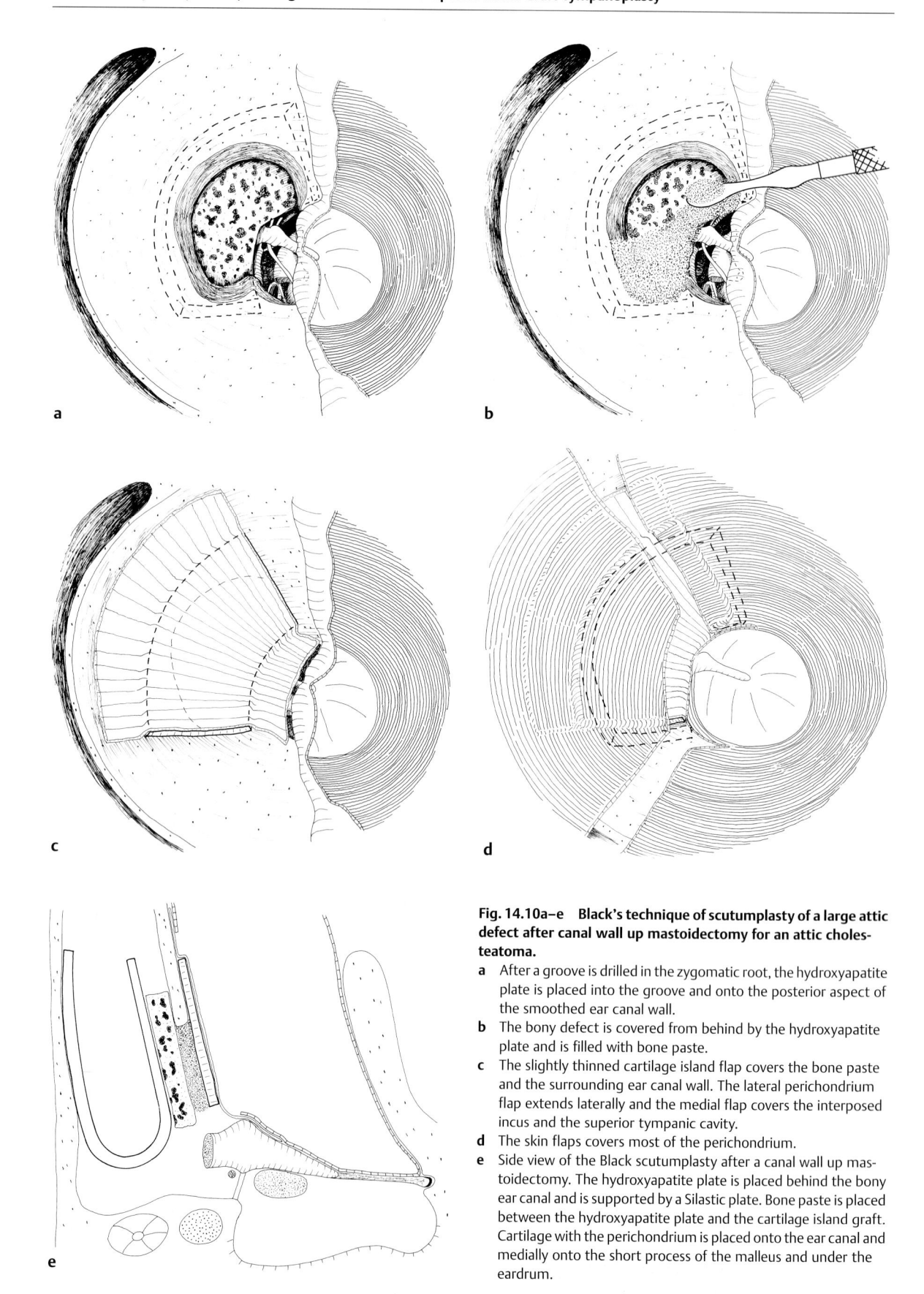

Fig. 14.10a–e Black's technique of scutumplasty of a large attic defect after canal wall up mastoidectomy for an attic cholesteatoma.

a After a groove is drilled in the zygomatic root, the hydroxyapatite plate is placed into the groove and onto the posterior aspect of the smoothed ear canal wall.

b The bony defect is covered from behind by the hydroxyapatite plate and is filled with bone paste.

c The slightly thinned cartilage island flap covers the bone paste and the surrounding ear canal wall. The lateral perichondrium flap extends laterally and the medial flap covers the interposed incus and the superior tympanic cavity.

d The skin flaps covers most of the perichondrium.

e Side view of the Black scutumplasty after a canal wall up mastoidectomy. The hydroxyapatite plate is placed behind the bony ear canal and is supported by a Silastic plate. Bone paste is placed between the hydroxyapatite plate and the cartilage island graft. Cartilage with the perichondrium is placed onto the ear canal and medially onto the short process of the malleus and under the eardrum.

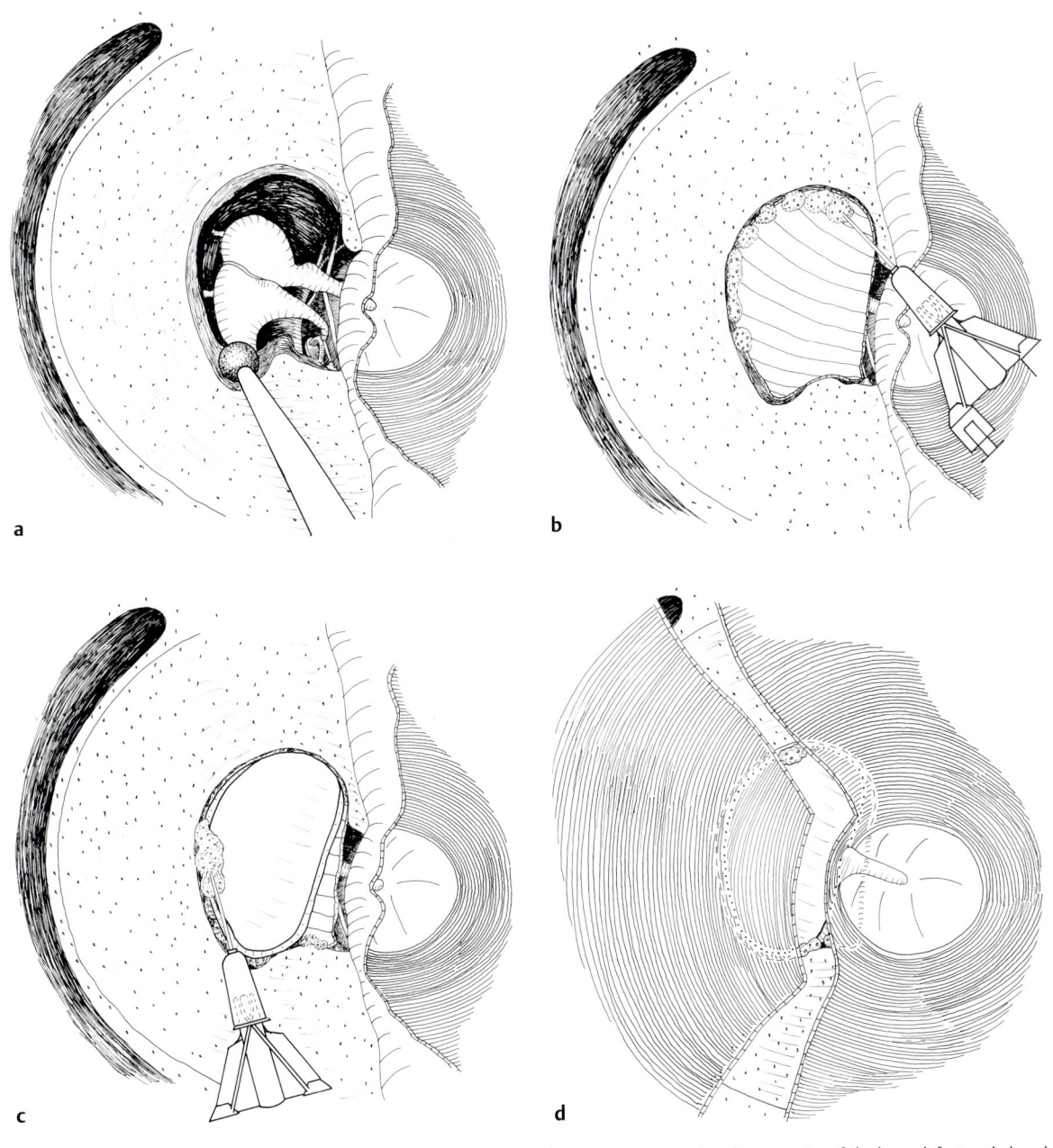

Fig 14.11a–d
The Honda scutumplasty with fascia, fibrin glue, and free concha cartilage graft.
a   An intact canal wall mastoidectomy and an atticotomy are performed and an attic cholesteatoma is removed. The ossicular chain is intact. A groove is drilled along the edge of the bony defect.
b   Fascia is trimmed to the exact size of the bony defect and placed onto the bony groove and glued to the bone all the way around the defect. Fascia also covers the mesotympanic region.
c   A concave piece of concha cartilage is trimmed and placed onto the groove of the bony defect. It is glued to the bone. The concave side of the cartilage graft faces the meatus.
d   The epithelial flaps are replaced.

Results of Surgery

McCleve (1969) obtained good primary results in 19 of 20 operated cases.

Adkins and Osguthorpe (1984) performed scutumplasty with superior cartilage island flap on 40 ears—17 after atticotomy and 23 after canal wall up mastoidectomy. One to six years after surgery satisfactory results were obtained in 38 patients. Further information on 17 of these cases 7–13 years after surgery, revealed one additional failure (Adkins 1990).

In a retrospective study of 84 patients being operated for cholesteatoma with canal wall up mastoidectomy who

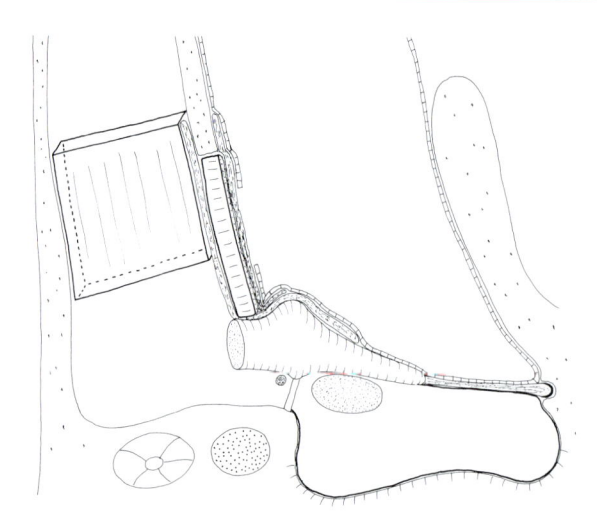

Fig. 14.12 Side view of Quinn's scutumplasty after the combined approach tympanoplasty. A piece of concha cartilage, with perichondrium attached on the concave side, is trimmed and placed between the edge of the bony defect and the neck of the malleus. The concave side of the composite graft faces the meatal site. The cartilage graft is covered with a large fascia ending medially on the malleus and laterally on the ear canal wall. On the attic side, the cartilage graft is covered by fascia, extending medially from the neck of the malleus and laterally to the bony ear canal wall. A piece of cartilage is placed perpendicular to the attic graft to act as a buttress.

could be followed, the scutum was not reconstructed in 52 patients. Of these, 53% developed retraction. Only a third of these patients required further surgery. Of the 32 patients who had the scutum reconstructed with cartilage, 34% developed retraction and only one-third of them required further surgery (Weber and Gantz 1998).

Black (1992) applied cartilage composite island grafts to 14 patients with scutum defects. In a short follow-up, even the bone paste had resorbed moderately and in some cases the cartilage island grafts were able to prevent recurrent cholesteatoma and the attic region was epithelialized.

Pfleiderer et al. (2003) performed primary attic reconstruction in a combined approach tympanoplasty (CAT) for cholesteatoma in 47 patients. During the period 1990–95 the cartilage was shaped as a "D" to fit the attic defect and was often reinforced with Silastic sheets. The cartilage graft was not a composite graft and perichondrium flaps were not involved in the closure of the attic defect. In the following period (1996–99) the preferred technique was bone paste repair mixed with tissue glue (Tissel). In 14 patients from the cartilage group, a "second look" procedure was performed with recurrence in 8 cases (57%). Among 29 patients treated with bone paste, recurrence was found at "second look" surgery in 6 ears (21%).

The results of the Quinn technique after 9 months are good on 16 patients (5 children and 11 adults) with mesotympanic or attic cholesteatoma operated with a combined approach tympanoplasty and a second-stage operation. At a mean follow-up of 19 months (range 10–53 months), failure of the attic reconstruction in two cases (13%), one clean retraction, and one recurrent attic cholesteatoma occurred. In one case (6%) a small residual cholesteatoma was found.

In a recent Polish study by Golabek and co-workers (2005), in 27 patients with attic cholesteatoma, a transmeatal atticotomy was performed and cholesteatoma was removed. The bony defect was covered with a typical attic cartilage–perichondrium composite island graft. At the follow up 3–6 years after surgery, the bony defect was closed in 89% of cases.

Lateral Attic Reconstruction (LAR) Technique: Preventive Surgery for Epitympanic Retraction Pockets

From a cohort of 25 adult patients with type 2 attic retraction pockets, Barbara (2008) randomly made two groups: The first group of 15 patients underwent LAR; in the second group of 10 patients, only observation was planned and this group was therefore used as control. In the classification of Charachon et al. (1992), the type 2 retraction is fixated to the incus body and malleus head, with stagnating and accumulating epithelial debris, indicating poor self-cleaning.

LAR Surgical Technique
After a retroauricular incision, an anteriorly based musculoperiostal flap is raised from the mastoid cortex. The ear canal is then entered posteriorly and the vascular strip area is isolated and elevated. After inspection of the attic area, a 5 mm × 5 mm piece of tragal cartilage with the perichondrium is harvested. From the 7-o'clock to 2-o'clock positions a tympanomeatal flap is elevated as far as the short process of the malleus. The flap is covered with an aluminum foil and an atticotomy is performed with exposure of the posterior part of the attic, exposing the malleus head and incus body, which are covered with the retraction membrane. The entire membrane is carefully elevated from the attic walls and the ossicles, and carefully removed, including the surrounding ear canal skin. This situation resembles **Fig. 14.11** or **Fig. 14.13a**, where I drill out a groove to support the cartilage graft. Barbara cuts a half-moon-shaped cartilage graft according to a preshaped Silastic dummy. The perichondrial flap of this cartilage–perichondrium composite island graft is used to repair Shrapnell's membrane defects and to facilitate re-epithelialization. The tympanomeatal flap repositioned over the epitympanic area.

Results of Surgery in the LAR Group
Patients were followed for 12 months postoperatively.
At the 1-year follow-up of the operated group, the hearing was the same as before the operation. Otomicroscopy showed a reconstructed attic. Tympanometry

showed type A of attic retraction in 60%, type B in 20%, and type C in 20% of 15 cases.

The control group, followed for 12 months, showed progress of the disease in 3 of 10 patients, with widening the bony epitympanic erosion. These patients will be operated.

Recently Pennings and Cremers (2009) proposed, in surgery of cholesteatoma in the anterior epitympanum, as part of a closed canal wall up procedure, **a postauricular approach atticomey: a modified closed technique with reconstruction of the scutum with cymbal cartilage**. However a second-look procedure is recommended because of a relatively high percentage of recurrent and residual disease.

Author's Comments and Proposals

There is great variability in the methods presented and none of the published methods are identical. The Adkins method, using a solid closure of the attic defect and the eardrum with a cartilage–perichondrium composite graft and covering of the entire attic region with a large fascia, seems very reliable and I would recommend it. Ideally of course we would have a prospective randomized study of two series: one series with the superior cartilage–perichondrium composite island graft without fascia and the other with identical cartilage island graft with fascia.

On the basis of personal experience, I recommend the following method of reconstruction of the scutum defect.

- Complete removal of the cholesteatoma, saving as much ear canal bone as possible. However, in an extension of the cholesteatoma to the anterior attic, much more radical removal of bone is necessary to view the cholesteatoma, especially in children (Duckert et al. 2002).
- Drilling a groove along the borders of the ear canal defect for the safe placement of the cartilage disk (**Fig. 14.13a**).
- Cutting and shaping the cartilage–perichondrium composite island graft after exact measurement of the diameters of the scutum defect. The perichondrium flap should be as large as possible, especially the lateral and medial parts, but the anterior and posterior parts may be smaller (**Fig. 14.13b**).
- The graft with the perichondrium folded inward is placed in the groove of the scutum defect. Any gaps between the cartilage and bone can be closed with small cartilage palisades (**Fig. 14.13c**). Palisades are placed between the malleus and the anterior wall of the tympanic cavity. Similar palisades are placed in the posterosuperior part of the tympanic cavity.
- The perichondrium flaps are folded out (**Fig. 14.13 d**).
- Then a large piece of fascia is used to cover the perichondrium (**Figs. 14.13e, f**), which helps further to prevent a later retraction (**Fig. 14.13 g**).

Difficulties in Comparison of the Various Series

The variety of cholesteatomas and other pathologies, requiring different surgeries with different prognoses and outcomes, explains why comparisons of results between the various series must be treated with caution, as the severity of the series is practically never sufficiently described. The use of various canal wall up and canal wall down methods and the various methods of reconstruction also make the comparisons between the various series difficult.

Different Techniques in Cholesteatoma Removal
Some surgeons will be very radical and remove all ossicles from the attic together with the cholesteatoma. Other surgeons will dissect the cholesteatoma matrix from the ossicles, keeping them intact. Such essential differences in the technique are usually not described and are not taken into consideration in the description of surgical procedure.

Different Approaches to the Attic
The attic can be approached (a) through the mastoid and the antrum in a classic **intact canal wall up mastoidectomy** as a transcortical atticotomy (Jansen 1963; House and Sheehy 1963; Smyth 1969), or (b) as a transmeatal atticotympanonotomy (Morimitsu et al. 1989), or (c) as an extensive transcanal atticotympanotomy (Rosborg 1993). These methods are thoroughly explained and illustrated in MMES_2, Chapter 6. (d) In a **modified combined approach mastoidectomy** (Tos 1978, 1982), transcanal atticotomy with or without preservation of a thin bony bridge is performed before mastoidectomy (MMES_2, Chapter 7).

Each of the atticotomies mentioned requires a specially shaped and usually large attic composite cartilage island graft for reconstruction of the attic and ear canal.

Several other **transmeatal atticotomies** have been published and are applied worldwide, such as tympanomeatoplasty with preservation of the bony bridge of Wigand (1970) (MMES_2, Chapter 9), transmeatal anterior atticotympanotomy, and the transcortical mastoidectomy of Farrior (MMES_2, Chapter10). Moreover, **transmeatal retrograde canal wall down mastoidectomy on demand** requires an extensive reconstruction of the attic with cartilage (MMES_2, Chapter 11). **Retrograde mastoidectomy on demand** by following the cholesteatoma in a posterior direction with limited bone work (Olaizola 1988) requires an extensive reconstruction of the attic and antrum with cartilage (MMES_2, Chapter 13).

Different Types, Location, and Extension of Cholesteatoma
Preoperative otomicroscopy performed by the surgeon reveals the type, location, and extension of the cholesteatoma, which is divisible into:

Attic cholesteatoma: starting with an attic retraction and bone resorption, while the tympanic cavity is not involved.

a

b

c

d

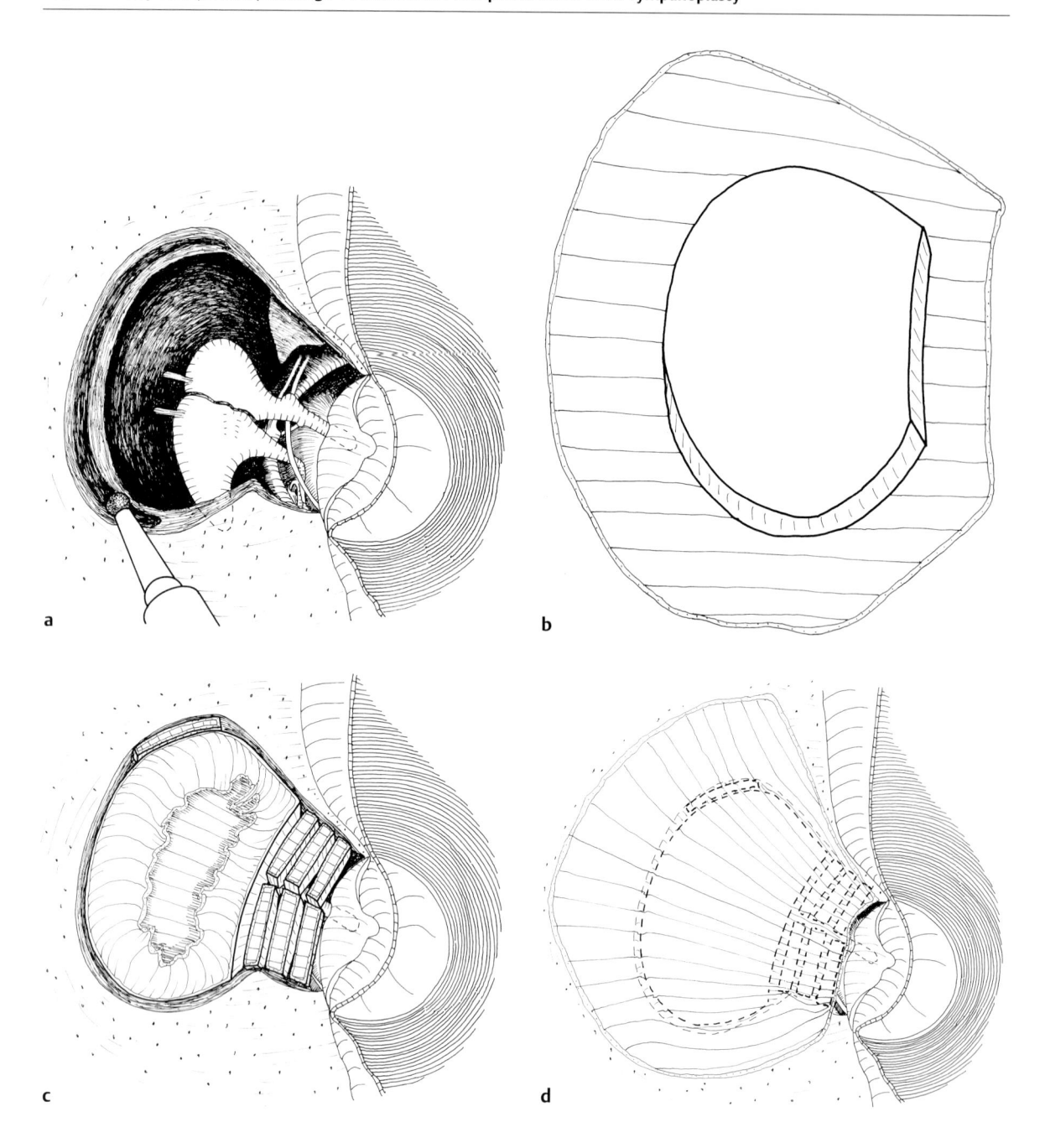

Sinus cholesteatoma: starting with a posterosuperior retraction of pars tensa, involving the tympanic sinuses and eventually continuing under the incus into the posterior attic and antrum. Hypotympanum, anterior tympanum, and anterior attic are not involved.

Entire tensa retraction cholesteatoma: starting with retraction of the entire pars tensa and involving the entire tympanic cavity, with common resorption of the long process of the incus, stapes crura, and malleus handle. The cholesteatoma may extend into the hypotympanic cells and the tympanic orifice, and up into the anterior and posterior attic.

The condition of the ossicles, eardrum, and middle ear mucosa are also important factors in comparing the results.

Tubal function testing (tympanometry, aspiration test, deflation test, nine-step test)—unfortunately neglected by most surgeons—should be included, especially when making a decision for cartilage tympanoplasty. At least tubal patency with Valsalva maneuver should be tested.

CT-scanning to determine extension of cholesteatoma and the pneumatization of the mastoid process is performed by most surgeons consistently but by some only occasionally.

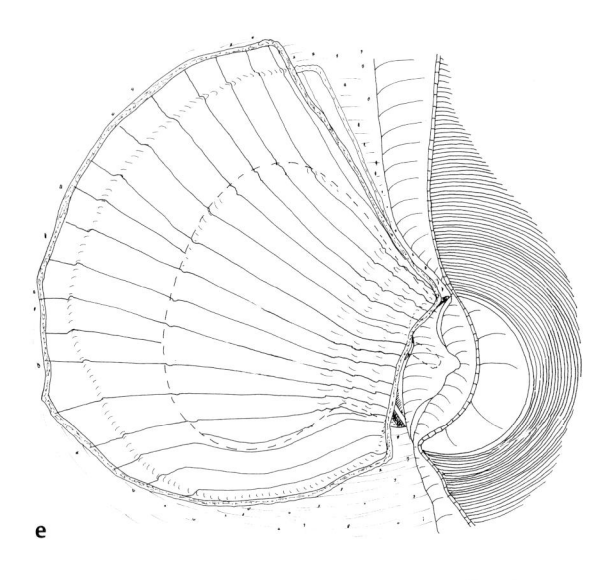

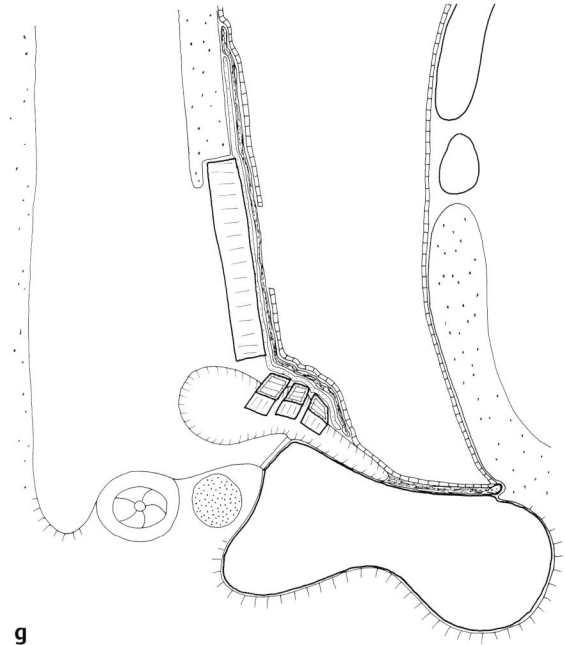

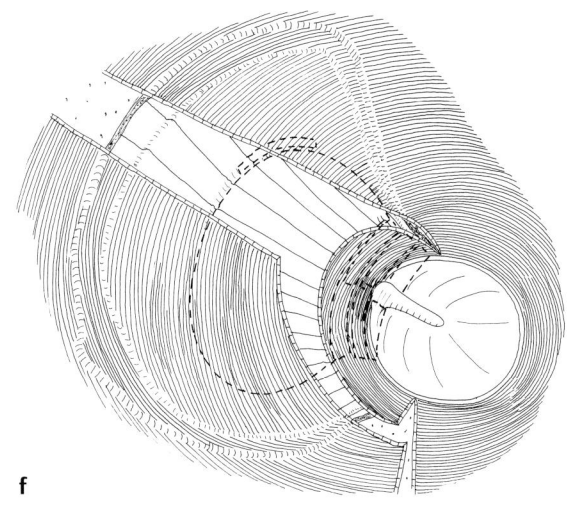

Fig. 14.13a–g The present author's proposal for closure of a large scutum defect with an attic island graft, cartilage palisades, and fascia.
a After canal wall up mastoidectomy and removal of an attic cholesteatoma with preservation of an intact ossicular chain, a groove is made on the surrounding bone of the scutum.
b The superior cartilage–perichondrium composite island graft is cut after exact measurement of the diameters and the shape of the scutum defect.
c A cartilage–perichondrium island graft is placed onto the bony groove of the scutum defect. A small cartilage palisade covers a small gap between the cartilage and the bone. Three cartilage palisades are placed between the neck of the malleus and the anterior border of the tympanic cavity, and three palisades are similarly placed posteriorly.
d A large perichondrium flap is folded out, covering the ear canal bone and the superior part of the tympanic cavity and the palisades.
e A large fascia covers the perichondrium flap and the ear canal bone.
f The epithelium and superior eardrum remnant are replaced. The ear canal skin flaps are replaced, covering the fascia.
g Side view of reconstruction of the scutum with an attic cartilage graft, cartilage palisades, and the fascia after intact canal wall up mastoidectomy and removal of an attic cholesteatoma. The cartilage graft is placed in the bony groove. Small palisades cover the superior part of the tympanic cavity. The inferior perichondrium flap covers the palisades and the superior part of the tympanic cavity, and the superior flap covers the superior wall of the ear canal. Fascia covers the large superior ear canal area and the perichondrium. Ear canal skin flaps and eardrum remnant cover the fascia.

Indications for Preventive Surgery of Epitympanic Retraction Pockets

Before "performing the surgery to prevent the surgery" of a moist attic retraction, I start to treat conservatively with repetitive suction of the debris and placement of a cotton or gauze, moistened with hydrocortisone–polymyxin ointment. Moist retractions will become dry. In case of recurrently moist retraction for a year, I recommend LAR (Lateral attic reconstruction) operation. The reason is the enormous difference between the incidence of attic cholesteatoma and the incidence of attic retraction.

Incidence of Cholesteatoma

There are only few papers on this topic in the literature. Among 191 patients with cleft palates, followed up for many years, the incidence of cholesteatoma was 9.2% (Harker and Severeid 1982). The main reason was poor tubal function.

An epidemiological study from Iowa (USA) showed an incidence of 6 cholesteatomas per 100 000 inhabitants (Harker 1977).

In our study from Copenhagen, based on surgery of 137 cholesteatomas in children and 603 in adults (Tos 1988) during a period of 14 years, from 1967 through 1980, in an area comprising 300 000 inhabitants, the annual incidence was 15.5% per 100 000 inhabitants (2.9% in children and 12.6% in adults). In a similar Finnish study (Kemppainen et al. 1999), based on surgery of 500 cholesteatomas during 1982–91, at the Tampere University and Mikkeli Central Hospital, the incidence of cholesteatoma was 9.2% per 100 000 inhabitants.

In our study the incidence per 100 000 inhabitants was separated for attic cholesteatoma (5.7%), for sinus cholesteatoma (5.7%), and for (entire) tensa cholesteatoma (4.1%), together 15.5% (Tos 1988).

Incidence of Attic Retractions

In our epidemiological studies at least one episode of secretory otitis media was found in 80% of Danish children with type B tympanometry (Tos 1983). As a consequence of secretorys otitis media, at the age of 6 years, 26.3% have had attic retractions (14.6% attic only, 11.7% attic and pars tensa). In our classification (**Fig. 14.2**) type 3, with some bone resorption, was found in 4.3% and type 4, with extended bone resorption, in 0.4% of the cohort of otherwise healthy Danish children. Bone resorption is a clear evidence of a period of active infection in these 4.7% of attic retractions (Tos et al. 1990b).

These results demonstrate that a severe attic retraction is about 1000 times more common than attic cholesteatoma. A preventive LAR surgery should in my opinion be performed in attic retractions with evident clinical symptoms that cannot be eliminated by conservative treatment.

References

Adkins WY. Composite autograft for tympanoplasty and tympanomastoid surgery. Laryngoscope 1990;100:244–247.

Adkins WY, Osguthorpe DJ. Use of a composite autograft to prevent recurrent cholesteatoma caused by canal wall defects. Otolaryngol Head Neck Surg 1984;92:319–321.

Barbara M. Lateral attic reconstruction technique: preventive surgery for epitympanic retraction pockets. Otol Neurotol 2008;29: 522–525.

Black B. Prevention of recurrent cholesteatoma: use of hydroxyapatite plates and composite grafts. Am J Otol 1992;13:273–278.

Charachon R, Barthez M, Lejeune JM. Spontaneous retraction pockets in chronic otitis media: medical and surgical therapy. Ear Nose Throat J 1992;71:578–583.

Duckert LG, Makielski KH, Helms J. Management of anterior epitympanic cholesteatoma: expectations after epitympanic approach and canal wall reconstruction. Otol Neurotol 2002;3:8–13.

Fleury P, Legent F, Lefebvre C. Techniques chirurgicales de l'oreile. Paris: Masson; 1974..

Golabek W, Zadrozniak M, Szymanski M, Morshed K, Zimolag-Kslazka K. Reconstruction of meatal wall with cartilage and perichondrium. Pol Merkur Lekarski 2005;19:411–412.

Harker LA. Cholesteatoma: an incidence study. In: McCabe, Sade, Abramson, eds. Cholesteatoma: First Internal Conference. Birmingham, AL: Aesculapius; 1977: 293–301..

Harker LA, Severeid LR. Cholesteatoma in the cleft palate patients; In: Sade J, ed. Cholesteatoma and Mastoid Surgery Amsterdam: Kugler: 1982:37–40..

Honda Y. My tympanoplasty. Otorhinolaryngology Tokyo 1992; 35(Suppl. 5):1–127.

House WF, Sheehy JL. Functional restoration in tympanoplasties. Arch Otolaryngol 1963;78:304–309.

Jansen C. Cartilage-Tympanoplasty. Laryngoscope 1963;73: 1288–301.

Kemppainen HO, Puhakka HJ, Laippala PJ, Sipilä MM, Manninen MP, Karma PH. Epidemiology and etiology of middle ear cholesteatoma. Acta Otolaryngol 1999;119(5):568–572.

Koury E, Faris C, Sharma S, Qiunn SJ. How we do it: Free conchal cartilage revisited for primary reconstruction of attic defects in combined approach tympanoplasty. Clin Otolaryngol 2005;30: 465–467.

McCleve DE. Tragal cartilage reconstruction of the auditory canal. Arch Otolaryngol 1969;90:35–38.

McCleve DE. Repair of bony canal wall defects in tympanomastoid surgery. Am J Otol 1985;6:76–79.

Milewski C. Ergebnisse der Tympanoplastik nach Verwendung von Knorpel-Perichondriumtransplantaten zum Trommelfellersatz unter ungünstigen Bedingungen. Laryngorhinootologie 1991; 70:402–404.

Morimitsu T, Nagai T, Nagai M. Pathogenesis of cholesteatoma based on clinical results of anterior tympanotomy. Auris Nasus Larynx 1989;16(Suppl. 1) S 9–14.

Olaizola F. Tympanoplasty: a 5-year review of results using the on demanda (AAD) technique. Am J Otol 1988;9:318–322.

Pennings RJ, Cremers CW. Postauricular approach atticotomy: a modified closed technique with reconstruction of the scutum with cymbal cartilage. Ann Otol Rhinol Laryngol 2009;118(3): 199–204.

Pfleiderer AG, Ghosh S, Kairinos N, Chaudri F. A study of recurrence of retraction pockets after various methods of primary reconstruction of attic mesotympanic defects in combined approach tympanoplasty. Clin Otolaryngol 2003;28:548–551.

Rosborg J. Long term results of anterior atticotomy in the treatment of attic cholesteaomas. In: Nakano Y, ed. Cholesteatoma and Mastoid Surgery; Proceedings of the Fourth International Conference. Amsterdam: Kugler; 1993:667–669.

Smyth G. Combined approach tympanoplasty. Arch Otolaryngol 1969;89:250–251.

Sudhoff H, Tos M. Pathogenesis of attic cholesteatoma. Clinical and immunohistochemical support for combination of retraction theory and proliferation theory. Am J Otol 2000;21:786–792.

Sudhoff H, Tos M. Pathogenesis of attic cholesteatoma. In: Magnan J, Chays A, eds. Cholesteatoma & Ear Surgery. Proceedings of the Sixth International Conference on Cholesteatoma and Ear Surgery. Marseille: Label Production Ed; 2001:13–22.

Stangerup SE, Tos M, Arnesen R, Larsen P. A cohort study of point prevalence of eardrum pathology in children and teenagers from age 5 to age 16. Eur Arch Otorhinolaryngol 1994;251:399–403.

Tos M. Die operative Therapie der chronischen Otitis und des Mittelohrcholesteatoms mit Erhaltung der hinteren Gehörgangswand ("Intact Wall Technique"). HNO 1978;26:217–223.

Tos M. Upon the relationship between secretory otitis in childhood and chronic otitis and its sequeale in adults. J Laryngol Otol 1981;95:1011–1022.

Tos M. Modification of combined approach tympanoplasty in attic cholesteatoma. Arch Otolaryngol 1982;108:772–778.

Tos M. Epidemiology and spontaneous improvement of secretory otitis. Acta Otorhinolaryngol Belg 1983;37:31–43.

Tos M. Incidence, etiology and pathogenesis of cholesteatoma in children. Adv Otorhinolaryngol 1988;40:110–117.

Tos M, Poulsen G. Screening tympanometry in newborn infants and during the first six months of life. Scand Audiol 1978;7:159–166.

Tos M, Poulsen G. Changes of pars tensa in secretory otitis. ORL 1979;41:313–328.

Tos M, Poulsen G. Attic retractions following secretory otitis. Acta Otolaryngol 1980;89:479–486.

Tos M, Poulsen G, Borch J. Tympanometry in two-year-old children. ORL J Otorhinolaryngol Relat Spec 1978;40:77–85.

Tos M, Poulsen G, Hancke AB. Screening tympanometry during the first year of life. Acta Otolaryngol 1979;88:388–394.

Tos M, Holm-Jensen S, Sørensen CH, Mogensen C. Spontaneous course and frequency of secretory otitis in four-year-old children. Arch Otolaryngol 1982a;108:4–10.

Tos M, Melchiors J, Thomsen J, Plate S. Changes of the drum in untreated secretory otitis and chronic tubal dysfunction. Acta Otolaryngol 1982b;(Suppl 386):149–151.

Tos M, Stangerup SE, Holm-Jensen S, Sørensen CH. Spontaneous course of secretory otitis and changes of the eardrum. Arch Otolaryngol 1984;110:281–289.

Tos M, Stangerup SE, Hvid G, Koks AU. Point prevalence of secretory otitis of different types. In: Bluestone CD, Casselbrandt ML, eds. Workshop on Epidemiology of Otitis Media. Ann Otol Rhinol Laryngol Suppl 1990a; 149:14–16..

Tos M, Hvid G, Stangerup S-E, Koks Andreassen U. Prevalence and progression of sequelae following secretory otitis. In: Bluestone CD, Casselbrant ML, eds. Workshop on Epidemiology of Otitis Media. Ann Otol Rhinol Laryngol Suppl 1990b;149:36–38..

Weber PC, Gantz BJ. Cartilage reconstruction of the scutum defects in canal wall up mastoidectomies. Am J Otolaryngol 1998;19: 178–182.

Wigand ME. Transcanal mastoidectomy restoring and aerated antrum. Arch Otolaryngol 1970;92:353–357.

15 Posterior Cartilage–Perichondrium Composite Island Graft Tympanoplasty

Definition

The posterior cartilage–perichondrium composite island graft (**Fig. 15.1a**) covers the posterior perforation, most often a perforation after removal of the posterior retraction. The large anterior perichondrium flap is originally placed under the malleus handle and the anterior part of the eardrum. The posterior perichondrium flap is placed onto the ear canal bone (**Fig. 15.1b**).

In reconstruction of a posterosuperior defect of the scutum caused by drilling or resorption of the scutum by sinus cholesteatoma, the cartilage disk is enlarged posteriorly to cover the scutum defect or even an aditotomy (**Fig. 15.2a, b**). Placement of another compound graft posteriorly to the posterior graft is also a possibility. The

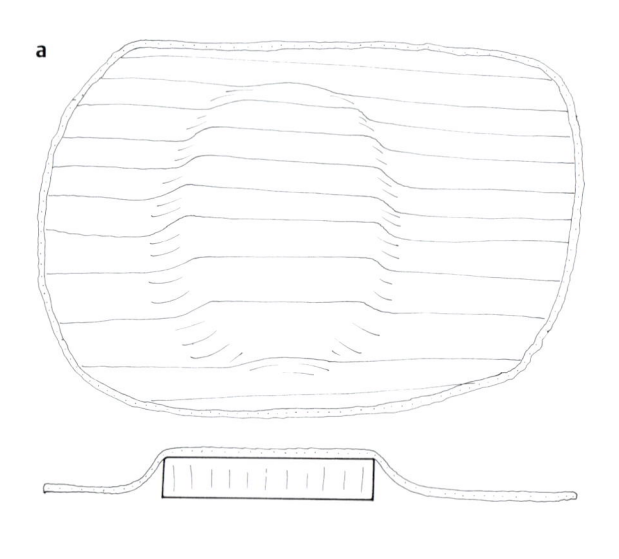

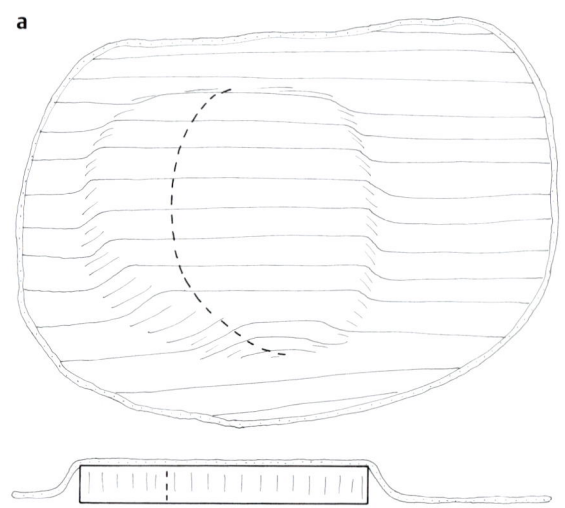

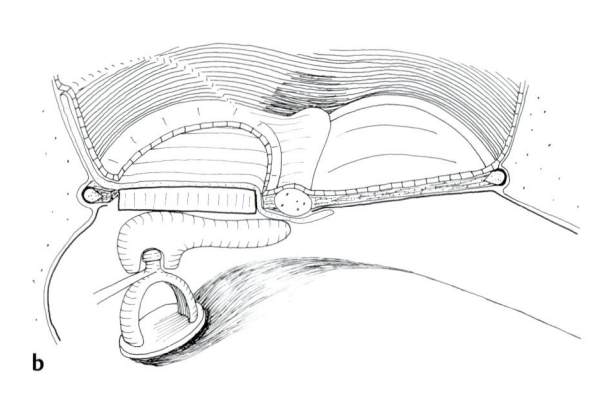

Fig. 15.1a, b The Linde posterior cartilage–perichondrium composite island graft.
a The cartilage disk is oval, the anterior perichondrium flap is largest, the superior flap is smallest.
b Side view with some perspective of Linde graft in tympanoplasty type 2 with interposition of a shaped autogenous incus.

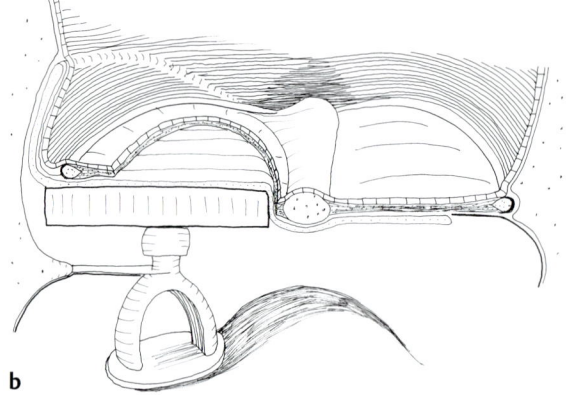

Fig. 15.2a, b The Linde graft for covering the posterior perforation and a defect of the posterosuperior bony scutum.
a The dotted line indicates the border between the tympanic graft and the scutum graft.
b Side view with some perspective of a large posterior cartilage–perichondrium composite island graft in a tympanoplasty type 2. The graft covers both the posterior perforation and the large defect of the scutum.

second graft can be completely separated from the posterior graft or it can be connected by the perichondrium (**Fig. 15.3**).

Linde (1973) was the first to present the posterior cartilage graft "as developed by the late Dr. Frederick Guilford." Guilford began using the cartilage perichondrium graft, obtained from the conchal region, in about 1967 and found the procedure worthwhile (Linde 1973).

The posterior island graft soon became popular, and several authors have presented their results and eventual modifications of the graft. Glasscock et al. (1982) applied a very long posterior perichondrium flap and a smaller anterior flap (**Fig. 15.4a, b**).

The French school uses the term "reinforcement" for tympanoplasty with cartilage–perichondrium grafts (Martin et al. 1973; Martin 1979; Florant et al. 1987), and uses only the posterior perichondrium flap, not the anterior flap (**Fig. 15.5a**). The cartilage disk may be thinned at the anterior edge and placed under the malleus handle (Roger et al. 1994), while the posterior perichondrial flap is placed onto the posterior ear canal wall. The cartilage disk is positioned onto the cartilage prosthesis (**Fig. 15.5b**). A similar graft is used by Gilain et al. (1997) and Gerard et al. (2003). These authors prefer tragus cartilage thinned to less than 0.5 mm.

Instead of applying a large cartilage disk with extensive drilling of the scutum (as in **Figs. 15.2a, 15.4a**), two minor disks—one for the posterior perforation, one for the scutum defect—may often provide an easier reconstruction.

In 122 patients with posterior retraction pockets, Page et al. (2008) used "chondroperichondrial graft" in retroauricular approach to reinforce the tympanic membrane and prevent a new retraction. The graft is larger than the retraction and is placed under the eardrum remnant. Presumably the ossicular chain was intact in all cases and in none was ossiculoplasty performed.

Harvesting and Shaping of the Graft

The posterior graft is relatively small and easy to shape. The cartilage with the perichondrium attached on both sides is harvested either from the concha or from the tragus, depending on the approach used (Linde 1973; Florant et al. 1987; Milewski 1991, 1993; Roger et al. 1994; Gerber et al. 2000; Couloigner et al. 2003). Some surgeons apply tragal cartilage regardless of the approach (Mikaelian 1986; Adkins 1990; Mills and Phill 1991; Gilain et al 1997; Gerard et al. 2003; Pfleiderer et al. 2003), and some others exclusively apply conchal cartilage (Puls 2003).

The methods of harvesting tragal cartilage, either through a skin incision performed on the tragal dome or—for cosmetic reasons—2–3 mm medial to the dome, have been illustrated in Chapter 3.

There is enough tragal cartilage for even the largest posterior island graft. Only in the case of a large sinus cholesteatoma extending into the antrum, requiring re-

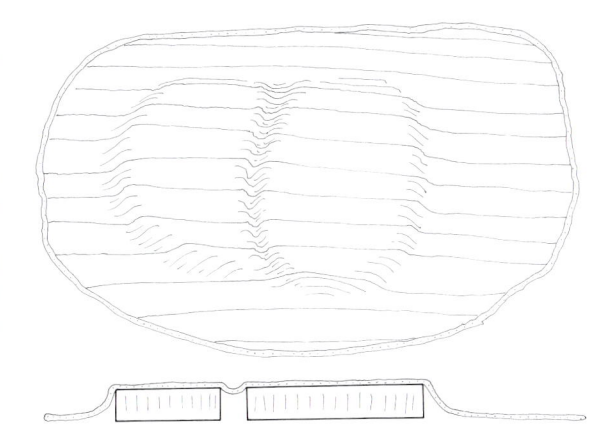

Fig. 15.3 The large scutum defect in an aditotomy can be covered by two cartilage disks connected with the perichondrium.

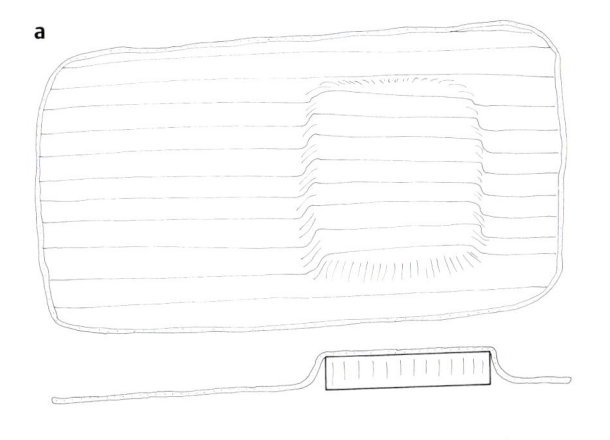

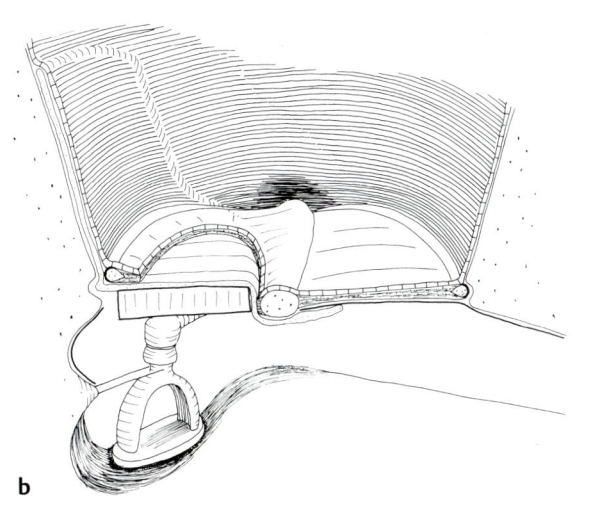

Fig. 15.4a, b The Glasscock posterior cartilage–perichondrium composite island flap.
a The Glasscock posterior cartilage–perichondrium composite island graft, with a very long posterior perichondrium flap.
b Side view of the Glasscock cartilage–perichondrium composite island graft with a large posterior perichondrium flap in a tympanoplasty type 1.

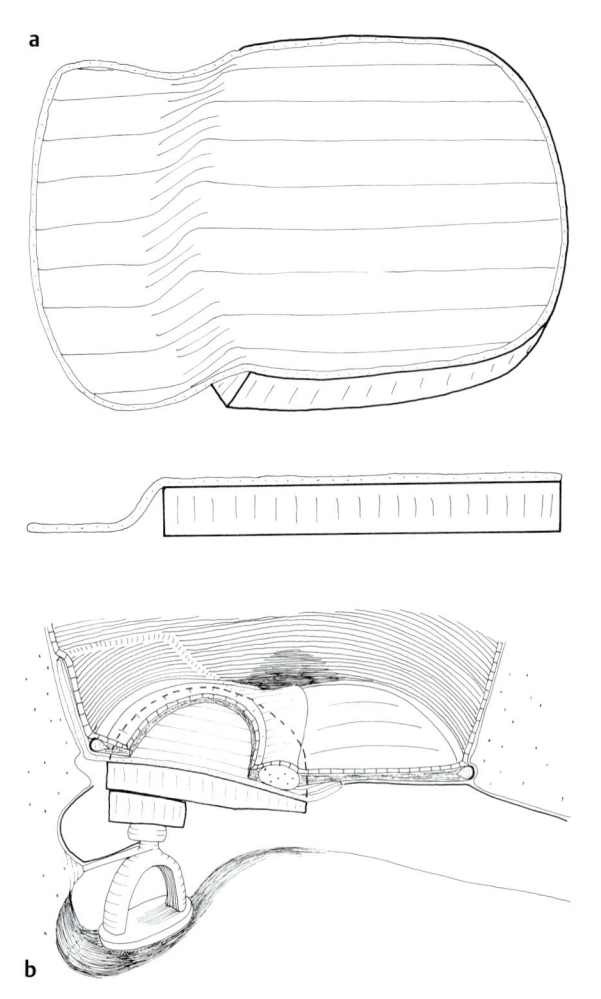

Fig. 15.5a, b Posterior cartilage–perichondrium island graft
a Posterior cartilage–perichondrium composite island graft with only a posterior perichondrium flap (Roger et al. 1994).
b Side view of a tympanoplasty type 2 with interposition of a rectangular cartilage prosthesis between the stapes head and the cartilage–perichondrium composite graft placed under the malleus handle.

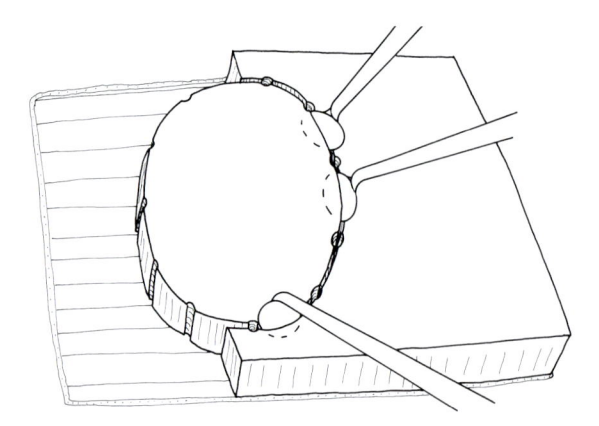

construction of the posterior and superior ear canal with cartilage grafts, will more cartilage be required than can be harvested from the tragus. In such cases, conchal cartilage must be used.

The use of homogenous cartilage grafts is permitted in Belgium (Gilain et al. 1997, Gerard et al. 2003) but unfortunately not in other countries.

Shaping of the Posterior Cartilage–Perichondrium Island Graft

Shaping of the posterior cartilage–perichondrium island graft is easy if the size of the cartilage disk is adequate. Using a large hook, the distance from the posterior edge of the malleus handle to the posterior bony annulus is measured. The superoinferior length of the perforation is measured in the same way. Another possibility is to cut an oval disk of Silastic, place it under the edge of the posterior perforation and then onto the harvested tragal cartilage to check its size.

The perichondrium is removed from the posterior (concave) side of the tragal cartilage. The desired shape and size of the cartilage disk is marked on the cartilage with needle sticks. Using a round knife, the cartilage is cut, leaving the perichondrium intact (**Fig. 15.6**). The longer perichondrium flap is placed onto the posterior ear canal bone, the shorter flap under the malleus handle and the anterior part of the eardrum.

Indications for Surgery

Many reports indicate that, due to the stiffness of the cartilage, the cartilage tympanoplasty obviates the postoperative retraction, but postoperative hearing may be poorer with the cartilage graft than with thin perichondrium or fascia grafts. However, in the conditions listed below treatment with fascia or perichondrium carries greater risk of development of postoperative retractions, leading to poorer hearing.

Fig. 15.6 Shaping an oval cartilage–perichondrium island graft from a piece of tragal cartilage. The perichondrium is removed from the posterior (concave) side. This side will face the tympanic cavity. Using a round knife the cartilage is gradually and gently cut down to the perichondrium all the way around the oval cartilage disk. The superfluous cartilage is elevated from the perichondrium flaps. The posterior flap is larger than the anterior flap.

- **Posterior retraction** is the most common indication for the posterior cartilage–perichondrium composite island graft.
- **Recurrent posterior retraction.**
- **Posterior perforation with negative Valsalva maneuver** and/or otherwise impaired tubal function.
- **Recurrent posterior perforation.**
- **Sinus precholesteatoma**, defined as posterosuperior retraction with infection and accumulation of debris within the retraction.
- **Sinus cholesteatoma**, defined as posterosuperior retraction extending to the tympanic sinuses filled with white cholesteatoma mass. The sinus cholesteatoma may extend as a retraction laterally or medially to the incus, to the posterior attic and antrum. The anterior attic, the anterior half of the tympanic cavity, and the hypotympanum are not involved in sinus cholesteatoma.

Surgical Techniques with Posterior Cartilage–Perichondrium Composite Island Graft

There are no major differences among surgeons when using the underlay technique for closing a posterior perforation with the posterosuperior cartilage–perichondrium island graft. Any differences are mainly in the length of the posterior and/or of the anterior perichondrium flap. Thus Linde (1973) prefers the anterior perichondrium flap longer than the posterior flap (see **Fig. 15.1a**). As already mentioned, some surgeons do not use the anterior flap (see **Fig. 15.5a**), and some place a slightly thinned cartilage disk under the malleus handle (see **Fig. 15.5b**).

Glasscock et al. (1982) prefer, in retroauricular approach, a very long posterior and a relatively large anterior perichondrium flap (see **Fig. 15.4a, b**).

There may also be differences in the approach. Most surgeons will use a retroauricular approach, some will use an endaural approach with intercartilaginous incision, and yet others, including the present author, use a transmeatal approach with a fixed ear speculum (see Chapter 3). The transmeatal approach is the best one for pathologies of the posterior part of the tympanic cavity.

Transmeatal Technique with Posterosuperior Island Graft

First, the edges of the posterior perforation are cleaned and the mucosa around the perforation is scarified. Then a circumferential incision between the 11-o'clock and 6-o'clock positions and a vertical incision through the fibrous annulus at the 9-o'clock position are made (**Fig. 15.7a**), allowing a swing-door technique, with elevation of the superior and inferior flap and a good overview of the posterior tympanic cavity (**Fig. 15.7b**). Gelfoam balls are placed into the tympanic cavity to support the perichondrium and thus help it adhere to the undersurface of the eardrum. The posterosuperior cartilage island graft is placed into the tympanic cavity at the level of the bony annulus. First the anterior, then the superior, and lastly the

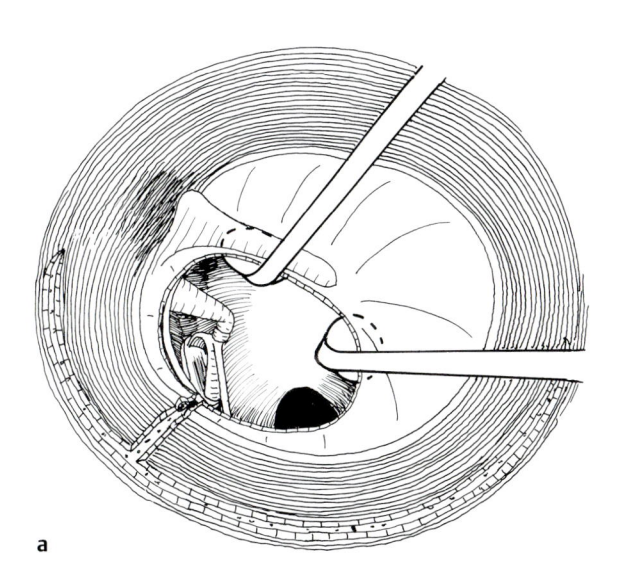

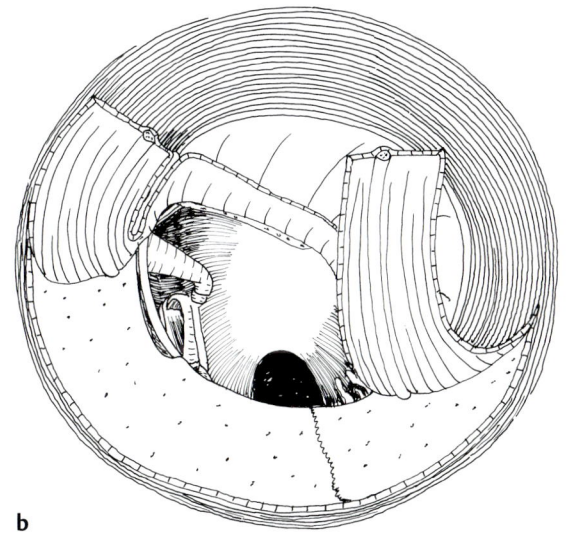

Fig. 15.7a–f Tympanoplasty type 1 with application of a posterior cartilage–perichondrium composite island graft in a posterior perforation and intact ossicular chain.
a A median circumferential incision and a radial incision at the 9-o'clock position are made. The fibrous annulus is cut. The edges of the perforation are removed. Using a round knife, the mucosa under the surface of the malleus handle and eardrum is scarified.
b In the swing-door technique the inferior and superior tympanomeatal flaps are elevated together with the epithelium surrounding the perforation.

Fig. 15.7c–f ▷

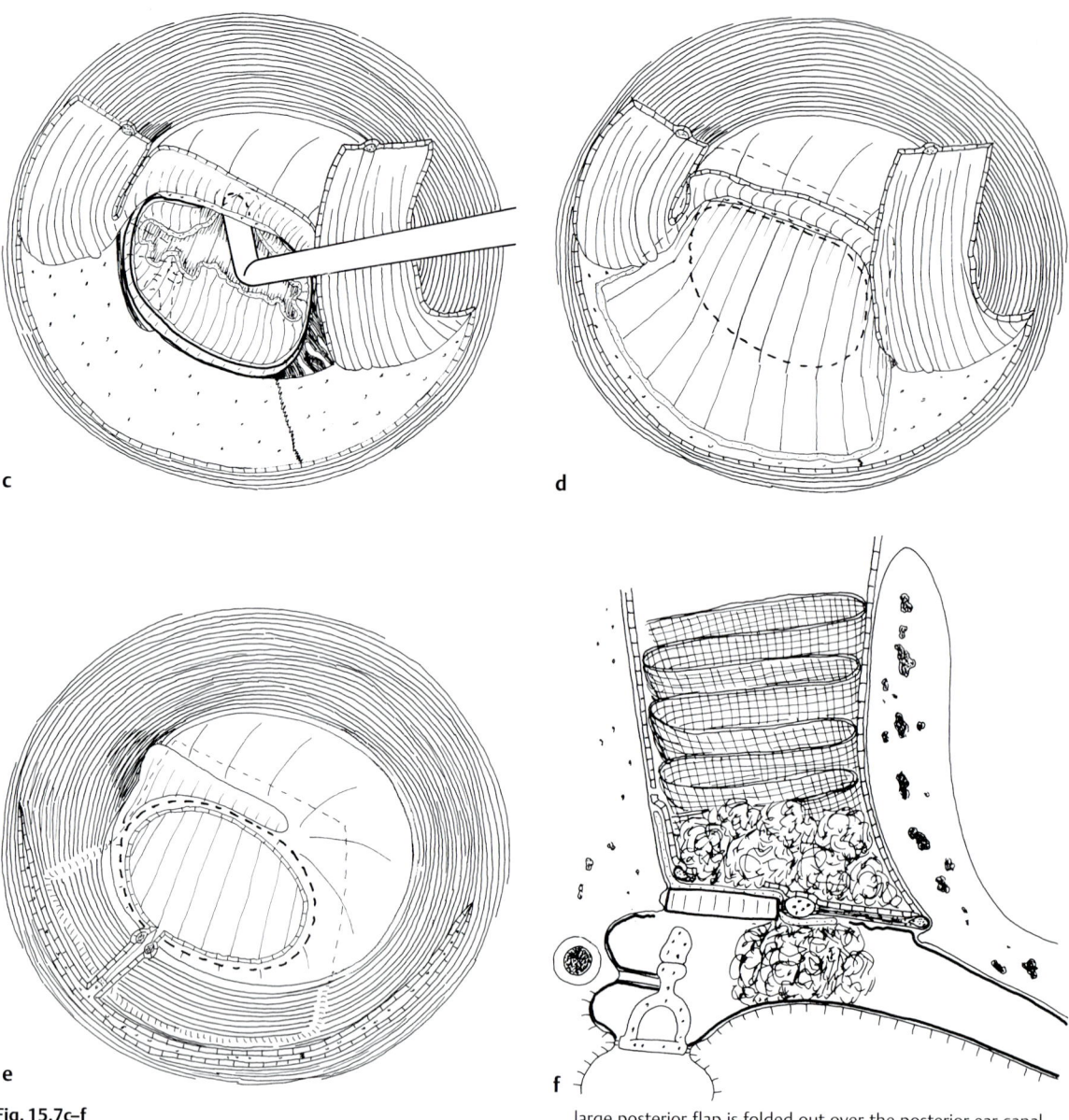

Fig. 15.7c–f

c The cartilage island graft with the unfolded perichondrium flaps is placed in the tympanic cavity at the level of the bony annulus. Using the incudostapedial knife, the anterior perichondrium flap is pushed under the malleus handle and under the anterior part of the denuded eardrum.

d The entire anterior perichondrium flap is positioned under the malleus handle and the anterior eardrum. The superior perichondrium flap covers the superior bony annulus; the inferior flap is placed under the inferior border of the perforation and the large posterior flap is folded out over the posterior ear canal bone.

e The tympanomeatal flaps are replaced.

f Side view of tympanoplasty type 1 with posterior cartilage–perichondrium composite island graft in a posterior perforation and intact ossicular chain. The anterior perichondrium flap is placed under the malleus handle and the anterior eardrum. It is supported by Gelfoam. The ear canal is packed with Gelfoam and gauze moistened with hydrocortisone ointment.

inferior part of the flap are pushed under the eardrum (**Fig. 15.7c**). The posterior perichondrium flap is placed onto the ear canal bone (**Fig. 15.7 d**). Lastly, the tympanomeatal flaps are replaced (**Fig. 15.7e**), and the ear canal is packed with Gelfoam balls and gauze (**Fig. 15.7 f**).

Transmeatal Removal of a Posterior Retraction

Using swing-door incisions, the retraction membrane is separated from the eardrum remnant, and from the anterior and posterior sides of the chorda tympani (**Fig. 15.8a**). In **Fig. 15.8b**, it is shown that the retraction extends far behind into the lateral tympanic sinus and down to the stapedial tendon. After careful and gradual separation of the retracted membrane, first from the inferior border of the eardrum and then from the undersurface of the malleus handle, drilling of the posterosuperior scutum is started with a diamond drill, saving the chorda tympani (**Fig. 15.8c**). After completion of removal of the scutum, the retracted membrane is carefully elevated from the lateral sinus, from the remnant of the long process of the incus, and from the stapedial tendon. Then the entire membrane is elevated and removed in toto (**Fig. 15.8d**). Finally, the last part of the membrane is elevated from the promontory (**Fig. 15.8e**). The incus is removed, shaped, and accommodated to the neck of the stapes and malleus handle as well as to the cartilage disk (**Fig. 15.8f**). The posterior cartilage island graft is placed into the tympanic cavity and the perichondrium flaps are placed under the eardrum remnant and onto the bone of the ear canal (**Fig. 15.8g**).

After replacement of the tympanomeatal flaps (**Fig. 15.8h**), the eardrum is covered with Gelfoam balls and gauze moistened with hydrocortisone–oxytetracycline and polymyxin B ointment for 3 weeks.

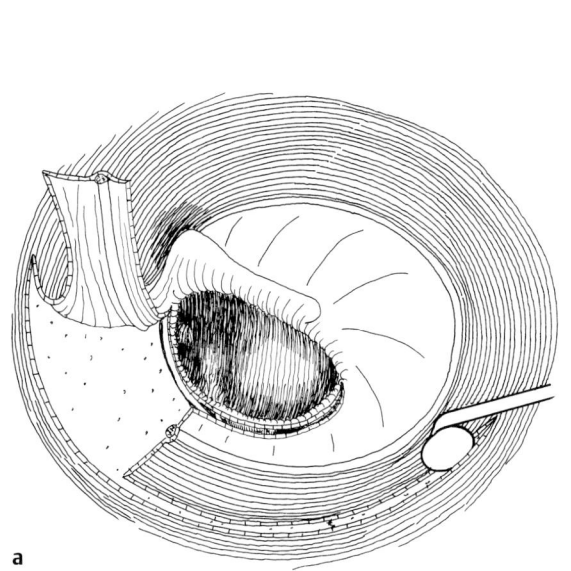

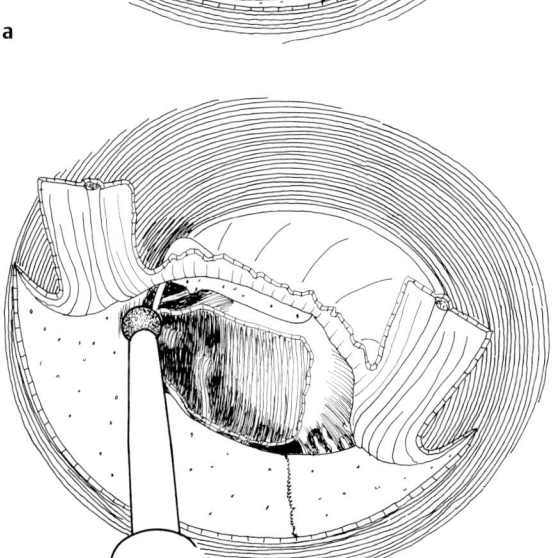

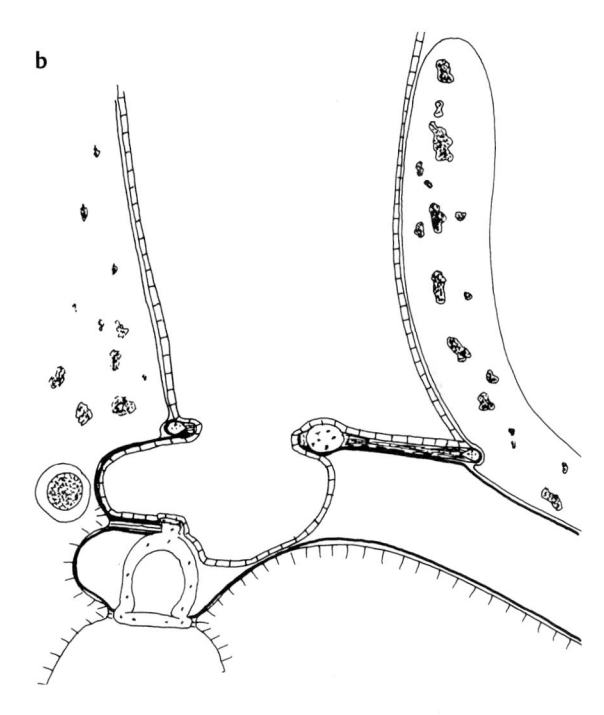

Fig. 15.8a–h Removal of a deep posterior retraction with resorption of the long process of the incus and the head of the stapes.

a Incisions for swing-door technique are made and the superior tympanomeatal flap is elevated.

b Side view of the posterior retraction. Anteriorly the retraction extends under the malleus handle; medially it is adherent to the promontory and stapes crura; superiorly it is adherent to the remnant of the incus and posteriorly it is adherent to the walls of the lateral sinus.

c The inferior tympanomeatal flap is elevated together with the bottom of the retraction. Anteriorly the retraction is elevated from the umbo. Posteriorly the drilling of the scutum is started, exposing the posterior border of the retraction.

Fig. 15.8d–h ▷

Fig. 15.8 d–h

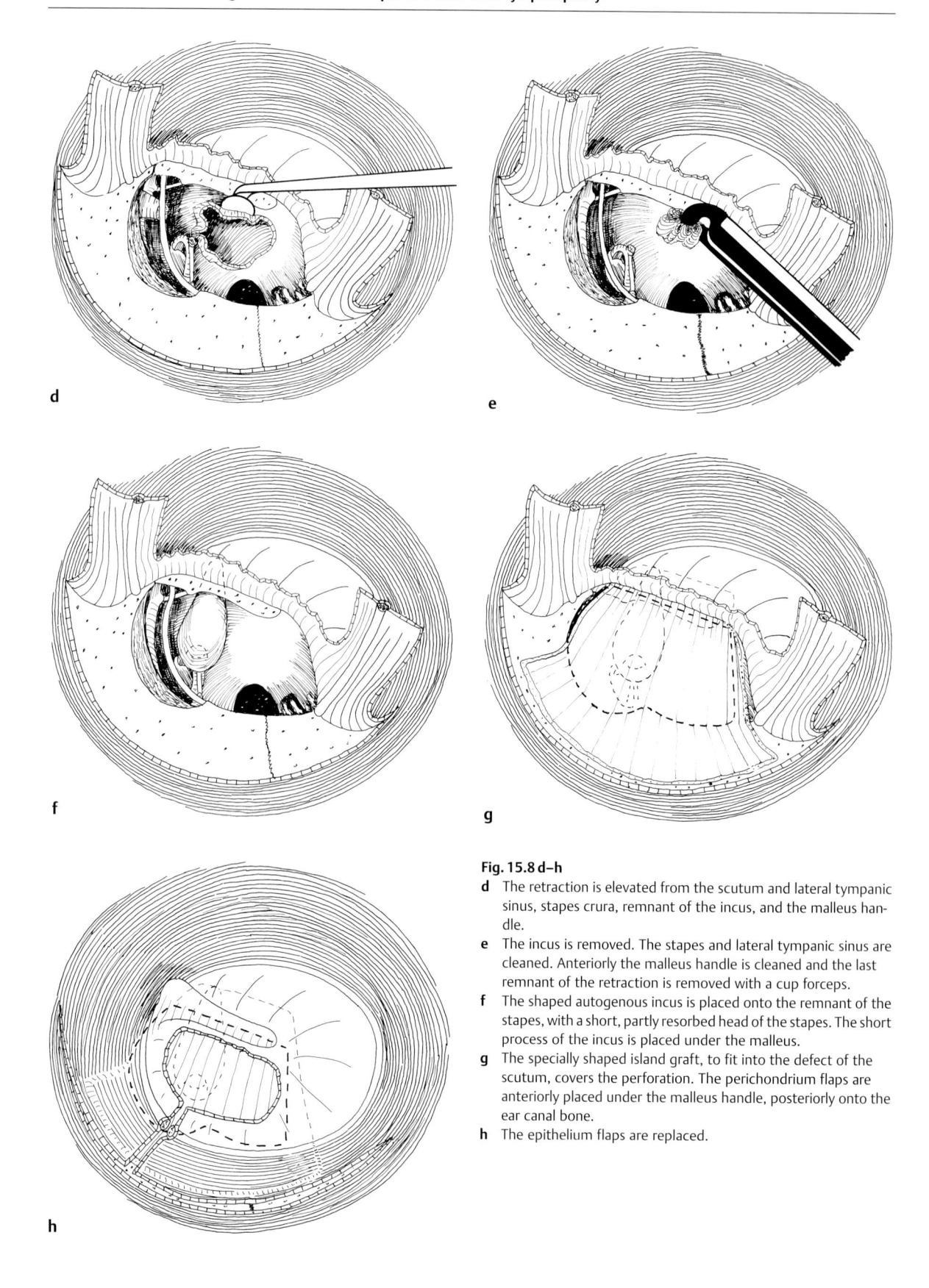

d The retraction is elevated from the scutum and lateral tympanic sinus, stapes crura, remnant of the incus, and the malleus handle.

e The incus is removed. The stapes and lateral tympanic sinus are cleaned. Anteriorly the malleus handle is cleaned and the last remnant of the retraction is removed with a cup forceps.

f The shaped autogenous incus is placed onto the remnant of the stapes, with a short, partly resorbed head of the stapes. The short process of the incus is placed under the malleus.

g The specially shaped island graft, to fit into the defect of the scutum, covers the perforation. The perichondrium flaps are anteriorly placed under the malleus handle, posteriorly onto the ear canal bone.

h The epithelium flaps are replaced.

Transmeatal Removal of the Sinus Cholesteatoma

The sinus cholesteatoma, with the initial pathology around the stapes and tympanic sinuses, is most often easiest to approach transmeatally, especially in children. This is also the minimally invasive approach.

If extensive drilling of the scutum is expected, a large circumferential incision and a vertical incision at the 9-o'clock position are made, with elevation of two large tympanomeatal flaps (**Fig. 15.9a**). The retraction is elevated and separated from the eardrum, saving as much epithelium as possible. Early identification of the chorda tympani and removal of the scutum provides a good view to the sinuses and exposure of the cholesteatoma, enabling safe removal of the cholesteatoma together with the incus (**Fig. 15.9b–d**). After shaping and reducing the incus and drilling a groove for the stapes head, the incus is positioned in such manner that the posterior cartilage graft is able to vibrate (**Fig. 15.9e**). The posterior cartilage disk is in contact with the incus and the malleus handle. The most posterior cartilage disk covers the scutum defect. Small cartilage palisades may close some defects around the cartilage disk (**Fig. 15.9e**). The perichondrium flaps cover small defects and suspend the posterior disk, allowing good vibration of the disk (**Fig. 15.9 f–h**). The graft covering the scutum defect should not and must not vibrate.

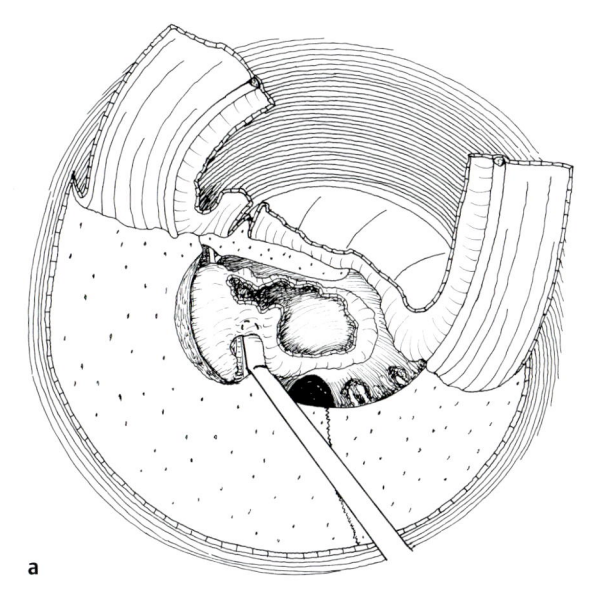

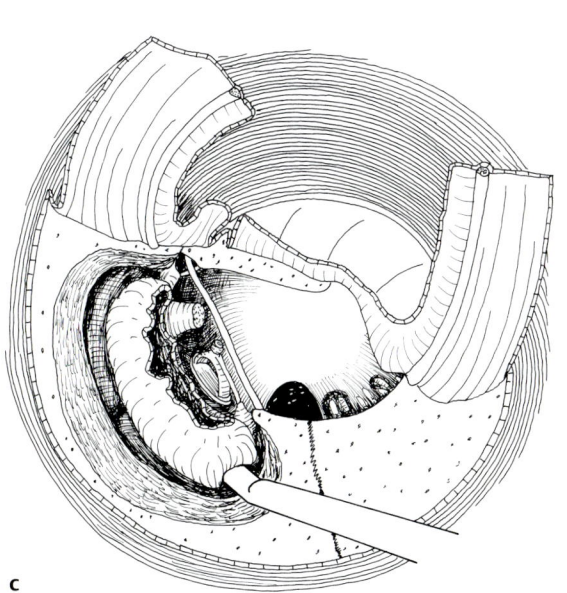

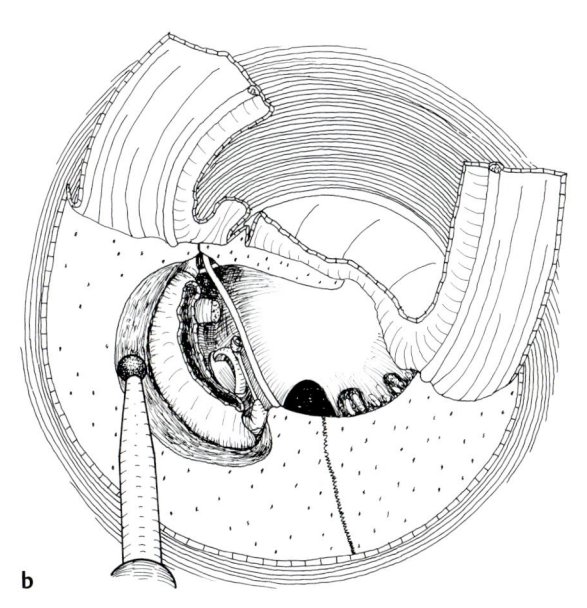

Fig. 15.9a–h Transcanal removal of a sinus chlolesteatoma extending into the aditus.

a After a large swing-door incision, the posterior, inferior, and anterior parts of the retraction are separated from the inferior part of the eardrum and the malleus handle. After drilling of the scutum, the extension of the sinus cholesteatoma into the lateral sinus is observed. The tympanic part of the cholesteatoma is elevated and can be separated from the remnant of the long process of the incus and from the stapes.

b Continued drilling and removal of the scutum exposes cholesteatoma covering the incus body.

c After further drilling, the upper border of the cholesteatoma and of the incus body are localized. The inferior part of the cholesteatoma is elevated from the medial wall of the tympanic sinus, allowing removal of the entire cholesteatoma together with the incus. The cholesteatoma membrane from the tympanic cavity is also removed.

Fig. 15.9d–h ▷

Fig. 15.9d–h

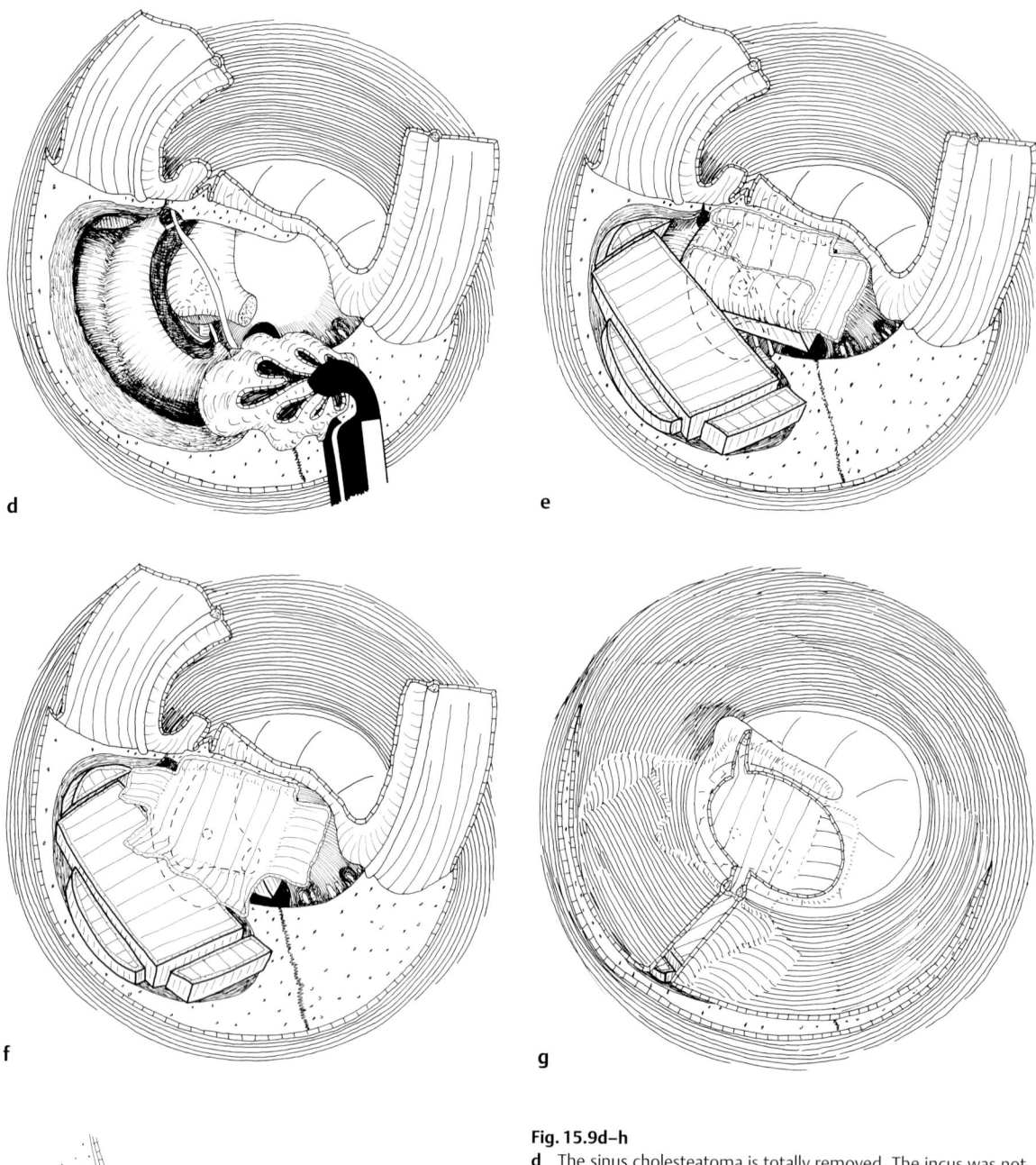

d The sinus cholesteatoma is totally removed. The incus was not affected by cholesteatoma; it is shaped and reduced, and a groove is made to be placed onto the stapes head. The short process is placed under the malleus handle.

e The posterior island graft is placed onto the diminished incus at the level of the malleus handle and the anterior perichondrium flap is placed onto the denuded malleus handle. The posterior scutum defect is covered more laterally by another composite cartilage graft and small palisades.

f The various perichondrium flaps are folded out.

g Epithelial flaps and the tympanomeatal flaps are replaced. The cartilage island graft is covered by the ear canal skin.

h Side view at the level of the stapes of reconstruction of the eardrum and the scutum with two island grafts. The reduced incus is positioned onto the stapes. The posterior cartilage–perichondrium graft covers the posterior perforation and is in contact with the incus. The anterior perichondrium flap covers the malleus. A separate composite cartilage–perichondrium graft covers the defect of the scutum region.

Removal of a Large Sinus Cholesteatoma

Most sinus cholesteatomas are localized within the tympanic sinuses, some extend to the posterior attic and aditus, but only few involve the antrum and the mastoid process. A popular procedure is to follow the cholesteatoma from the tympanic sinuses backward by removal of the scutum, remove the cholesteatoma, and then reconstruct the scutum with cartilage grafts. If the sinus cholesteatoma is large and involves the antrum, the same principle can be applied and the reconstruction with cartilage can be performed.

In retroauricular approach, the tympanic cavity is entered by elevating a large inferior and a large superior tympanomeatal flap and gradually removing as much of the posterior scutum as necessary (**Figs. 15.10a–c**) to reveal the extent of the cholesteatoma. After removal of the defective incus and resection of the malleus head (**Figs. 15.10d, e**), the entire cholesteatoma is exposed and opened and its mass is reduced by suction, allowing easy and safe elevation and removal of the entire cholesteatoma matrix. After placement of a Kurz titanium TORP prosthesis of Dresden type (**Fig. 15.10f**), the posterior cartilage–perichondrium island graft covers the head of the prosthesis (**Fig. 15.10g**). The bony defect of the scutum is covered by another island graft and by small palisades. The various perichondrium flaps are replaced (**Fig. 15.10h**).

Several other methods are illustrated in the Manual of Middle Ear Surgery, Vol. 2 (Tos 1995), such as classic canal wall up method (see Chapter 6), modified canal wall up method (see Chapter 7) or various canal wall up mastoidectomies (see Chapters 8 to 10), and canal wall down methods (see Chapters 11 to 13).

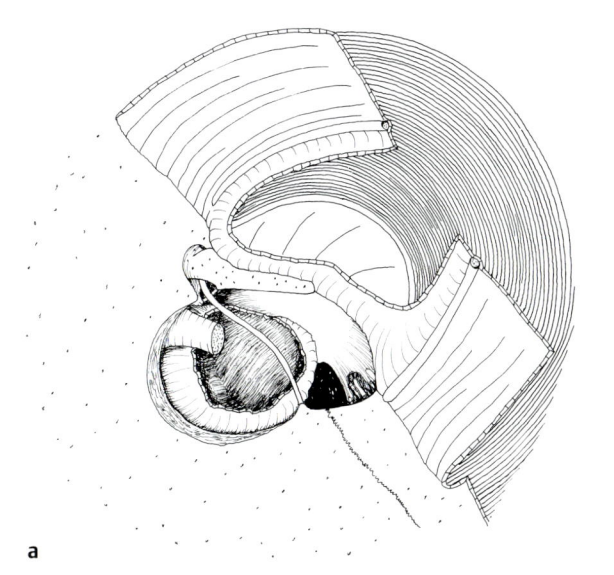

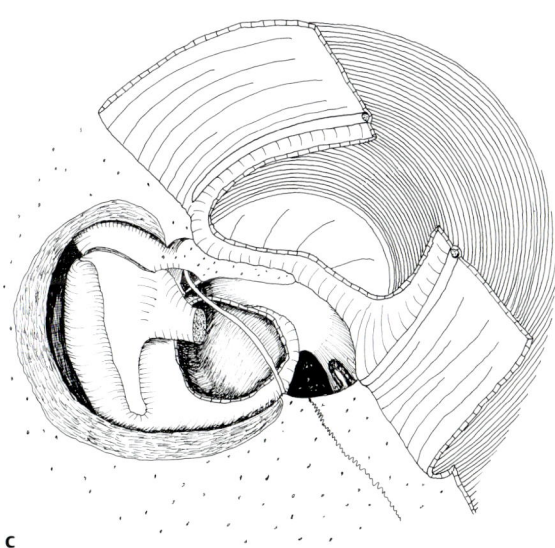

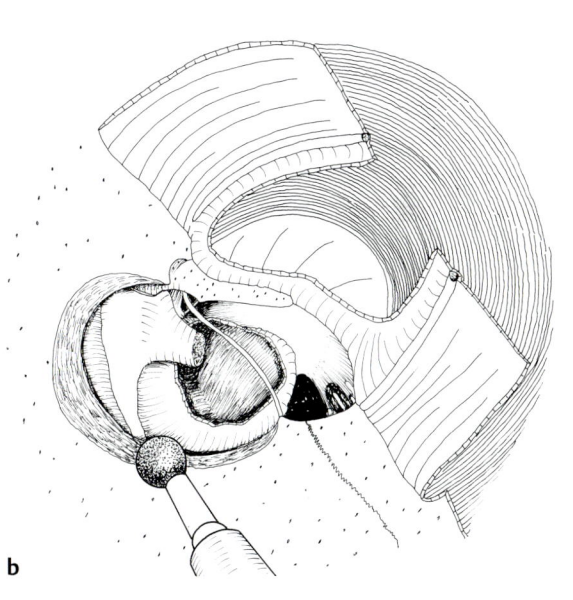

Fig. 15.10a–h Removal of a sinus cholesteatoma extended into the posterior attic and aditus.
- **a** In retroauricular approach, a superior and inferior tympanomeatal flap is elevated and the retraction is separated from the eardrum and the malleus handle. Sinus cholesteatoma covers the footplate and extends under the incus toward the attic. A part of the scutum is removed.
- **b** Further drilling toward the attic reveals the cholesteatoma sac medial to the incus body and head of the malleus.
- **c** Further drilling reveals the superior border of the cholesteatoma, lying under the incus.

Fig. 15.10d–h ▷

Fig. 15.10d–h

d The incus is removed; the cholesteatoma extends under the malleus head. A hole is made in the cholesteatoma matrix and the cholesteatoma mass is suctioned out. The malleus head is resected and removed.

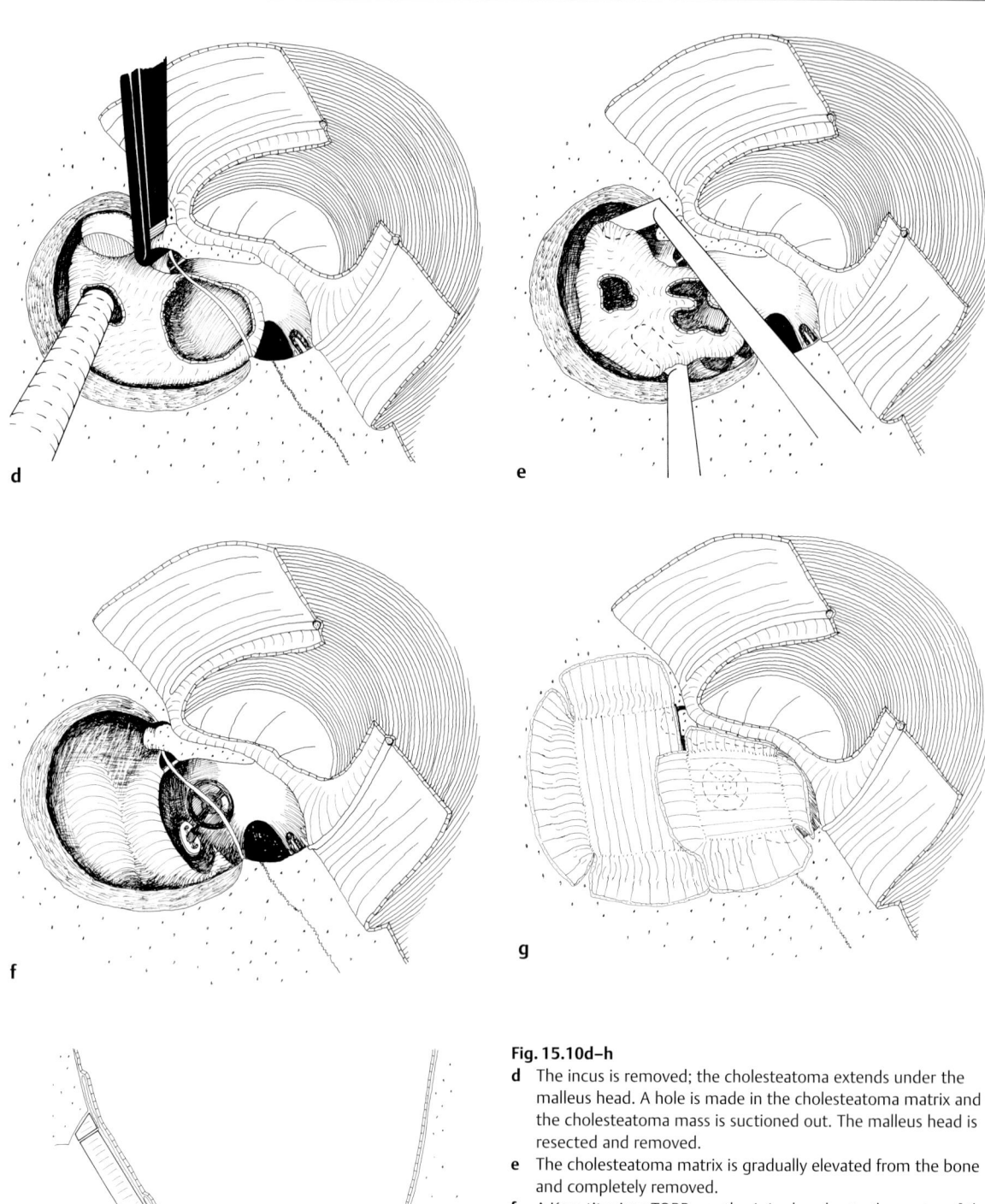

e The cholesteatoma matrix is gradually elevated from the bone and completely removed.

f A Kurz titanium TORP prosthesis is placed onto the center of the footplate.

g The posterior island graft is placed onto the head of the titanium prosthesis and parallel to the malleus handle. Another island graft covers the defect of the scutum. Small palisades are placed around the island graft and are covered by the perichondrium flaps.

h Side view of aditotomy and tympanoplasty type 3 with a Kurz titanium TORP prosthesis, after removal of a sinus cholesteatoma and reconstruction of the eardrum with the posterior island graft and a large scutum island graft. The posterior graft is suspended under the malleus handle and under the anterior part of the eardrum. The posterior perichondrium flap covers the scutum graft and the ear canal bone.

Retrograde Atticoantrotomy in a Large Sinus Cholesteatoma

In a retroauricular approach with elevation of two large tympanomeatal flaps, the posterior retraction is separated from the eardrum and the malleus handle (**Fig. 15.11a**) and then the sinus cholesteatoma are followed toward the aditus and antrum by removal of the posterior and superior scutum and ear canal wall until the borders of the cholesteatoma are completely exposed (**Fig. 15.11b**). The incus is removed, the malleus head is resected, the cholesteatoma mass is reduced (**Fig. 15.11c**), and the matrix is removed (**Fig. 15.11 d**). After completion of removal of the cholesteatoma, a titanium TORP prosthesis is placed onto the footplate and covered with a posterior island flap. The perichondrium flaps are folded out onto the malleus handle and under the inferoposterior eardrum (**Fig. 15.11e**). The antrum and attic are covered with a large concha cartilage island graft, surrounded by perichondrium flaps covering the ear canal walls and the posterior graft (**Fig. 15.11 f, g**). In the side view, the horizontal graft covers the posterior perforation, the vertical graft composite graft covers the missing posterior ear canal bone (**Fig. 15.11h**).

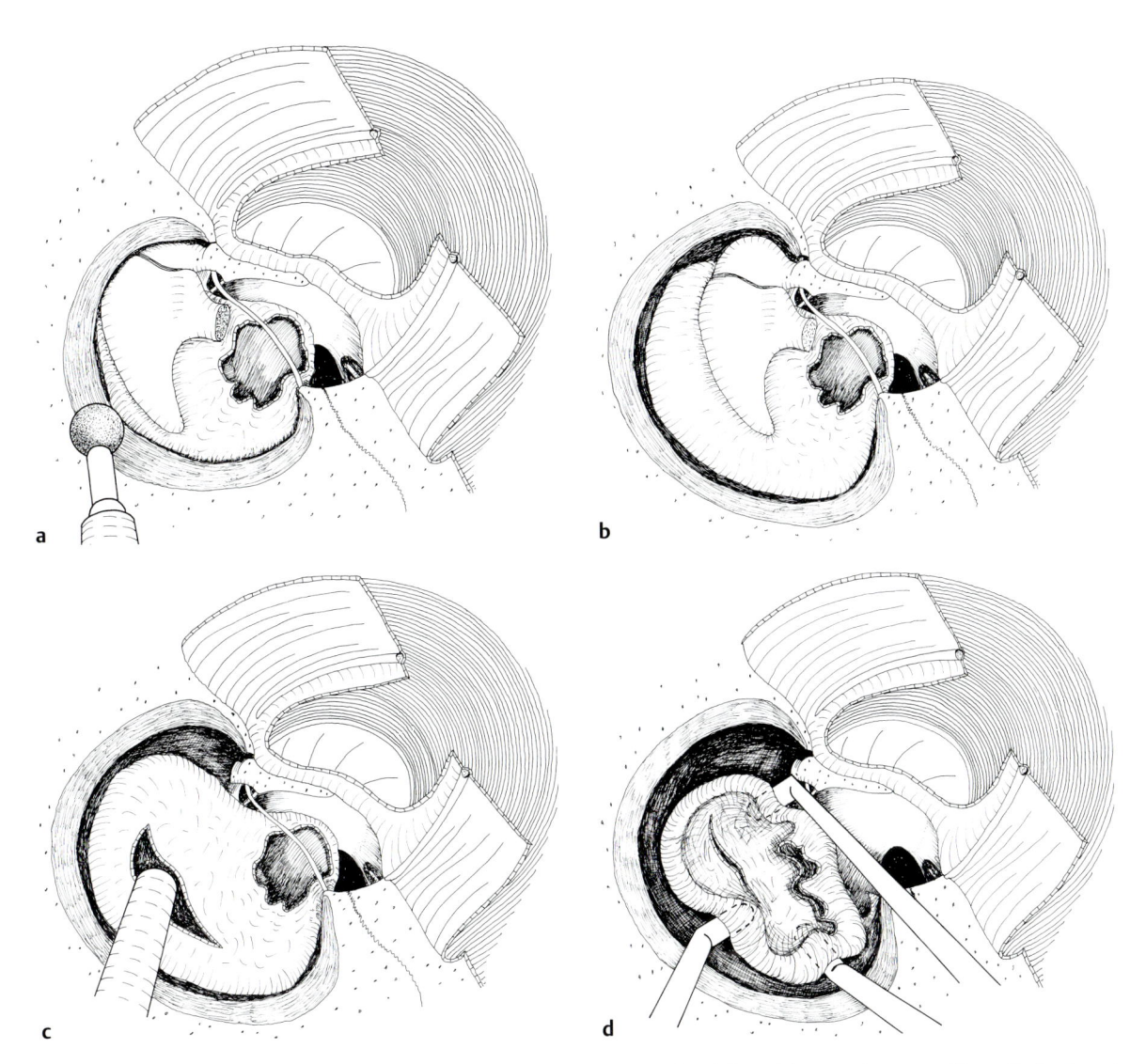

Fig. 15.11a–h Removal of a large sinus cholesteatoma with retrograde atticoantrotomy.
- **a** In retroauricular approach, the tympanomeatal flaps are elevated, the posterior retraction is separated from the eardrum, the malleus handle, and the posterior bony annulus. Only the footplate is present. The cholesteatoma is partly removed from the tympanic cavity and followed toward the antrum by removal of the scutum and the ear canal wall.
- **b** By further drilling of the posterior ear canal bone, the borders of the cholesteatoma are reached. An atticoantrotomy is performed and the cholesteatoma is gradually removed.
- **c** The incus is removed, the malleus head is resected, and a hole is made in the cholesteatoma matrix for suctioning out of the cholesteatoma mass and reduction of the cholesteatoma.
- **d** The cholesteatoma matrix is elevated in the anterior and superior parts of the attic; it is further elevated in the inferior part of the aditus.

Fig. 15.11e–h ▷

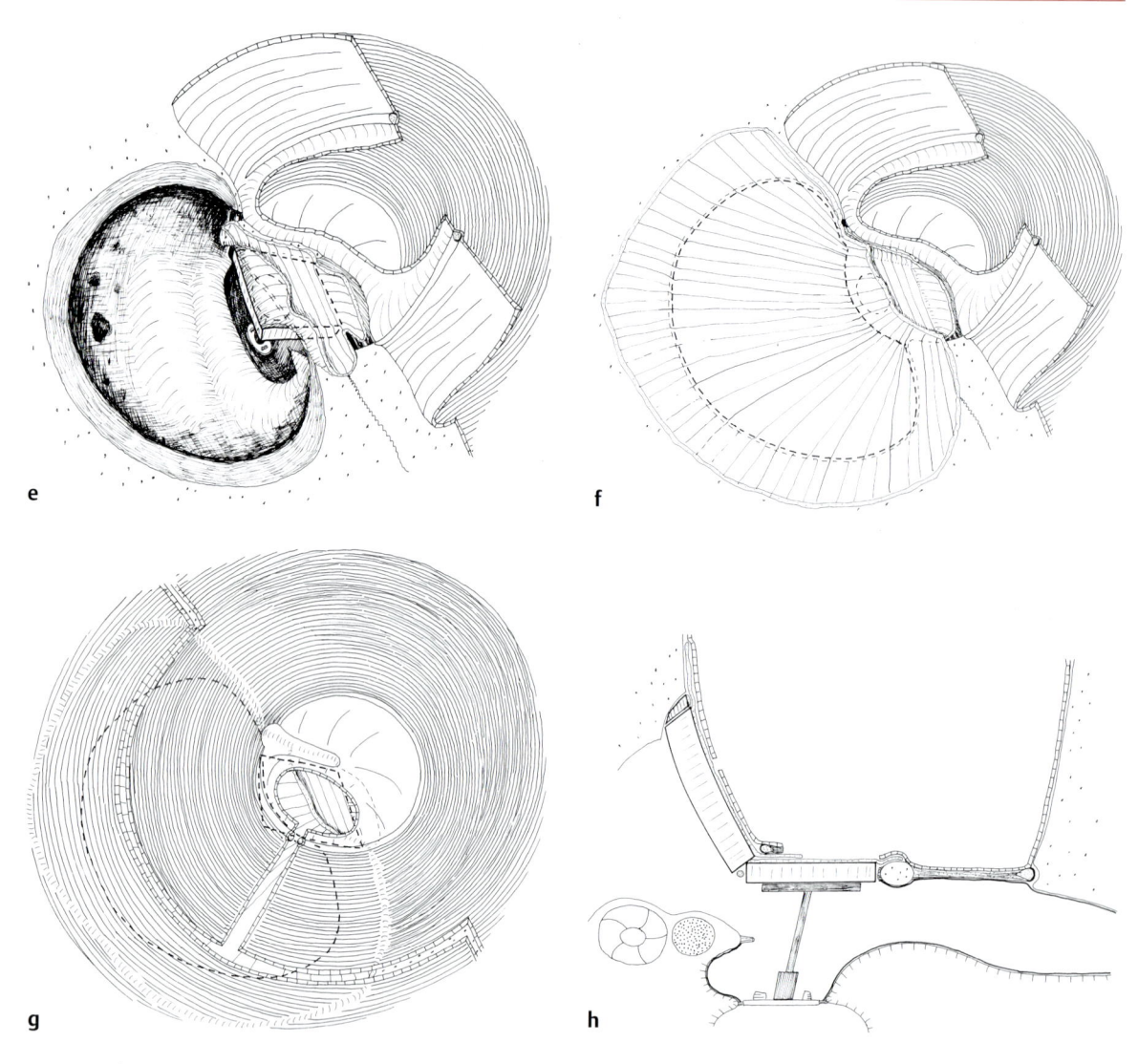

Fig. 15.11e–h

e The cholesteatoma is completely removed. A Kurz titanium TORP is placed onto the footplate, and the posterior island graft is placed onto the head of the prosthesis. Its anterior perichondrium flap is placed onto the denuded malleus handle and the neck of the malleus.

f A large cartilage–perichondrium composite island graft, tailored exactly to the scutum defect and the posterior island graft and with large perichondrium flaps, is placed onto the edges of the drilled ear canal wall. The surrounding perichondrium is placed onto the ear canal bone and onto the posterior island graft.

g The eardrum remnant with the epithelium and the large superior and inferior tympanomeatal flaps are replaced. The elevated ear canal skin is replaced.

h Side view of a retrograde atticoantrotomy with removal of a large sinus cholesteatoma and posterior retraction, reconstructed with tympanoplasty type 3 with a Kurz titanium columella placed onto the footplate and covered with a posterior cartilage island graft. The bony defect of the ear canal wall is covered with a large cartilage–perichondrium composite island graft with large perichondrium flaps. Small bony defects around the graft are covered with small palisades.

Posterior Ear Canal Wall Reconstruction with a Composite Cartilage Titanium Mesh Graft

Total reconstructions of the posterior ear canal wall with fascia, cartilage, muscles, bone, Proplast, glass ceramic material (Ceravital), glass ionomer cement and hydroxyapatite, are thoroughly described and illustrated in Vol. 2 of my *Manual of Middle Ear Surgery* (Tos 1995). Accordingly, ear canal wall reconstructions with cartilage have been described in this book only in some specific situations. In Chapter 4 the superior and posterior defects of the ear canal wall were covered with palisades (see **Figs. 4.8a–c** and **4.10a–d**); in Chapter 6, with broad cartilage palisades (see **Fig. 6-6a–e**). In Chapter 7 the defect of the posterior scutum was covered with cartilage strips (see **Figs. 7.16a–c, 7.17, 7.18a–c**). In Chapter 14 several reconstructions of the superior ear canal defects with cartilage-perichondrium composite grafts are presented. In this chapter and in Chapter 16, small and large ear canal wall defects are reconstructed with cartilage–perichondrium composite grafts.

Among methods with total reconstructions of the ear canal wall, only the new method of Sudhoff et al. (2006), with cartilage titanium mesh graft will be described, in five stages:

1. Measurement of the appropriate length and broadness of the ear canal and cutting of the titanium mesh. The mesh is bent by manual manipulation and cut, using a special wire scissors (Spiggle & Theis, Overath, Germany), into the final, moderately curved shape.
2. The final shaping of the mesh is made by placing the mesh into the cavity and gradually forming it into its final shape and its final position. The mesh is then removed, to be covered outside the cavity with full-thickness cartilage graft.
3. A large piece of shaped concha cartilage is placed and adapted to the medial concave side of the titanium mesh, fixed with a clamp, and sutured to the mesh with resorbable sutures. The uncovered lateral areas of the concave mesh are covered with other, but smaller cartilage pieces and sutured to the mesh.
4. The already shaped mesh is placed, as a composite cartilage–titanium mesh graft, slightly anterior to the facial ridge and extending depth-wise to the former bony tympanic annulus. The lateral part of the titanium mesh is attached to the remaining parts of the adjacent superior and inferior cortical bone
5. The mesh is subsequently covered with a large piece of the temporal muscle fascia and then laterally fixed with two 3 mm titanium screws. Finally, a retroauricular split-thickness skin graft is placed onto the fascia.

The indication for surgery of 15 patients was extended recurrent cholesteatoma after previous canal wall up surgery in 10 cases; draining radical cavities in four cases; and after extended external ear canal cholesteatoma in one case.

In a postoperative period of 9–13 months, out of 15 operated patients one patient had two revisions, one patient had one revision.

Titanium mesh has previously been used for reconstruction of mastoid cortex in 14 patients with good effect (Jung and Park 2004) and together with bone paste for reconstruction of ear canal wall after previous canal wall down mastoidectomy in nine patients, without any complications. At the second-look operation the posterior canal was stable in all cases and the medial part of the mesh was covered with mucosa (Zini et al. 2002).

Cartilage Ossiculoplasty and Myringoplasty by Lever Method

In reconstruction of a canal wall down mastoidectomy after removal of cholesteatoma, Yamane et al. (2008) used a new ossicular chain reconstruction by lever method. The facial ridge is lowered. A 5 mm × 3 mm piece of cartilage is harvested from the cymba and trimmed like a rod with scissors; a small pit adjusted to the size of the head of the stapes is made using a Skeeter drill. The length of the short arm of the cartilage posterior to the stapes head is 1 mm; anterior to the stapes head it is 3–4 mm. This means that the ratio of short arm to long arm length is a approximately 1:3. The edge of the short arm is placed on the lowered facial ridge; the pit is put on the head of the stapes, but the long arm must be separate from the tympanic ring to make a lever. Small pieces of chopped cortical bone are put on the edge of the short arm of the cartilage and fixed on the facial ridge using fibrin glue. Obliteration of the attic and of the antrum as well as reconstruction of the ear canal wall is done with chopped cortical bone and fibrin glue. The remaining part of the cavity is obliterated by the temporal muscle. Temporal muscle fascia covers the reconstructed ear canal, the long cartilage arm, and the remaining defect perforation of the tympanic membrane.

The tympanic membrane can also be reconstructed with cartilage palisades, cartilage stripes, or thin foils.

Results of Surgery with the Posterior Island Graft

Linde (1973) followed up all eight patients treated with posterior island graft. All patients had posterior retraction with dehiscent bone of the posterior scutum, four patients had iatrogenic dehiscent scutum because of previous surgery, and one patient had sinus cholesteatoma. None of the patients developed a postoperative retraction. Linde recommended vigorous insufflation treatment with Valsalva and Politzer maneuvers. When conservative treatment fails and the retraction is adherent to the incudostapedial joint, surgery should be performed because bone destruction of the long process of the incus can appear within few weeks. Thus Linde recommends early surgery of posterior retraction.

Glasscock et al. (1982) report on 75 cartilage tympanoplasties with the posterior island graft with at least 6 months' follow-up. There was one graft failure and no evidence of recurrent cholesteatoma or tympanic membrane retraction. This technique "has greatly decreased the incidence of the recurrent drum retractions in the posterosuperior quadrant of the tympanic membrane and the stiffness of the drum has not affected hearing results. In essence, the cartilage replaces the fibrous layer of the drum and acts somewhat like a tympanosclerotic plaque."

Mikaelian (1986) placed a composite graft of tragus cartilage–perichondrium onto the stapes head in 18 patients, and achieved long-term air–bone gap closure within 0–10 dB in 72 % of the cases. The perforations were closed completely and the ears healed within 4 weeks.

As well as the attic island graft, Adkins (1990) applied posterior cartilage island grafts, with one failure among 55 posterior cartilage island grafts.

East and Mangham (1991) placed a posterior cartilage–perichondrium island graft onto the head of the PORP prosthesis in tympanoplasty type 2 (15 ears) and onto the head of the TORP prosthesis in tympanoplasty type 3 (3 ears). The hearing results 2 years after surgery were significantly better than in a similar group in which the prosthesis was covered with bone paste. The mean postoperative air–bone gap was 15 dB with cartilage covering, compared with 24 dB. The prostheses should be quite short to allow placement of a full-thickness cartilage graft. There were no extrusions of the prostheses in the cartilage group, compared with five extrusions in the bone paste group.

Milewski (1991, 1993) presented far the largest series for that time, of 550 patients with tympanoplasty, most reconstructed with cartilage–perichondrium islands grafts. He stressed the importance of exact shape and size of the cartilage disk, with some convexity toward the tympanic cavity and a large perichondrium flap. Milewsky found a high rate of epithelialization of the graft within 3 weeks and did not observe major curling of the grafts within 2 years after surgery. The rate of healing of the graft was 92%, despite 219 patients having been operated previously elsewhere. Unfortunately, the results of posterior and total graft were not separated, nor were cases with palisades separated. In 146 cases with primary tympanoplasty and intact ossicular chain, the air–bone gap was closed within 10 dB in 41%, within 11–30 dB in 54%. In 51 revision cases with intact ossicular chain the closure within 10 dB was 51%, that within 11-30 dB was 34%.

Mills and Phill (1991) applied posterior island graft in 6 cases suitable for surgery out of 77 patients (93 ears) with retractions. Preoperatively, one patient had grade 2 retraction, five patients had grade 3 or 4. One year after surgery, one patient had grade 3, three patients had grade 2. Mills recommends long- term follow up of patients with retraction.

In 21 patients with posterior retraction treated with posterior island graft, Harner (1995) found one graft failure and an improvement of mean air–bone gap from 19 to 14 dB. Harner concluded that posterior cartilage island graft is the best currently available treatment.

Matthew Yung (1997) elevated the posterior retraction in 32 cases. He placed a piece of Silastic sheet onto the promontory and a posterior compound island graft to cover the posterosuperior part of the tympanic cavity. During a follow-up period of 3–8 years, 81% of the patients were free of recurrence of the retraction pocket. The results were much better for posterior than for total retraction of the eardrum.

Gerber et al. (2000), compared 11 patients treated by posterior island cartilage–perichondrium graft with a similar group of patients treated with fascia graft and found no difference in postoperative hearing. Thus, when indicated, the cartilage–perichondrium graft can be used for prevention of recurrence.

In 56 children (60 ears), with a mean age of 10 years, the posterosuperior retraction was treated either with posterior or with total pars tensa cartilage–perichondrium graft, with 8% recurrence rate (Couloigner et al. 2003). The authors found recurrence to be less common (6%) when total pars tensa graft was used than when posterior island graft was used (22%).

Page et al. (2008) found a mean preoperative hearing of 23 dB in 122 patients at five frequencies (250–4000 Hz). In 98 patients, with at least one year follow-up, the mean hearing was 13.71 dB. No resorption of the cartilage was found, even after 14 years' observation. The surgery was presumably preventive, to elevate and reinforce the retraction and prevent further extension of the retraction and bone resorption of the incus and the stapes. Preoperative hearing was not bad; the postoperative hearing was very good.

The results of cartilage ossiculoplasty by the lever method in 24 cholesteatoma patients were good at 2.1–3.2 years after surgery. Average postoperative air–bone gaps of less than 10, 15, 20, 25, and 30 dB were found in 4.2%, 37.5%, 70.8%, 91.6% and 100% respectively, and the mean postoperative air–bone gap was 17.2 dB (Yamane et al. 2008).

However, the good long-term results of the lever method may deteriorate for the following reasons: It is well-known that cartilage columellae become fibrotic after some years, causing deterioration of the initially good hearing. Cartilage columellae have been abandoned today (see Chapter 27). The stiff and rigid long cartilage arm may became fibrotic and may vibrate without movement of the stapes. In contrast, the fibrosis of the stiff cartilage composite island graft is an advantage for hearing, which may improve with time (Hitari et al. 2004; Hitari 2006; see Chapter 27).

Author's Comments and Recommendations

The published results are good, with good hearing results and good stability of the posterior compound graft. The shaping and placement of the posterior graft is easy. Care should be taken when an interposition prosthesis and columella are used. They may be too high and may hamper placement of the cartilage graft.

In this chapter the transmeatal approach is used to illustrate some cartilage methods. Although the tympanoplasty may also be performed with the retroauricular or the endaural approach, I consider the transmeatal approach in posterior pathology to be the approach of choice. It is the most direct and minimally invasive approach. Treatment of the pathology caused by posterior retraction is focused around the stapes, similarly to otosclerosis. No-one will perform a stapedectomy in the retroauricular approach!

It is heartening to see that several authors have compared the results of posterior island graft with other treatments: a comparison of results in cases with impaired tubal function and cases with poor tubal function also needs to be carried out.

In our epidemiological studies of secretory otitis and eardrum sequelae of three cohorts of healthy Danish children from birth to 16 years of age (Tos 1985, Tos 1986; Tos et al. 1984, 1988, 1990; Stangerup et al. 1994), we have distinguished from early age of the patients between posterior atrophy and total atrophy, and/or between the posterior and total retraction of pars tensa. It was evident already in early childhood that a posterior atrophy will persist either with or without retraction.

When to Operate a Posterior Retraction?

The Present Author's Classification of Posterior Retraction

On the basis of a recent classification of posterior retraction in six stages by the present author, the following management is proposed for each stage.

- **Stage 1: Atrophy and slight retraction of the posterosuperior quadrant of the eardrum.** Retraction does not touch the incus (**Fig. 15.12a**). In this stage, surgery is not indicated.
- **Stage 2: Retraction has progressed to the long process of the incus**, but it is not fixated to the ossicle (**Fig. 15.12b**). The atrophic part of the eardrum can be elevated by Valsalva maneuver or with the Siegle otoscope. Surgery is not necessary in stage 2. Valsalva maneuver is recommended.
- **Stage 3: Myringoincudopexy. Retraction is adherent and fixated to the long process of the incus and the lenticular process.** This stage is most important and indicates irreversibility and progression of the retraction. The retraction may be adherent only to the lateral aspect of the long process of the incus, or it can partly or totally surround and adhere to the lenticular process, creating new small retractions around the three sides of the lenticular process (**Fig. 15.12c**) In case of poor self-cleaning, stagnation of the debris and infection within the retraction will appear, causing small cholesteatomas with proliferation of the epithelium and resorption of the long process of the incus and the lenticular process (**Figs. 15.13a–c**). Surgery is indicated in stage 3, especially in case of poor self-cleaning from the small retractions. The transcanal approach is best in this stage, but sinus cholesteatoma with retraction into the facial recess (**Fig. 15.13a, b**) demands removal of the scutum in the retroauricular or endaural approach.
- **Stage 4: Myringostapediopexy.** The long process of the incus with the lenticular process is resorbed and the retraction is adherent to the head of the stapes (**Fig. 15.12d**). Myringostapediopexy may become a stable connection between the stapes head (**Fig. 15.14a**) or even between the stapes neck and the eardrum (**Fig. 15.14b**). The self-cleaning and the epithelial migration may in some cases function well without accumulation of the keratin and debris in the retraction. In most cases however the retraction will extend medially along the stapes neck, with formation of a retraction around the head and neck of the stapes (**Fig. 15.14c, d**). Within the retraction, poor epithelial migration and poor self-cleaning may cause infection of the epithelial membrane, cholesteatoma formation, and bone resorption, resulting in disappearance of the head and neck of the stapes. Surgery is indicated in all situations, especially in case of poor self-cleaning of the retraction. Transcanal approach is sufficient in most situations of stage 4.
- **Stage 5: Myringocruropexy, without stapes head and stapes neck** This stage includes retraction with **intact stapedial arch** (**Fig. 15.12e**), which may in some cases remain stable and self-cleaning, and various defects of stapes crura (**Fig. 15.15a–d**). Transcanal surgery with removal of the retraction, ossiculoplasty and reconstruction of the eardrum with the posterior composite graft is indicated.
- **Stage 6: Myringoplatinopexy, with total resorption of the crura and the retraction membrane covering the entire footplate (Fig. 15.12f).**

At each stage, the retraction may be dry and self-cleaning, without evident progression, or it may be moist with disturbed self-cleaning and accumulation of the debris within the retraction; infection and proliferation of the squamous epithelium to cholesteatoma may occur. Similar transcanal surgery as for stage 5 is indicated.

The present classification includes the posterior retraction only. The previous classification of the retractions include both the posterior retraction and the total retraction (Sade and Berco 1976; Ohnishi et al.1985; Charachon 1988; Gersdorff and Garin 1994; Bours et al. 1998).

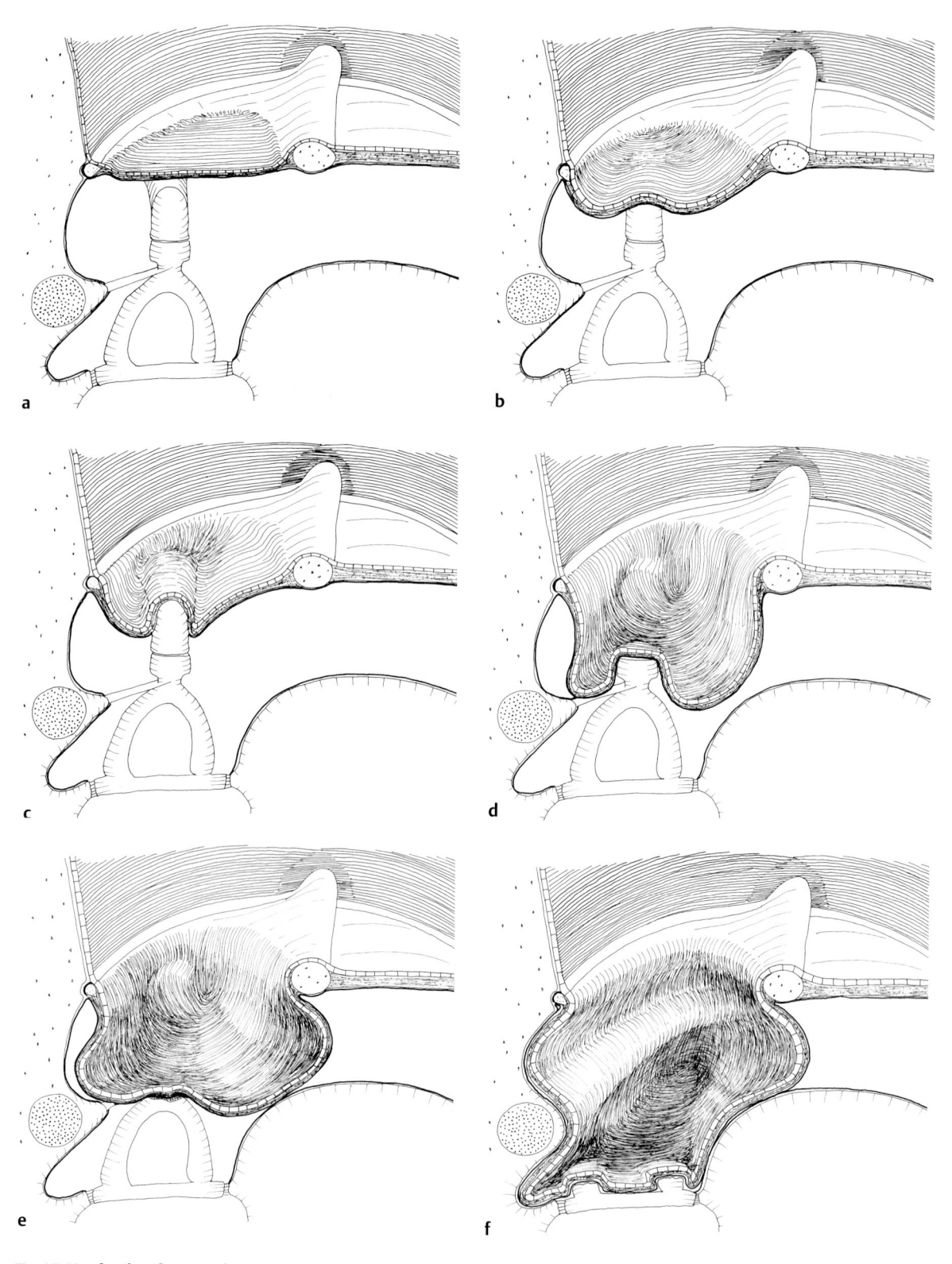

Fig. 15.12a–f Classification of posterior tensa retraction by the present author.

a Stage 1: Atrophy and slight retraction of the posterior pars tensa. The incus is not touched.
b Stage 2: Retraction onto the incus, but the membrane is not fixated.
c Stage 3: Myringoincudopexy. The membrane is fixated to the long process of the incus and the lenticular process.
d Stage 4: Myringostapediopexy, with resorbed long process of the incus and lenticular process. The retraction membrane surrounds the head and neck of the stapes.
e Stage 5: Myringocruropexy, with missing stapes head and stapes neck. Retraction is adherent to the stapes arch or stapes crura at any level.
f Stage 6: Myringoplatinopexy with completely resorbed stapes crura.

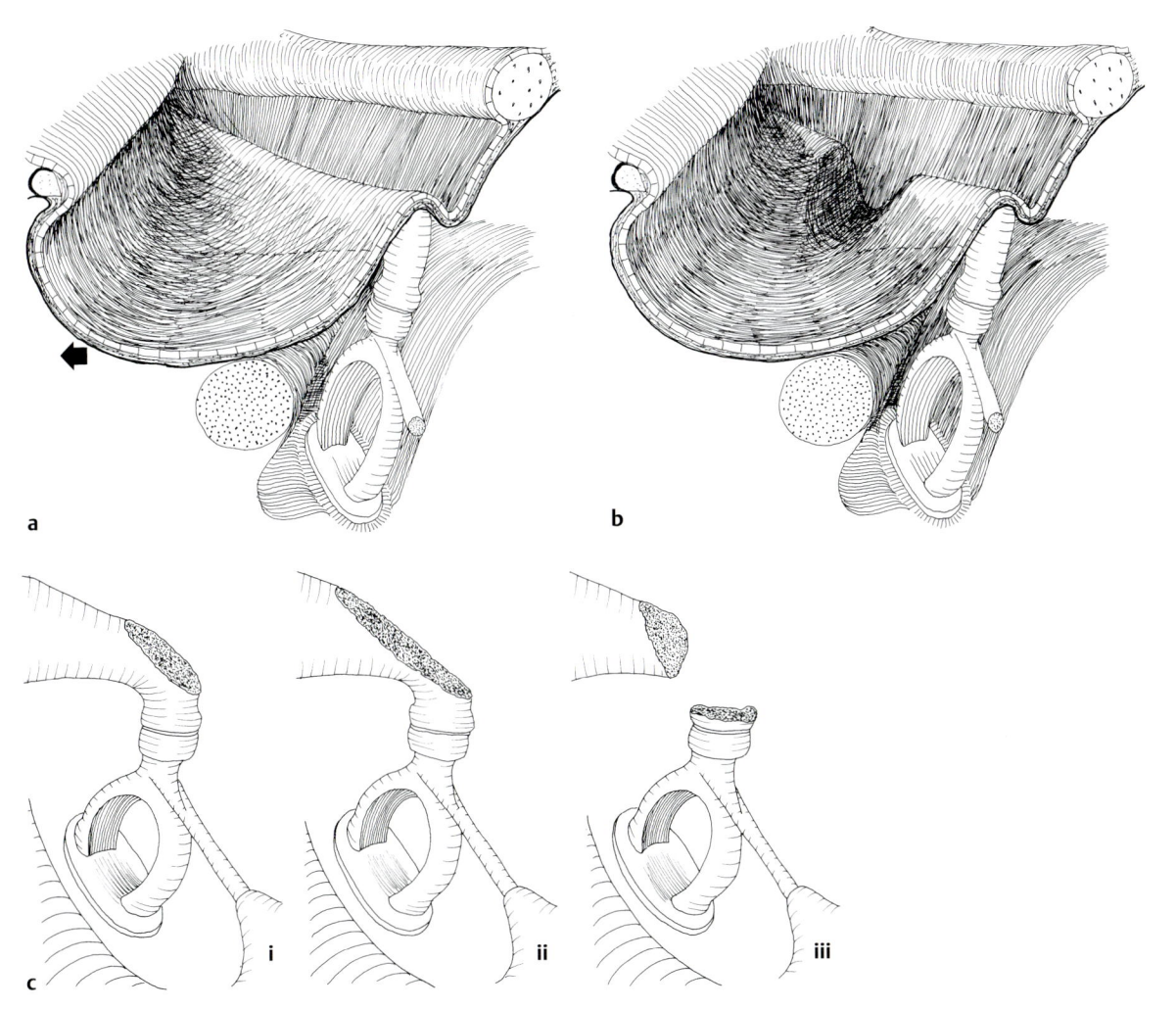

Fig. 15.13a–c Various sitations in myringoincudopexy.
a The long process of the incus and the lenticular process are surrounded by the retraction membrane, which extends posteriorly into the lateral tympanic sinus and toward the short process of the incus (arrow).
b The long process is resorbed by the cholesteatoma; the lenticular process is still intact but is surrounded by the retraction membrane. The retraction is not self-cleaning
c Various shapes of partially resorbed long process of the incus and lenticular process during and after the stage of myringoincudopexy. **(i) and (ii)** Partly resorbed long process of the incus and the lenticular process, and **(iii)** totally resorbed lenticular process, all caused by a cholesteatoma.

Pathogenesis of Sinus Cholesteatoma

Based on epidemiological, clinical and immunohistochemical studies we (Sudhoff and Tos 2007) proposed a four-step pathogenesis of sinus cholesteatoma, combining the retraction and proliferation theory. The basic mechanism is the same as in attic cholesteatoma (Sudhoff and Tos 2000), but the anatomical conditions, especially the shape and severity of retractions around the incudostapedial joint and around the stapes differ from the attic cholesteatoma.

The retraction pocket stage of posterior pars tensa of various depths, and various abilities for self-cleaning of the retraction. If self-cleaning is disturbed, accumulation of debris and keratin, crust formation, and infection behind the crest will occur. This local infection can induce proliferation of the epithelium with cone formation. In sinus cholesteatoma, a retraction can be formed around the long process of the incus (**Fig. 15.12c, 15.13a, b**), around the head and neck of the stapes (**Fig. 15.12 d, 15.14c, d**), and around the stapes crura (**Fig. 15.15a–d**). Furthermore, the retractions with poor self-cleaning can be found in the tympanic sinuses (**Fig. 15.13c, 15.15a–d, 15.12f**).

The proliferation stage of the retraction pocket, with change in the keratinocyte proliferation and cone formation on the bottom of the retraction, local release of collagenases, which degrade the basement membrane and cause its focal disruptions. Due to proliferation of basal cells an active down-growth and elongation of the cones appears. Within the elongated epithelial cone, the process

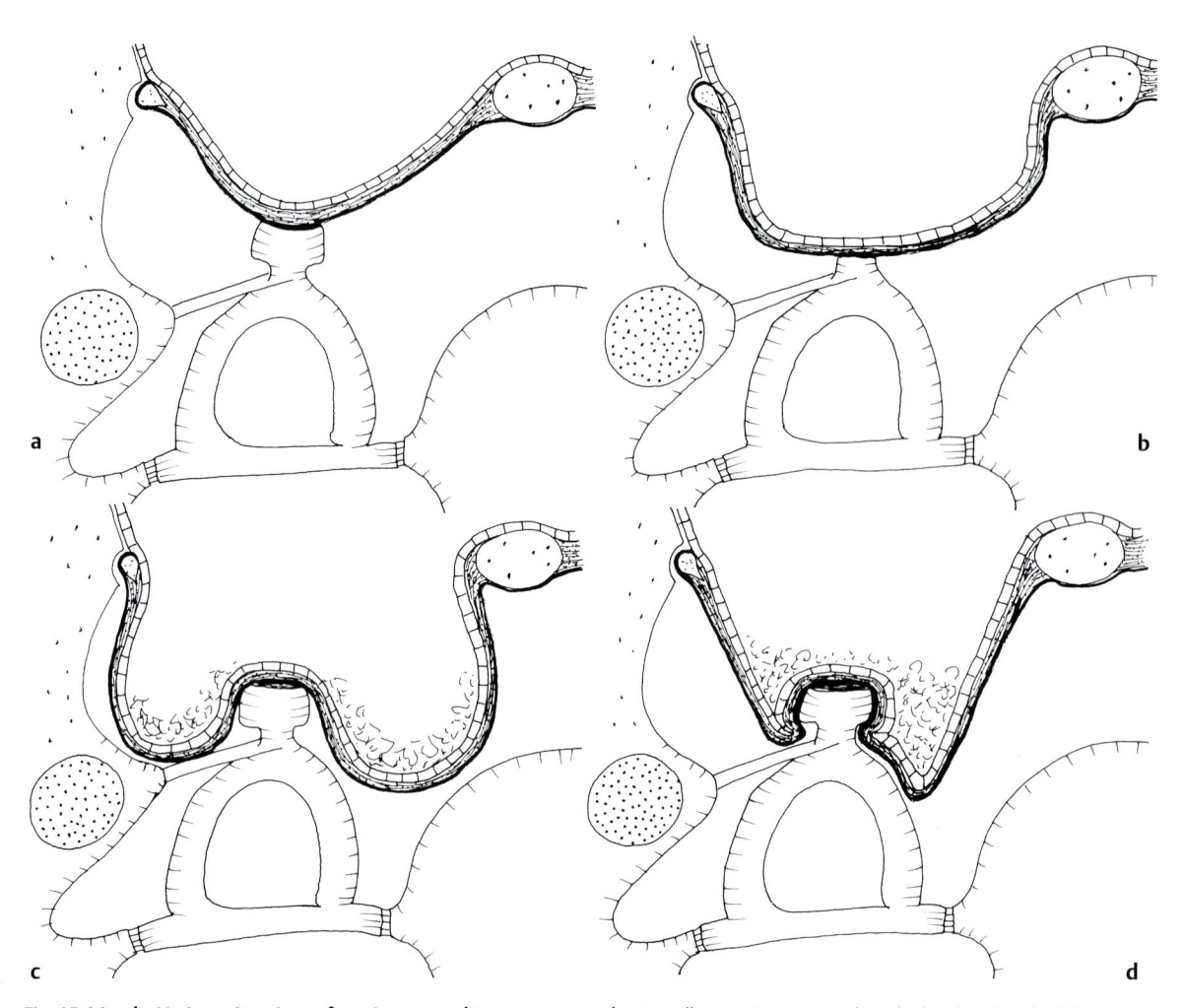

Fig. 15.14a–d Various situations of myringostapediopexy.
a A stable and self-cleaning pexy to the stapes head
b Stable pexy to the neck of the stapes with good self-cleaning.
c Extension of the retraction around the head and neck of the stapes with poor self-cleaning.
d A small retraction surrounding the head and neck of the stapes with poor self cleaning, indicating a precholesteatoma with bone resorption.

of keratinization is altered, resulting in an accumulation of the keratin in the center of the cone, creating microcholesteatomas within the cones.

The expansion stage. Fusion and expansion of several micro-cholesteatomas and further expansion to the periphery will cause disappearance of the overlying keratinized epithelium. The cholesteatoma has opened to the bottom of the retraction, which has thereby grown in depth by the length of the one cone. This results in a new surface of the retraction pocket. As the process of proliferation in the bottom of the cones continues, a new accumulation of the keratin in the cone will soon be formed in the same manner as described before. These processes are continued repeatedly, allowing further expansion of cholesteatoma and retraction.

The bone resorption stage. Once the expansion stage is established a further well-known complication of cholesteatoma will appear—bone resorption. Active ingrowth of the cholesteatoma continues, and bone resorption of the adjacent ossicles and scutum will be initiated. In sinus cholesteatoma the first appearance of bone resorption will take place at the long process of the incus and the lenticular process, then the stapes head and stapes crura and the scutum will be resorbed gradually or stepwise (**Fig. 15.12c–f**). The basic processes of bone resorption are the same in sinus cholesteatoma as in attic cholesteatoma (Sudhoff and Tos 2000).

When to Operate a Posterior Perforation?

Posterior perforation is most often a final sequela of the posterior atrophy of the eardrum, with or without a retraction. Often a strip of epithelium with a very thin lamina propria extends from the upper border of the perforation down to the long process of the incus, indicating a previous retraction.

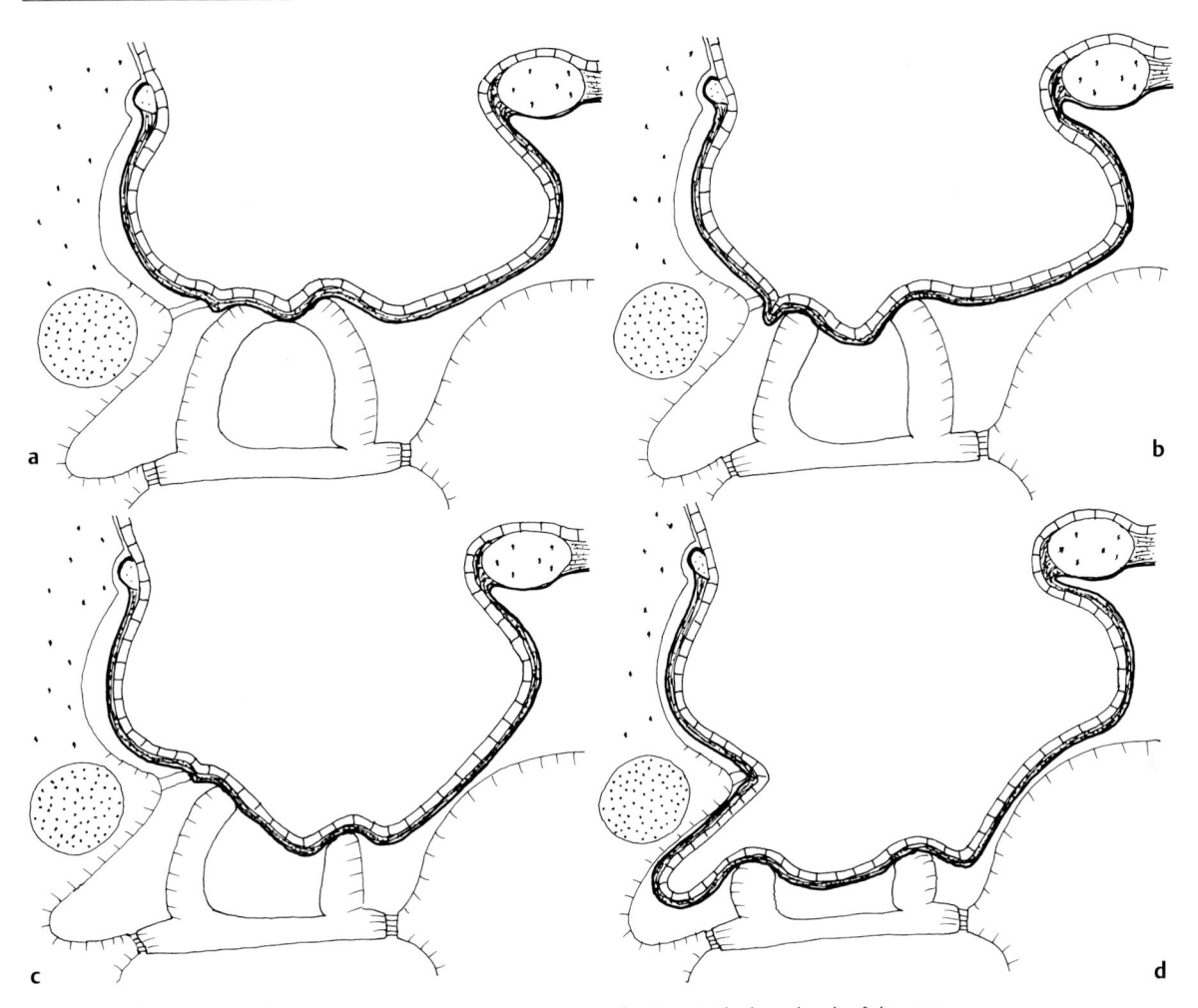

Fig. 15.15a–d Examples of myringocruropexy.
a Myringocruropexy to a slightly defective stapedial arch.
b,c Pexy to the lateral ends of the crura.
d Pexy to the medial ends of the crura.

The good results with posterior island graft in intact ossicular chain and the easy procedure indicate surgery. Even a retraction with fixated myringoincudopexy and a small perforation should be operated. The surgery should be undertaken by a transcanal underlay procedure, applying a posterior cartilage–perichondrium composite island graft.

Posterior perforation with defective ossicular chain is a very common situation, caused by bone resorption of the long process of the incus during the postretraction stages 3 and 4 and by resorption of the stapes in retractions of types 5 and 6. Reconstruction of the ossicular chain in tympanoplasty type 2 with interposition of the incus or in type 3 with placement of a columella covered with the posterior cartilage–perichondrium composite island graft are good solutions.

References

Adkins WY. Composite autograft for tympanoplasty and tympanomastoid surgery. Laryngoscope 1990;100:244–247.

Bours AF, Decat M, Gersdorff M. Our classification of tympanic retraction pockets. Acta Otorhinolaryngol Belg 1998;52:25–28.

Charachon R. Classification des poches de retraction. Rev Laryngol Otol Rhinol (Bord) 1988;109:205–208.

Couloigner V, Molony N, Viala P, Contencin P, Narcy P, Van Den Abbeele T. Cartilage tympanoplasty for posterosuperior, retraction pockets of the pars tensa in children. Otol Neurotol 2003; 24:264–269.

East CA, Mangham C. Composite tragal perichondrial/cartilage autografts vs. cartilage and bone pasta grafts in tympanoplasty. Clin Otolaryngol 1991;16:540–542.

Florant A, Trang M, Jaulin JF, BarilC, RoulleauP. Poches de retraction tympaniques bilan a 3 ans de notre attitude therapeutique a propos de 106 cas. [Tympanic retraction pockets. Evaluation after 3 years of our therapeutic regimen. Apropos of 106 cases] Ann Otolaryngol Chir Cervicofac 1987;104:519–533.

Gerard JM, Decad M, Gersdorff M. Tragal cartilage in tympanic membrane reconstruction. Acta Otorhinolaryngol Belg 2003;57: 147–150.

Gerber MJ, Mason JC, Lambert PR. Hearing results after primary cartilage tympanoplasty. Laryngoscope 2000;110:1994–1999.

Gersdorff M, Garin P. L'endoscopie de l'oreille modifie-t-elle la classification des poches de rétraction et les indications opératoires? Rev Laryngol Otol Rhinol (Bord) 1994;115:367–368.

Gilain C, Gersdorff M, Decat M, Garin P, Phillips C. The relevance of using tragal cartilage in tympanoplasty. Acta Otorhinolaryngol Belg 1997;51:195–196.

Glasscock ME 3 rd, Jackson CG, Nissen AJ, Schwaber MK. Postauricular undersurface tympanic membrane grafting: a follow-up report. Laryngoscope 1982;92:718–727.

Harner SG. Management of posterior tympanic membrane retraction. Laryngoscope 1995;105:326–329.

Hitari F. Posttransplantacni histomorfologicke elasticke chrupavky po myingoplastice. [Posttransplant histomorphological changes of elastic cartilage after myringoplasty] Thesis. Medical School Olomouc; 2006..

Hitari F, Klacansky J, Novotny J, Proskova M, Chrapkova P. Posttransplantacne zmeny elastickej chrupky. Choroby hlavy a krku (Head and Neck Diseases) 2004;3/4:39–43.

Jung TT, Park SK. Reconstruction of mastoidectomy defect with titanium mesh. Acta Otolaryngol 2004;124:440–442.

Linde RE. The cartilage perichondrium graft in the treatment of posterior tympanic membrane pockets. Laryngoscope 1973;83:747–753.

Martin H. A propos de la chirurgie de renforcement du tympan. [Reinforcing surgery of the tympanum] J Fr Oto-Rhino-Laryngol 1979;28:195–196.

Martin H, Cajgfinger H, Gignoux B, Ondot J. De la chirurgie de renforcement tu tympan [Surgical reinforcement of the tympanum]. Ann Otolaryngol Chir Cervicofrac 1973; 90: 119–122.

Mikaelian DO. Perichondrial–cartilage island graft in one stage tympano-ossiculoplasty. Laryngoscope 1986;96:237–239.

Milewski Chr. Ergebnisse der tympanoplastik nach Verwendung von Knorpel-Perichondriumtransplantaten zum Trommelfellersatz unter ungünstigen Bedingungen. Laryngorhinootologie 1991; 70:402–404.

Milewski C. Composite graft tympanoplasty in the treatment of ears with advanced middle ear pathology. Laryngoscope 1993;103:1352–1356.

Mills RP, Phill M. Management of retraction pockets of pars tensa. J Laryngol Otol 1991;105:525–528.

Ohnishi T, Shirahata Y, Fukami M, Hongo S. The atelectatic ear and its classification. Auris Nasus Larynx 1985;12(Suppl. 1):211–212.

Page C, Charlet L, Strunski V. Cartilage tympanoplasty: postoperative functional results. Eur Arch Otorhinolaryngol 2008;265(10):1195–1198.

Pfleiderer AG, Ghosh S, Kairinos N, Chaudhri F. A study of recurrence of retraction pockets after various methods of primary reconstruction of attic and mesotympanic defects in combined approach tympanoplasty. Clin Otolaryngol 2003;28:548–551.

Puls T. Tympanoplasty using conchal cartilage graft. Acta Otorhinolaryngol Belg 2003;57:187–191.

Roger G, Bokowy C, Coste A, . Tympanoplastie avec greffon chondroperichondral. Indications, techniques et results A propos dune serie de 127 tympanoplasties. Ann Otolaryngol Chir Cervicofac 1994;111:29–34.

Sade J, Berco D. Atelectasis and secretory otitis media. Ann Otol Rhinol Laryngol 1976;85(Suppl 25):66–72.

Stangerup SE, Tos M, Arnesen R, Larsen P. A cohort study of point prevalence of eardrum pathology in children and teenagers from age 5 to age 16. Eur Arch Otorhinolaryngol 1994;251:399–403.

Sudhoff H, Tos M. Pathogenesis of attic cholesteatoma: clinical and immunohistochemical support for combination of retraction theory and proliferation theory. Am J Otol 2000;21:786–792.

Sudhoff H, Tos M. Pathogenesis of sinus cholesteatoma. Eur Arch Otorhinolaryngol 2007;264(10):1137–1143.

Sudhoff H, Brors D, Al-Lavati A, Gimenez E, Dazert S, Hildmann H. Posterior canal wall reconstruction with a composite cartilage titanium mesh graft in canal wall down tympanoplasty and revision surgery for radical cavities. J Laryngol Otol 2006;120:832–836.

Tos M. Atelectasis, retraction pockets and cholesteatoma. Ann Otol Rhinol Laryngol 1985;94(Suppl 120):49–51.

Tos M. Sequelae after secretory otitis. Proceedings of the Annual Meeting of Clinical Otolarynologists of Japan, Niigata. 1986: 57–71.

Tos M. Manual of Middle Ear Surgery. Vol. 2. Mastoid Surgery and Reconstructive Procedures. New York, Stuttgart: Thieme; 1995..

Tos M, Stangerup SE, Holm-JensenS, SorensenCH. Spontaneous course of secretory otitis and changes of the eardrum. Arch Otolaryngol 1984;110:281–289.

Tos M, Stangerup SE, Hvid G, Andreassen UK. Epidemiology and natural history of secretory otitis. In: Lim D, Bluestone CD, Klein JO, Nelson JD, eds. Recent Advances in Otitis Media. Philadelphia: BC Decker; 1988:29–34..

Tos M, Hvid G, Stangerup SE, Andreassen UK. Prevalence and progression of sequelae following secretory otitis. Ann Otol Rhinol Laryngol 1990;99(149):36–48.

Yamane H, Takayama M, Sunami K, . Cartilage ossiculoplasty by lever method. Acta Otolaryngol 2008;128:744–749.

Yung MW. Retraction of pars tensa—long term results of surgical treatment. Clin Otolaryngol Allied Sci 1997;22:323–329.

Zini C, Quaranta N, Piazza F. Posterior canal wall reconstruction with titanium micro-mesh and bone pate. Laryngoscope 2002;112:753–756.

16 Superior and Posterior Cartilage–Perichondrium Composite Island Graft Tympanoplasty

Definition

Attic retraction or attic cholesteatoma may coexist with a posterior retraction of the pars tensa. In such cases a cartilage–perichondrium composite graft can be shaped in such a way that both the attic and pars tensa retractions can be covered with a single graft.

Levinson (1987) uses a single large piece of tragal cartilage with perichondrium and tailors it to graft the defect at the attic and the superior tensa area (**Fig. 16.1**).

Poe and Gadre (1993) fashion the tragal cartilage–perichondrium graft in a different way to repair the posterosuperior quadrant of the pars tensa and the pars flaccida. Their cartilage–perichondrium composite graft has two cartilage islands (**Fig. 16.2**). The larger cartilage island covers the defect in the posterosuperior tensa, and the smaller covers the defect in the attic region.

Harvesting and Shaping of the Graft

Levinson harvests the tragal cartilage with an incision 3 mm medial to the dome, for cosmetic reasons. A large piece of cartilage, covered on both sides with the perichondrium, is removed. The perichondrium on the convex (anterior) side is removed and saved should additional grafting material be needed. After working out the size of the graft needed, the cartilage is cut and thinned with a scalpel using a "shaving" technique (**Fig. 16.3a–c**).

Poe and Gadre (1993) harvest the tragal cartilage using a similar incision, but they remove only the posterior perichondrium together with the tragal cartilage. The anterior perichondrium of the tragal cartilage is left in situ.

As well as the cartilage graft, a piece of areolar tissue from the temporal fascia is also harvested using a retroauricular incision and will be used as a medial surface graft.

The shaping of the double-island composite graft is rather complicated. The graft is placed with the cartilage facing up. First, a rectangular-shaped cartilage island is fashioned (to repair the posterosuperior tensa), and then a separate boat-shaped cartilage island (to repair the attic) (**Fig. 16.4a**). The cartilage between the tensa and the attic island is removed. Care is taken to leave sufficient length of perichondrium at the superior and posterior sides of the cartilage islands to form a flap to lie on the bony canal wall. It is important that the shaping of the graft is carried out at the end of drilling, just before its placement (**Fig. 16.4b**), because the surgeon cannot know how much bone from the ear canal has to be removed during removal of the deep retraction or large cholesteatoma.

Indications

The indication for surgery is decided by the main disease in two situations:

1. **Sinus disease as the main pathology.** In such situation the primary pathology may be a posterosuperior tensa

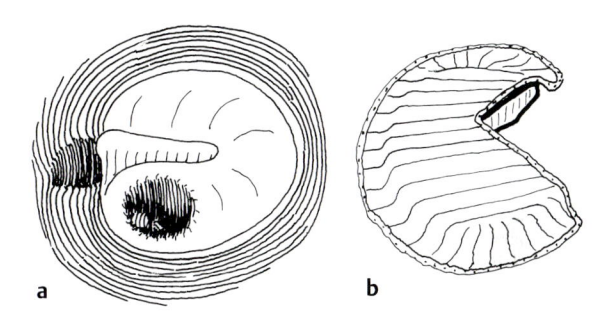

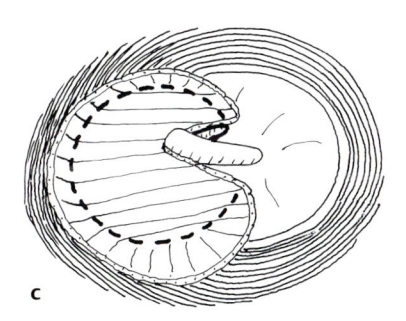

Fig. 16.1a–c Cartilage–perichondrium composite graft of Levinson, tailored to cover the attic retraction and posterosuperior retraction of the pars tensa.
a Attic retraction and posterosuperior retraction of pars tensa.
b The cartilage–perichondrium composite graft is tailored, and has the shape of a "Pac Man."
c The graft covers the attic region and the superior half of the tympanic cavity.

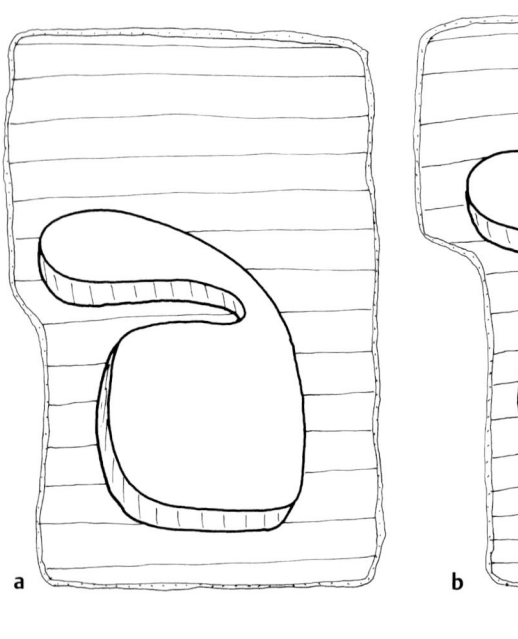

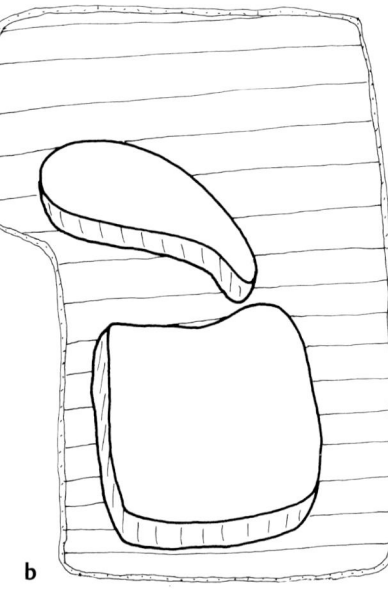

Fig. 16.2a,b Cartilage–perichondrium composite graft of Poe and Gadre.

a The cartilage is shaped as one piece. The rectangular portion of the cartilage covers the posterosuperior tensa retraction, the boat-shaped portion covers the attic retraction.

b The cartilage is divided into two separate islands, the larger piece covers the posterosuperior retraction, the smaller island covers the attic retraction.

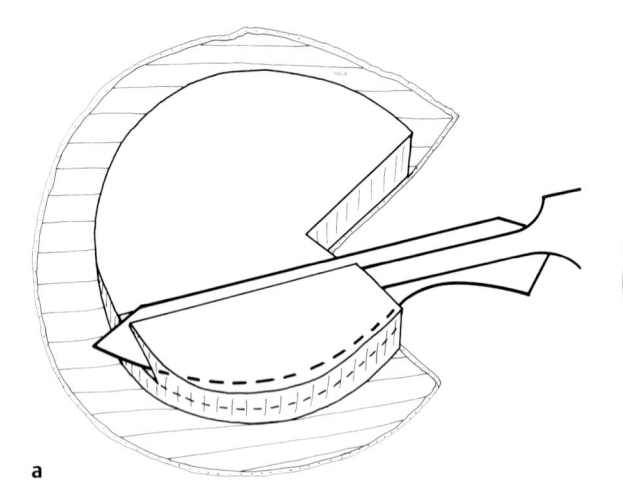

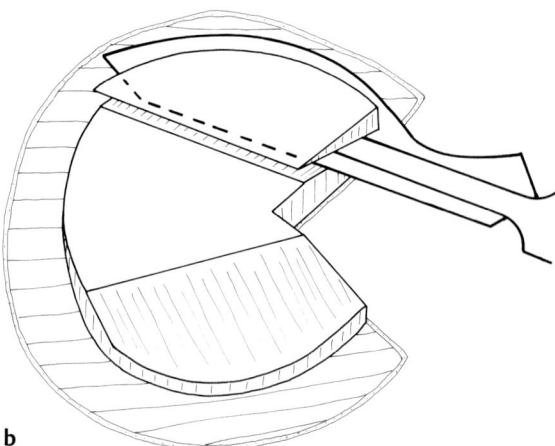

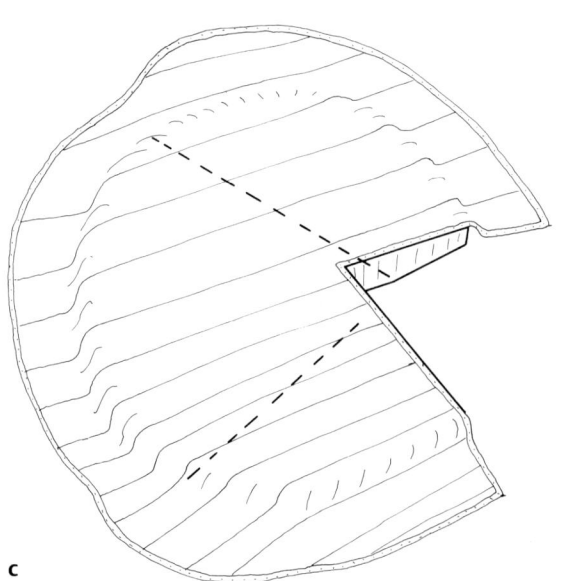

Fig. 16.3a–c Shaping and thinning of the large Levinson cartilage–perichondrium composite graft for the attic and posterosuperior tensa area.

a The graft is shaped and cut to cover a large superior scutum defect and a large posterosuperior and a large anterosuperior defect of the pars tensa. It is positioned with the perichondrium on the table. The anterior part of the graft is thinned.

b The posterior part of the graft is thinned.

c The thinned perichondrium–cartilage composite graft is placed into the middle ear. The larger posterior portion of the graft covers the posterior tensa defect, and the superior portion covers the scutum defect. The perichondrium flaps surrounding the cartilage island are relatively small. The convex side of the cartilage island without the overlying perichondrium faces the tympanic cavity. The dotted lines indicate where the thinning of the cartilage begins.

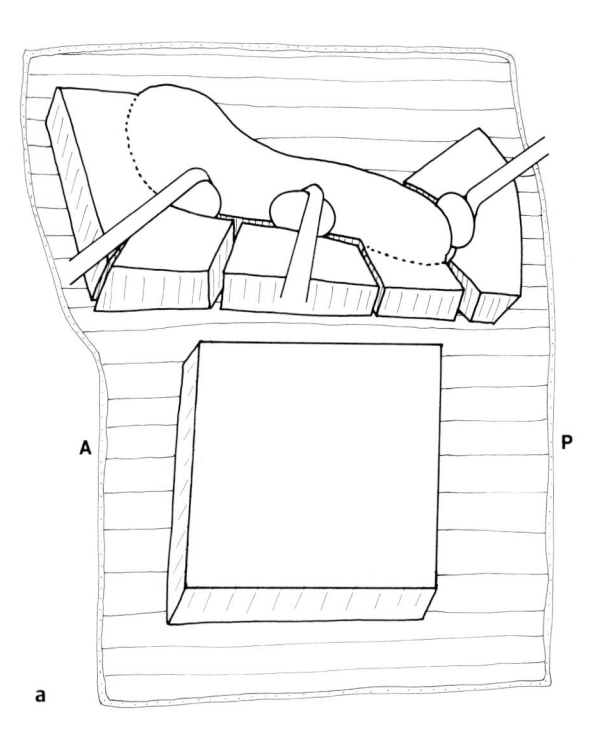

Fig. 16.4a, b Shaping of the Poe-Gadre double cartilage–perichondrium composite island graft.

a The tragal cartilage graft is placed with the cartilage side facing up. First, a rectangular island pars tensa graft is created remembering to include the anterior (A) and posterior (P) perichondrium flaps. Using a round knife, the superfluous cartilage is removed piece by piece from the separate boat-shaped cartilage island, saving the underlying perichondrium.

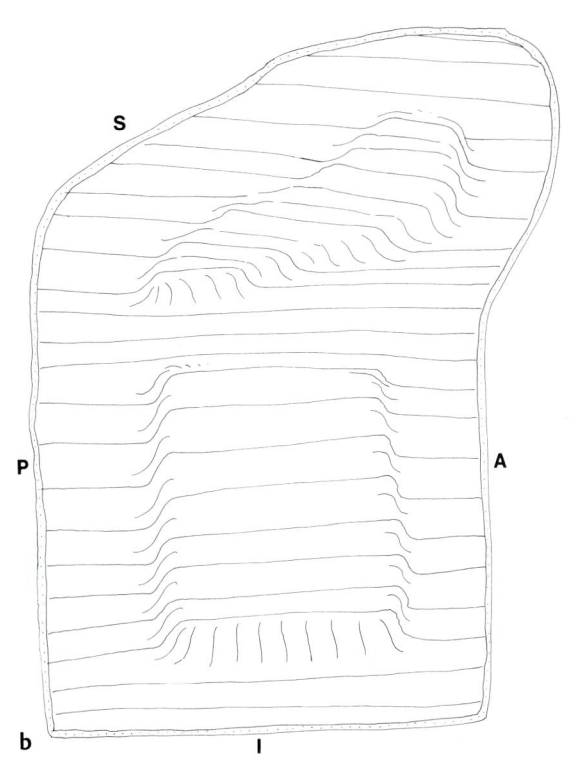

b The completed double graft, with two cartilage islands, surrounded by the anterior (A), inferior (I), posterior (P), and superior (S) perichondrium flaps, before insertion in the tympanic cavity. The rectangular cartilage island graft is placed into the posterosuperior part of the tympanic cavity as an underlay graft and is suspended by the surrounding perichondrium flaps. The boat-shaped cartilage island graft is placed onto the bony ear canal wall to cover the attic defect.

retraction with sinus cholesteatoma. The secondary pathology is an attic retraction of various grades of severity. The attic retraction will usually not cause any symptoms, but will often be adherent to the incus body. At the time of surgery on the posterosuperior tensa retraction and/or sinus cholesteatoma, the long process of the incus will often be found to be resorbed. In removing the incus remnant, the adherent membrane of the attic retraction will be torn. This may well require removal of the attic retraction pocket, but such event is relatively rare.

2. **Attic disease as the main pathology.** In such situation the primary pathology may be an infected and deep attic retraction, attic precholesteatoma, or attic cholesteatoma. The second pathology is a posterosuperior tensa retraction. The posterosuperior retraction may be adherent to the long process of the incus—myringoincudopexy. Often the long process of the incus is also resorbed, and the retracted eardrum is adherent to the stapes head—myrigostapediopexy. In case of further retraction and resorption of the stapes crura, a myringocruropexy may occur, and in total resorption of the crura a myringoplatinopexy. If the ossicular pathology results in a hearing loss, surgery on the posterosuperior tensa retraction may be necessary.

Surgical Methods

Technique of Levinson

Levinson (1987) prefers a transcanal approach, but endaural or retroauricular approaches can also be used. A large circumferential incision between the 5-o'clock and 2-o'clock positions and a radial incision at the 9-o'clock position are made (**Fig. 16.5a**) to facilitate the swing-door technique. The incisions give a good exposure of the attic bone. A large posterosuperior meatal flap is elevated (**Fig. 16.5b**), and an inferior tympanomeatal flap is also elevated. The epithelium at the edge of the posterior retraction is elevated and preserved. The squamous keratinized epithelium of the posterior retraction pocket is then carefully elevated and dissected away from the stapes, incus, and posterior and medial walls of the tympanic cavity (**Fig. 16.5c–f**).

The bone overhanging the attic retraction is removed, initially exposing the lateral wall of the retraction pocket (**Fig. 16.5 f, g**). Further drilling around the anterior, superior, and posterior aspects of the retraction pocket (**Fig. 16.5h, i**) provides a complete exposure and the removal of the retraction. A large Levinson cartilage–perichondrium composite graft is needed to reconstruct the defect at the scutum and the posterior perforation area (**Fig. 16.5j, k**).

It is difficult to predict extension and depth of the retraction and the amount of drilling required to remove all the pathology. Accordingly, the harvested piece of cartilage must be large enough, and the shaping of the graft should be done when the size of the defect is known. The

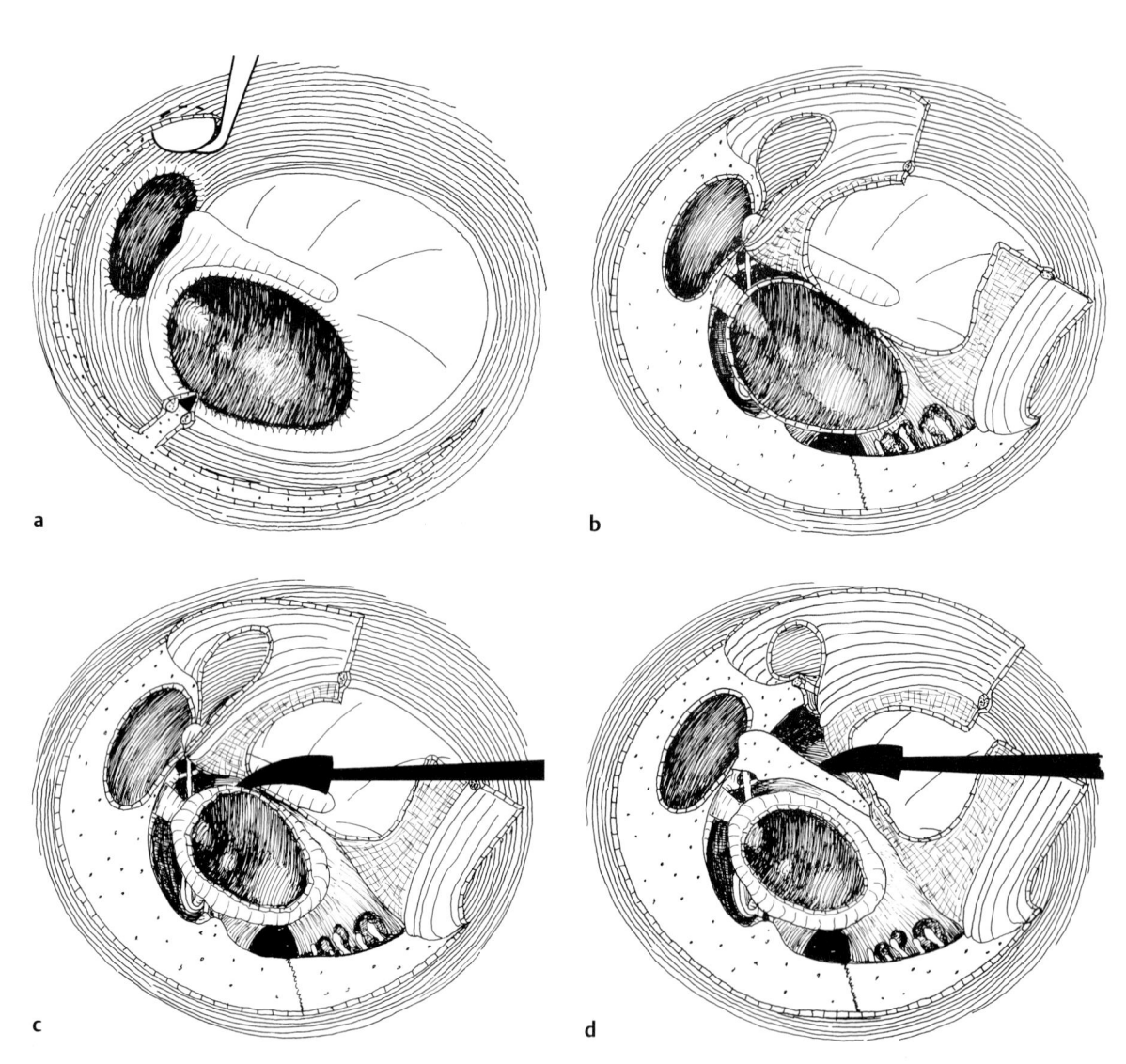

Fig. 16.5a–k Removal of an unstable attic retraction with the attic pre-cholesteatoma as the main disease and a dry posterosuperior tensa retraction.

a The Levinson "Pac Man" cartilage–perichondrium composite graft is used to cover the attic and the posterosuperior tensa defects, with resorption of the long process of the incus. A circumferential incision between the 5-o'clock and 2-o'clock positions and a radial incision at the 9-o'clock position are made.

b The posterosuperior tympanomeatal flap is elevated together with the fibrous annulus and the flap is separated from the posterior tensa retraction and the attic retraction. The inferior tympanomeatal flap is also elevated and separated from the inferior and anterior border of the posterior tensa retraction.

c Using a sickle knife, the borders of the retraction pockets are elevated. Epithelium of the retraction along the malleus handle is elevated as well and the posterior side of the malleus handle is cleaned.

d The anterosuperior part of the eardrum is elevated with its fibrous annulus and then detached from the malleus handle, but not from the umbo. All epithelium from the short process of the malleus is dissected away and the malleus handle is freed from the retraction pocket.

Fig. 16.5e–k

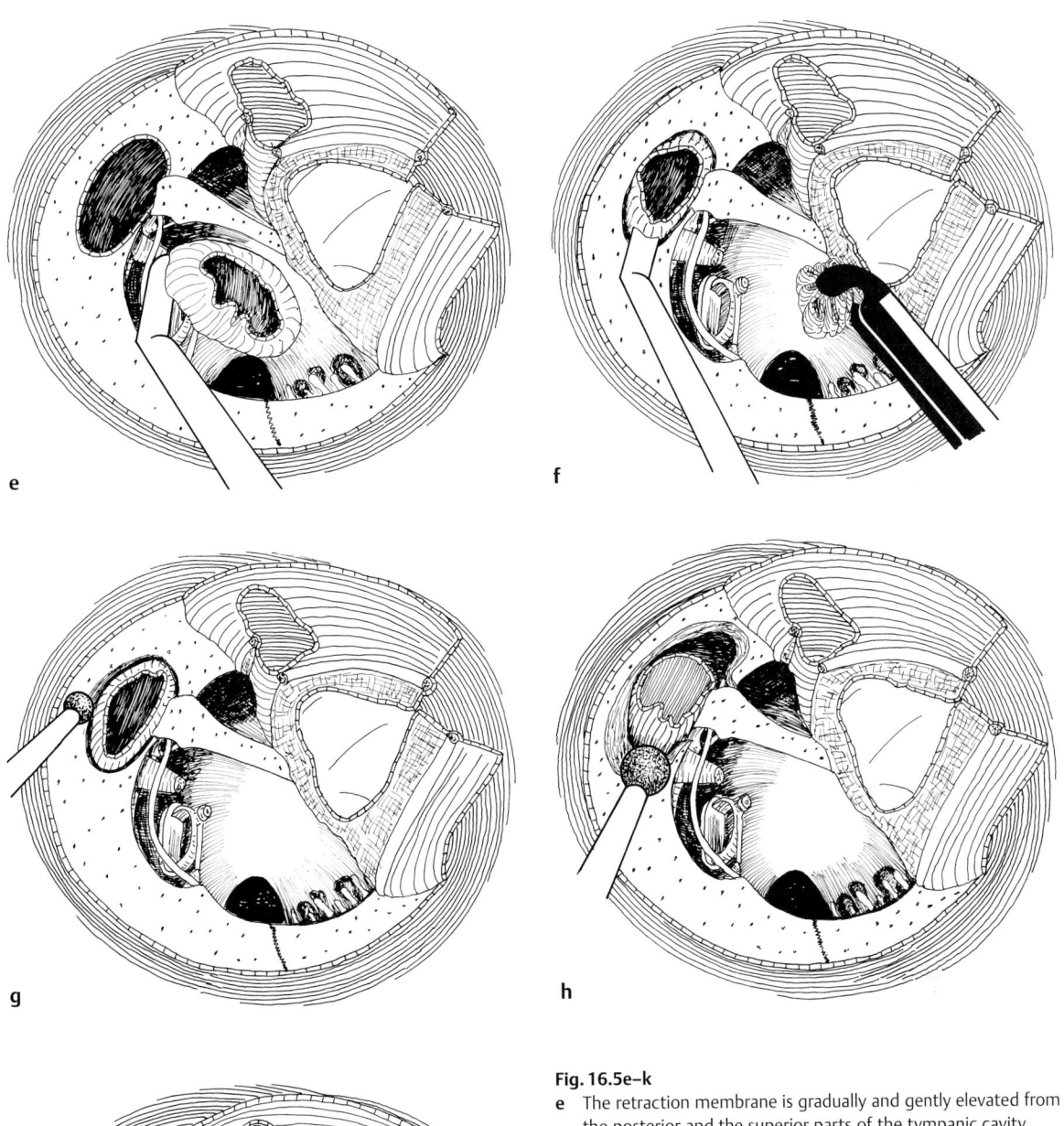

e The retraction membrane is gradually and gently elevated from the posterior and the superior parts of the tympanic cavity.

f The squamous epithelium is dissected away from the remnant of the long process of the incus and the stapes. The last part of the posterior tensa retraction pocket is removed with forceps. The edge of the attic retraction is then carefully elevated.

g Gradual drilling of the bone around the attic retraction is carried out in order to expose the whole retraction pocket before it can be safely removed.

h The anterior part of the attic retraction is exposed, but not the posterior part: further drilling posteriorly is necessary.

i The bone at the attic around the attic retraction is carefully removed, to allow good access to the attic retraction pocket. The incus remnant is removed and re-shaped. A groove for the head of the stapes is drilled in the reduced incus body and the incus is interposed between the stapes head and the cartilage graft.

Fig. 16.3j–k ▷

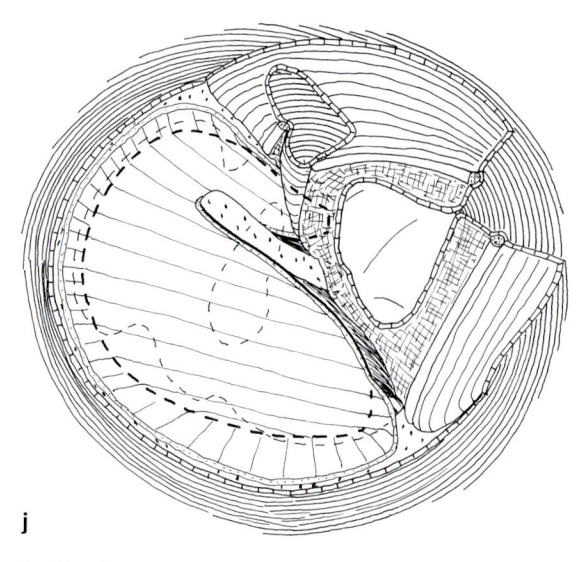

Fig. 16.5j, k

j A large Levinson cartilage–perichondrium composite graft covers the attic bony defect and the posterosuperior tensa perforation. Part of the perichondrium flap around the cartilage is placed on the bony ear canal, the other parts are tucked under the inferior margin of the perforation and placed along the malleus handle.

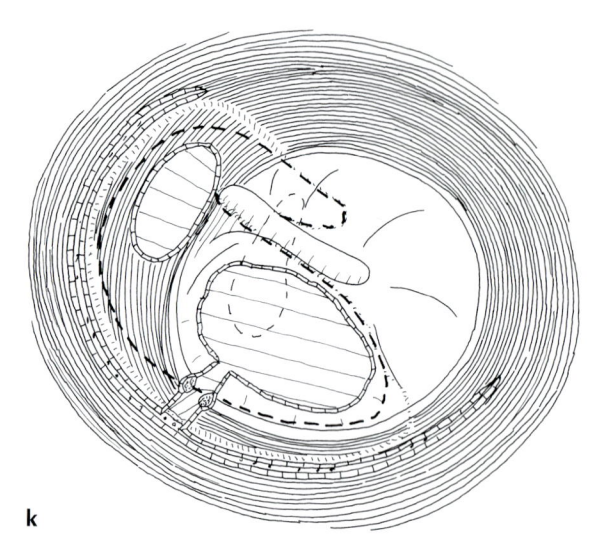

k The tympanomeatal flaps are replaced.

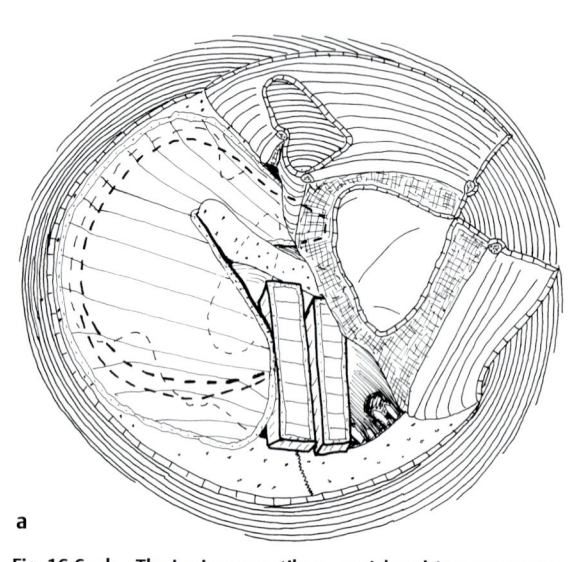

Fig. 16.6a, b The Levinson cartilage–perichondrium composite graft may be too small to cover the attic bony defect and repair the whole posterior perforation.

a In such situation cartilage palisades are placed to cover the inferior part of the perforation. The perichondrium flaps of the Levinson graft are placed on the ear canal bone.

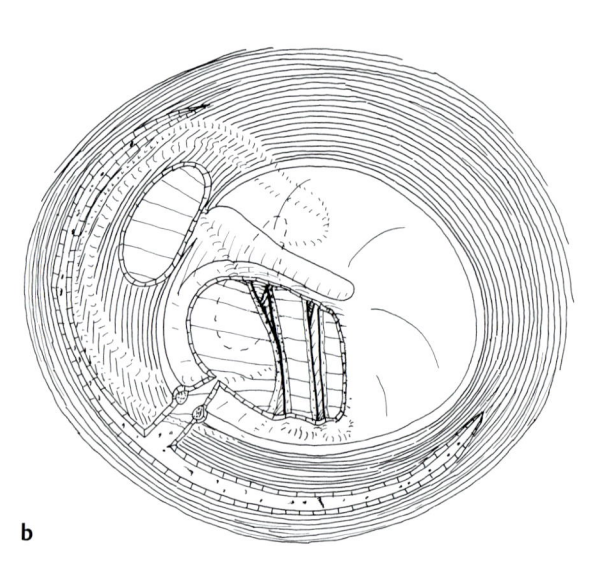

b The tympanomeatal flaps with the elevated epithelium from the retraction are replaced, partly covering partly the cartilage palisades.

reconstruction of the tympanic membrane can be supplemented by small cartilage palisades should a single Levinson graft not be big enough to repair the whole defect (**Fig. 16.6a, b**).

Technique of Poe and Gadre

Poe and Gadre (1993) combine a posterior cartilage–perichondrium composite island graft with an underlay fascia graft. In a case with a total perforation and a small attic retraction (**Fig. 16.7a**), the attic retraction is elevated first.

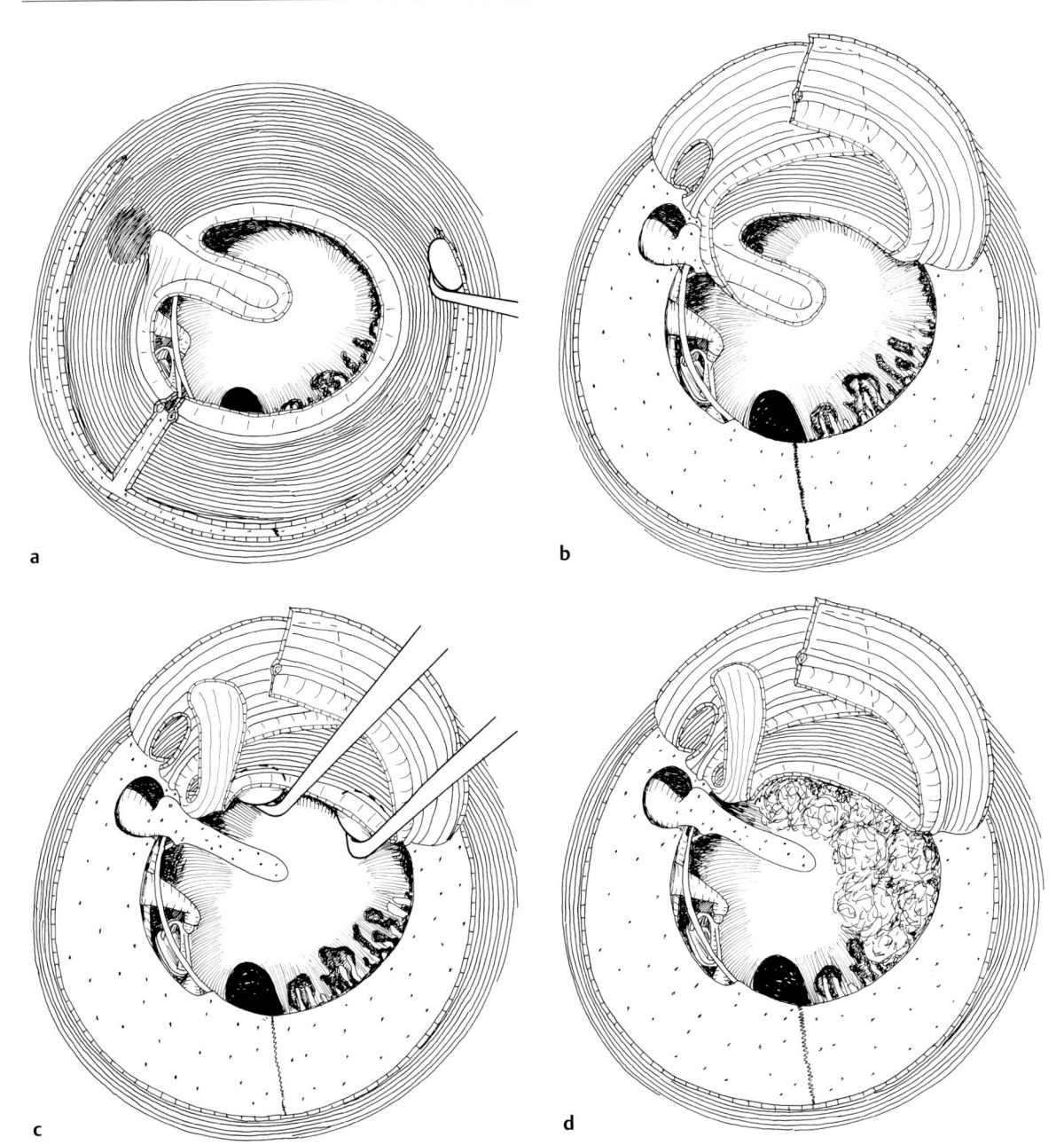

Fig. 16.7a–j The Poe-Gadre technique of placing the double-island cartilage–perichondrium composite graft in a case of total perforation of pars tensa with intact ossicular chain and a small retraction of the Shrapnell membrane.

a Using a retroauricular approach, a circular incision between the 1-o'clock and 5-o'clock positions and a radial incision at the 9-o'clock position are made, allowing a swing-door technique. The edge of the perforation is excised with its squamous epithelium.

b First the superior tympanomeatal flap is elevated up to the short process of the malleus. The attic retraction pocket is carefully dissected off, taking care that no squamous epithelium is left around the neck and the short process of the malleus. The inferior tympanomeatal flap is also elevated.

c The tympanic membrane is dissected off the malleus handle in the form of a malleus flap. The mucosa on the undersurface of the anterior eardrum remnant and bony annulus is partly removed to facilitate placement of the fascia as an underlay graft.

d Gelfoam balls are placed into the anterior and inferior parts of the tympanic cavity to support a large fascia graft.

Fig. 16.7e–j ▷

Then the total perforation is closed with a temporalis fascia graft (**Fig. 16.7b–f**).

The posterior half of the fascia graft is further reinforced using a cartilage–perichondrium composite graft (**Fig. 16.7f**). First, the posterior half of the fascia is elevated, and the rectangular-shaped cartilage–perichondrium composite graft is placed in the posterosuperior defect of the pars tensa. The smaller boat-shaped part of the graft is

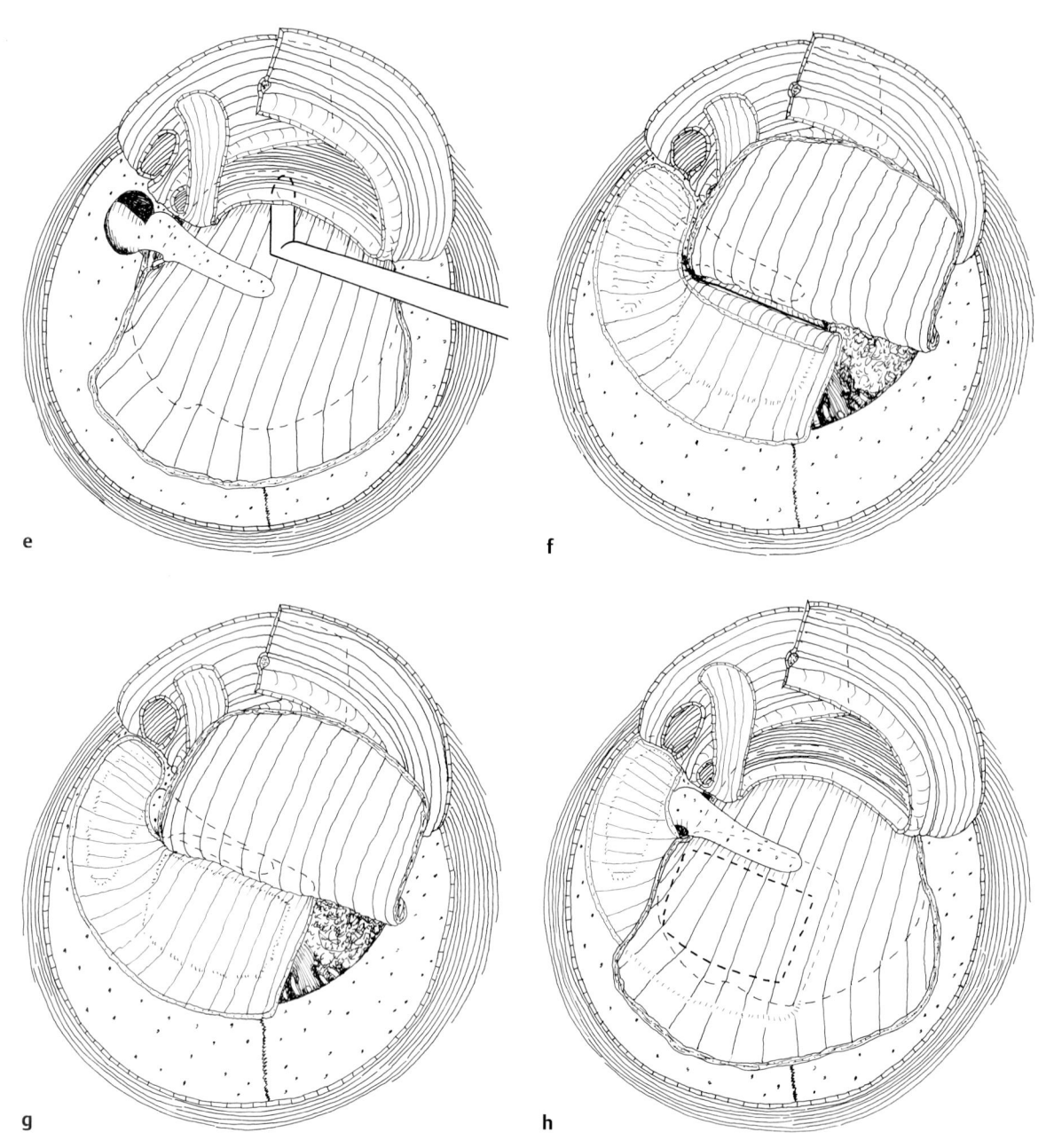

Fig. 16.7e–j

e The temporal fascia graft is placed as an underlay graft with its anterior part tucked under the eardrum remnant.

f The posterior half of the fascia graft is elevated and folded forward. The double-island cartilage–perichondrium composite graft is positioned. The rectangular cartilage island is placed into the posterosuperior part of the tympanic cavity, between the malleus handle and the posterior bony annulus.

The smaller boat-shaped cartilage island is placed over the scutum defect to cover the opening after removal of the attic retraction pocket.

g The perichondrium flaps are replaced: The anterior flap is placed under the fascia and the malleus handle; the posterior perichondrium flap is placed on the ear canal bone; the superior flap is placed on the bony scutum.

h The posterior half of the fascia graft is replaced over the perichondrium surface of the composite graft and the bony ear canal wall.

then positioned onto the scutum defect to cover the small attic retraction. The anterior perichondrium flap of the composite graft is placed under the malleus handle; the superior and posterior perichondrium flaps are placed over the bony ear canal (**Fig. 16.7 g**). The fascia graft (**Fig. 16.7h**) and the tympanomeatal flaps are then replaced (**Fig. 16.7i, j**).

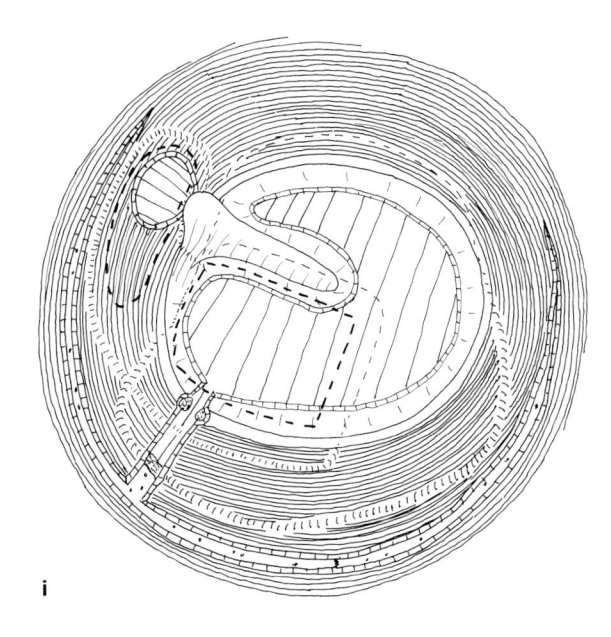

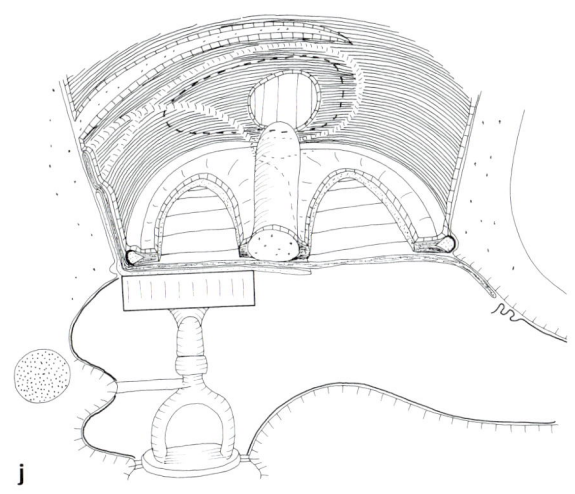

Results of Surgery

Only three surgical teams have described their surgical techniques and published the results.

Levinson Series

Levinson reported on 85 ears of 75 patients, with a minimum follow-up period of one year. All patients had a posterior marginal retraction and/or a deep attic retraction—"a blind pocket that [makes it] difficult to determine the extent of the disease into the facial recess and/or epitympanum."

In addition, all the patients fulfilled one or more of the following criteria:

1. Presence of overt cholesteatoma
2. Recurrent or persistent otorrhea
3. Persistent granulation tissue
4. Conductive hearing loss (negative Rinne)
5. Irreversible eustachian tube dysfunction (i. e., cleft palate, skull base fracture involving the eustachian tube).

Operative Findings

- Effusion 7%, granulation 59%, cholesteatoma 19%.

Ossicular pathology
- Total erosion of long process of the incus 29%
- Stapes erosion 1%
- Ossicular fixation 2%
- The ossicular chain was intact in 71% of the 85 ears!

Postoperative Findings

Hearing improved after surgery, with an air–bone gap within 0–10 dB in 66% of patients compared with 27% before the operation (**Table 16.1**).

There was no graft failure or recurrence of the retraction pocket at the original location. In 11 ears, retraction pockets were found in new locations (attic 6, anterior pars tensa 4, inferior pars tensa 1). Middle ear effusion was found in 6 ears, residual cholesteatoma was identified on second-look tympanoplasty in 5 ears.

Fig. 16.7i, j
i The tympanomeatal flaps and the malleus flap are replaced.
j Side view with some perspective showing a tympanoplasty type 1 for a total perforation with fascia, buttressed in the posterosuperior part of the pars tensa with a double cartilage–perichondrium graft. In the same session a small attic retraction was removed and covered with the same double cartilage–perichondrium island graft. A large fascia covers the total perforation as an underlay graft. The cartilage–perichondrium island graft is placed under the posterosuperior part of the fascia and is suspended by the perichondrium flaps. Superior part of the graft covers an attic retraction.

Table 16.1 Percentage of preoperative and postoperative air–bone gaps for different sizes of air–bone gap (out of 85 ears)

Air–bone gap group	Preoperative (%)	Postoperative (%)
0–10 dB	27	66
11–20 dB	33	20
21–30 dB	24	8
>30 dB	17	6

Two Separate Grafts of Couloigner

Couloigner et al. (2003) use two separate cartilage–perichondrium composite island grafts. One is rectangular-shaped to close the posterosuperior tensa perforation, the other is smaller and covers the bony defect after removal of the attic retraction.

Table 16.2 Percentage of preoperative and postoperative air–bone gap for different sizes of air–bone gap (out of 24 ears)

Air–bone gap group	Preoperative (%)	Postoperative (%)
0–10 dB	25	46
11–20 dB	38	38
> 20 dB	38	17

Series of Poe and Gadre

Over a period of 3.5 years, 150 tympanoplasties with intact external auditory canals were carried out in the Lahey Clinic Medical center. Of these, 39 ears were grafted with a cartilage–perichondrium composite graft. In the first 15 ears, only a posterosuperior rectangular graft, was applied. In the other 24 ears, the cartilage graft was fashioned to reinforce both the posterosuperior pars tensa and the pars flaccida. In most cases a single graft with two separate cartilage islands (**Fig. 16.2b**) was used, so that each cartilage island could vibrate freely. The results of these 24 ears that had pars flaccida and posterior pars tensa reinforced by cartilage is summarized. The average follow-up period was 13.7 months.

Postoperative Complications
(The number of ears is given in parentheses.)
- Pars flaccida retraction pocket (1)
- Retraction between cartilage and malleus (1)
- Cartilage graft failure (0)
- Anteroinferior retraction (0)
- Anteroinferior perforation (1)
- Secretory otitis requiring ventilation tubes (2)
- Cartilage dislodged (0)

After surgery, the hearing was moderately improved (**Table 16.2**): 46% of patients had an air–bone gap closure within 0–10 dB, compared with 25% before the operation.

Poe and Gadre noted fewer postoperative complications in the group that had both attic and posterosuperior pars tensa repaired using separate cartilage islands than in the group that had only the posterosuperior pars tensa graft. The postoperative hearing was the same in the two groups (Poe and Gadre 1993).

Pediatric Series with Two Separate Cartilage–Perichondrium Composite Island Grafts

Couloigner et al. (2003) reported the use of two separate cartilage–perichondrium composite grafts in 8 children. They used a posterior composite island graft for the posterior tensa retraction or perforation, and a separate small attic island graft for the attic retraction.

For another 8 children who had a posterior tensa retraction, a total tensa composite island graft and a separate attic composite island graft were used for the attic retraction. In these 16 children, only 2 (12%) developed a recurrent retraction.

Couloigner et al. did not specify the type or size of the attic retractions or whether they were symptomatic. It was apparent that operation on the attic retractions was for prophylactic reasons. Out of 65 children with a posterior retraction, 16 also had an attic retraction. It is possible that most of these attic retractions were small and asymptomatic (of grades 1 or 2) and might never progress to a cholesteatoma.

Author's Comments and Recommendations

Vibratile and Non-vibratile Island Grafts

The cartilage–perichondrium composite island graft, such as the posterosuperior tensa graft (Chapter 15) or the total pars tensa graft (Chapter 17), is suspended by the surrounding perichondrium flaps and is therefore vibratile. The superior (or attic) cartilage–perichondrium graft is presumably not vibratile. The attic island graft is not supposed to be vibratile; its purpose is to permanently prevent the attic retraction. The cartilage is firmly fixed to the scutum bone by the surrounding perichondrium, and is not in contact with the ossicles. Even if the medial edge of the superior graft may in some cases be in contact with the neck of the malleus, there will presumably be only minimal or no vibration of the superior graft.

The Levinson large "Pac Man" graft (**Fig. 16.3**) is anchored at the attic region (**Fig. 16.6a, b**) and could hinder the vibratory ability of the posterior graft. I believe that the good hearing results reported in Levinson's series (see **Table 16.1**) were most probably due to vibration at the malleus handle and the inferior half of the eardrum, especially because 71% of the ears in his series had an intact ossicular chain. A type 1 tympanoplasty may well give a more predictable improvement of the air–bone gap. Furthermore, the placement of the "Pac Man" graft involves elevation of the anterosuperior part of the eardrum and detachment from the malleus handle.

Dividing the single large "Pac Man" graft into two pieces—a superior attic graft and a posterosuperior tensa graft—may make the placement of each graft easier and more precise, especially connecting the graft to the inferior margin of a posterior perforation, as illustrated in **Fig. 16.6a**.

Poe and Gadre (1993) preferred separate cartilage islands within a single cartilage–perichondrium composite graft (**Fig. 16.2b**). Such a graft is easier to position onto the scutum defect and this attic portion of the graft is not vibratile.

Couloigner et al. (2003) used two separate composite island grafts to repair the attic and posterosuperior part of the pars tensa. I use and recommend this method for following reasons: It is easier to shape two smaller grafts than one large graft. It is also easier to exactly position two small grafts than one "Pac Man" graft. The vibratility of the smaller posterosuperior island graft is better than that of a large graft fixed firmly in the attic.

Prevalence and Classification of Attic Retractions

The purpose of the following comments, based on our long-term studies, is to show that small attic retractions of grades 1 and 2 are common (**Fig. 14.2**), and they are usually harmless and asymptomatic. They are extremely unlikely to progress to an attic cholesteatoma. I therefore do not recommend "prophylactic" surgery on such small, asymptomatic retractions pockets merely for the fear that they could develop into attic cholesteatomas. The risk of leaving behind squamous epithelium and causing residual cholesteatoma is hundreds of times greater than that of a small attic retraction developing into attic cholesteatoma.

Our epidemiological research involved long-term observation of secretory otitis and revealed a surprisingly high prevalence of attic retractions. These are mainly small and harmless retractions, and only very few progress to attic cholesteatoma.

Classification and Grading of Attic Retractions
Classification and grading of attic retractions is absolutely necessary in longitudinal epidemiological studies. We have proposed and used the following grading (Tos and Poulsen 1980), dividing attic retractions into four grades or types (**Fig. 14.2**):
- **Grade 1** represents a slight retraction with air present between the Shrapnell membrane and the neck of the malleus.
- **Grade 2** indicates a retraction extending to the neck of the malleus, and no air space is visible behind the retraction. The Shrapnell membrane may be adherent to the neck of the malleus, but this is not always the case.
- **Grade 3** indicates a retraction beyond the bony annulus, but on tilting the head of the patient, the bottom of the retraction can still be seen and air can be seen in the attic. There may also be some resorption of the bony annulus, whereas the area of the Shrapnell membrane is enlarged.
- **Grade 4** indicates pronounced bone resorption at the scutum and the Shrapnell membrane is adherent to the head of the malleus and body of the incus, which are clearly visible. However, due to the bone resorption the bottom of the retraction is still visible.

When the bottom of the retraction pocket cannot be seen with an otomicroscope, an endoscope can sometimes provide a clear overview of the retraction. Such a condition may be termed grade 5 retraction.

Table 16.3 Prevalence (%) of various types (or grades) of attic retractions in cohort 3 of healthy Danish children as sequelae of chronic secretory otitis and tubal dysfunction (Tos et al. 1989)

Type (grade) of retraction	5 years (444 ears)	6 years (444 ears)	7 years (444 ears)	8 years (414 ears)	9 years (406 ears)	10 years (470 ears)
1	9.2	14.9	11.5	9.2	11.1	10.6
2	7.0	9.2	13.7	8.5	9.6	11.1
3	1.1	2.3	3.4	5.8	4.4	4.3
4	0.7	1.3	0.9	0.5	0.3	0.4
Total attic	18.0	27.7	29.5	24.0	25.4	26.4
Attic only	14.9	19.8	21.6	15.2	15.5	14.7
Tensa only	5.7	9.2	9.2	6.5	7.4	6.4

Epidemiological Studies of Middle Ear Diseases
Epidemiological studies of middle ear diseases were carried out at our department during the 1970s and 1980s using tympanometric and otomicroscopic screenings of three cohorts of otherwise healthy children.
- **Cohort 1** was of children at birth, and they were examined with tympanometry and otoscopy. These investigations were repeated every 3 months during the first 2 years and then every year until the age of 8 years (Tos 1983; Tos et al. 1988). At the yearly investigations, otomicroscopy was also performed.
- **Cohort 2** was of children starting at the age of 2 years. They were observed every 3 months until the age of 4 years, and then every year until they were 11 years old (Tos et al. 1978; Tos 1984).
- **Cohort 3** was of children starting at the age of 4 years. They were observed every 3 months until the age of 5 years and then every year until age of 16 years (Tos et al. 1990; Stangerup et al. 1994).

We document that during childhood 90 % of otherwise healthy Danish children (80 % of ears) have had secretory otitis in at least one period. We further observed in all three cohorts that one-third of the ears have had some forms of sequelae of the eardrum, either of the pars tensa alone or together with attic retraction, or attic retraction alone (**Table 16.3**).

The Prevalence of Attic Retractions
The prevalence of attic retractions was very high in cohorts 1 and 2, and was even higher in cohort 3 (**Table 16.4**). About 25 % of healthy Danish children had some degree of attic retraction, but very few of them progressed to attic cholesteatoma. The prevalence of small and harmless retractions of types 1 and 2 was very high, at 20 % and the majority did not progress to a more severe grade.

At 16 years of age, 20 % of the teenagers from cohort 3 had an attic retraction (Tos et al. 1990; Stangerup et al. 1994).

Table 16.4 Prevalence (%) of attic retractions in cohort 3 of otherwise healthy teenagers (Stangerup et al. 1994) and the incidence of attic retractions in two clinical series of secretory otitis treated with grommets and adenoidectomy (Tos et al. 1989)

Retraction grades	Randomized cohort 3			Treated secretory otitis		
	Age 11 years (374 ears)	Age 12 years (294 ears)	Age 16 years (320 ears)	Series 1 3–8 years (527 ears)	Series 1 10–16 years (362 ears)	Series 2 11–18 years (178 ears)
1	10.4	6.8	6.6	12.7	9.4	13.5
2	8.3	6.5	9.4	17.3	9.9	14.6
3	2.4	5.8	2.8	3.4	5.8	4.5
4	0.0	0.3	1.3	0.8	1.7	1.7
Attic cholesteatoma				0.2	0.6	1.7
Total	21.1	19.4	20.1	34.4	27.4	36.0

Incidence of Attic Retractions in Clinical Series of Secretory Otitis Treated with Adenoidectomy and Grommets, and Followed with Reevaluations

Clinical series 1 originally involved 278 children with secretory otitis treated during the period 1970–1975 with grommet insertion and adenoidectomy. The children were followed and first recalled for assessment in 1977/78, 3–8 years postoperatively, and again in 1984, 10–16 years after the initial treatment.

Clinical series 2 originally involved 220 children with secretory otitis, treated with grommet insertion and adenoidectomy during 1967–1974. They were reassessed 0.5–7 years after the operation, and again in 1985, 11–18 years after the initial treatment. This is our earliest series with most pathology, when the more severe and protracted cases were selected for surgery.

We observed high prevalence of grade 1 and grade 2 attic retractions among healthy teenagers (cohort 3, **Table 16.4**). The incidence of grades 1 and 2 attic retractions was even higher in adults who had had secretory otitis in their childhood. Although both groups had had secretory otitis and chronic tubal dysfunction, the severity and duration of the disease was more severe and more long lasting in the clinical series than in the cohorts.

The prevalence of more severe attic retractions (grades 3 and 4) in cohort 3 was the same—about 5%—from the age of 6 years to 16 years (**Tables 16.3** and **16.4**). In the clinical series the incidence of grade 3 and grade 4 retractions was slightly higher than the prevalence of grades 3 and 4 attic retractions in cohort 3, although the difference was not significant.

Two of the 278 children in series 1 developed cholesteatoma (0.6%), whereas 3 out of 178 ears developed cholesteatoma (1.7%), indicating a progression of some attic retractions to cholesteatoma.

Attic Precholesteatoma

Attic precholesteatoma is a condition with disturbed migration of the surface epithelial cells in the attic retraction pocket. This affects the self-cleaning property and eventually leads to accumulation of keratin within the retraction pocket.

Most grade 3 and 4 retractions are dry and maintain their self-cleaning. When the self-cleaning property is disturbed, the retraction pocket can become infected, leading to proliferation of the epithelial cells and formation of cholesteatoma.

The precholesteatoma condition can be treated conservatively by regular suction clearance of the retraction and local medical treatment using hydrocortisone–oxytetracycline and polymyxin eardrops or other steroid/antibiotic preparations.

Pathogenesis of Attic Cholesteatoma

The Retraction Theory (Bezold 1890) and the Papillary Proliferation Theory (Lange 1925; Ruedi 1979) cannot individually fully explain the pathogenesis of attic cholesteatoma. On the basis of epidemiological, clinical, and immunohistochemical studies, Sudhoff and Tos (2000, 2001) could explain the pathogenesis of attic cholesteatoma by combining the retraction and the papillary proliferation theories. We proposed four stages in the development of cholesteatoma.

Retraction Stage

As demonstrated in **Tables 16.3** and **16.4**, the prevalence and incidence of grades 1 and 2 attic retractions were relatively high, between 16% and 25% in cohort 3 and between 19% and 30% in the clinical series. The prevalence and incidence of more severe attic retractions (grades 3 and 4) was between 2% and 5% in cohort 3 and between 4% and 6% in the clinical series (**Tables 16.3** and **16.4**). In a small number of attic retractions, the keratinized epithelium proliferates, leading to the **interruption of the self-cleaning mechanism.**

Several **external factors** can induce or trigger the proliferation of the keratinized epithelium within the retraction pocket, such as external otitis with a high epithelial turnover. Cerumen lodged at the entrance of the retraction pocket or other blockage of debris transport can also cause an interruption of keratin migration. The resultant accumulation of keratin and debris within the retraction may lead to localized infection behind the crust. This local infection can in turn induce cone proliferation within the squamous epithelium. Clinically this condition can be regarded as precholesteatoma.

There are also **internal factors**, such as acute otitis media, that can also cause a high turnover of the epithelium, an increase in desquamation, and accumulation of keratin and debris within the retraction pocket. Dysfunction of the eustachian tube can also cause the retraction pocket to progress further.

Proliferation Stage

Local inflammation within the retraction will alter and increase the keratinocyte proliferation and lead to cone formation. The basal keratinocytes proliferate, which enhances proliferation of basal cells and results in active downgrowth and elongation of the cones. Within the prolonged cone the keratinization is altered, which results in an accumulation of keratin in the center of the cone and causes microcholesteatoma in the cone. Under the pressure of the keratin, the microcholesteatoma will expand in size and gradually fuse with the adjacent cones and lead to expansion of the cholesteatoma.

Expansion Stage

Fusion of several microcholesteatomas leads to expansion toward the surface lining of the retraction pocket. It may lead to the disappearance of the overlying keratinized epithelium. The cholesteatoma is then opened into the bottom of the retraction pocket, which in effect has grown deeper by one length of the cone. The surface of the retraction pocket is replaced in each cycle. As the process of proliferation of basal cells in the depth of the cones continues, new microcholesteatomas will continue to form, thus creating a vicious circle in the bottom of the retraction pocket: (1) Proliferation of keratinocytes at the bottom of the epithelial cones, expanding the cones in depth. (2) Increase of keratinocyte differentiation, leading to keratin formation and keratin lakes within the cones—microcholesteatomas. (3) expansion and fusions of the microcholesteatomas.

Bone Resorption

The fourth stage of cholesteatoma is bone resorption, which is most often a complication of cholesteatoma.

The Incidence of Cholesteatoma

In our surgical series the incidence of cholesteatoma is 15.5 cholesteatomas per year per 100 000 inhabitants. This calculation is based on 740 cholesteatomas operated in Gentofte hospital, Copenhagen, during 16 years in a population of 300 000 inhabitants. There were only 5.7 attic, 5.7 sinus, and 4.1 entire tensa retraction cholesteatomas per year per 100 000 inhabitants (Tos 1988). In a study in Iowa (Harker 1977), 6 cholesteatomas per 100 000 inhabitants per year were found. In a Finnish study (Kemppainen et al. 1999) based on 500 cholesteatomas operated during 1982–91 in two hospitals from the Tampere region, an annual incidence of 9.2 cholesteatomas per 100 000 inhabitants was found.

These figures indicate that attic retractions are more than 1000 times more common than attic cholesteatoma. Accordingly, prophylactic surgery should not be undertaken for small and asymptomatic attic retractions.

References

Bezold F. Cholesteatom, Perforation der Membrana flaccida und Tubenverschluss. Z Hals Nasen Ohrenheilkd 1890;20:5–29.

Couloigner V, Molony N, Viala P, Contencin P, Narcy P, Van Den Abbeele T. Cartilage tympanoplasty for posterosuperior retraction pockets of the pars tensa in children. Otol Neurotol 2003; 24:264–269.

Harker LA. Cholesteatoma: an incidence study. In: McCabe B, Sade J, Abramson J, eds. Cholesteatoma: First International Conference. Amsterdam: Kugler; 1977:308–312.

Kemppainen HO, Puhaka HJ, Laippala PJ, Sipilä MM, Manninen MP, Karma PH. Epidemiology and aetiology of middle ear cholesteatoma. Acta Otolaryngol 1999;119:568–572.

Lange W. Über die Entstehung der Mittelohrcholesteatoma. Z Hals Nasen Ohrenheilkd 1925;11:250–271.

Levinson RM. Cartilage-perichondrium composite graft tympanoplasty in the treatment of posterior marginal and attic retraction pockets. Laryngoscope 1987;97:1069–1074.

Poe DS, Gadre AK. Cartilage tympanoplasty for management of retraction pockets and cholesteatomas. Laryngoscope 1993;103: 614–618.

Ruedi L. Pathogenesis and surgical treatment of middle ear cholesteatoma. Acta Otolaryngol Suppl 1979;361:1–45.

Stangerup SE, Tos M, Arnesen R, Larsen P. A cohort study of point prevalence of eardrum pathology in children and teenagers from age 5 to age 16. Eur Arch Otorhinolaryngol 1994;251:399–403.

Sudhoff H, Tos M. Pathogenesis of attic cholesteatoma: clinical and immunohistochemical support for combination of retraction theory and proliferation theory. Am J Otol 2000;21:786–792.

Sudhoff H, Tos M. Pathogenesis of attic cholesteatoma. In: Magnan J, Chays A, eds. Cholesteatoma and Ear Surgery. Marseille: Label Production; 2001: 13–22.

Tos M. Epidemiology and spontaneous improvement of secretory otitis. Acta Otorhinolaryngol Belg 1983;37:31–43.

Tos M. Epidemiology and natural history of secretory otitis. Am J Otol 1984;5:459–462.

Tos M. Incidence, etiology and pathogenesis of cholesteatoma in children. Adv Otorhinolaryngol 1988;40:110–117.

Tos M, Poulsen G. Attic retractions following secretory otitis. Acta Otolaryngol 1980;89:479–486.

Tos M, Poulsen G, Borch J. Tympanometry in two-year-old children. Alteration of tympanograms at reevaluation. ORL 1978;40: 206–215.

Tos M, Stangerup SE, Hvid G, Andreassen UK. Epidemiology and natural history of secretory otitis. In: Lim D, Bluestone CD, Klein JO, Nelson JD, eds. Recent Advances in Otitis Media. Philadelphia: BC Decker; 1988: 29–34.

Tos M, Stangerup SE, Larsen PL, Siim C, Hvid G, Andeassen UK. The relationship between secretory otitis and cholesteatoma. In: Tos M, Thomsen J, Peitersen E, eds. Cholesteatoma and Mastoid Surgery. Amsterdam: Kugler; 1989:25–30.

Tos M, Hvid G, Stangerup SE, Andreassen UK. Prevalence and progression of sequelae following secretory otitis. Ann Otol Rhinol Laryngol 1990;99(149):36–48.

17 Total Pars Tensa Cartilage–Perichondrium Composite Island Graft Tympanoplasty

Definitions

The total pars tensa cartilage–perichondrium composite island graft consists either of one round disk (see **Fig. 17.1a**) or of two semicircular cartilage disks, or even of four disks, covered laterally by the perichondrium. The perichondrium also surrounds the cartilage as a 1–4 mm wide peripheral flap, which will be placed onto the denuded ear canal bone. The cartilage disk is suspended by the perichondrium flap.

There are principally four different shapes of the total pars tensa graft:
1. The round cartilage disk of 7–9 mm in diameter surrounded by the perichondrium (**Fig. 17.1a**).
2. The round cartilage disk with notches of various sizes and shapes to accommodate the malleus handle (**Fig. 17.2b**).
3. The Dornhoffer graft, which is primarily round, but with a 2 mm wide vertical strip of cartilage removed, creating a graft with two semicircular cartilage disks connected by strip of perichondrium (**Fig. 17.1c**).
4. The Jahnke graft with four 1.5–2.0 mm cartilage sections, separated by 0.2–0.4 mm belts without cartilage (**Fig. 17.1 d**). The grafts can be further shaped in relation to the actual situation. The belts without cartilage in the Jahnke graft can easily be enlarged and accommodated to the malleus handle. The various wedges can also be enlarged (Neumann and Jahnke 2005).

The Tolsdorff and the Nitsche Grafts

Tolsdorff (1983) was the first to apply a cartilage–perichondrium graft of diameter 6–10 mm to close large perforations of the pars tensa in cases with a disrupted ossicular chain. The graft is composed of three layers: there is a large perichondrium flap on the concave (ear canal) side of the cartilage disk, to be placed onto the ear canal bone; and the cartilage disk is covered with perichondrium on the tympanic side as well (**Fig. 17.2**). Tolsdorff believed that the presence of perichondrium on both sides improves nutrition of the cartilage.

Nitsche (1985) applied a round cartilage–perichondrium graft covered with perichondrium on the canal side only. Nitsche was also the first to use grafts with a notch to accommodate the malleus handle (**Fig. 17.3**).

Harvesting and Shaping of the Cartilage Graft

Tolsdorff (1983) used tragus cartilage, and made an incision on the tragus dome (see **Fig. 26.2a**); he elevated the subcutaneous tissue on both sides and removed a large piece of the tragus, together with the dome (see **Fig. 26.2b, c**). Often the scar and some deformity is visible, so most surgeons incise 2 mm medial to the dome of the tragus. The cartilage incision goes through both sides of the perichondrium and the cartilage. A 15 mm × 15 mm piece of the cartilage can be removed, leaving the tragal dome intact (see **Fig. 3.21**).

Nitsche (1985) applied the endaural approach of Heermann with an intercartilaginous incision of type B and harvested the tragal cartilage through the intercartilaginous incision. With a pair of scissors the subcutaneous tissue is cleaned from the posterior side of the tragus and then from the anterior side (**Fig. 17.4a**). The tragus cartilage is pulled through the intercartilaginous incision in superior direction and cut inferiorly and medially (**Fig. 17.4b, c**). A reasonably large piece of tragal cartilage can be harvested.

Dornhoffer (1997) prefers a large tragus cartilage because it is thinner than the conchal cartilage. He makes a large incision 2 mm medial to the dome. To maximize the length and width of the harvested cartilage, it is necessary to make the inferior cut as low as possible (**Fig. 17.5a**) The cartilage is then grasped and retracted inferiorly, which delivers the superior edge of the cartilage from the incision area (**Fig. 17.5b**). The superior edge and the superior portion are then dissected out while retracting, which produces a graft 15 mm long and 10 mm wide in children and somewhat larger in adults (**Fig. 17.5c**).

Shaping of the Tolsdorff Graft

The characteristic of the Tolsdorff graft is the perichondrium on both sides of the cartilage disk (**Fig. 17.2**). After exact measurement of the diameters of the tympanic cavity at the level of the bony annulus, the size of the cartilage disk is decided. Often it measures 9 mm. The surrounding perichondrium on the concave side of the tragus graft is elevated all the way around (**Fig. 17.6**) and the superfluous cartilage with the perichondrium from the opposite side is

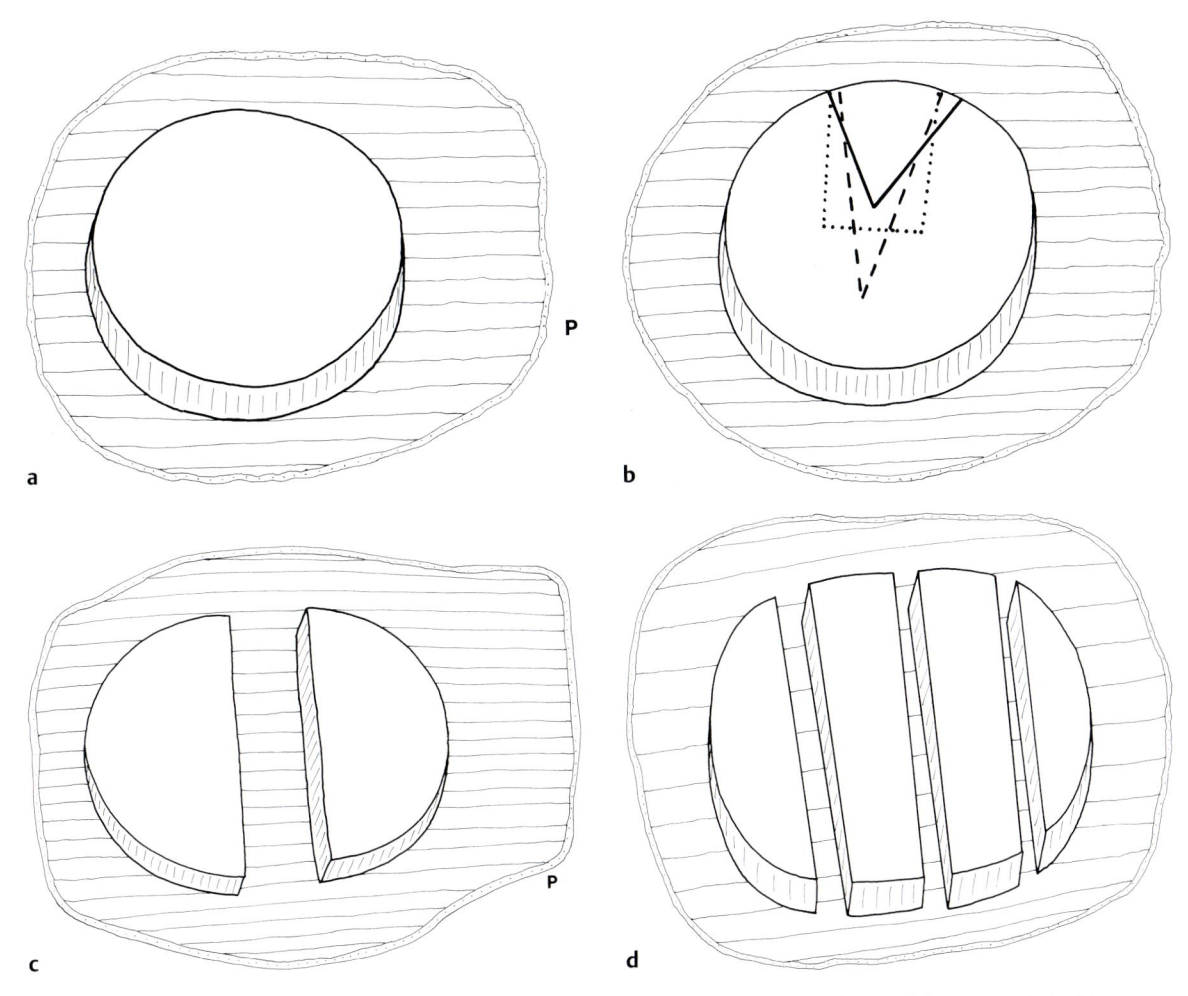

Fig. 17.1a–d Four shapes for the total pars tensa graft.
a   A large round cartilage–perichondrium composite graft with a diameter of 9 mm for closure of a total perforation. On the ear canal side, the cartilage disk is covered by the perichondrium surrounding the cartilage as a peripheral perichondrium flap. The posterior (P) perichondrium flap is usually larger than the anterior.
b   Three examples of the shape of the notch in a round cartilage disk: short V-shaped (solid line); long V-shaped (dashed line); rectangular (dotted line).
c   The Dornhoffer cartilage–perichondrium composite island graft, consisting of two semicircular cartilage disks for closure of a total perforation. Between the two disks there is a belt of 1–2 mm without cartilage, to accommodate the malleus. On the ear canal side the perichondrium covers the cartilage and continues in a peripheral flap that is considerably larger posteriorly (P) than anteriorly.
d   The Jahnke total pars tensa cartilage–perichondrium composite graft. It consists of four cartilage belts, separated by three 0.2–0.4 mm wide belts without cartilage. On the ear canal side the cartilage is covered by the perichondrium, which extends as a 1–1.5 mm wide peripheral flap.

removed piece by piece. The perichondrium on the convex (tympanic) side of the cartilage disk is not removed and serves to provide nutrition for the epithelium. The cartilage disk is suspended on the relatively large perichondrium flap (**Fig. 17.2**). Tolsdorff did not create a wedge for the malleus handle: he consequently removed the entire malleus!

Shaping of the Dornhoffer Graft

First the perichondrium from the anterior (convex) side of the graft is removed. Using a thin needle, a round disk with a diameter of 9–10 mm is marked. The disk is shaped in the anterior part of the graft, allowing a 1 mm long anterior and 5 mm long posterior perichondrium flap. With a round knife, the superfluous cartilage is removed (**Fig. 17.7a**). Finally, to accommodate the entire malleus handle, a strip of cartilage 2–3 mm in width is removed from the centre of the round disk (**Fig. 17.7b**). The creation of two cartilage

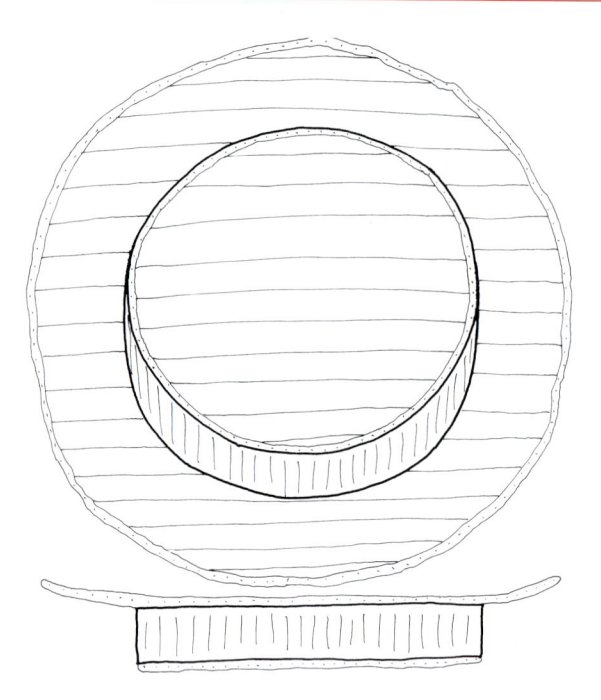

Fig. 17.2 The first total pars tensa perichondrium–cartilage composite island graft of Tolsdorff. The graft is harvested from the tragus and is covered on both sides with the perichondrium, which extends on the ear canal side as a perichondrium flap.

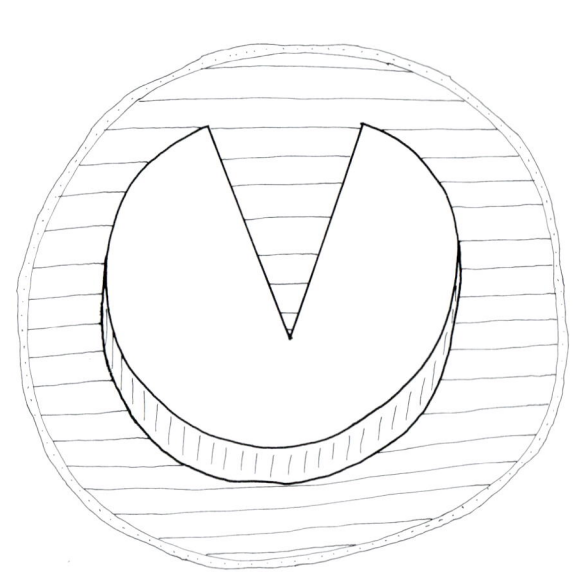

Fig. 17.3 The first total pars tensa cartilage–perichondrium composite graft of Nitsche, with the notch to accommodate the malleus handle. The cartilage is covered with the perichondrium on the ear canal side only, and the perichondrium extends as a peripheral flap.

islands in this manner is necessary to enable the reconstructed tympanic membrane to bend and conform to its normal conical shape. Sometimes Dornhoffer (1999, 2000) removes an upper posterior wedge to accommodate an eventual ossiculoplasty (**Fig. 17.7c**). The entire graft is placed in an underlay fashion, with the cartilage toward the promontory and the perichondrium adjacent to the tympanic membrane remnant, both of which are medial to the malleus (**Fig. 17.7 d**).

Klacansky Small Total Pars Tensa Composite Island Graft

Professor Jyraj Klacansky of Olomouc, Czech Republic, is in my opinion the most experienced cartilage tympanoplasty surgeon in Europe. Since the early 1990s he has performed about 7000 cartilage tympanoplasties, using mainly the total pars tensa composite island graft with a V-shaped notch, similar to the graft shown in **Fig. 17.1b** (Klacansky et al. 1998). In the earlier years the cartilage disks were

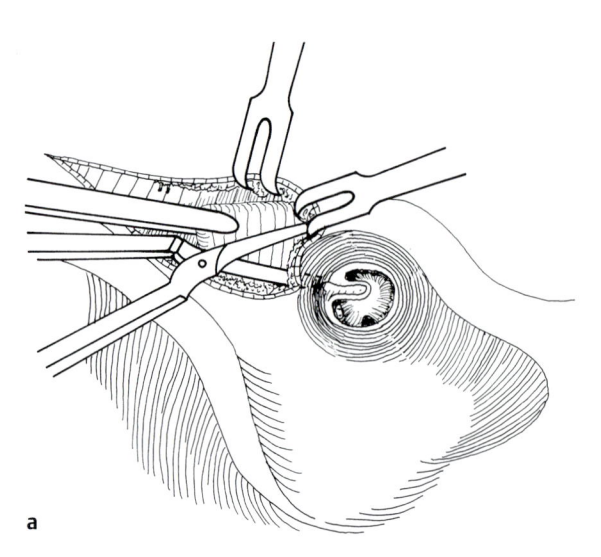

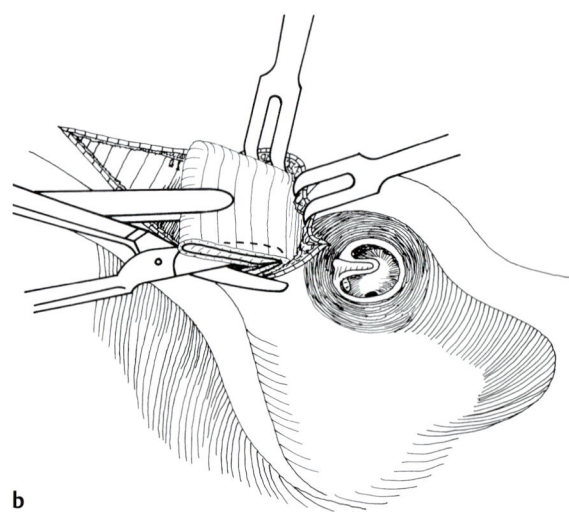

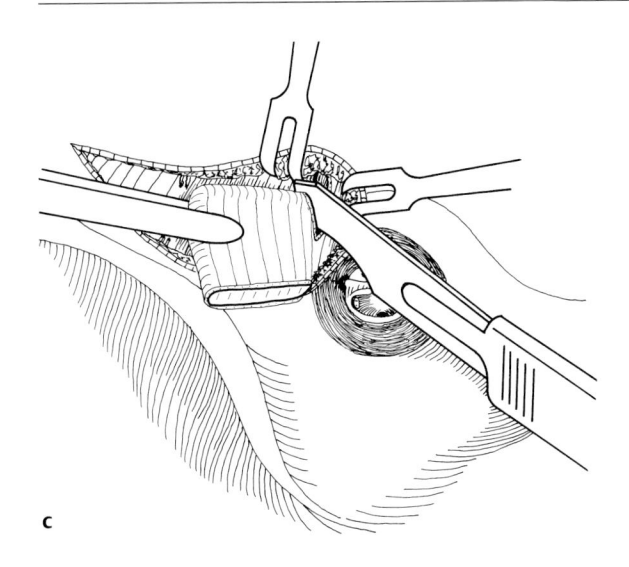

Fig. 17.4a–c Harvesting the tragus cartilage through the intercartilaginous incision in Hermann B endaural approach (Nitsche 1985).
a The superior edge of the tragus is first separated from the fibrous tissue of the intercartilaginous region. Then the tragus is grasped and pulled in superior direction, and the subcutaneous tissue is elevated from the dome anteriorly and posteriorly.
b The cartilage is cut along the medial border using a pair of scissors.
c A vertical incision made with a scalpel in the inferior part of the tragus completely mobilizes the tragal graft.

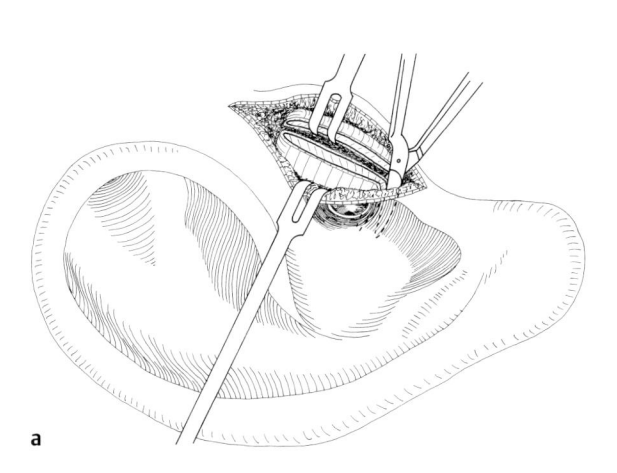

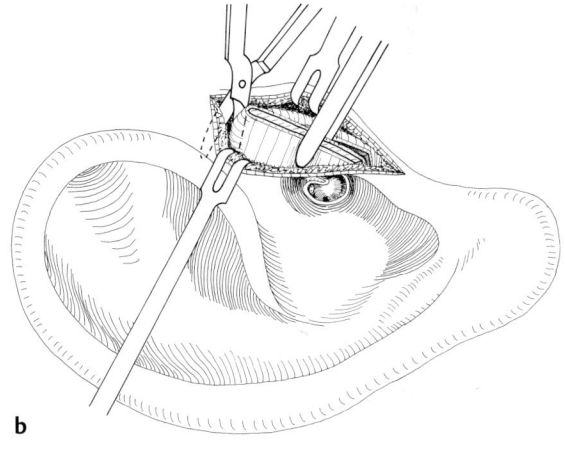

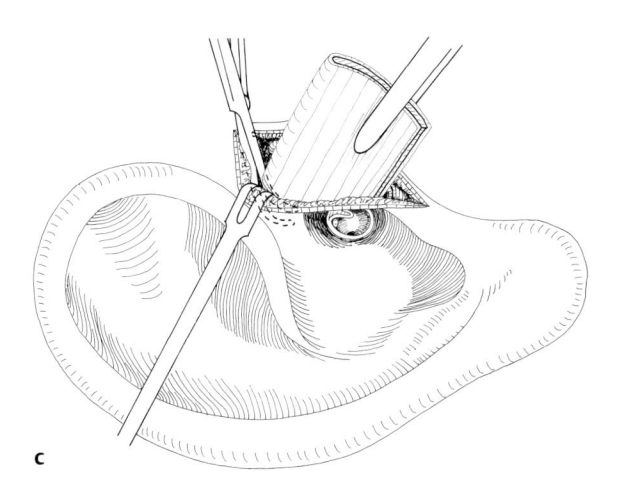

Fig. 17.5a–c Harvesting a large tragal graft to shape a Dornhoffer pars tensa cartilage–perichondrium composite graft.
a A skin incision is made and an incision through the cartilage with the perichondrium is made 2 mm medial to the tragal dome. The subcutaneous tissue is elevated on both sides of the tragus using a pair of scissors. Inferior vertical cuts are made with scissors to cut the cartilage as deeply as possible.
b The tragus is grasped with a pincette and pulled in lateral and inferior directions, which delivers the superior portion from the incisure. The superior edge of the tragus is separated from the fibrous tissue of the area of incisure.
c With scissors, medial cuts are made as deep as possible to separate the tragal graft completely.

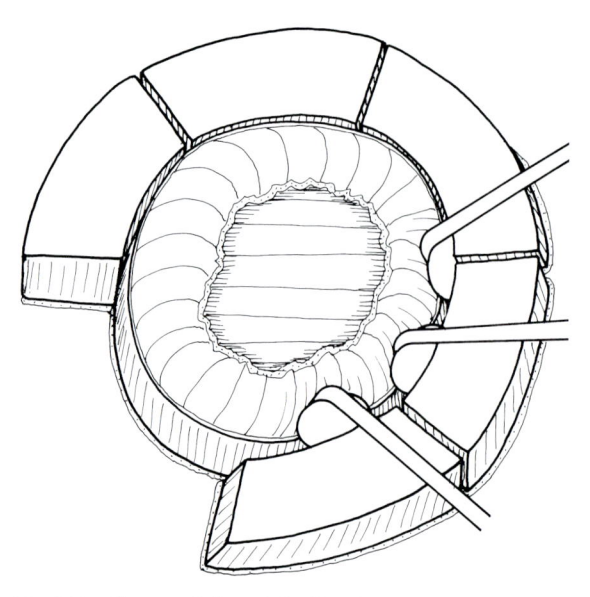

Fig. 17.6 Shaping of the Tolsdorff graft to close a total perforation. The tragal graft is placed with the convex (anterior) side on the table. The diameter of the cartilage disk is decided to be 9 mm. All the superfluous peripheral perichondrium is elevated, leaving the perichondrium attached to the 9 mm cartilage disk. Using a round knife, the cartilage and the perichondrium peripheral to the border of the cartilage disk are gradually removed all the way around, resulting in the graft shown in **Fig. 17.2**.

8–9 mm in diameter; since 2000 they have been only 6–7 mm because better hearing was obtained than with the larger graft (J. Klacansky, personal communication, 2008). The wedge is still the same, allowing the center of the disk to ride on the umbo and consequent better vibration of the graft. After elevation of the eardrum epithelium and the ear canal skin, the perichondrium flap is placed onto the denuded eardrum and onto the bony annulus.

Other Pars Tensa Composite Grafts

Spielmann and Mills (2006) used the "Mercedes-Benz" graft in four patients to reinforce the total retractions (**Fig. 17.8a**).

Shin et al. (2007) introduced the wheel-shaped cartilage–perichondrium composite graft (**Fig. 17.8b**). The graft is very flexible, with the possibility of placing a ventilation tube in one of the four cartilage segments. The edges of the four segments have direct contact with the umbo, transferring the vibrations to the malleus handle.

Indications for Surgery

The total pars tensa cartilage–perichondrium composite graft is used in ears with pathology involving the entire pars tensa and the entire tympanic cavity. The pathologies recommended for treatment with the pars tensa cartilage–perichondrium composite graft are:

- Total tensa retraction
- Atelectasis
- Adhesive otitis media
- Tensa retraction cholesteatoma
- Total perforation with poor tubal function or negative Valsalva
- Total perforation with thick moist middle ear mucosa
- Large perforation after several grommet insertions
- Recurrent total retraction
- Recurrent surgery in reconstruction of any major perforation
- Total perforation with the reconstruction of an old radical cavity

Surgical Techniques

Several techniques or modifications related to the shape of the composite island grafts have been published. The total pars tensa cartilage–perichondrium composite graft seems to be the most commonly used composite graft.

The Nitsche On-lay Technique

Nitsche (1985) operated all cases under local anesthesia, using the endaural approach with Heermann B, intercartilaginous incision (see MMES_1, Figs. 27–47). The description of the technique is poor; in total and subtotal perforation Nitsche (1985) used a **special on-lay technique** with outward elevation of the epithelium. The operation starts with the removal of the edges of the perforation and an incision across the malleus handle, allowing elevation of a malleus epithelium flap (**Fig. 17.9a**). The malleus flap is elevated first. To facilitate the elevation of the epithelium from the lamina propria and the fibrous annulus, five small radial incisions of the epithelium are made along the perforation (**Fig. 17.9b, c**). The Nitsche composite island graft with a V-shaped wedge (see **Fig. 17.3**) is placed onto the umbo (**Fig. 17.9d**) and the perichondrium flap is folded out onto the lamina propria, the fibrous annulus, and the ear canal bone (**Fig. 17.9e**). Perichondrium of the wedge covers the malleus handle, tightly closing the superior half of the eardrum (**Fig. 17.9f**). After replacement of the epithelial flaps and the malleus flap (**Fig. 17.9g**), this on-lay technique seems to be very convincing from the anatomical point of view, with double covering of the perforation: first the perichondrium flap, then the epithelial flaps (**Fig. 17.10**).

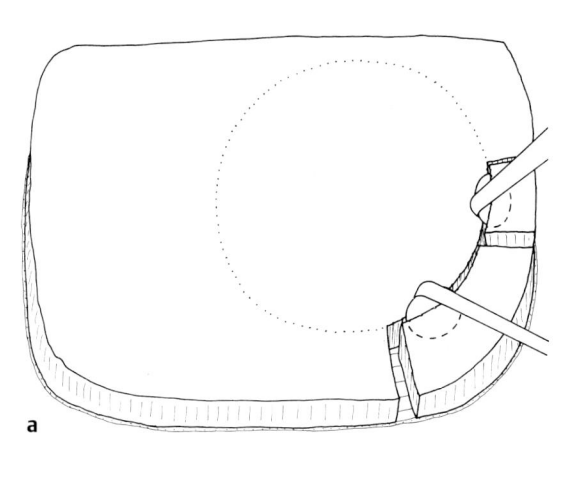

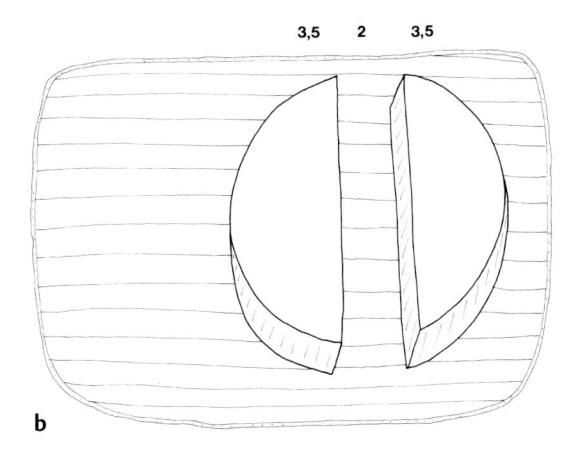

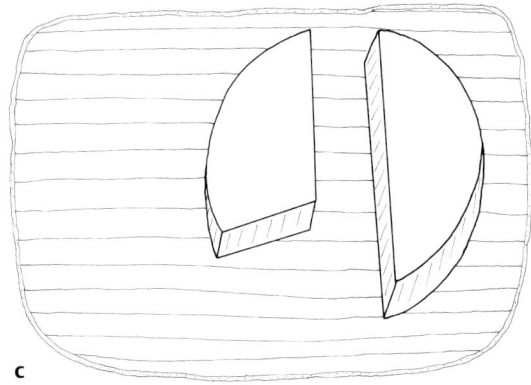

Fig. 17.7a–d Shaping of the Dornhoffer graft.

a Shaping of the graft starts with removal of the perichondrium from the convex anterior side. To achieve a large posterior perichondrium flap, the cartilage disk is cut asymmetrically on the large piece of the tragal cartilage. The exact position and size of the cartilage disk is indicated with a pick and the superfluous cartilage is then removed.

b The diameter of the overall cartilage disk is 9 mm. In the middle a 2 mm wide belt of the cartilage is removed, completing the shaping of the graft. The largest width of each of the two semicircular pieces is 3.5 mm. The anterior, inferior, and superior perichondrium flaps are short, the posterior flap is long.

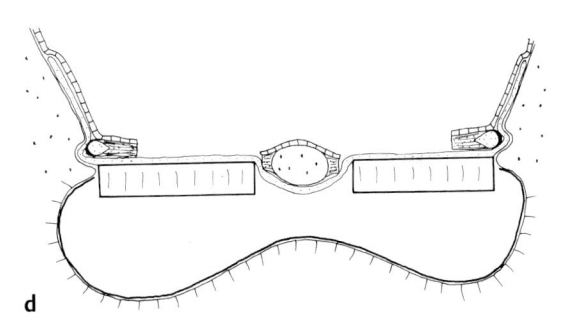

c A wedge of cartilage is removed from the superior end of the posterior semicircle, to accommodate ossiculoplasty. After placement of the graft into the tympanic cavity, the position of the missing wedge will be in the posterosuperior area.

d Side view of underlay placement of the Dornhoffer cartilage–perichondrium composite graft in a total perforation with intact ossicular chain. The perichondrium flap is placed onto the anterior, inferior, and posterior ear canal bone. The cartilage disk is placed at the level of the bony annulus. The central belt of perichondrium is placed under the malleus handle.

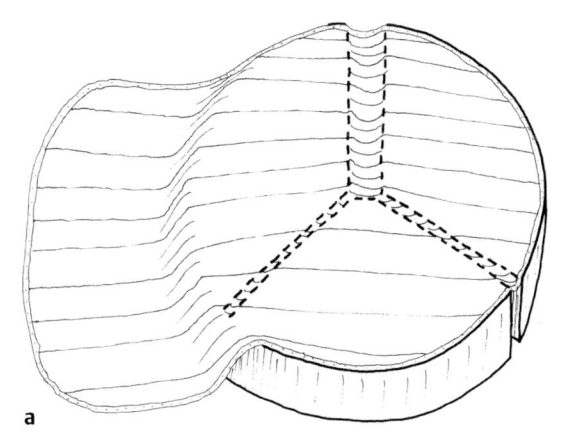

Fig. 17.8a, b Other pars tensa composite grafts.

a The "Mercedes-Benz" graft. A channel is created by removal of a strip of cartilage from the superior edge of the graft, extending inferiorly to its centre to accommodate the malleus handle. Two radial incisions are made from the inferior end of this channel. This means that the graft becomes conical (Spielmann and Mills 2006).

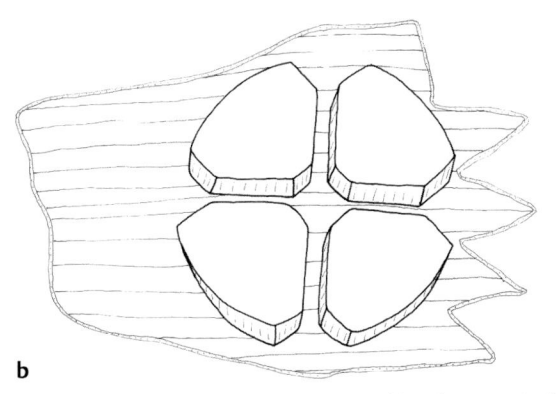

b The cartilage–perichondrium half-thickness composite graft for the prevention of development of retraction pockets (the "wheel" graft) (Shin et al. 2007).

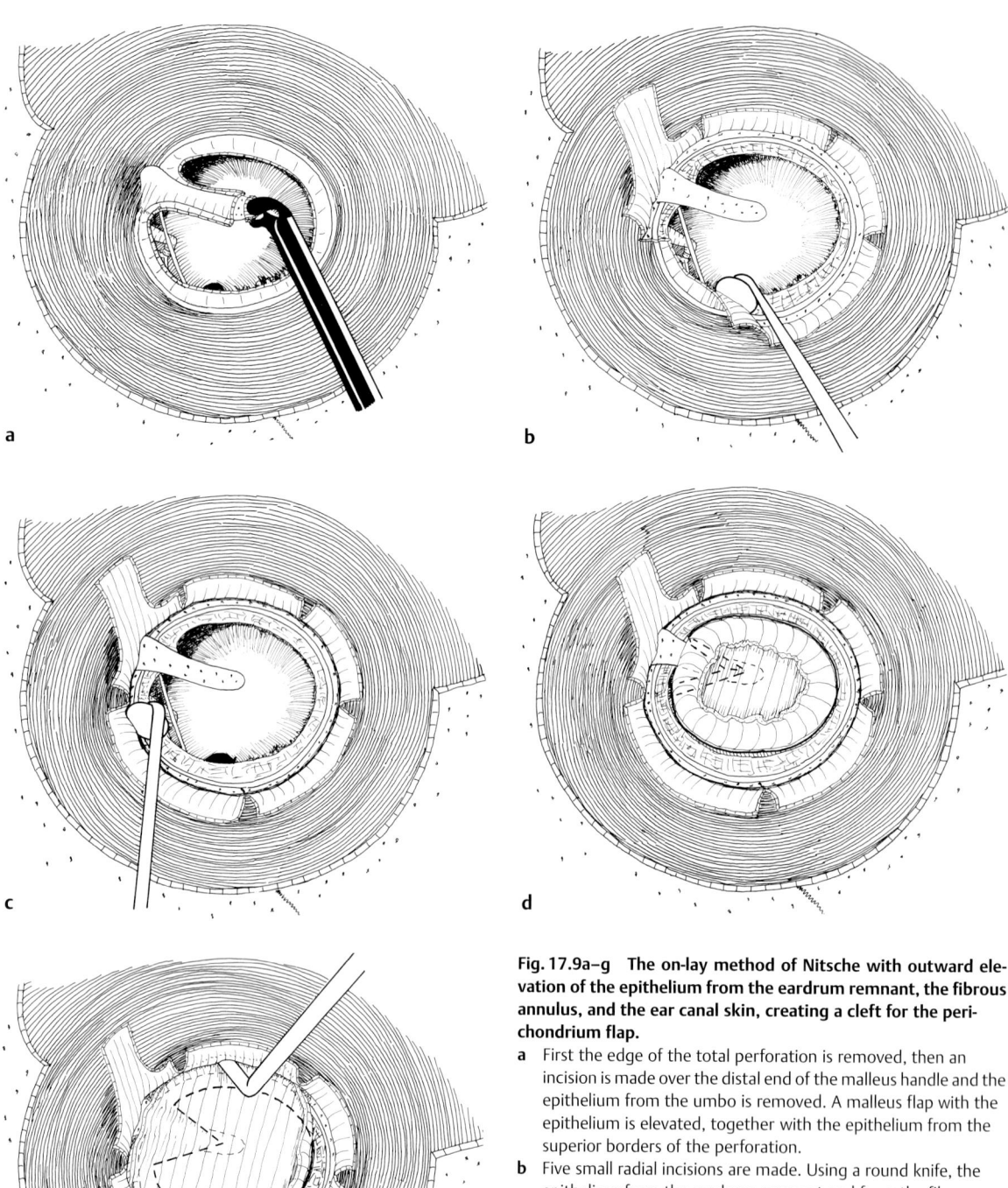

Fig. 17.9a–g The on-lay method of Nitsche with outward elevation of the epithelium from the eardrum remnant, the fibrous annulus, and the ear canal skin, creating a cleft for the perichondrium flap.

a First the edge of the total perforation is removed, then an incision is made over the distal end of the malleus handle and the epithelium from the umbo is removed. A malleus flap with the epithelium is elevated, together with the epithelium from the superior borders of the perforation.

b Five small radial incisions are made. Using a round knife, the epithelium from the eardrum remnant and from the fibrous annulus together with the ear canal skin is elevated all the way around, creating a cleft between the bone and the ear canal skin.

c Elevation of the eardrum epithelium and the ear canal skin is completed. A belt of the denuded ear canal bone and a cleft between the denuded bone and elevated ear canal skin are created all the way around.

d A cartilage disk with the perichondrium flap and a wedge for the malleus handle is placed into the tympanic cavity at the level of the lamina propria of the eardrum remnant and the fibrous annulus.

e The peripheral perichondrium flap is folded out, covering the lamina propria of the eardrum remnant, the fibrous annulus, and the denuded bone. The perichondrium is pushed into the cleft between the bone and the skin of the ear canal. The perichondrium of the wedge covers the malleus handle.

The Tolsdorff Technique

Tolsdorff applied the graft exclusively in connection with TORP and PORP, and, in case of defective ossicular chain, he always removed the remaining incus and the entire malleus, including the malleus handle.

First the edges of the total perforation are removed. In a retroauricular approach, with a large circumferential incision with a radial swing-door incision at the 9-o'clock position, two large tympanomeatal flaps are elevated. The undersurface of the eardrum remnant and the mucosa of the anterior and the inferior bony annulus are scarified, to facilitate attachment of the perichondrium flap (**Fig. 17.11a**). Superiorly, a malleus epithelium flap, together with the Shrapnell membrane as well as the epithelium along the fibrous annulus is elevated. The defective incus and the intact malleus are removed (**Fig. 17.11b**). In the 1980s Tolsdorff placed a polyethylene PORP; I recommend a titanium PORP (**Fig. 17.11c**). The island graft is placed onto the head of the prosthesis. It is positioned under the anterior scarified eardrum remnant. The anterior perichondrium flap is pushed under the anterior and inferior annulus (**Fig. 17.11 d**). Superiorly, the perichondrium flap is placed onto the bone, under the Shrapnell membrane and in the cleft between the bone and the skin. After replacement of the tympanomeatal flaps and the malleus flap (**Fig. 17.11e, f**), the epithelialization of the eardrum will take place.

The Würzburg Clinic Techniques

During the 1980s and 1990s, the Würzburg Clinic, Germany, under the leadership of professor Jan Helms, was the world-leading clinic in otosurgery, including cartilage tympanoplasty, in particular using cartilage–perichondrium composite grafts and palisades. Results of large series of ears, operated and reconstructed with cartilage–perichondrium composite grafts or with cartilage palisades, have been published by Milewski and co-workers (Milewski 1989,1991,1992, 1993; Milewski et al 1996). Many otologists from all over the world have visited the clinic, some for extended periods, and some, like Larry Duckert from the University of Washington, have been included in a scientific collaboration with the Würzburg Clinic on the problem of cartilage shield T-tube tympanoplasty (Duckert et al. 1995, 2003).

The most important part of the cartilage shield T-tube tympanoplasty, described in Chapter 20, is the elaboration of the appropriate cartilage–perichondrium composite graft and placement of the anterior perichondrium flap. The flap can be placed either under the anterior bony annulus, as shown in the Tolsdorff technique (**Fig. 17.11 f**) or onto the anterior bony annulus and onto the ear canal bone.

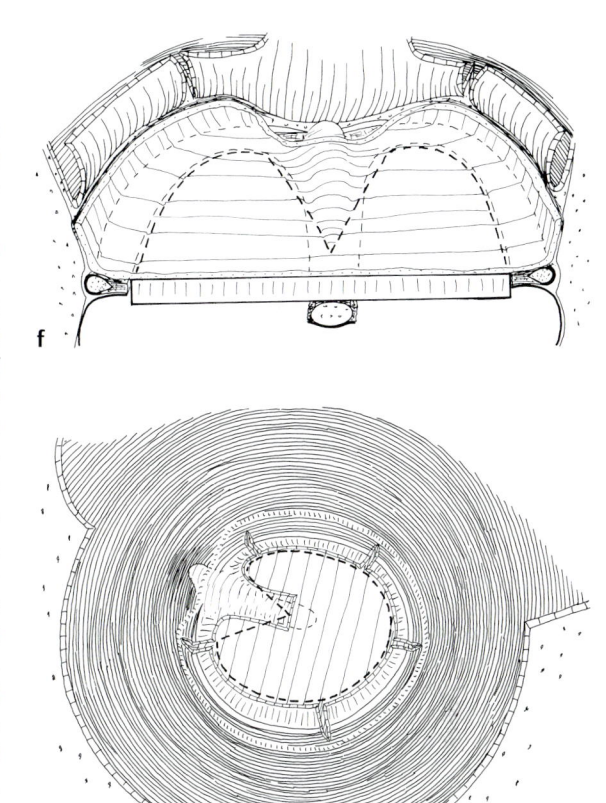

Fig. 17.9f, g
f Side view with some perspective to illustrate the on-lay placement of the perichondrium flap onto the fibrous annulus.
g The malleus flap, the ear canal skin, and the epithelium of the eardrum remnant are replaced.

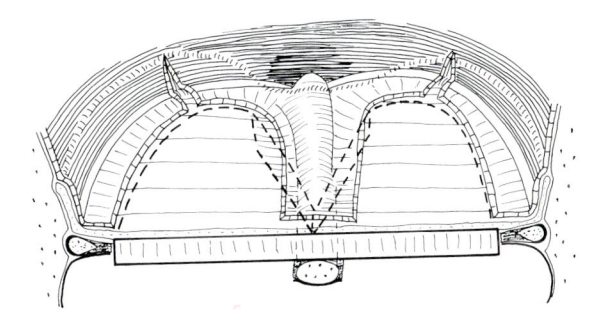

Fig. 17.10 Side view with some perspective, at the level of the umbo, of the on-lay cartilage–perichondrium composite island graft (Nitsche method). The cartilage disk is positioned at the level of the eardrum remnant; at the umbo region the cartilage disk is placed onto the umbo. The cartilage disk is suspended by the peripheral perichondrium flap, which covers the eardrum remnant, the fibrous annulus, and the ear canal bone.

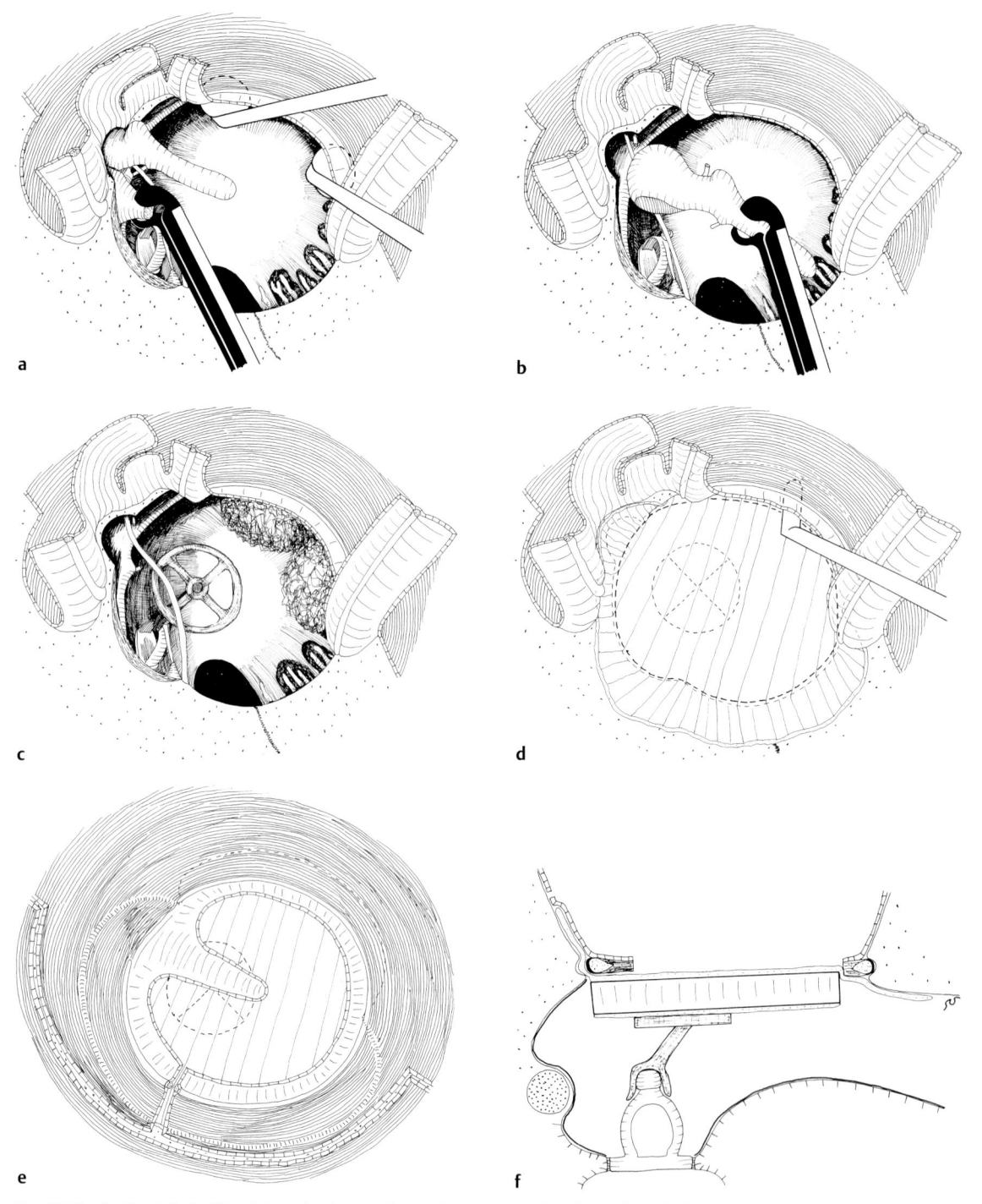

Fig. 17.11a–f The Tolsdorff technique in closure of a total perforation with the cartilage–perichondrium composite island graft and removal of the malleus.

a The inferior and superior tympanomeatal flaps and the malleus flap are elevated and the undersurface of the eardrum is scarified. The defective incus is removed.

b The ligaments of the malleus are cut and the entire malleus is pulled out and removed, saving the chorda tympani. The superior skin flaps are further elevated.

c A titanium PORP prosthesis is placed onto the head of the stapes. The head of the PORP is orientated toward the center.

d The composite graft with the perichondrium on both sides is placed onto the titanium prosthesis and suspended by the perichondrium flap, which is pushed under the anterior and inferior eardrum remnant. Superiorly and posteriorly the perichondrium is placed onto the ear canal bone.

e The malleus flap and the superior and posterior flaps are replaced.

f Side view of the Tolsdorff cartilage–perichondrium composite graft placed onto the Kurz titanium PORP prosthesis. The malleus and the incus are removed. The prosthesis is placed onto the stapes head; the island graft is placed onto the head of prosthesis; the anterior perichondrium flap is placed under the bony annulus, and the posterior flap is placed onto the bony annulus.

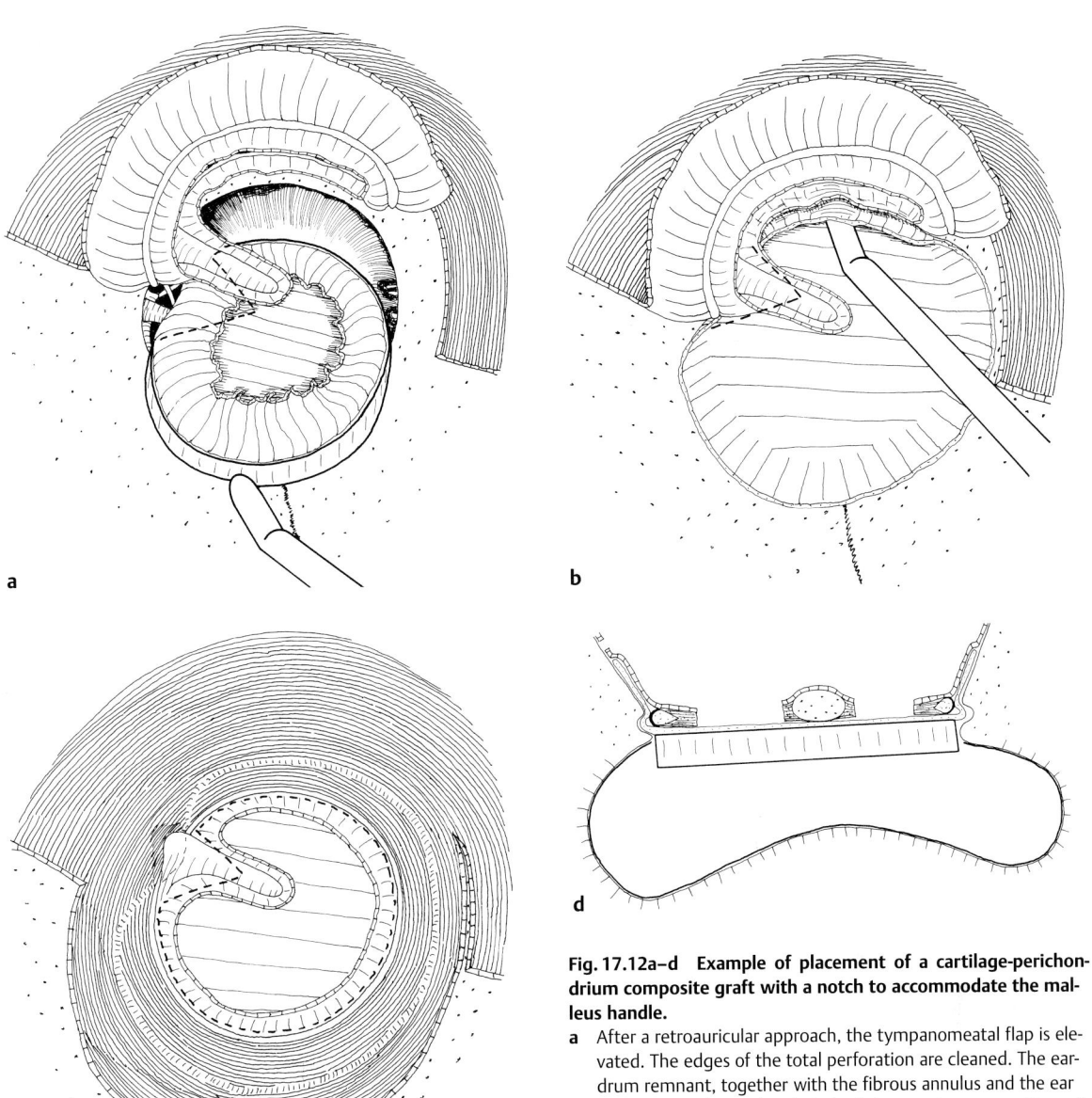

Fig. 17.12a–d Example of placement of a cartilage-perichondrium composite graft with a notch to accommodate the malleus handle.

a After a retroauricular approach, the tympanomeatal flap is elevated. The edges of the total perforation are cleaned. The eardrum remnant, together with the fibrous annulus and the ear canal skin, is elevated and a belt of the anterior ear canal bone is exposed. The composite graft is pushed under the malleus handle into the tympanic cavity.
b The posterior and inferior perichondrium flap is folded out; the anterior flap is pushed under the skin and under the elevated fibrous annulus.
c The tympanomeatal flap and the eardrum remnant are replaced.
d Side view, inferior to the notch, of the composite graft, placed under the malleus handle, closing a total perforation. The graft is suspended by the perichondrium flap, and placed onto the denuded anterior and posterior ear canal bone. The eardrum remnant is replaced.

Placement of the Perichondrium Flap onto the Bony Annulus

In order to suspend the composite graft from the bony annulus by the flap, the inferior and anterior eardrum remnants, with the fibrous annulus and some ear canal skin, have to be elevated (**Fig. 17.12a**). After placement of the composite graft under the malleus handle, the larger posterior perichondrium flap is easily folded out, but the anterior flap is pushed under the skin onto the denuded bone (**Fig. 17.12b**). After replacement of the eardrum remnant and the tympanomeatal flap (**Fig. 17.12c, d**), the reconstruction of the eardrum is solid and the epithelialization of the graft will be rapid.

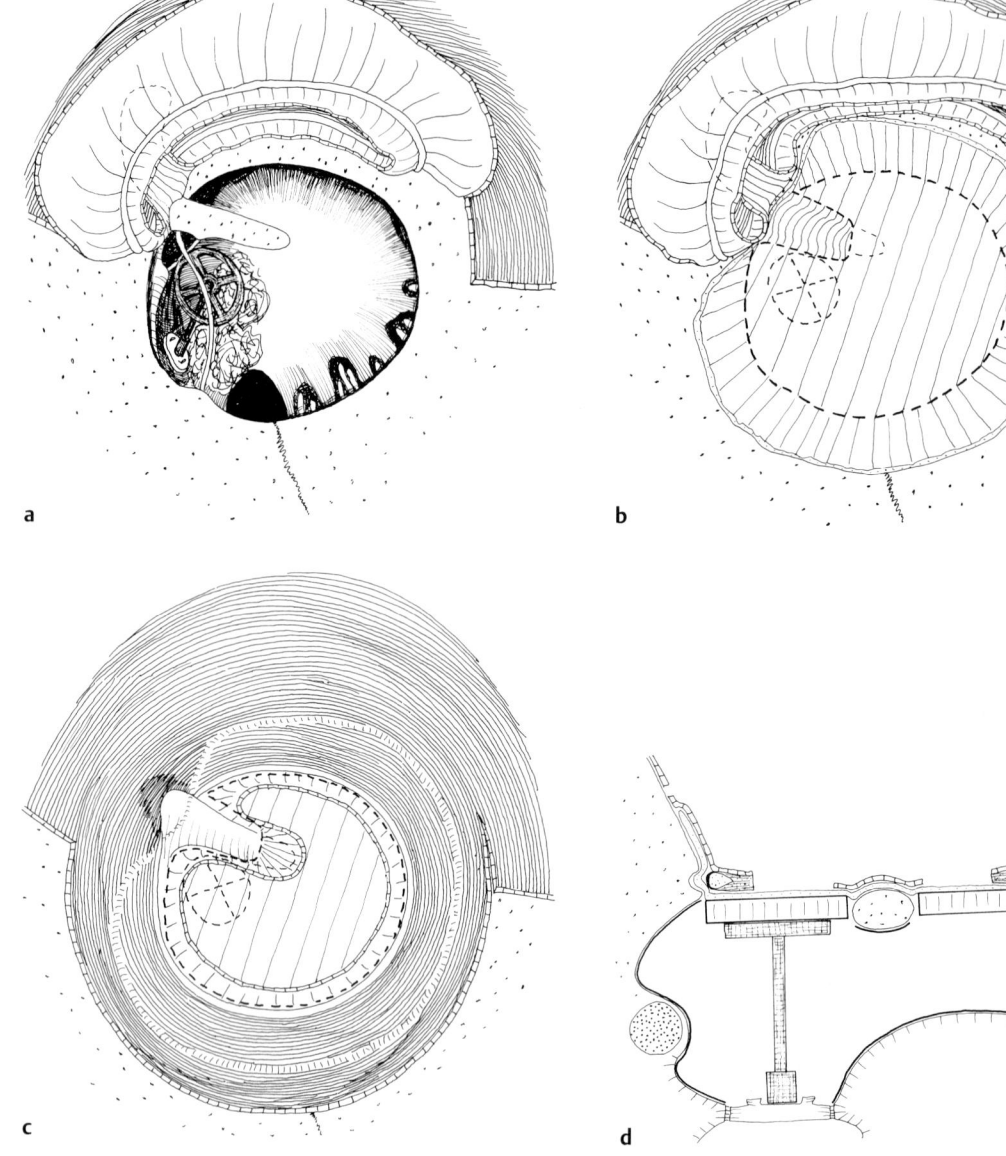

Fig. 17.13a–d Placement of the cartilage-perichondrium composite graft onto the malleus handle and the head of the titanium columella to close a total perforation.

a The edges of the total perforation are cleaned and the malleus flap is elevated. In a retroauricular approach, a large tympanomeatal flap is elevated. The inferior and anterior eardrum remnants with the fibrous annulus and the adjacent anterior ear canal skin are elevated, exposing the ear canal bone. A Kurz titanium columella is placed onto the footplate. The chorda and Gelfoam balls stabilize the columella.
b The composite graft with a notch to accommodate the superior part of the malleus handle is placed onto the umbo and the lower part of the malleus handle. The perichondrium flaps are folded out onto the anterior inferior, posterior, and superior parts of the ear canal bone. The perichondrium of the notch region covers the malleus.
c The malleus flap and the tympanomeatal flap with the eardrum remnant are replaced.
d Side view of tympanoplasty type 3 with a Kurz titanium columella and a cartilage–perichondrium composite graft placed onto the malleus handle. The perichondrium flap is placed onto the bone and covered by the skin.

The composite graft can also be placed onto the malleus handle, then the epithelium flap is elevated first from the malleus handle (**Fig. 17.13a**). After the placement of the island graft, with a notch, onto the head of the titanium columella, onto the inferior part of the malleus handle, and onto the umbo (**Fig. 17.13b**), the perichondrium flap covers the malleus, the entire bony annulus, and the adjacent ear canal bone. After replacement of the malleus flap and the eardrum remnant (**Fig. 17.13b, c**), the conditions for are good for rapid epithelialization.

The influence of the Würzburg ENT Clinic and of Professor Jan Helms on the development of techniques using the tensa cartilage–perichondrium island graft is seen in cartilage shield T-tube tympanoplasty (Duckert et al. 1995, 2003). This method is based on stable fixation of the total tensa cartilage–perichondrium composite graft with an implanted T-tube. These methods are thoroughly described in Chapter 20 (**Fig. 20.2** and **Figs. 20.12–20.19**), with some innovative improvements, such as:

- **Widening of the anterior annular sulcus,** in cases with atrophic, flat, or missing annular sulcus, by drilling a groove along the anterior bony sulcus, using a diamond drill (**Figs. 20.14, 20.15**).
- **Placement of the anterior perichondrium flap into the tympanic cavity.** This can be done by drilling a deep groove into the tympanic cavity, and leaving the anterior bony annulus intact (**Fig. 20.16a–d**).
- **Fixation of the anterior perichondrium flap in the deep anterior sulcus.** I propose additional obliteration of the deep new anterior sulcus with small palisades, fixating the inserted anterior perichondrium flap (**Fig. 20.16e, f**).

The Dornhoffer Technique

Dornhoffer (1997, 1999, 2000, 2003, 2006) often uses a retroauricular approach, with elevation of a large tympanomeatal flap, together with the elevation of the anterior eardrum remnant and the anterior fibrous annulus and a small belt of ear canal skin (**Fig. 17.14a**). Gelfoam balls are placed into the anterior part of the tympanic cavity, to support the graft. The Dornhoffer composite island graft is placed into the tympanic cavity. The central perichondrium is placed under the malleus handle. The large posterior perichondrium flap is folded out (**Fig. 17.14b**). The small anterior flap is carefully pushed under the elevated anterior ear canal skin and fibrous annulus (**Fig. 17.14c**) and then the anterior eardrum remnant and the posterior tympanomeatal flap with the eardrum is replaced (**Fig. 17.14 d**). A side view of this reconstruction has been illustrated previously (see **Fig. 17.7 d**).

Results of Surgery with the Total Tensa Composite Graft

Tolsdorff (1983) reported very good results among 87 ears operated during 4 years in the late 1970s for total perforation and defect ossicular chain. The tympanoplasty involved either a TORP or PORP prosthesis covered with the entire tensa composite cartilage–perichondrium graft. Apart from two extrusions of the prosthesis caused, at the beginning, by the use of too small cartilage grafts without perichondrium, no other extrusions of the prostheses, no recurrent perforations, and no retractions were observed.

In 28 patients the hearing was tested 3 years after surgery with very good results: 71 % had a complete closure of the air–bone gap. In 29 % of patients an air–bone gap of 9 dB was found in PORP cases and of 11 dB in TORP cases. The mean improvement of the air–bone gap was 24 dB in PORP patients and 22 dB in TORP patients.

No hearing results were presented for the other 59 patients.

It is important to compare cases in which the malleus was removed with cases with an intact malleus.

The First Würzburg Series (1982–1987)

The first reports on a large series with cartilage tympanoplasty were presented by Milewski (1989, 1991, 1992, 1993) on 550 patients, operated on the Würzburg Clinic, during the period from 1982 to 1987. In 331 patients the surgery was primary surgery and in 219 patients it was revision surgery.

Primary Surgery

The cartilage–perichondrium composite island graft technique was used in approximately half of the cases; in the other half the underlay palisade technique was used.

In 146 patients with **intact ossicular chain**, a postoperative air–bone gap in the range 0–10 dB was found in 41 %. The air–bone gap was poorer than 30 dB in 5 % of patients.

Among 185 patients with **disrupted ossicular chain**, the postoperative air–bone gap was in the range of 0–10 dB in 20 %, and poorer than 30 dB in 19 % of the patients.

Revision Surgery

Among 51 patients with **intact ossicular chain**, the air–bone gap improved to 0–10 dB in 51 %, and was poorer than 30 dB in 15 %.

Among 168 patients with **active chronic otitis media, or cholesteatoma and defective ossicular chain**, the air–bone gap was in the range 0–10 dB in 11 %, and poorer than 30 dB in 34 % of the patients.

Recurrent Perforations

In **dry ears**, recurrent perforation was found in 8.5 % with intact ossicular chain and in 3.5 % with disrupted ossicular chain and type 3 tympanoplasty. In **discharging ears**, the respective percentages were 28 % and 11 %. The poor anatomical results are mainly caused by severe pathology, with 219 revision cases.

There were no major differences between results with the composite island graft and with palisades.

The Second Würzburg Series (1989–1994)

Milewski et al. (1996) reported 5-year results in 415 patients after operation with total tensa cartilage–perichondrium island graft, performed during the period from January 1989 to June 1994.

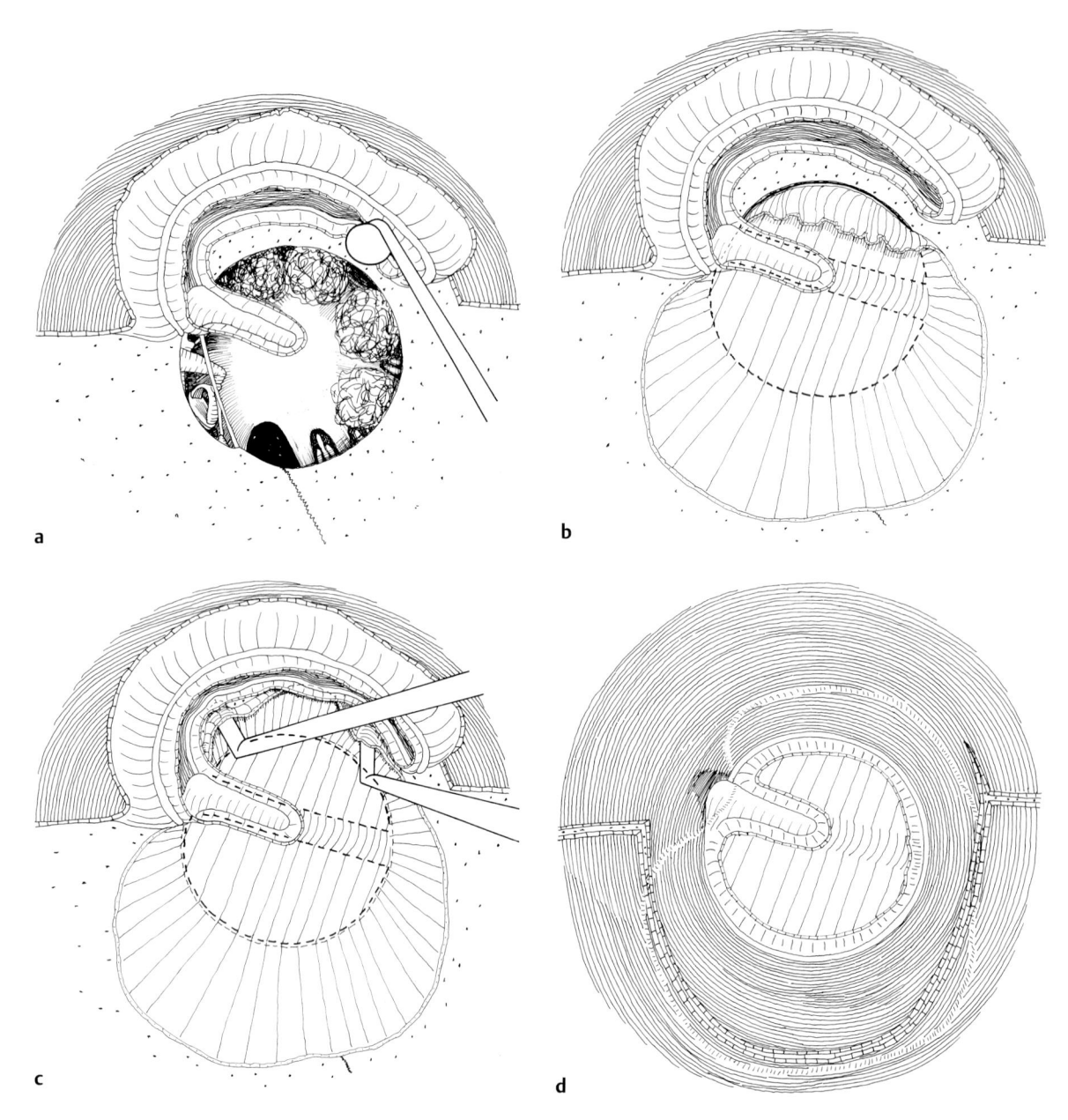

Fig. 17.14a–d The Dornhoffer cartilage–perichondrium composite island graft technique in a total perforation and an intact ossicular chain.

a In the retroauricular approach, the edges of the perforation are cleaned and a large tympanomeatal flap is elevated all the way around, exposing the bony annulus. Gelfoam balls are placed into the tympanic cavity.

b The Dornhoffer composite graft is placed into the tympanic cavity, with the central perichondrium strip under the malleus handle. The large posterior perichondrium flap is folded out over the posterior ear canal bone.

c The anterior perichondrium is folded out over the denuded anterior bony annulus and the anterior sulcus.

d The tympanomeatal flaps are replaced

Anatomical Results

Of 415 patients, 42 (10%) developed recurrent perforation. Among 45 patients with total perforation, 13.9% developed recurrent perforation. In 47 ears where the head of the prosthesis was not covered, re-perforation was found in 4.2%.

Audiological Results

Mean postoperative air–bone gap improved at most frequencies in all five groups of patients. The best improvement in air–bone gap was at the frequency 2000 Hz. Accordingly, the improvement of the air–bone gap will be illustrated for 2000 Hz only as preoperative/postoperative air–bone gap in dB.

1. Intact ossicular chain, 63 patients, 19/13 dB.
2. Island graft directly onto the stapes head, 24 patients, 26/15 dB
3. PORP onto the stapes head, 75 patients, 22/13 dB.
4. PORP and ear canal reconstruction, 58 patients, 20/17 dB
5. PORP and radical cavity, 45 patients, 23/18 dB
6. TORP, columella, 24 patients, 30/15 dB.

Thus, the best hearing was achieved, as expected, in closure of a total perforation in an intact ossicular chain, with a mean postoperative air–bone gap of 13 dB.

In the group with the PORP prosthesis, the postoperative air–bone gap was also good at 2000 Hz, but it was lower for the other frequencies, as it was in the series with intact ossicular chain.

The good air–bone gap after surgery in tympanoplasty with TORP was surprising.

The influence on postoperative hearing of the "on-lay in-lay" placement of the graft is also interesting. The perichondrium flap is placed onto the denuded lamina propria, but the cartilage disk is placed into the perforation, which is similar to the method initiated for small and middle-sized perforations (see Chapter 24).

The Dornhoffer Series

Dornhoffer's first report on total pars tensa cartilage–perichondrium composite graft in 22 patients with **total perforation and intact ossicular chain** showed improvement of the mean air–bone gap at frequencies 500, 1000, 2000, and 4000 Hz from a preoperative value of 17.9 dB to the 7.7 dB 13 months postoperatively. Preoperatively, 9% of patients had an air–bone gap of 0–10 dB, postoperatively 77%. In comparison with 20 similar patients with closure of the total perforation with perichondrium, the improvement of the postoperative air–bone gap was better in the cartilage group, but not significantly better mainly because of the small series (Dornhoffer 1997).

In a later report of 1000 cartilage tympanoplasty cases, Dornhoffer (2003) reported series of three types of tympanoplasty. The perforation was closed, either with total pars tensa island graft or with mosaic cartilage tympanoplasty (Chapter 9). The mean observation period was 2.7 years, range 3 months to 7 years.

Boone et al. (2004) showed good results in revision tympanoplasty cases using the Dornhoffer graft in 95 patients, with successful closure of perforations in 95% of cases.

Tympanoplasty Type 1 with Intact Ossicular Chain

In 226 available cases (out of 319), the mean preoperative PTA-ABG was 16.1 dB, and the postoperative value was 11.3 dB. Surgery was revision surgery in 28% of the ears.

Tympanoplasty Type 2 with a PORP Prosthesis Placed onto the Stapes

In 252 available cases (out of 499), the mean preoperative PTA-ABG was 26.7 dB, and the postoperative value was 14.5 dB. Revision cases accounted for 43%.

Tympanoplasty Type 3 with a TORP Prosthesis Placed onto the Footplate

In 158 available cases (out of 282), the mean preoperative PTA-ABG was 34.4 dB, and the postoperative value was 16.6 dB. Revision cases accounted for 72%.

Overall Hearing Outcome

In 712 available cases, the mean preoperative PTA-ABG was 25.7 dB, and the postoperative value was 14.1 dB, representing a statistically significant improvement in hearing for the total and also separately for the three tympanoplasty types. Revision cases accounted for 48%.

Complications

Perforations 2.2%; conductive hearing loss requiring revision surgery 3.3%; postoperative tube insertion 4.4%; intraoperative tube insertion 6.0%; prosthesis extrusion 0.5%. Recurrent cholesteatoma was seen in 1.6%, or in 3.6% of the 220 cases where the cholesteatoma was the primary surgical indication. In three cases a delayed, slight facial nerve paresis was seen that recovered spontaneously.

Outcomes by Surgical Indication

Cholesteatoma

Out of the 636 cases included for assessment, 220 were cholesteatomas (100 in children 120 in adults). Of these cholesteatoma cases, 40% were revision cases. The average follow-up time was 4 years 11 months. The average preoperative PTA-ABG was 26.5 dB, and the postoperative value was 14.6 dB. Recurrent cholesteatoma was found in 3.6% of cases. Revisions because of conductive hearing loss (mainly because of displacement of the prosthesis), was performed in 1.8% of cases.

Perforation

Perforation was the reason for operation in 215 cases (129 children, 86 adults); 45% of cases were revision surgery.

The preoperative PTA-ABG was 21.7 dB, and the postoperative value was 11.9 dB. Recurrent perforation was found in 4.2 % of ears. Most perforations were found between the anterior border of the perforation and the anterior annulus. Two ears showed complete dissolution of the cartilage graft; they were later reconstructed using cartilage palisades.

Atelectasis

Atelectasis was a surgical indication in 98 cases; 21 % were revision cases. Preoperative PTA-ABG was 20.2 dB, and the postoperative value was 14.2 dB. Complications were few: perforation in 1 %, conductive hearing loss in 2 %. An intraoperative ventilation tube was inserted in 12 % of cases.

Audiological Indications

One hundred and three cases (36 children and 67 adults) were operated to improve hearing; 77 % were revision surgeries. There had been various types of previous surgery, most often canal wall down surgery without reconstruction. The average preoperative PTA-ABG was 33.6 dB, and the postoperative value was 14.6 dB. Recurrent conductive hearing loss was found in 11 %, in half of them the cartilage island graft was used in a missing malleus situation (Dornhoffer 2003).

In all four disease conditions, the improvement of hearing was statistically significantly improved, and there were relatively few complications.

During a 2-year period 1996–1997, Klacansky et al. (1998) operated 372 patients: 77 with palisades, 47 with the annular graft, and 248 with total pars tensa cartilage–perichondrium composite island graft. In all cases the cartilage grafts were incorporated and could be re-used in case of a surgical revision. Marginal crevices were found in 25 cases (7.5 %). The defect can be eliminated by a special packing, as shown in **Fig. 18.19j**.

Pediatric Series

El-Hennawi (2001) placed the total Dornhoffer composite graft under the eardrum remnant in 30 children with various types and sizes of perforations. There were 8 anterior, 6 subtotal, 10 central (inferior) and 6 posterior perforations. El-Hennawi placed the perichondrium under the eardrum and the two semilunar cartilage disks under the perichondrium. The take rate 2 years after surgery was 86.6 % and the hearing 1 year after the operation was improved by more than 10 dB in 90 % of children, without relation to the size or type of the perforation.

In 28 children with a posterior perforation, Couloigner et al. (2003) used the total pars tensa cartilage–perichondrium composite graft placed under the eardrum and the perichondrium flap on the anterior and posterior ear canal wall. With such total reinforcement of the entire tympanic membrane, the recurrence rate was 6 %. The authors found better results in posterior retraction using total composite graft and total reinforcement of the eardrum than using a posterior composite graft. Similar results were found by Roger et al. (1994) and by Charachon et al. (1996).

In an "Ear Camp" for children in Namibia, 38 children were operated for total perforations using a total cartilage–perichondrium composite graft similar to the Dornhoffer graft with a notch (see **Fig. 17.7c**) to accommodate the malleus handle and the posteriosuperior ossiculoplasty. Preoperatively, all ears had perforation and were discharging; postoperatively, perforation of the eardrum was found in total in five ears caused by continuing discharge. The average hearing gain at 250–4000 Hz was 15 dB (Lehnerdt et al. 2005).

Comparison of the Cartilage–Perichondrium Graft with the Fascia Graft

Kirazli et al. (2005) carried out the first comparison of the results of the total pars tensa graft in two groups of patients with identical pathology. One group of 15 ears with intact ossicular chain and a subtotal perforation was treated with total cartilage–perichondrium composite underlay graft. In the other group, of 10 similar ears, the perforation was closed by the underlay fascia graft. The mean postoperative gain of the air–bone gap for the four frequencies 500, 1000, 2000, and 4000 Hz, was 11.9 dB for the cartilage group and 11.5 dB for the fascia group. The composite graft was shaped from a large piece of tragus cartilage with the dome and with perichondrium on both sides. The perichondrium from the convex side was elevated to the dome and served as a large posterior flap. The graft had a rectangular notch, shown in **Fig. 17.1b** as a dotted line. Kirazli et al. concluded that cartilage is the ideal grafting material in problem cases; the comparability of its acoustic properties, especially in the form of cartilage island, to those of fascia will allow more liberal application in less severe cases, in which functional outcome is more essential.

Shin et al. (2007) used their "wheel" graft in 47 patients to prevent retraction in connection with one stage intact canal wall mastoidectomy for total or near-total perforation, cholesteatoma, and chronically discharging ears. The half-thickness tragus–perichondrium composite graft (see **Fig. 17.8b**) is placed under the eardrum and the perichondrium is placed onto the bony annulus in the same manner as in the Dornhoffer technique (**Fig. 17.14a–d**). Postoperative retractions developed in 6.7 % of cases; postoperative protrusion of the PORP prosthesis and lateral healing of the eardrum were each found in one case. The average air–bone gap decreased from 30.0 dB to 24.0 dB. The mean air conduction thresholds decreased from a preoperative level of 47.3 dB to a level of 35.7 dB.

Series with Posterior and Total Pars Tensa Grafts

Several authors have reported results with posterior pars tensa composite grafts and with total pars tensa composite grafts (Florant et al. 1987; Mills 1991; Roger et al. 1994; Yung 1997). The results for posterior pars tensa grafts are briefly described in Chapter 15. The results with total composite grafts were acceptable, but Yung (1997) found poorer results with total pars tensa grafts than with posterior pars tensa grafts.

Author's Comments and Recommendations

The composite grafts with cartilage-free belts, such as the Dornhoffer graft and the Jahnke graft, are flexible during insertion and can easily accommodated to the size of the cavity and to the malleus handle. Dornhoffer apparently did not find particular retractions along the malleus handle.

Dornhoffer (2003) indicates poorer results in placement of the cartilage island graft in situations with the malleus absent. My opinion is the same, and the results of reconstruction of the eardrum with missing malleus have always been poorer in any type of grafting. Thus, the malleus handle should be and can be preserved in any situation.

It is interesting that the half-thickness "wheel" composite graft of Shin et al. (2007) has the poorest postoperative hearing. Experimental research suggests that the hearing should be better with the half-thickness graft than with a full-thickness graft.

It is a pity that the largest series of Milewski and of Dornhoffer did not separate the results achieved with total pars tensa composite graft from those with cartilage palisades. We do not yet know which method is the better, but it will always be difficult to collect comparable clinical series.

I fully agree with the conclusion of Kirazli et al. (2005). We know that cartilage is more resistant than fascia. We also know that the risk of recurrent retraction is larger after grafting of a retraction with fascia than after grafting with cartilage. If the postoperative hearing after grafting with cartilage is as good as after fascia, the indications for cartilage tympanoplasty may become wider and more liberal.

References

Boone RT, Gardner EK, Dornhoffer JL. Success of cartilage grafting in Revision tympanoplasty without mastoidectomy. Otol Neurotol 2004;25:678–681.

Couloigner V, Molony N, Viala P, Contencin P, Narcy P. Van Den Abbeelet. Cartilage tympanoplasty for posterosuperior retraction pockets of the pars tensa in children. Otol Neurotol 2003;24:264–269.

Charachon R, Lavieille JP, Boulat E, Verdier N. Le traitement chirurgical des poches de retraction. Revue Officielle de la Société Francaise d'ORL 1996;36:18–20.

El-Hennawi DM. Cartilage perichondrium composite graft (CPCG) in pediatric tympanoplasty. Int J Pediatr Otorhinolaryngol 2001;59:1–5.

Dornhoffer JL. Hearing results with cartilage tympanoplasty. Laryngoscope 1997;107:1094–1099.

Dornhoffer JL. Surgical modification of the difficult mastoid cavity. Otolaryngol Head Neck Surg 1999;120:361–367.

Dornhoffer JL. Surgical management of the atelectatic ear. Am J Otol 2000;21:315–321.

Dornhoffer J. Cartilage tympanoplasty: indications, techniques, and outcomes in a 1000 patient series. Laryngoscope 2003;113:1844–1856.

Dornhoffer JL. Cartilage tympanoplasty. Otolaryngol Clin North Am 2006;39:1161–1176.

Duckert LG, Müller J, Makielski KH, Helms J. Composite autograft "shield" reconstruction of remnant tympanic membranes. Am J Otol 1995;16:21–26.

Duckert LG, Makielski KH, Helms J. Prolonged middle ear ventilation with the cartilage shield T- tube tympanoplasties. Otol Neurotol 2003;24:153–157.

Florant A, Trang M, Jaulin JF, Baril C, Roulleau P. Poches de retraction tympaniques-bilan a 3 ans de notre attitude therapeutique. A propos de 106 cas. [Tympanum retraction pockets: results of treatment, 106 cases with 3-year follow-up]. Ann Otolaryngol Chir Cervicofac 1987; 104:519–533.

Kirazli T, Bilgen C, Midilli R, Ôğüt F. Hearing results after primary cartilage tympanoplasty with island technique. Otolaryngol Head Neck Surg 2005;132(6):933–937.

Klacansky J, Kucera J, Starek I. Rekonstrukcija blanky bubienka chrupkovymi transplantati. [Reconstruction of the eardrum with cartilage transplants] Otolaryngol (Prague) 1998;47:59–63.

Lehnerdt G, van Delden A, Lautermann J. Management of an "Ear Camp" for children in Namibia. Int J Pediatr Otorhinolaryngol 2005;69:663–668.

Milewski C. Fascia or perichondrium/cartilage in tympanoplasties. A comparative study regarding hearing results and recurrence of perforations in 1529 cases. In: Tos M, Thomsen J, Peitersen E. Cholesteatoma and Mastoid Surgery. Kugler: Amsterdam; 1989:1201–1204.

Milewski C. Ergebnisse der Tympanoplastik nach Verwendung von Knorpel-Perichondriumtransplantaten zum Trommelfellersatz unter ungünstigen Bedingungen. Laryngorhinootologie 1991;70:402–404.

Milewski C. Perichondrium–cartilage composite grafts in tympanomastoid surgery. In: Nakano Y, ed. Cholesteatoma and Mastoid Surgery. Amsterdam: Kugler; 1992:611–613..

Milewski C. Composite graft tympanoplasty in the treatment of ears with advanced middle ear pathology. Laryngoscope 1993;103:1352–1356.

Milewski C, Giannakopoulos N, Müller J, Schön F. Das Perichondrium-Knorpelinsel-Transplantat vom Tragus in der Mittelohrchirurgie. HNO 1996;44:235–241.

Mills RP. Management of retraction pockets of the pars tensa. J Laryngol Otol 1991;105(7):525–528.

Neumann A, Jahnke K. Trommelfellrekonstruktion mit Knorpel. Indikationen, Techniken und Ergebnisse. HNO 2005;53:573–586.

Nitsche O. Tragusperichondrium und -Knorpel bei der Tympanoplastik. Bericht über 2500 Operationen durch niedergelassenen HNO-Arzt. HNO 1985;33:455–457.

Roger G, Bokowy C, Coste A. Tympanoplastie avec greffon chondro-perichondral. Indications, techniques et results A propos dune serie de 127 tympanoplasties. Ann Otolaryngol Chir Cervicofac 1994;111:29–34.

Spielmann P, Mills R. Surgical management of retraction pockets of the pars tensa with cartilage and perichondrial grafts. J Laryngol Otol 2006;120:725–729.

Shin S-H, Lee W-S, Kim H-M, Lee H-K. Wheel shaped cartilage-perichondrium composite graft for the prevention of retraction pocket development. Acta Otolaryngol 2007;127:25–28.

Tolsdorff P. Tympanoplastik mit Tragusknorpel-Transplantat: "Knorpeldeckel-Plastik. Laryngol Rhinol Otol (Stuttg) 1983;62:97–102.

Yung MW. Retraction of pars tensa—long term results of surgical treatment. Clin Otolaryngol 1997;22:323–329.

18 Annular Cartilage–Perichondrium Composite Graft Tympanoplasty

Definition

The annular cartilage–perichondrium composite graft is a 1.5–3 mm wide, horseshoe-shaped (**Fig. 18.1**) or circular (**Fig. 18.2**) or U-shaped (**Fig. 18.3**) cartilage ring attached to perichondrium, which continues as a circumferential peripheral extension. The cartilage ring of the annular graft is placed either onto the fibrous annulus or onto the bony annulus or into the tympanic cavity at the level of the bony annulus. The central perichondrium serves as the eardrum and is placed either under or onto the malleus handle. The peripheral perichondrium is placed onto the bone of the ear canal, suspending and stabilizing the cartilage ring.

The shape of the cartilage used differs according to the pathology in the middle ear: In the case of total perforation and missing malleus and incus, a complete circular annular graft can be applied to include the region of the Shrapnell membrane as well (**Fig. 18.2**). In a subtotal or inferior perforation a U-shaped annular graft (**Fig. 18.3**) may be used.

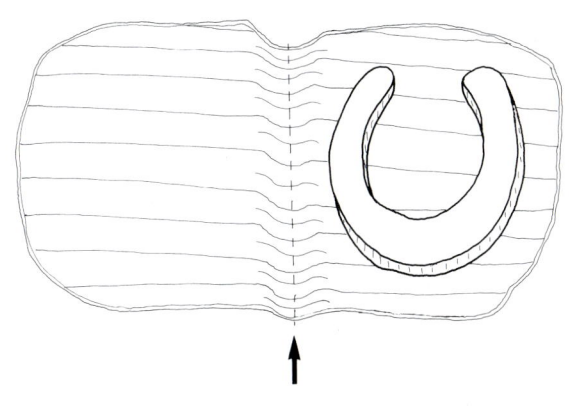

Fig. 18.1 Horseshoe-shaped annular cartilage-perichondrium composite graft (Goodhill 1967). The very first compound cartilage-perichondrium graft. A large piece of tragal cartilage with the perichondrium attached on both sides is removed. Perichondrium from one side is elevated and removed along the dashed line. Cartilage around the periphery is removed using a round knife, creating the outer borders of the graft. The inner borders are created similarly.

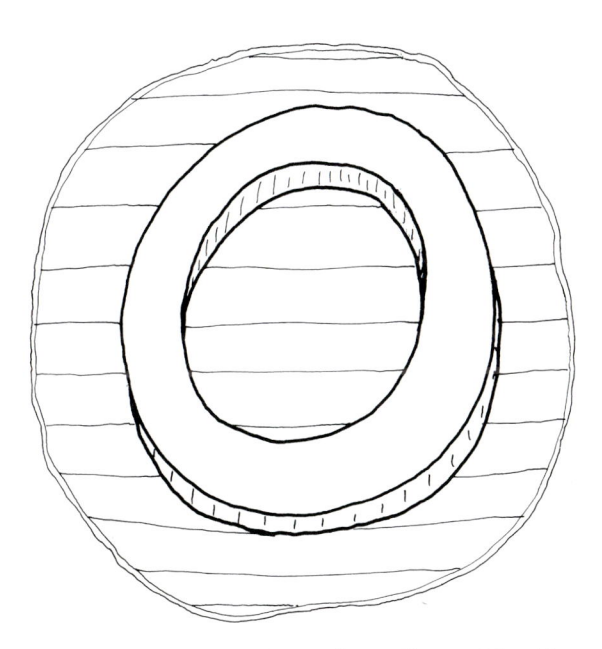

Fig. 18.2 A complete circular annular cartilage-perichondrium graft, used in the case of a total perforation with missing malleus and incus.

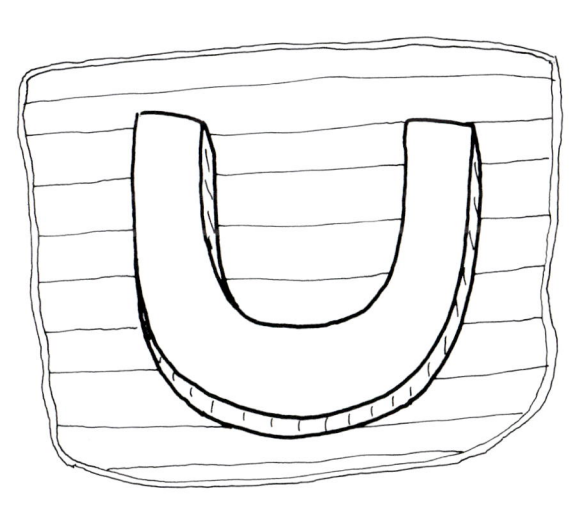

Fig. 18.3 A U-shaped annular graft to be used in a subtotal perforation.

Previous Applications of the Annular Graft

Goodhill (1967) was the first surgeon to apply an annular graft. In fact the very first composite cartilage–perichondrium graft was the annular graft (Chapter 1, **Fig. 1.12**). Goodhill called it a cartilage batten "which will aid in maintaining a lateral position for the eardrum graft, since the peripheral cartilage segment will be placed in contiguity with the bony annulus, thus the medial aspect of the perichondrium graft covers the stapedial capitulum and contacts no other surfaces of the medial tympanic wall" (see **Fig. 1.13**). Instead of a tympanoplasty type 4, in the case of a missing stapedial arch, Goodhill placed a solid cartilage columella between the footplate and the perichondrium.

I consider the term *annular cartilage–perichondrium graft*, as used by Klacansky et al. (1998) since 1996, to be the most appropriate, reflecting its annular shape and its placement onto the fibrous or bony annulus. In Germany, Slovakia, and the Czech Republic, the cartilage tympanoplasty is popular in several ENT hospitals. During 1996 and 1997, Klacansky and co-workers in the ENT Clinic in Olomouc, Czech Republic, performed cartilage tympanoplasty on 372 patients. In 77 patients, the eardrum was reconstructed with cartilage palisades; in 248 patients with a total pars tensa perforation, a combined cartilage–perichondrium island graft was used; and in 47 patients an annular cartilage–perichondrium graft was used (Klacansky et al. 1998).

Borkowski et al. (1999) used the term *Spannring* to indicate the function of minimizing shrinkage of the perichondrium and thus preventing it from herniating into the tympanic cavity.

Harvesting and Shaping of the Annular Graft

Goodhill (1967) used the entire tragal cartilage with the tragal dome, covered on both sides with perichondrium (**Fig. 18.1**). On the concave side, the perichondrium is elevated from the cartilage. By gradual trimming of the cartilage, the outer border of the cartilage island is formed, creating a horseshoe shaped piece with a diameter of 11 mm but leaving the surrounding perichondrium intact. Then the central component of cartilage is gradually removed using the round knife, leaving a 0.5–2 mm peripheral belt of cartilage, with the perichondrium intact. Finally the peripheral perichondrium flap is trimmed leaving a 1–2 mm belt as a graft.

Klacansky et al. (1998) incises 3 mm medial to the dome through the skin, tragal cartilage, and the perichondrium. An 11 mm × 11 mm piece of tragal cartilage with perichondrium attached on both sides is excised. The perichondrium from the convex (lateral) side is removed. This side will later face the tympanic cavity. The cartilage is placed with the concave (medial) side onto a plate. Using a sterile metal inner tracheal cannula with a diameter of 9 mm and pressing it gently onto the 11 mm × 11 mm cartilage–perichondrium plate (**Fig. 18.4a [A]**), the outer border of the annular graft is fashioned. By performing a similar procedure with a metal tracheal cannula of a 7 mm diameter, the inner border of the graft is fashioned (**Fig. 18.4a [B]**).

The cartilage ring can also be cut in a similar fashion using an ear speculum with a diameter of 9 mm (**Fig. 18.4b [A]**) and a smaller ear speculum 0.7 mm diameter (**Fig. 18.4b [B]**). The peripheral cartilage around the outer cut and the central cartilage inside the inner cut are then easily removed, keeping the central perichondrium intact (**Fig. 18.4c**).

A third method of making an annular graft is to use the corneal trephine (Klacansky et al. 1998).

The Klacansky Chondrotome

The chondrotome devised by Klacansky is a 10 cm long metal tube of outer diameter 13 mm, comprising two telescoping cylinders with sharp edges at one end (**Fig. 18.5a**). The larger, outer and slightly longer cylinder has a diameter of 9 mm. The smaller, inner and slightly shorter cylinder measures 7 mm in diameter (**Fig. 18.5b**). The chondrotome is first placed with the outer cylinder on the tragal cartilage. With slight pressure the outer border of the annulus graft is thus cut (**Fig. 18.6 [A]**). Then the inner cylinder is pressed down (arrow in **Fig. 18.6 [B]**) to cut the inner border of the graft. The remnant cartilage is discarded (**Fig. 18.4c**).

Borkowski et al. (1999) harvest the graft by a retroauricular approach, using a round piece of conchal cartilage 11 mm × 11 mm, together with the perichondrium attached on the concave (medial) side. The graft is placed with its concave side, covered with the perichondrium, on a plate and then a 1.5 mm wide belt of cartilage is removed, leaving the perichondrium intact as a flap (**Fig. 18.7a**). With a round knife, the cartilage from the central part of the disk is removed, leaving a 1 mm wide cartilage ring with an intact perichondrium within the ring (**Fig. 18.7b, c**). In case of a disrupted ossicular chain, a small island of cartilage is left attached to the perichondrium to cover the head of the PORP or TORP.

These cartilage islands are created on the left or right side of the graft, depending on the ear to be operated on (**Fig. 18.7d**).

Circular Graft and U-Graft

In cases of missing malleus handle or missing entire malleus, a circular annular graft is applied covering the region of the Shrapnell membrane as well (**Fig. 18.2**). In cases of missing malleus handle, the incudostapedial joint may be

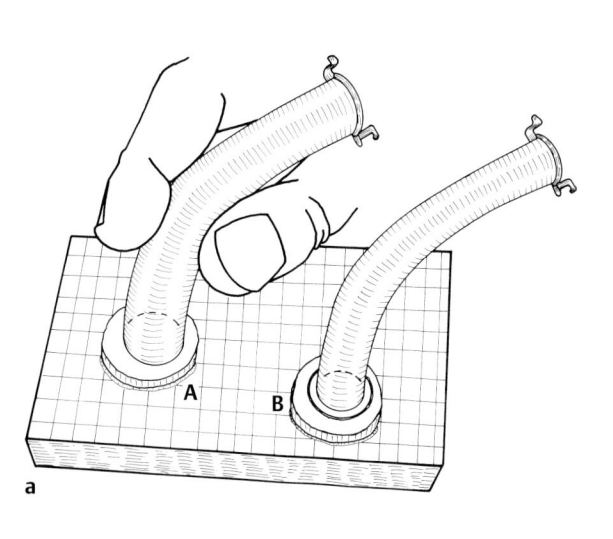

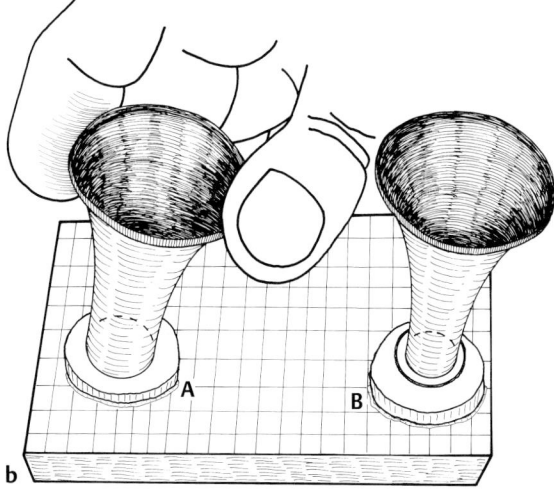

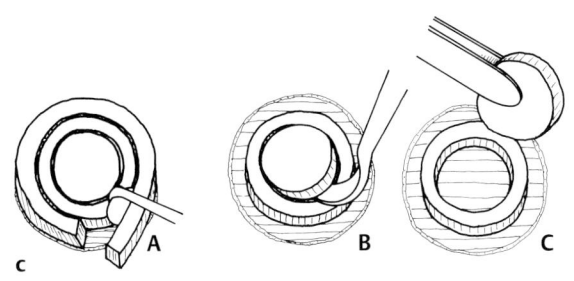

Fig. 18.4a–c Cutting an annular graft.
a Cutting the tragal cartilage with the perichondrium on the convex side lying on the underlying plate and using a tracheal cannula. A cannula of 9 mm diameter is used to cut the outer border of the annular ring graft (**A**). A cannula of 7 mm diameter cuts the inner border (**B**).
b Cutting the tragal cartilage with an ear speculum to prepare the annular graft. The outer border is cut with a speculum of 9 mm diameter (**A**). The inner border of the annular graft is cut with an ear speculum of 7 mm diameter (**B**).
c Removal of the peripheral cartilage around the annular graft and the central cartilage from the center of the graft.
   A The peripheral cartilage around the outer cut is removed all the way around with a round knife, keeping the perichondrium intact and thus creating the peripheral perichondrium flap.
   B The central cartilage island attached to the central perichondrium is carefully elevated in toto using a curved elevator and keeping the central perichondrium intact.
   C The annular graft made. The upper part of the cartilage ring can be removed depending on the pathology. The central island cartilage may be used in ossiculoplasty or in the obliteration of the attic.

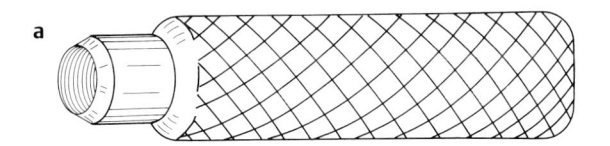

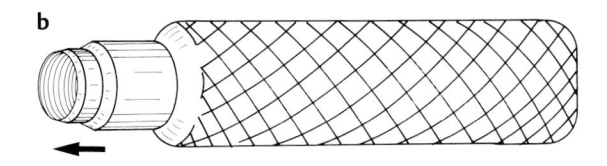

Fig. 18.5a, b The Klacansky chondrotome for cutting the annular graft.
a At one end two sharp cylinders are visible. The wider cylinder measures 9 mm in diameter and cuts the outer border of the cartilage annular graft.
b The narrower inner cylinder of diameter 7 mm is pushed out (arrow) to cut the inner border of the annular graft.

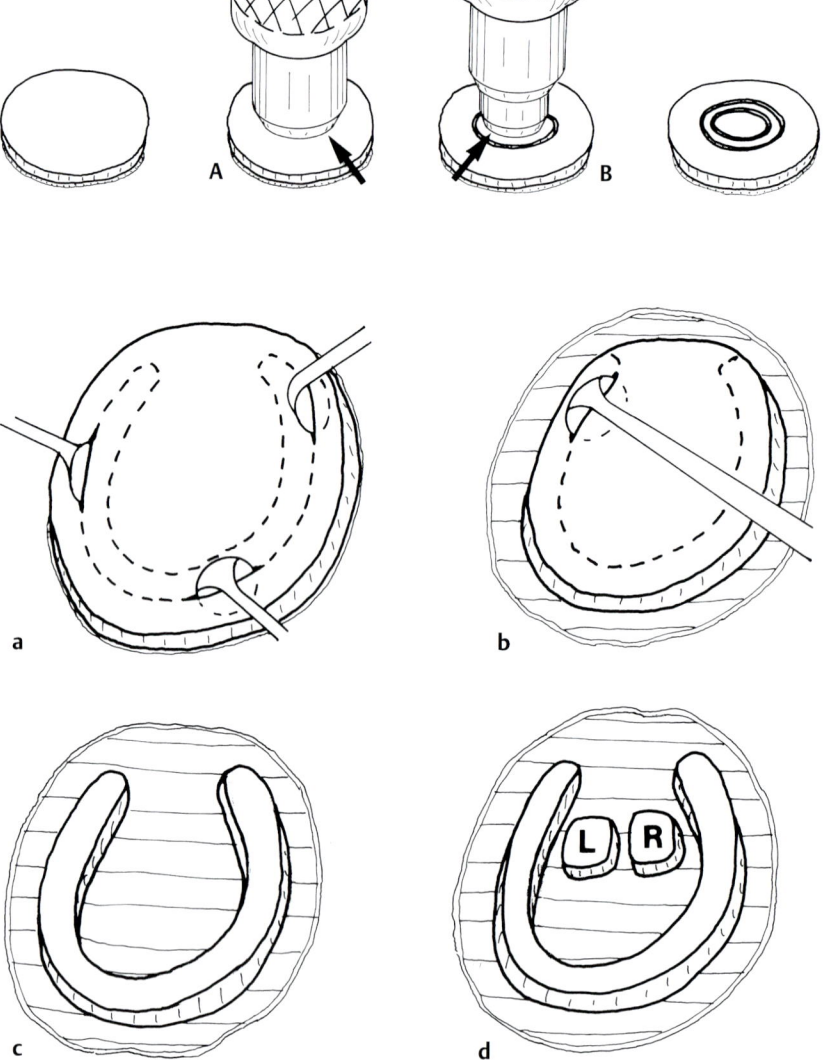

Fig. 18.6 Cutting the annular graft with the Klacansky chondrotome. The outer border (**A**, arrow) of the annular graft is cut with the wider cylinder. The narrower cylinder is pushed forward, cutting the inner border (**B**, arrow) of the annular graft.

Fig. 18.7a–d Shaping the annular cartilage–perichondrium composite graft from a round piece of conchal cartilage of 11 mm × 11 mm (Borkowski et al. 1999).
- **a** Removal of the cartilage along the outer dotted line, leaving a 1–1.5 mm broad belt of perichondrium. The round knife is the safest instrument to keep the perichondrium intact.
- **b** Using a round knife, the cartilage is removed along the inner dotted line, resulting in a horseshoe-shaped cartilage–perichondrium graft. This inner cartilage can be removed as one round piece, which may be used in covering the attic.
- **c** The graft is completed and can be used for a total perforation and an intact ossicular chain.
- **d** In case of a missing incus but with an intact stapes, a tympanoplasty type 2 can be performed by placing a rectangular piece of cartilage onto the head of the stapes. In the case of the right ear, the right cartilage prosthesis may be made and vice versa. (The right and left cartilage additions are my own proposals.)

intact and mobile or it may be disrupted with the stapes present or missing. Thus several types of tympanoplasty may be performed using the circular annular graft.

With the entire malleus missing and the incus also not present, a U-shaped annular graft (**Fig. 18.3**) is applied in a subtotal perforation or a large inferior perforation with protruding umbo.

Indications for Application of Annular Grafts

Goodhill's indication for the application of annular grafts was to avoid the retraction of the perichondrium or fascia in ears with large perforations and total or subtotal perforations with signs of previous or persisting indication of poor tubal function, such as previous eardrum retraction, a negative Valsalva maneuver, a thick tympanic mucosa, a poor outcome of aspiration or deflation tests and a history of previous recurrent grommet insertions.

Other indications are: retraction of the entire pars tensa, pars tensa retraction cholesteatoma, other types of cholesteatoma, atelectasis, adhesive otitis media, postoperative retraction, and revision surgery.

Surgical Techniques with Annular Grafts

Three different techniques have been published: the Goodhill on-lay technique, the Klacansky technique with removal of the fibrous annulus and the entire remnant of the eardrum, and the Borkowski underlay technique.

Goodhill's On-lay Annular Graft Technique

Goodhill (1967) employed the on-lay technique in all situations. A circumferential incision of the ear canal skin is made slightly lateral to the fibrous annulus (**Fig. 18.8a**). Superiorly, Goodhill used a horizontal incision of the epithelium along the upper border of the total perforation. In my practice I have for many years favored the on-lay technique (Tos 1980) with elevation of three superior skin flaps (**Fig. 18.8b, c**). This modification is an addition to Goodhill's technique. After elevation of the superior skin flaps, the annular graft is placed onto the eardrum remnant and fibrous annulus (**Fig. 18.8d**). The peripheral perichondrium is placed onto the bone and adapted to the edges of the skin (**Fig. 18.8e**). The central perichondrium is placed under the malleus handle. Sometimes Goodhill covered the denuded malleus handle with another small piece of perichondrium as a "perichondrial sandwich," providing further firmness after repositioning of the epithelial flaps and also aiding faster epithelialization (**Fig. 18.8 f, g**).

Annular Graft in Tympanoplasty Type 2 with Interposition Techniques

Several methods with interposition of a prosthesis between the head of the stapes and the eardrum and/or the malleus handle are available. The prostheses are made of different materials and are of different sizes and shapes, and they make contact with the annular graft in the posterosuperior part of the tympanic cavity.

Several solutions are available:
1. The posterosuperior end of the cartilage ring may be cut and removed.
2. The posterosuperior end of the cartilage ring may be trimmed and made smaller.
3. The prosthesis may be shaped and adapted to the smaller space.

Interposition of an Autogenous Incus

When the long process of the incus is missing, the most common ossiculoplasty is interposition of the incus (**Fig. 18.9a, b**). In the on-lay technique the annular graft is placed on the eardrum remnant and onto the fibrous annulus, allowing more space for the incus prosthesis (**Fig. 18.10a–c**). If the posterior part of the incus is protruding too much, this part of the bone can be drilled off.

Downsizing the Annular Graft

Often the annular graft has to be trimmed and downsized at its superoposterior end to allow interposition of the ossicle, bone, or cartilage between the head of the stapes and the eardrum and malleus handle. The posterosuperior end of the cartilage is removed and the remaining cartilage between the 9-o'clock and 10-o'clock positions is also made smaller (**Fig. 18.11**).

Placement of Small Cartilage Palisades in Case of Excessive Bone Removal of the Posterosuperior Annulus

To avoid retraction behind the annular graft and around the interposed incus, some small cartilage palisades are placed posterior and superior to the interposed incus (**Fig. 18.12a, b**). After placement of the annular graft, the palisades are covered with the perichondrium (**Fig. 18.12c**). After replacement of the epithelial flaps (**Fig. 18.12 d**), the reconstruction is resistant to retraction (**Fig. 18.12e**).

Other Ossiculoplasties in Tympanoplasty Type 2

Other ossiculoplasties in tympanoplasty type 2 can be used with the annular graft, such as a shaped autogenous incus, malleus head, cortical bone, homologous incus and malleus (MMES_1, Figs. 735–783). Additional application of small cartilage palisades posterior and superior to the interposed ossicle support the annular graft, especially if the upper end of the graft is shortened (**Fig. 18.13a–d**). The palisades prevent any retraction and act as an extension of the annular graft. They support the ossiculoplasty as well (**Fig. 18.13e, f**). Such a combined reconstruction is rather firm, as can be appreciated in the side view (**Fig. 18.13 g**).

Interposition Techniques with Cartilage

Interposition techniques with cartilage have been illustrated in mmES_1, Figs. 790–798. Most of the techniques can be used together with the annular graft, especially the interposition of tragal cartilage plates between the stapes head and the eardrum (**Fig. 18.14a–d**). The height of the stapes and depth of the tympanic cavity determine whether one or two plates of cartilage are needed.

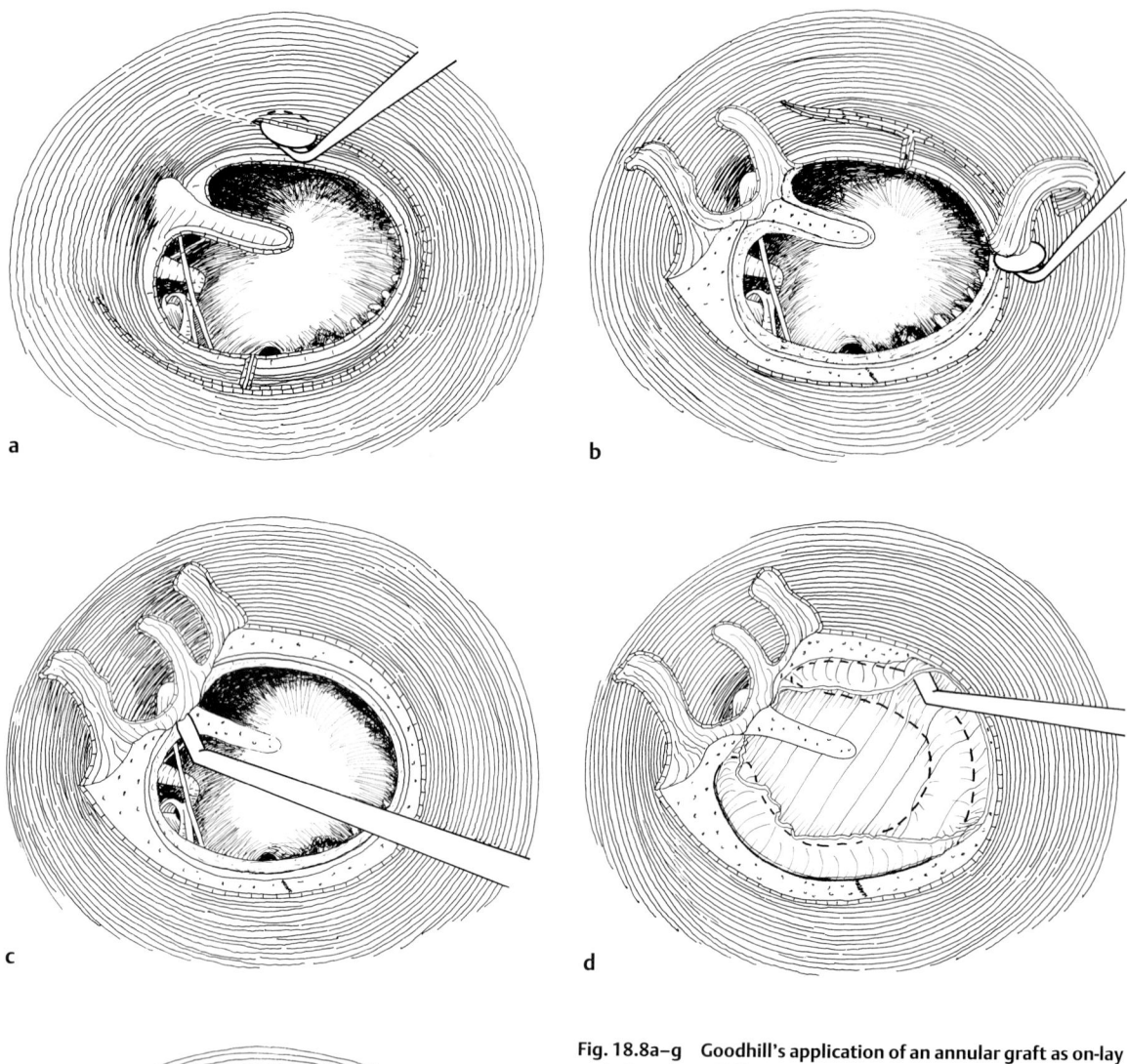

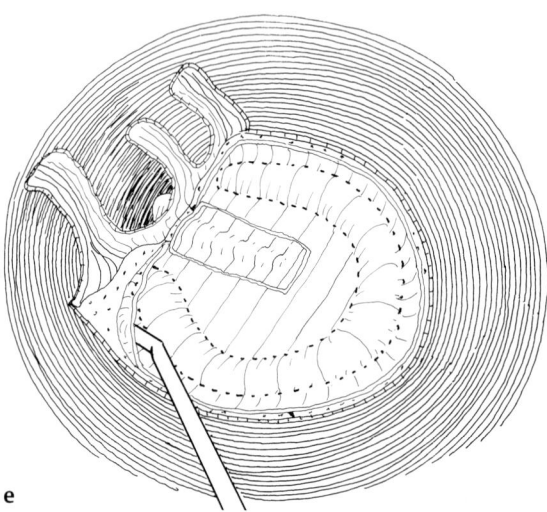

Fig. 18.8a–g Goodhill's application of an annular graft as on-lay technique (Goodhill 1967) combined with elevation of three superior epithelial flaps (Tos 1980) in a case with total perforation and intact ossicular chain.

a The epithelium is removed from the edges of the perforation and a medial circumferential incision of the ear canal skin is made. A small radial incision at the 9-o'clock position is also made.

b The posterosuperior skin flap and the malleus flap are raised, leaving the fibrous annulus intact. At the 3-o'clock position a small radial incision of the epithelium is made. The strip of ear canal skin between the 3-o'clock and 9-o'clock positions is removed and the lamina propria is cleaned of epithelium.

c The third superior epithelial flap—the anterosuperior flap—is elevated and the malleus is cleaned of epithelium.

d The annular graft is placed onto the fibrous annulus in an inferosuperior direction, allowing the perichondrium to be placed under the malleus handle. Anteriorly and inferiorly the perichondrium is spread over the denuded bone and smoothed out to the skin.

e A piece of perichondrium is placed over the malleus handle, a procedure Goodhill often used, forming a "perichondrial sandwich." The perichondrium is adapted to the skin along the posterior and superior incisions.

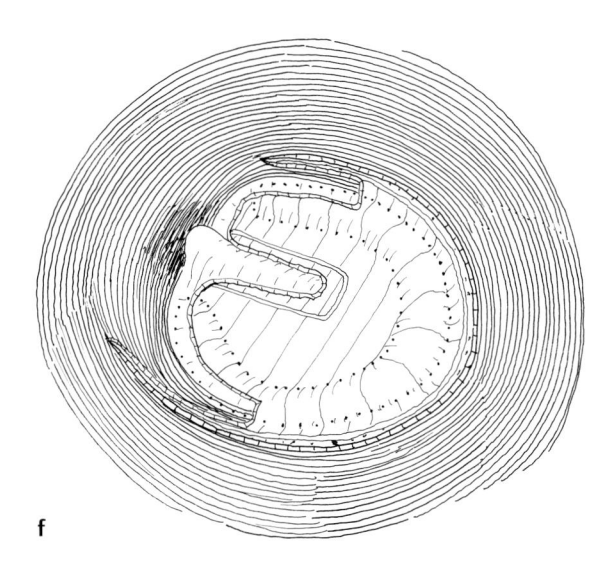

Fig. 18.8f, g

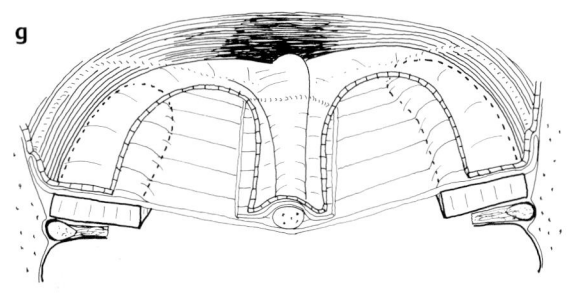

f The epithelial flaps, in particular the three superior flaps, are replaced, allowing faster epithelialization of the perichondrium.

g Cross-sectional view of Goodhill's annular cartilage graft technique. The cartilage ring is placed onto the fibrous annulus and the remnant of the eardrum. The annular graft perichondrium is placed under and a piece of perichondrium is placed over the malleus handle ("perichondrial sandwich"). The three superior epithelial flaps are next replaced.

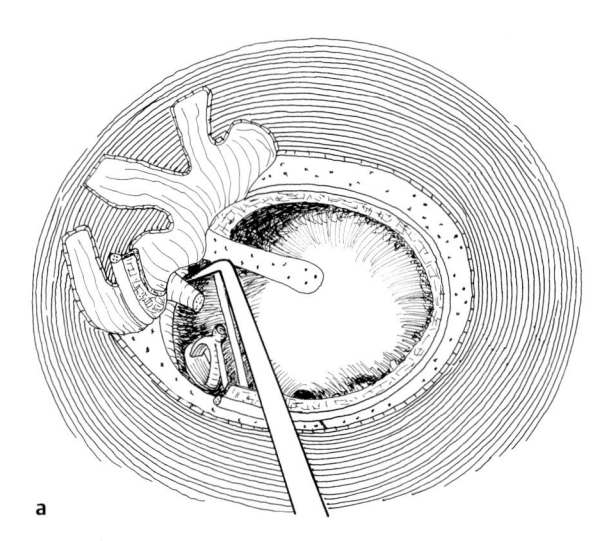

Fig. 18.9a, b   Interposition of an autogenous incus. Application of an annular graft as on-lay technique, combined with the application of the three superior epithelial flaps in a case of total perforation, interrupted ossicular chain and intact stapes.

a To view the stapes superstructure and the footplate, the fibrous annulus is cut at the 9-o'clock position and temporarily elevated. After cleaning of the epithelium from the edges of the perforation and after elevation of the superior epithelial flaps, the defective long process of the incus is rotated in a posterior direction and the incus is removed.

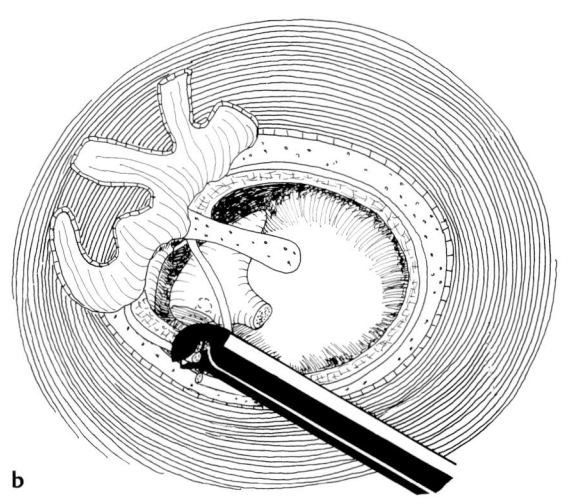

b The incus body with a small depression for the stapes head is placed onto the stapes with the short process pointing under the malleus handle in an anterior direction. The remnant of the long process points inferiorly. The chorda tympani fixates the incus. The elevated fibrous annulus is replaced on the bony annulus with a cup forceps.

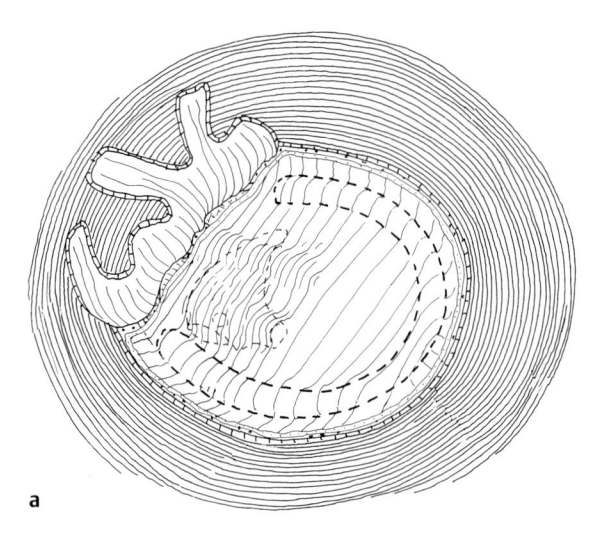

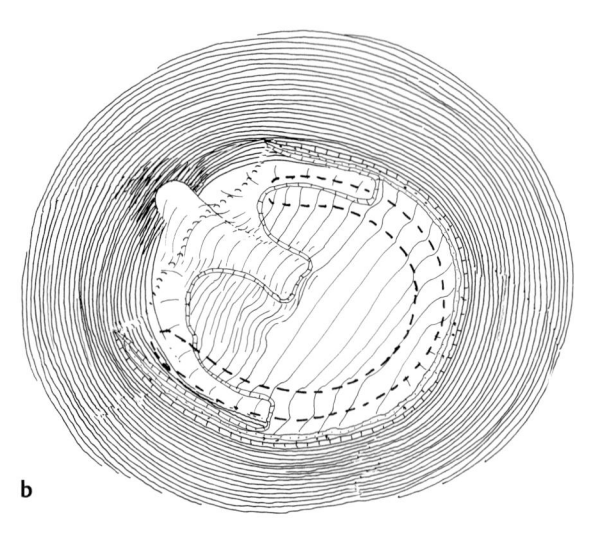

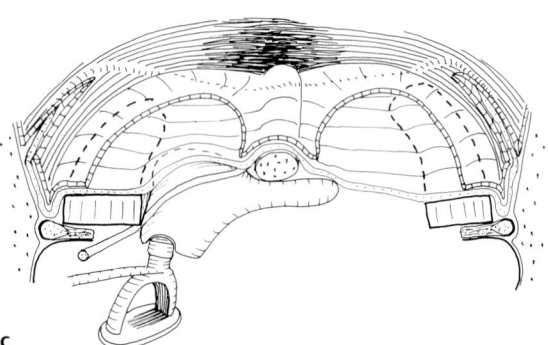

Fig. 18.10a–c Interposition of an autogenous incus. Application of an annular graft as on-lay technique, combined with the application of the three superior epithelial flaps in a case of total perforation, interrupted ossicular chain and intact stapes.

a   The annular graft is placed onto the fibrous annulus and onto the deepithelialized remnant of the eardrum. The perichondrium is placed onto the malleus handle and on the interposed incus.
b   The epithelial flaps are replaced and the perichondrium is smoothed out to the ear canal skin, completing the tympanoplasty type 2.
c   Cross-sectional view of the annular on-lay graft and the classic incus interposition between the intact stapes and the eardrum. The perichondrium covers the ear canal bone, the cartilage, the incus, and the malleus handle.

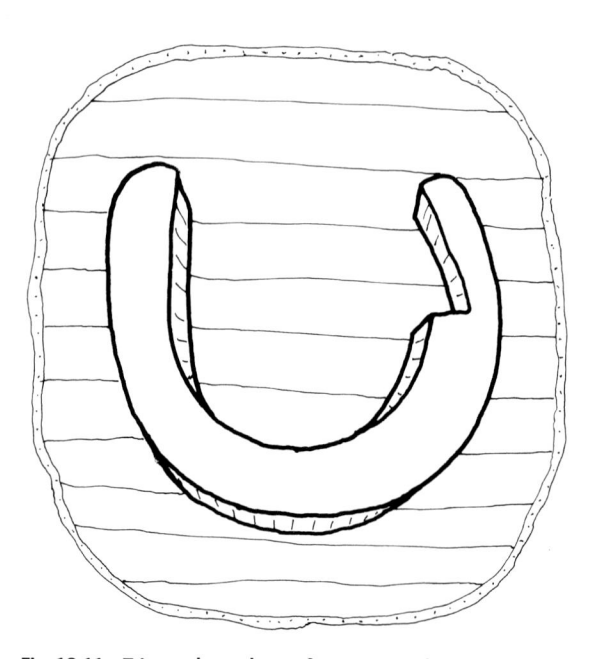

Fig. 18.11 Trimmed annular graft in cases with tympanoplasty type 2 with incus interposition and tympanoplasty type 3 with columella. The posterosuperior part of the annular graft cartilage, between the 9-o'clock and 10-o'clock positions, is either removed or downsized.

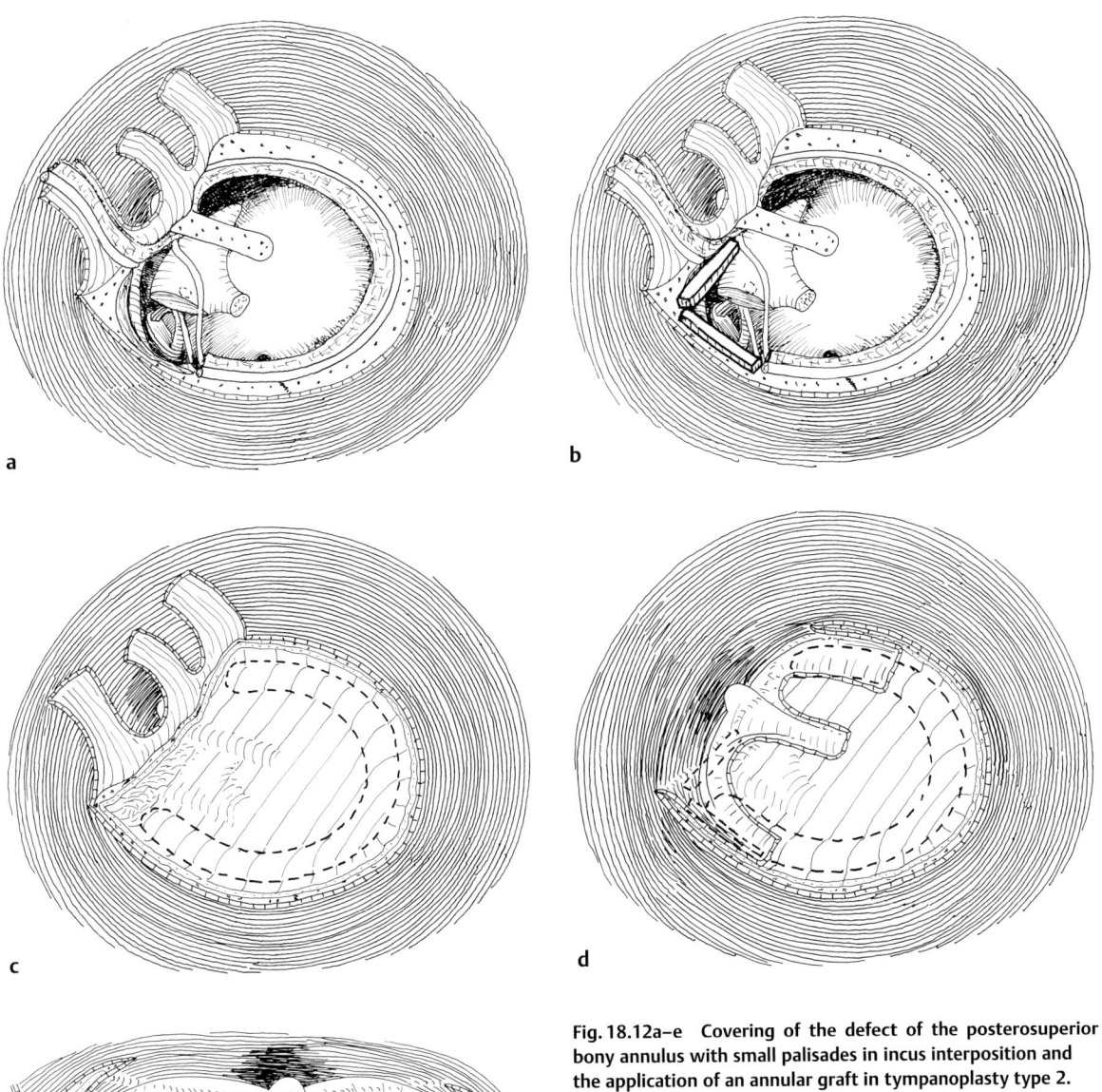

Fig. 18.12 a–e Covering of the defect of the posterosuperior bony annulus with small palisades in incus interposition and the application of an annular graft in tympanoplasty type 2.

a The bony defect posterior to the interposed incus cannot be covered with the annular graft alone.
b Two small palisades are placed, one posteriorly in the inferosuperior direction and another superiorly in the anteroposterior direction, close to the bony edges of the defect.
c The elevated fibrous annulus is replaced and the annular graft is placed onto the eardrum remnant and fibrous annulus. The perichondrium covers the denuded bone and the malleus handle.
d The flaps are replaced.
e Cross-sectional view illustrating additional covering of the posterosuperior bony defect with small cartilage palisades. Two palisades are placed onto the posterior bony defect. The small palisades are placed superiorly along the interposed incus.

Fig. 18.13a–g Underlay placement of an annular graft in a total perforation with keratinized squamous epithelium in the tympanic sinus and a defective incus.

a Retroauricular approach and removal of the epithelium from the edges of the perforation.
b A large tympanomeatal flap is elevated and the incus is removed. Extensive removal of the posterosuperior ear canal bone is completed and tympanic sinuses are cleared of keratinized epithelium. Anteriorly, further elevation of the fibrous annulus is performed. The removed incus is reshaped and reduced and replaced as a prosthesis between the stapes head and malleus handle.
c To cover the posterosuperior bony defect, two small palisades are placed in superoinferior direction. Another two small palisades are placed superior to the incus.
d The annular graft is placed into the tympanic cavity at the level of the bony annulus and the perichondrium is folded out. The posterior limb of the cartilage ring is shorter than the anterior ring.
e Anteriorly, the perichondrium is pushed under the fibrous annulus using an incudostapedial knife.

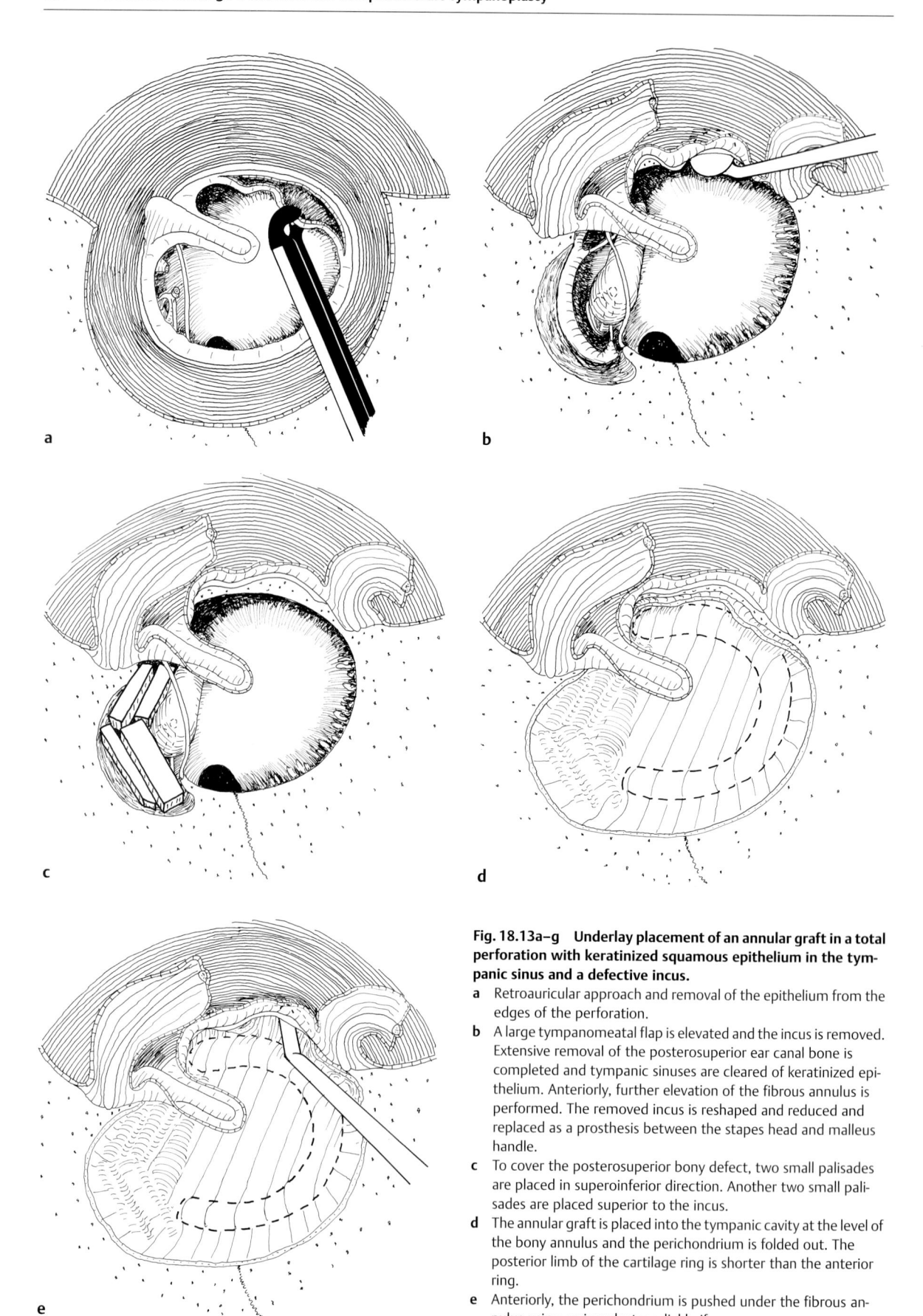

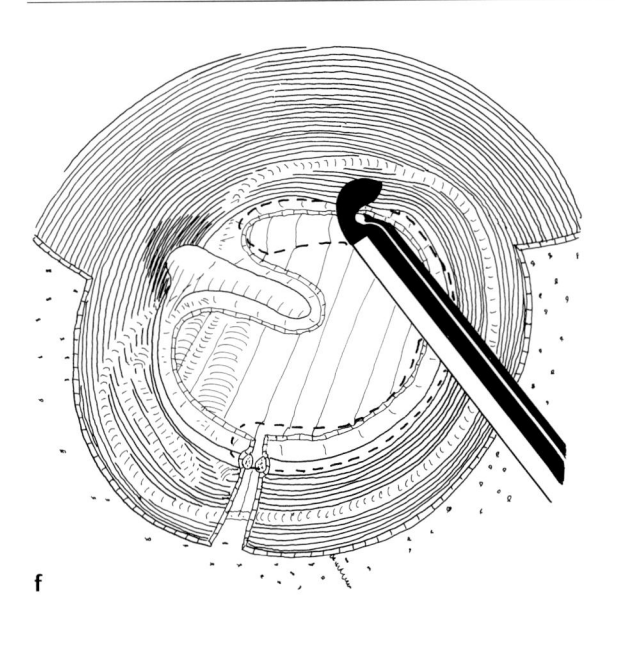

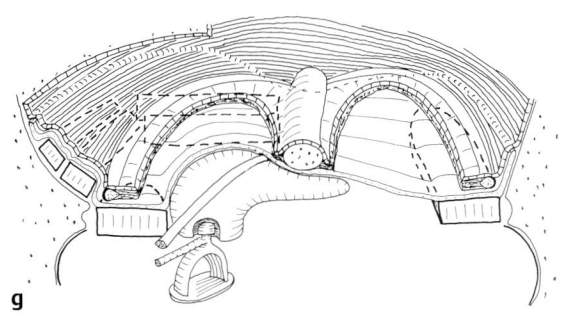

Fig. 18.13f, g

f The posterior tympanomeatal flap is replaced. Using a forceps, the anterior fibrous annulus along with the eardrum remnant is replaced.

g Cross-sectional view of tympanoplasty type 2 with a shaped incus, posteriorly shortened annulus graft and cartilage palisades. Posteriorly, two palisades cover the bony defect. The annular graft is in the tympanic cavity at the level of the bony annulus. The perichondrium is under the malleus handle.

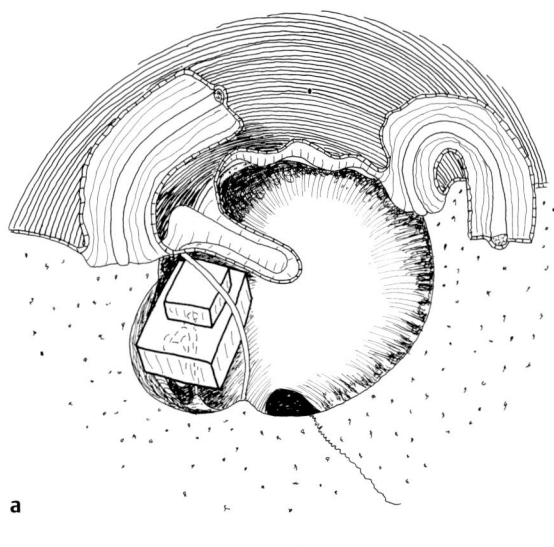

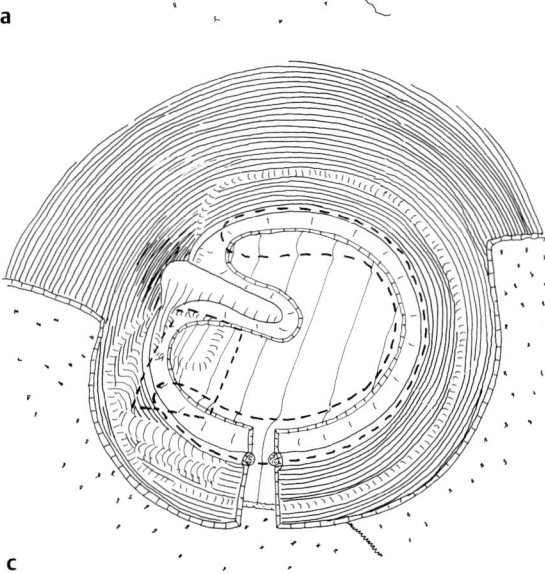

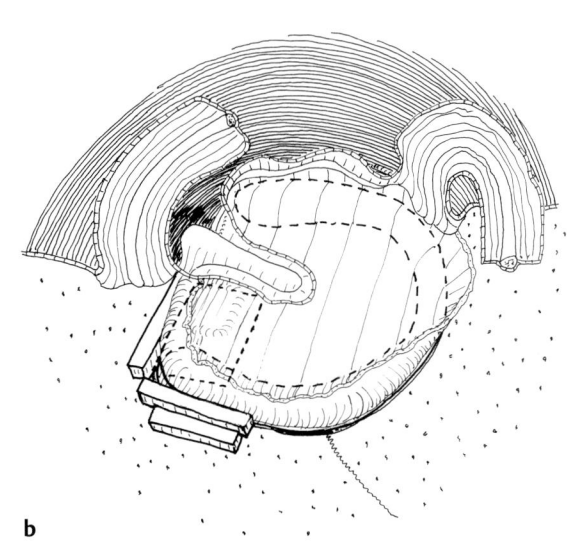

Fig. 18.14a–d Tympanoplasty type 2 with interposition of tragal cartilage between the stapes head and the eardrum with an annular graft and cartilage palisades in the case of a total perforation, missing incus, and superoposterior bony defect.

a Via a retroauricular approach a tympanomeatal flap is elevated by the swing-door technique. The edges of the perforation are removed. Anteriorly, the fibrous annulus is elevated. A larger piece of tragal cartilage is placed onto the stapes head and a smaller rectangular piece is placed onto the larger piece of cartilage. The chorda tympani stabilizes both cartilage plates.

b Posteriorly, two small cartilage palisades cover the bony defect. Superiorly, a small palisade is placed between the malleus handle and the posterior bony annulus. The annular graft is placed into the tympanic cavity. Posteriorly, it is positioned onto the large cartilage plate.

c The perichondrium is folded out posteriorly and superiorly, covering the palisades and the denuded bone. The tympanomeatal flaps are replaced.

Fig. 18.14d ▷

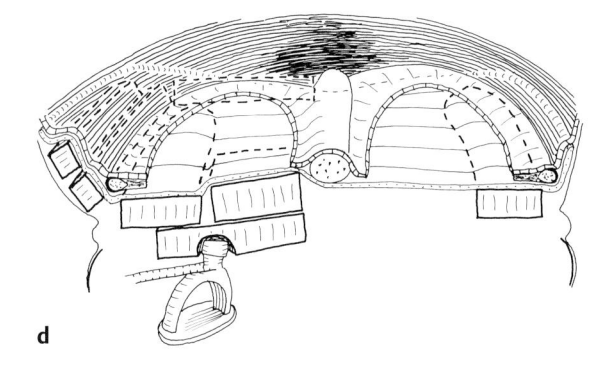

Interposition of the Helix Spine

An interesting technique is interposition of the shaped helix spine between the stapes head and the eardrum as a tympanoplasty type 2 (**Fig. 18.15a**). In such cases the annular graft is slightly reduced because the helix spine occupies some space in the stapes region (**Fig. 18.15b–d**).

Fig. 18.14d

d Cross-sectional view of interposition with cartilage plates and annular graft. The annular graft is in the tympanic cavity at the level of bony annulus. The perichondrium is under the malleus handle. Posteriorly, the larger cartilage plate is under the annular graft.

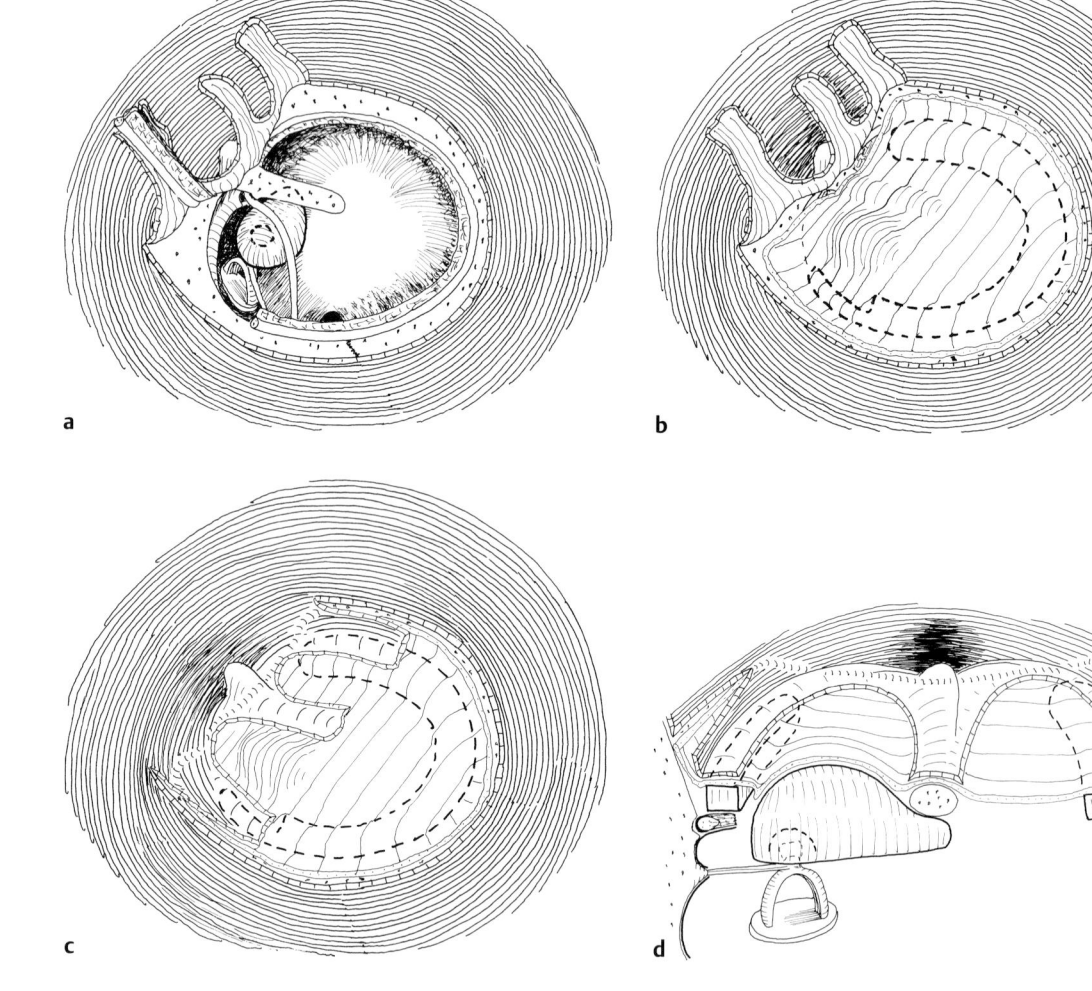

Fig. 18.15a–d Interposition of a shaped helix spine in case of a total perforation and missing incus.

a A depression for the stapes head is drilled on the inner surface of the cartilage and the prosthesis is placed onto the stapes head and fixed with the chorda tympani. The thinner anterior part is placed under the malleus handle.

b The trimmed annular graft is placed onto the eardrum remnant and the fibrous annulus. The peripheral perichondrium is folded out. The central perichondrium is in close contact with the prosthesis and malleus handle.

c The epithelial flaps are replaced.

d Cross-sectional view of the trimmed annular graft and the interposed helix spine cartilage prosthesis at the level of stapes crura. The cartilage prosthesis has good contact with the annular graft perichondrium.

Interposition with Prostheses Made of Biocompatible Materials

Interposition in type 2 tympanoplasty (the PORPs) with prostheses made of biocompatible materials, such as polyethylene, Teflon, porous plastic, bio-inert ceramics, bioactive glass ceramics, calcium phosphate ceramics, hydroxyapatite, and glass ionomer cement has been used previously, but these prostheses are seldom used today. These PORPs are described in detail and illustrated in MMES_1, Figs. 805–844. Because of their tendency to extrusion they should be covered with cartilage plates. An annular graft may be used in these circumstances. This annular graft may be broader in its posterosuperior section to cover the posterior part of the prosthesis. The anterior part of the prosthesis, up to the malleus handle, may be covered with a cartilage plate.

Interposition with Prostheses Made of Metals

Prostheses made of metals, such as the different steel wire prostheses, gold prostheses, and titanium prostheses, used for interposition in type 2 tympanoplasty should again be covered with cartilage plates (MMES_1, Figs. 845–495). The annular graft can be easily applied in these cases.

Interposition of Titanium PORP Prosthesis and Annular Graft

A clip prosthesis of the Dresden type is placed on the stapes and clamped onto the stapes head (**Fig. 18.16a**) in the situation with a total perforation and missing incus. A cartilage plate covers the round titanium plate. (**Fig. 18.16b**). The annular graft is placed onto the eardrum remnant covering the cartilage plate and the malleus handle (**Fig. 18.16c, d**). The reconstruction is thus firm (**Fig. 18.16e**).

Annular Graft in Tympanoplasty Type 3 with a Columella

Columella Made of Autogenous Incus

In the case of a total perforation and missing stapes crura, an autogenous incus columella is the most common, cheapest, and most stable prosthesis (**Fig. 18.17a**). Because the incus columella can be shaped to connect the footplate and the malleus handle, there is also enough space available for the annular graft (**Fig. 18.17b–d**). The many variations in the shaping and placement of the incus columella are shown in MMES_1, Figs. 981–992. The annular graft can be used with all variations of shaping of the autogenous incus.

Other Bony Grafts Shaped as Columellae in Tympanoplasty Type 3 and Annular Graft

An allogenous incus or malleus or autogenous cortical bone can be shaped as a columella in the various ways described in MMES_1, Figs. 993–1004. These prostheses can be employed with the annular graft. A columella of an allogenous stapes, placed with the capitulum on the footplate (MMES_1, Figs. 1007–1019) can also be used with the annular graft.

Cartilage Columellae and Annular Graft

Cartilage columellae have been used since the beginning of the tympanoplasty era (Utech 1959, 1961). They are easy to harvest and shape. Through the years many different types of columellae have been used; they are illustrated in MMES_1, Figs.1020–1035. It has been shown that in the long term the histopathological fate of long cartilage prostheses is unpredictable. For the L-shaped prostheses, Steinbach and Pusalkar (1981) and Steinbach et al. (1992) found that the columellae fractured at the angle between the vertical and horizontal limbs. They found fibrous degeneration and the disappearance of the cartilage in many columellae, and the sound conduction thus decreased gradually with time. As a result, cartilage columellae have been more or less abandoned and should not be used with the annular graft.

Columellae Made of Biocompatible Materials and Annular Graft

Columellae made of polyethylene, compact Teflon, and porous plastic have been abandoned. Plastic-Pore, proplast, malleable polycel, Frialit ceramic, hydroxyapatite, bioactive glass ceramic materials, and Ceravital (illustrated in MMES_1, Figs. 1036–1060) are still used in many countries, but the platforms have to be covered with a cartilage plate or with cartilage–perichondrium composite grafts. With a cartilage covering, they can be used together with the annular graft.

Columellae Made of Metals and Annular Graft

Metallic wire columellae (MMES_1, Figs. 1062–1067) are not compatible with the annular graft. Gold prostheses are seldom used today. Titanium prostheses can be used with the annular graft but they have to be covered with cartilage. The titanium prostheses are widely used.

Titanium Columellae in Tympanoplasty Type 3 and Annular Graft

Measurement of the distance from the footplate to the actual position of the platform of the prosthesis is important. The Fisch malleable measuring rod, used in stapes surgery, can be helpful. The foot of the prosthesis is placed on the centre of the footplate between the malleus handle

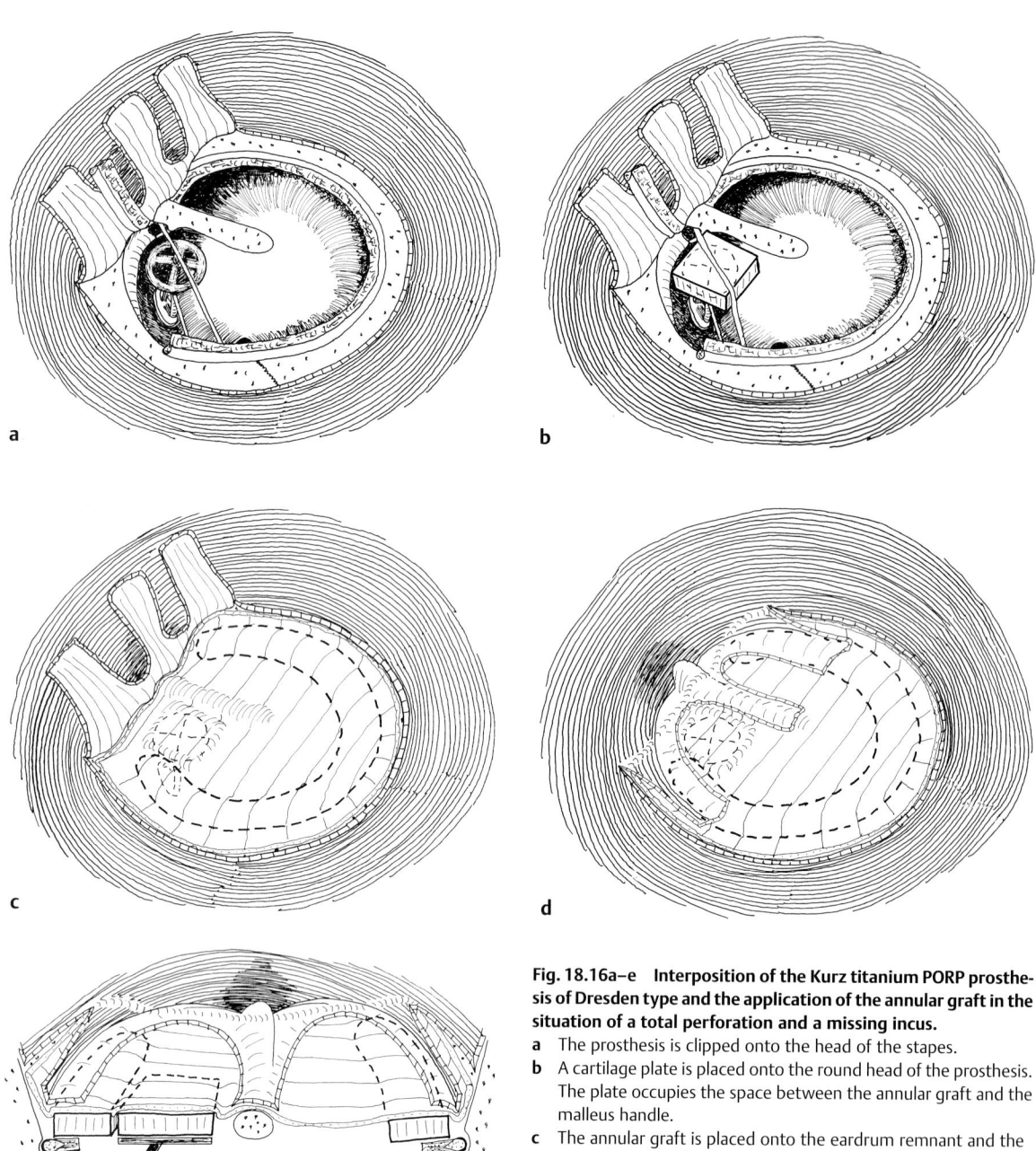

Fig. 18.16a–e Interposition of the Kurz titanium PORP prosthesis of Dresden type and the application of the annular graft in the situation of a total perforation and a missing incus.

a The prosthesis is clipped onto the head of the stapes.
b A cartilage plate is placed onto the round head of the prosthesis. The plate occupies the space between the annular graft and the malleus handle.
c The annular graft is placed onto the eardrum remnant and the central perichondrium covers the cartilage plate and the malleus handle. The peripheral perichondrium is folded out, covering the denuded bone and the superior region of the eardrum.
d The epithelial flaps are replaced and the peripheral perichondrium is adapted to the borders of the epithelium.
e Cross-sectional view of the interposition of a Kurz titanium PORP prosthesis of Dresden type and placement of an annular graft. The cartilage plate covers the round titanium head and is positioned between the annular graft and the malleus. The central perichondrium covers the plate and the malleus handle.

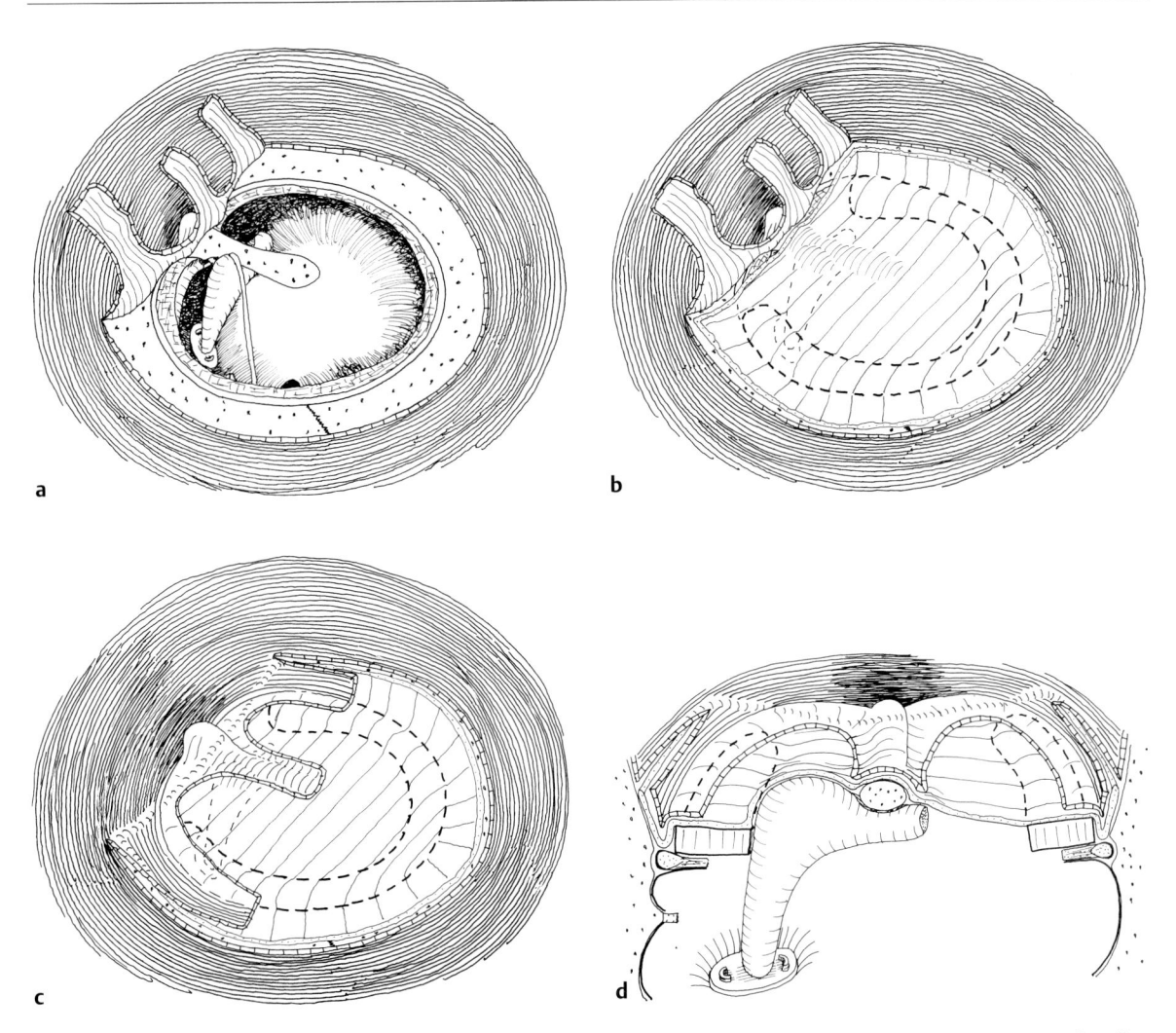

Fig. 18.17a–d Annular graft in case of a total perforation and missing stapes crura.

a The superior epithelial flaps are elevated and the autogenous incus is placed with its short process onto the middle of the footplate. The incus body is grooved to fit under the malleus handle.

b The annular graft is placed onto the fibrous annulus and the eardrum remnant. The perichondrium is folded out onto the bone and adapted to the edges of the ear canal skin. The perichondrium covers the malleus handle and the incus columella.

c The epithelial flaps are replaced and the perichondrium is further adapted to the edges of the skin, completing the tympanoplasty type 3.

d Cross-sectional view at the level of the footplate of tympanoplasty type 3 with an incus columella and an on-lay annular cartilage-perichondrium graft. Perichondrium covers the ear canal bone, the incus columella, and the malleus handle.

and the footplate (**Fig. 18.18a**). The cartilage plate is placed onto the platform (**Fig. 18.18b**), allowing space for the annular graft. The annular graft is placed onto the fibrous annulus and the perichondrium onto the malleus handle (**Fig. 18.18c, d**).

The side view (**Fig. 18.18e**) illustrates that the columella is slightly oblique, and the annular graft is positioned more laterally than in the Klacansky method without fibrous annulus and in the Borkowski underlay method.

Fig. 18.18a–e The Kurz titanium columella in tympanoplasty type 3 with a total perforation and missing stapes crura.

a The columella is placed onto the central part of the footplate. The head of the columella is positioned at the level of the inner border of the malleus handle.
b The head of the columella is covered with a cartilage plate.
c The annular graft is placed onto the remnant of the eardrum. The perichondrium covers the cartilage plate, the malleus handle, and the denuded bone.
d The epithelial flaps are replaced and the perichondrium is adapted to the edges of the epithelium.
e Cross-sectional view of the tympanoplasty type 3 with titanium columella and annular graft at the level of the head of the titanium prosthesis. The annular graft and the cartilage covering the prosthesis are on the same level as the malleus handle.

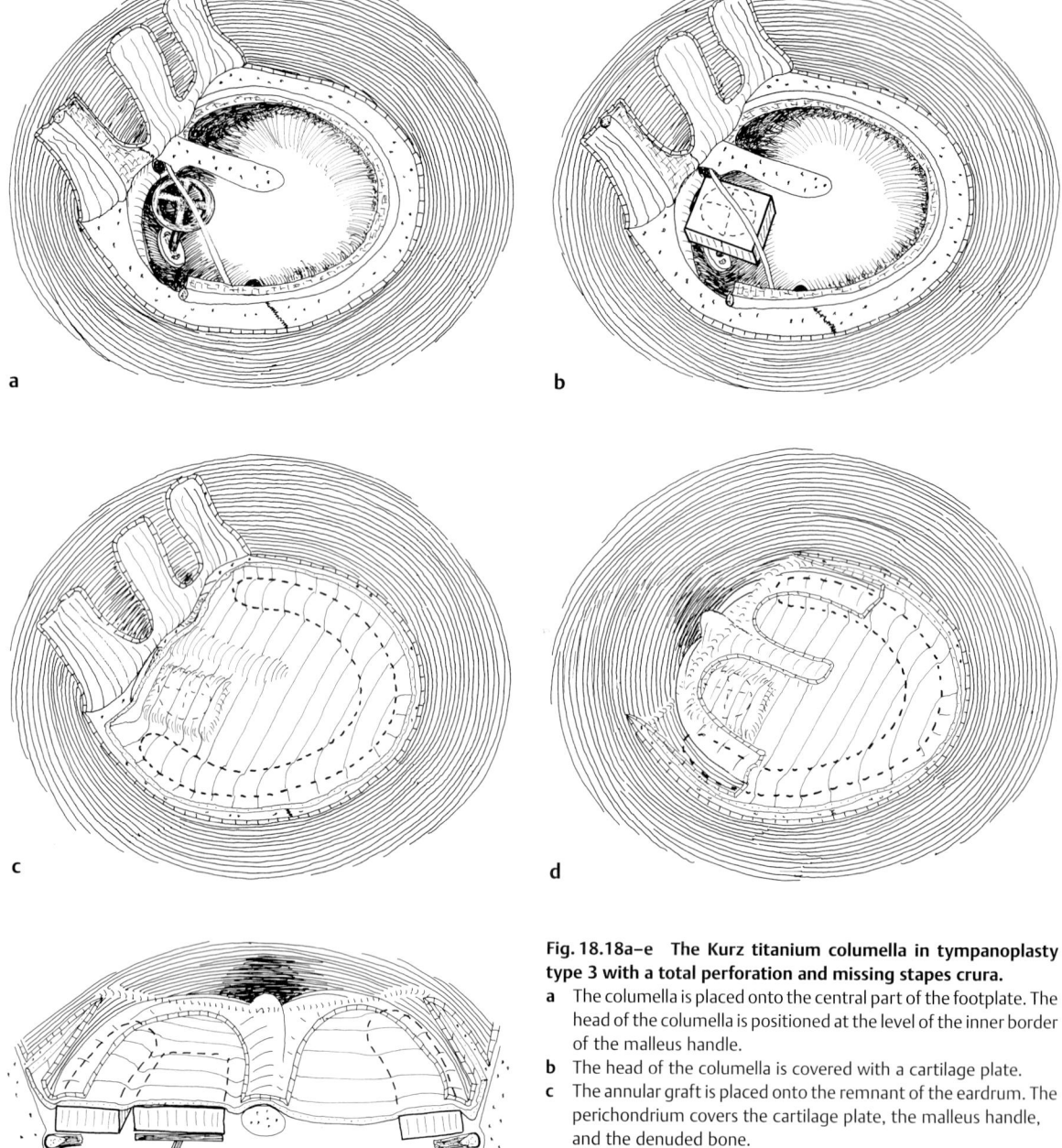

The Klacansky Annular Graft Technique with Removal of Fibrous Annulus and Eardrum Remnant

Since 1996 Klacansky has removed the entire fibrous annulus, along with the eardrum remnant and the attached ear canal skin. A medial circumferential incision of the ear canal skin is made (**Fig. 18.19a**) and the ear canal skin, the fibrous annulus, and the eardrum remnant are elevated from the tympanic sulcus and the bony annulus (**Fig. 18.19b, c**) and removed as a single component (**Fig. 18.19 d**). After cleaning of the malleus handle and elevation of the epithelial flap (**Fig. 18.19e**), the annular graft is placed into the tympanic cavity at the level of the bony annulus (**Fig. 18.19 f**). The surrounding peripheral perichondrium is folded out onto the denuded bone and adapted to the borders of the ear canal skin. Superiorly, the perichondrium is pushed, with an incudostapedial knife, up under the epithelium (**Fig. 18.19 g**) and the malleus flap is replaced (**Fig. 18.19h**).

The annular graft lies in the tympanic cavity at the level of the bony annulus and is thus suspended along with the perichondrium (**Fig. 18.19i**).

The ear canal is packed with the Klacansky packing, consisting of small balls of gauze connected with a silk thread (**Fig. 18.19j**).

Further Development of the Klacansky Annular Graft

Klacansky believes (personal communication, 2008) that in his hands the annular graft is the best graft, because it uses the cartilage as the frame only. Most of the graft consists of the stretched perichondrium (**Fig. 18.19k [i]**). The cartilage frame is smaller in comparison with the first annular grafts (**Figs. 18.3** and **18.8 d**). Such a graft is a combination of two properties, of soft and hard parts of the graft. Therefore, the hearing may become good early after the surgery, in contrast to hearing in total pars tensa cartilage–perichondrium composite grafts.

With intact malleus handle, the superior piece of the cartilage ring is removed to accommodate the superior part of the malleus handle. The next common modification is leaving a superoposterior cartilage plate (**Fig. 18.19k [ii]**) to accommodate the tympanoplasty type 2 with interposition between the stapes head and the annular graft, or tympanoplasty type 3 with placement of a columella between the footplate and the annular graft (**Fig. 18.19k [iii]**) The third variation is to leave half of the cartilage plate connected with the annulus graft (**Fig. 18.19k [iv]**). By rotation of the annular graft, the plate may cover the posterior half of the tympanic cavity, the superior, the anterior or the inferior half of the tympanic cavity.

The Borkowski Underlay Annular Graft Technique

Borkowski, Sudhoff, and Luckhaupt (1999) employ a classic underlay technique using a retroauricular approach, starting with the removal of the edges of the perforation (**Fig. 18.20a**) and the mucosa under the anterior remnant of the perforation and also the anterior wall of the tympanic cavity (**Fig. 18.20b**) to allow sufficient contact between the graft perichondrium and the denuded anterior wall of the tympanic cavity. After elevation of the posterior tympanomeatal flap (**Fig. 18.20c**) the annular graft is placed in the tympanic cavity (**Fig. 18.20d**). Anteriorly, the peripheral perichondrial flap is pushed under the bony annulus onto the denuded anterior wall of the tympanic cavity. The posterior and inferior parts of the perichondrial flap are folded out onto the denuded bone and adapted to the edges of the epithelium. After replacement of the tympanomeatal flap (**Fig. 18.20e**), the side view shows the annular flap in the tympanic cavity being suspended all the way round by the perichondrium (**Fig. 18.20f**), except for the anterior section of the perichondrium, which is attached to the undersurface of the anterior wall of the tympanic cavity.

Placement of the Annular Graft in the Underlay Technique with Elevation of the Anterior Fibrous Annulus

Instead of placing the anterior perichondrium under the anterior fibrous and bony annulus along the denuded anterior wall of the tympanic cavity (**Fig. 18.21a**), the anterior fibrous annulus with the eardrum remnant may be elevated (**Fig. 18.21b, c**), thus allowing the placement of the perichondrium flap onto the denuded bone (**Fig. 18.21d–f**). The stability of the suspension of the anterior part of the annular graft is thus secured (**Fig. 18.21g**).

Retracted Malleus Handle and Annular Graft

A particular function of the annular graft is to suspend the elevated malleus handle to the desired level during the critical postoperative period. The central perichondrium, being placed under the malleus handle, prevents immediate re-retraction, especially in the on-lay technique, with the annular graft being placed onto the fibrous annulus and onto the eardrum remnant.

a

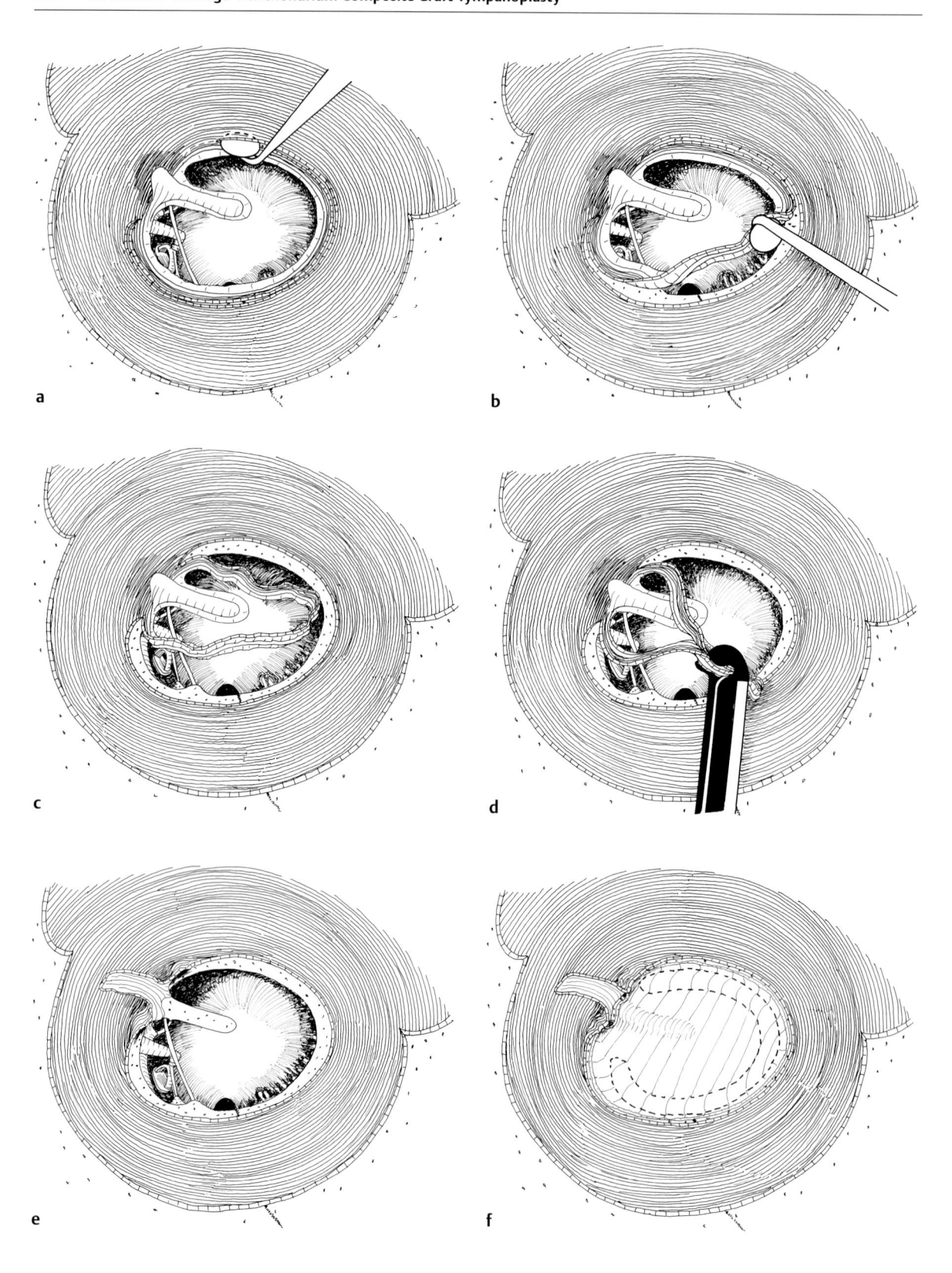

b

c

d

e

f

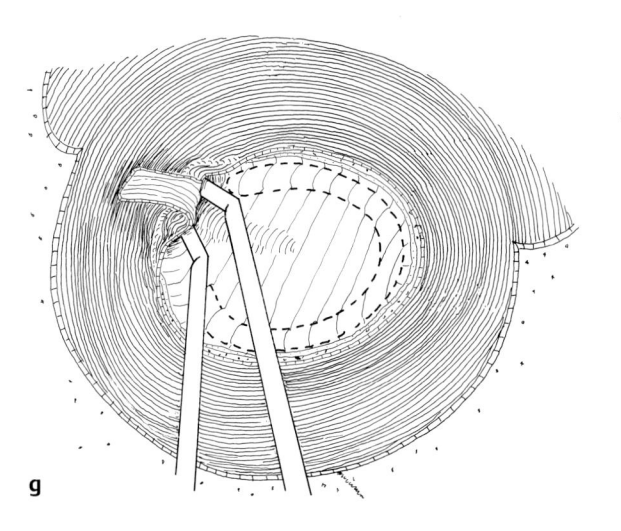

Fig. 18.19a–k The Klacansky method of annular graft with removal of the fibrous annulus and eardrum remnant and placement of an annular cartilage–perichondrium graft in the case of a total perforation and intact ossicular chain.

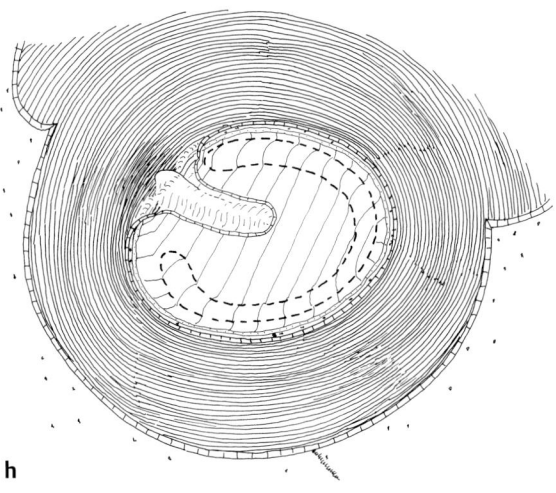

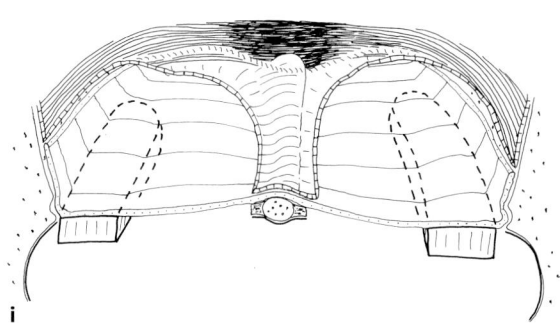

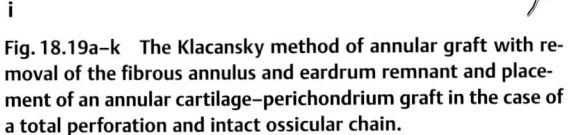

a   A medial circumferential incision of the ear canal skin between the 11-o'clock and 1-o'clock positions is made slightly lateral to the fibrous annulus.
b   Posteriorly, the ear canal skin with the fibrous annulus and the remnant of the eardrum is elevated, exposing the bony annulus.
c   The fibrous annulus is elevated all the way round, including the superior region. The bony annulus is exposed round the entire circumference.
d   The fibrous annulus and the eardrum remnant are removed, exposing the entire bony annulus.
e   The epithelium covering the malleus handle is elevated as a flap up to the short process. The superior edges of the epithelium are elevated slightly, preparing the surface for the perichondrium.
f   The annular graft is placed into the tympanic cavity at the level of the bony annulus. The central perichondrial part of the graft is placed onto the malleus handle. The peripheral perichondrium flaps are placed onto the bony annulus and denuded ear canal bone. This perichondrium is adapted to the borders of the ear canal skin. Superiorly, the perichondrium is placed under the elevated skin flaps.
g   Further elevation of the superior eardrum epithelium and placement of the borders of the perichondrium under the epithelium using an incudostapedial knife.
h   The small superior epithelial flaps and the malleus flap are replaced and the perichondrium is adapted to the edges. The annular cartilage graft is suspended by the perichondrium flaps.
i   Cross-sectional view of the Klacansky annular graft. The cartilage ring is placed at the level of bony annulus and is suspended by the perichondrium placed onto the denuded bone of the ear canal and the malleus handle.
j   The Klacansky packing of the ear canal. A black silk thread is tied to several consecutive small balls of gauze moistened with hydrocortisone–oxytetracycline. The gauze balls are placed onto the perichondrium along the bony annulus, fixing it along the ear canal bone.

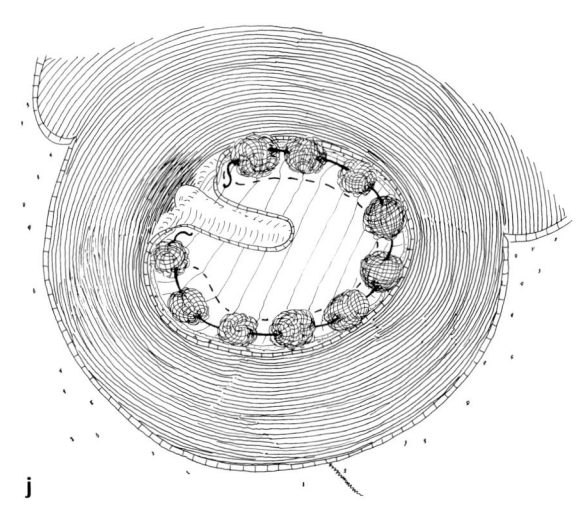

Fig. 18.19k ▷

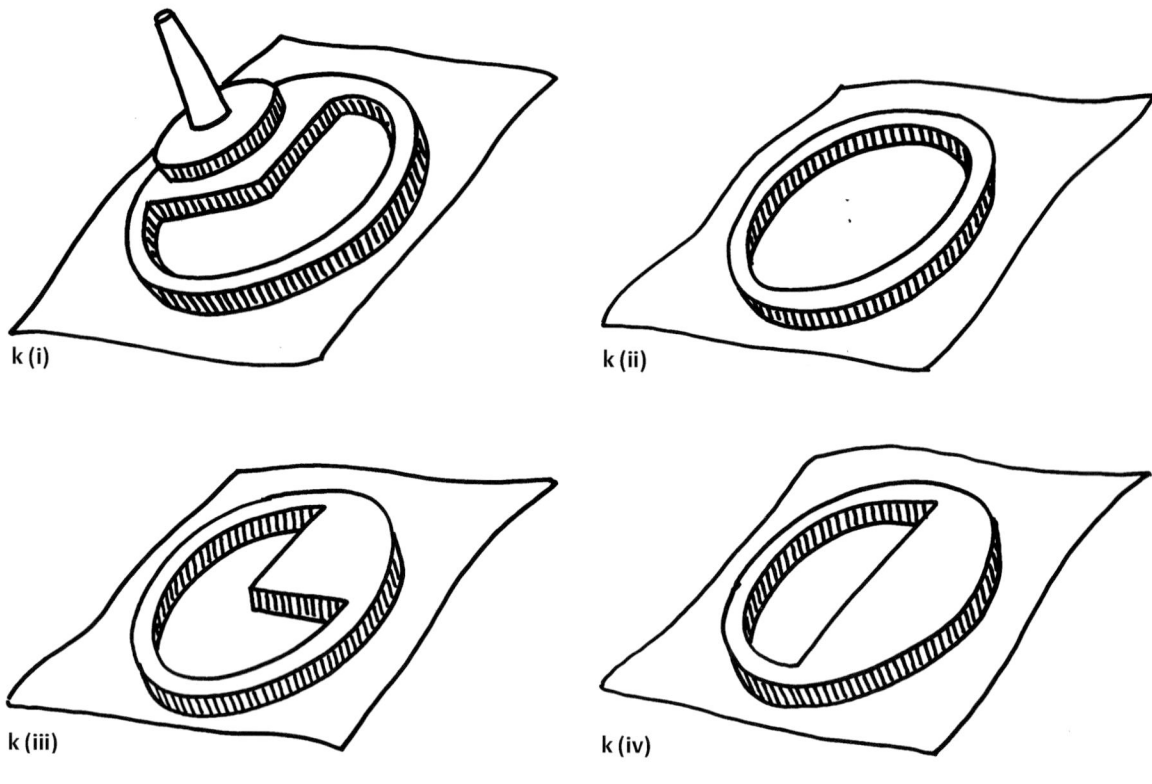

Fig. 18.19
k The Klacansky annular grafts. (The four figures ar those of Klacansky.) **i** The superoposterior cartilage plate covers the columella in tympanoplasty type 3. **ii** The round annular graft, less than 1 mm wide, with the stretched central perichondrium and a surrounding peripheral perichondrium flap. **iii** The annular graft is connected to a superoposterior cartilage plate. **iv** The annular graft is connected with a large cartilage plate, covering half of the tympanic cavity.

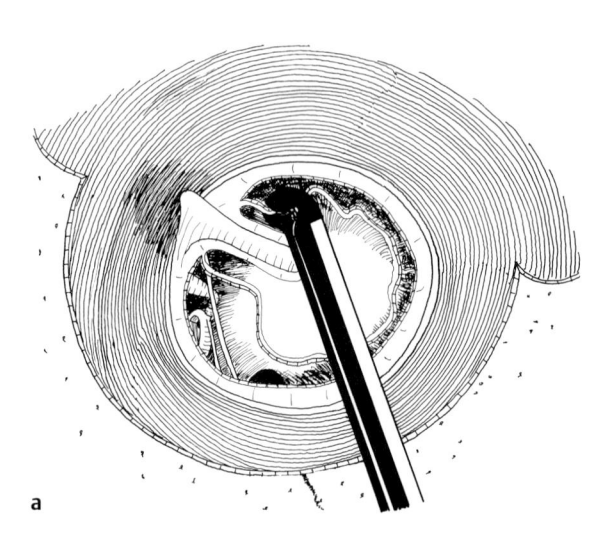

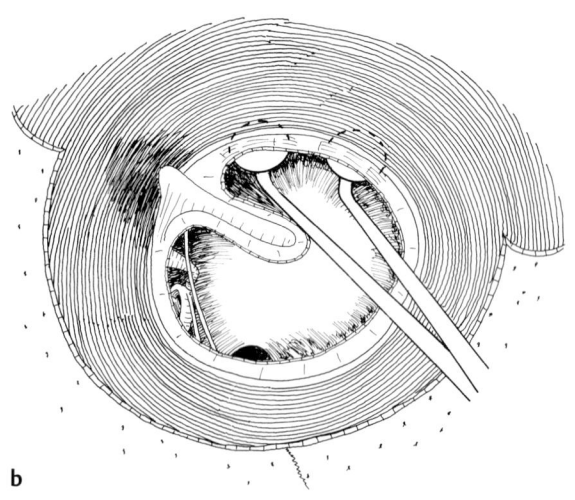

Fig. 18.20a–f The Borkowski underlay placement of the annular graft in a total perforation and an intact ossicular chain.
a Via a retroauricular approach, the edges of the perforation are removed.
b The mucosa under the anterior remnant of the perforation and under the fibrous annulus is removed to promote the attachment of the anterior perichondrium to the anterior wall of the tympanic cavity.

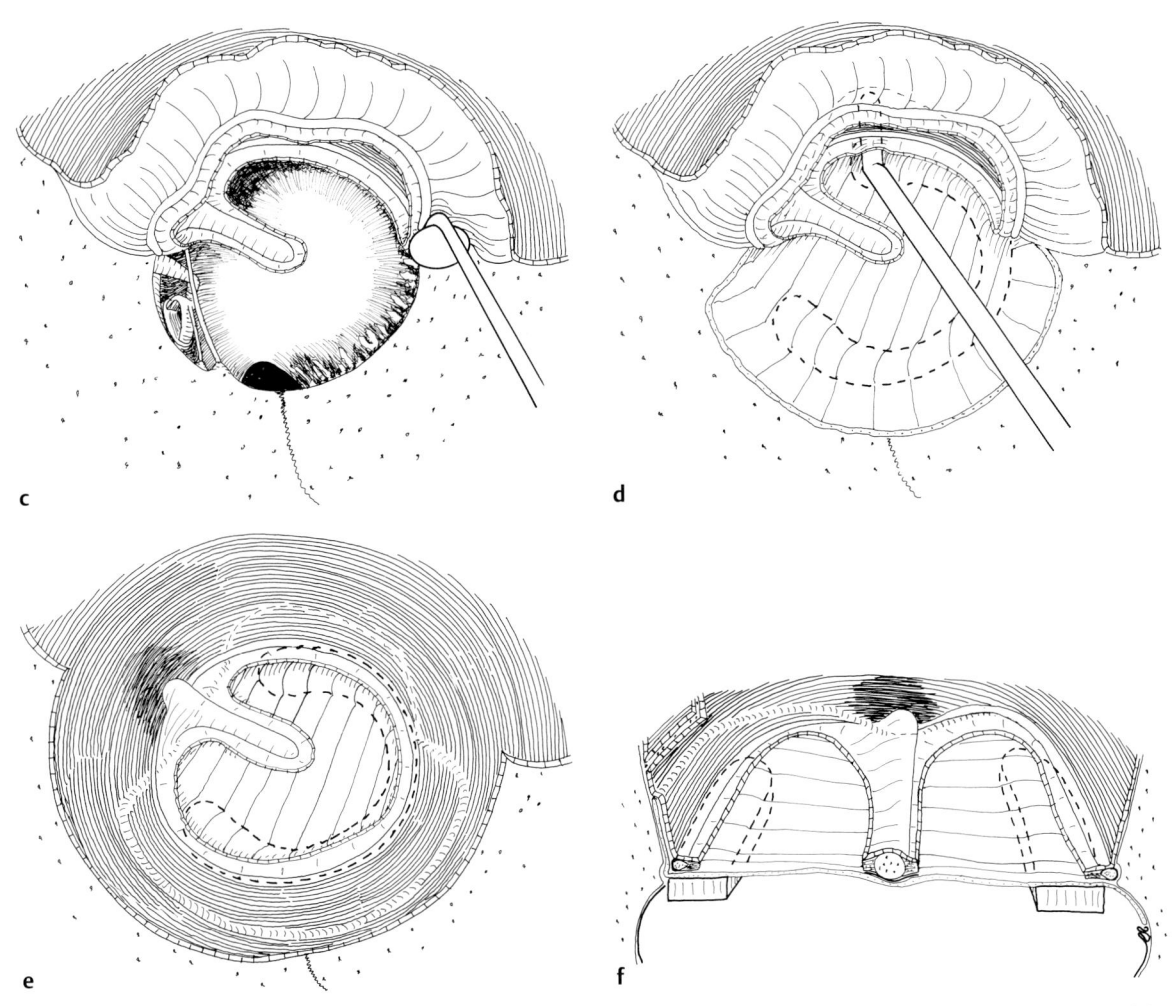

Fig. 18.20c–f

c The tympanomeatal flap with the fibrous annulus and the remnant of the eardrum is elevated.

d Anteriorly, the annular graft is placed under the eardrum remnant. Using an incudostapedial knife, the anterior perichondrial flap is pushed as much anteriorly as possible to be able to suspend the annular graft. Posteriorly and inferiorly, the cartilage is easily positioned in the tympanic cavity at the level of the bony annulus. Posteriorly, the graft is firmly suspended by the perichondrium being folded out onto the denuded bone.

e The tympanomeatal flap is replaced. The fibrous annulus and the remnant of the eardrum are placed onto the perichondrium flap.

f Cross-sectional view showing the position of the annular graft. Anteriorly, the perichondrium lies close on the denuded area of the anterior wall of the tympanum. The cartilage ring is in the tympanic cavity at the level of the bony annulus. The perichondrium lies under the malleus handle and under the fibrous annulus.

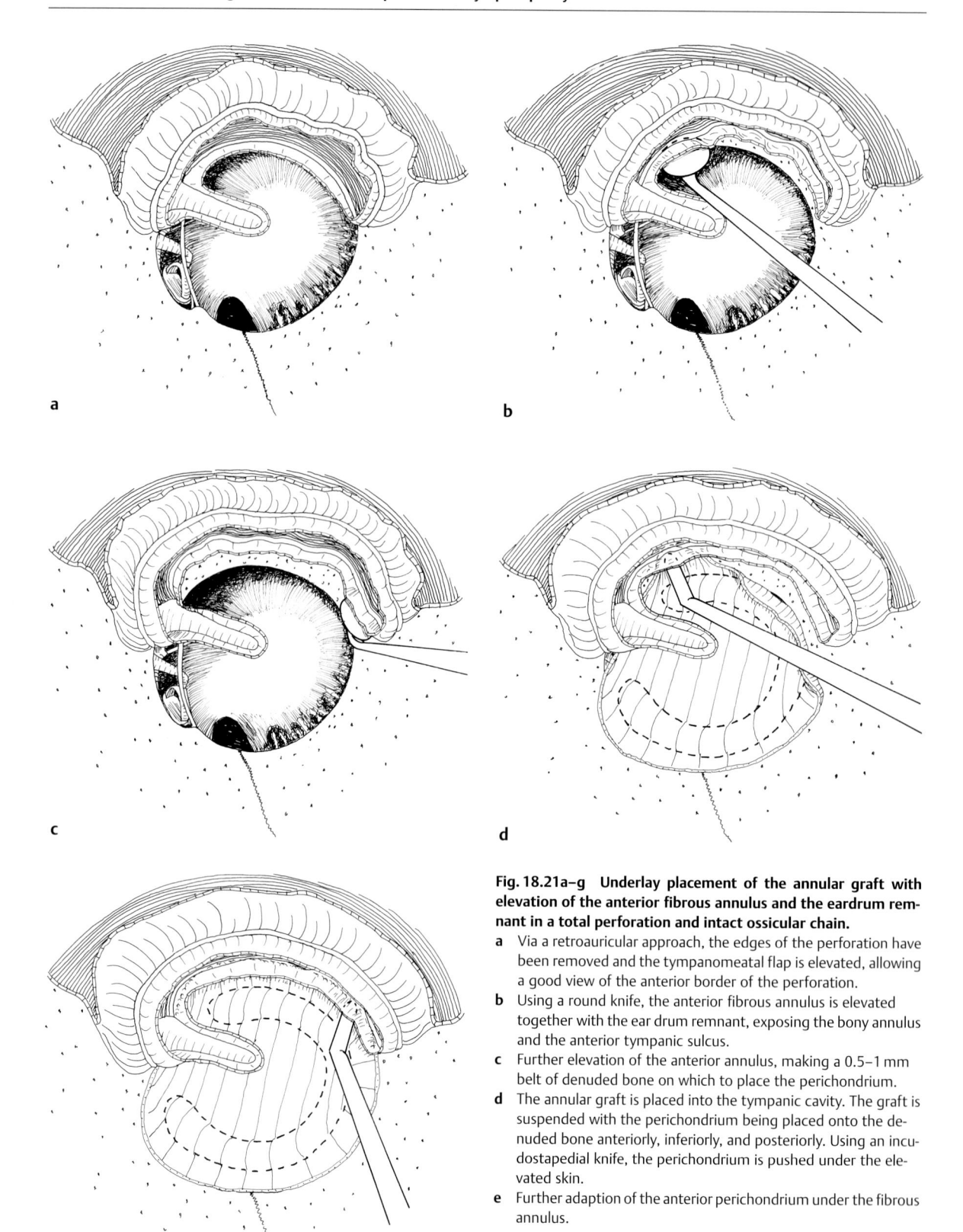

Fig. 18.21a–g Underlay placement of the annular graft with elevation of the anterior fibrous annulus and the eardrum remnant in a total perforation and intact ossicular chain.

a Via a retroauricular approach, the edges of the perforation have been removed and the tympanomeatal flap is elevated, allowing a good view of the anterior border of the perforation.
b Using a round knife, the anterior fibrous annulus is elevated together with the ear drum remnant, exposing the bony annulus and the anterior tympanic sulcus.
c Further elevation of the anterior annulus, making a 0.5–1 mm belt of denuded bone on which to place the perichondrium.
d The annular graft is placed into the tympanic cavity. The graft is suspended with the perichondrium being placed onto the denuded bone anteriorly, inferiorly, and posteriorly. Using an incudostapedial knife, the perichondrium is pushed under the elevated skin.
e Further adaption of the anterior perichondrium under the fibrous annulus.

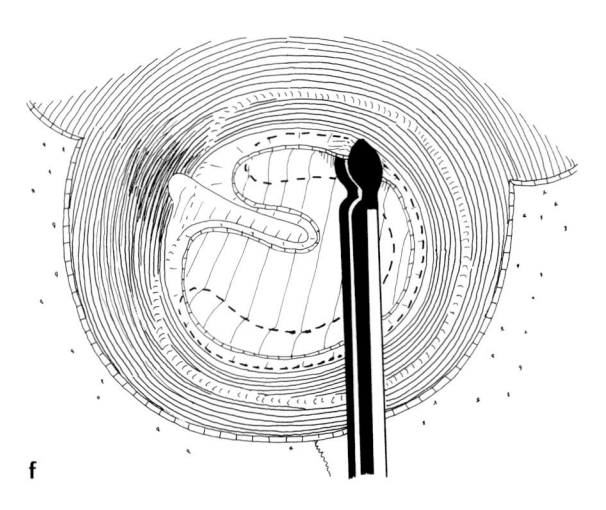

Fig. 18.21f, g
f The anterior fibrous annulus and the eardrum remnant are replaced in the original position. After placement of the perichondrium, the posterior flap is also replaced.
g Cross-sectional view of underlay annular graft with the elevation of the anterior fibrous annulus and the placement of the perichondrium onto the bony annulus. The cartilage graft is placed in the tympanic cavity at the level of the bony annulus. The anterior peripheral perichondrium is placed onto the bony annulus and is covered with the fibrous annulus and eardrum remnant. The central perichondrium is under the malleus handle.

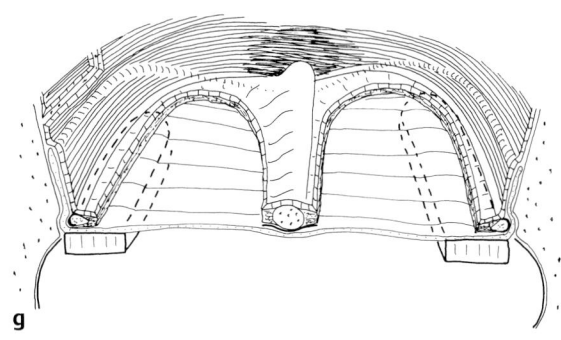

Pathogenesis of Retracted and Adherent Malleus Handle

On the basis our long-term epidemiological and clinical studies of secretory otitis media in children, the following stages of ear drum changes are observed in secretary otitis: (1) Diffuse atrophy with retraction of the malleus and myringoincudopexy that often progresses to resorption of the long process of the incus, resulting in myringostapediopexy. (2) Further retraction of the atrophic eardrum and malleus handle, causing contact between the umbo and the mucosa of the promontory. (3) In cases of acute suppurative otitis media, the atrophic pars tensa may become necrotic, resulting in a total perforation. At this time or on a later occasion, adhesions may occur between the promontory and the umbo in some cases.

These pathogenic changes may occur during the whole of childhood and may result in the following conditions seen at surgery: (1) Total perforation with retraction of the malleus handle with or without adhesions to the umbo. (2) Total perforation with retraction of the malleus handle and evidence of previous retraction such as (a) keratinized epithelium under the border of the perforation, (b) keratinized epithelium between the posterosuperior annulus and the incudostapedial joint. (3) Total perforation with retraction of the malleus handle and missing long process of the incus. (4) Total atelectasis of the eardrum, which, during the course of surgery and after removal of the adherent eardrum, will result in a total perforation.

Retracted and Adherent Malleus Handle and Annular Graft with Intact Ossicular Chain

Surgery of the retracted malleus handle with an intact incudostapedial joint should be delicate. Forceful manipulation of the malleus handle may cause disruption of the joint between the incus and the head of the malleus. A slight elevation and closure of the perforation using an annular graft placed under the malleus is the safest solution (**Fig. 18.22a, b**). After removal of the mucosa of the promontory and cleaning of the malleus handle, a small piece of Silastic is used to cover the mucosal defect to prevent refixation of the umbo. The annular graft is placed onto the eardrum remnant, with the central perichondrium under the malleus handle (**Fig. 18.22c**). The laterally placed annular graft, with the perichondrium placed under the malleus handle and reinforced by the perichondrial sandwich (**Fig. 18.22d, e**), is a good solution to this problem (**Fig. 18.22f**).

Retracted and Adherent Malleus Handle and Annular Graft in Tympanoplasty Type 2 with Interposition of a Prosthesis between Stapes and Eardrum

Elevation of the retracted and adherent malleus handle when the incus is missing is easier and safer than in cases with an intact ossicular chain, because the more forceful elevation of the malleus handle does not influence the stapes; the malleus handle can be elevated to the optimal level (**Fig. 18.23a**) and a shaped incus interposed between stapes head and the malleus handle (**Fig. 18.23b**). After placement of the annular graft, the perichondrium lies on the elevated malleus handle (**Fig. 18.23c–e**).

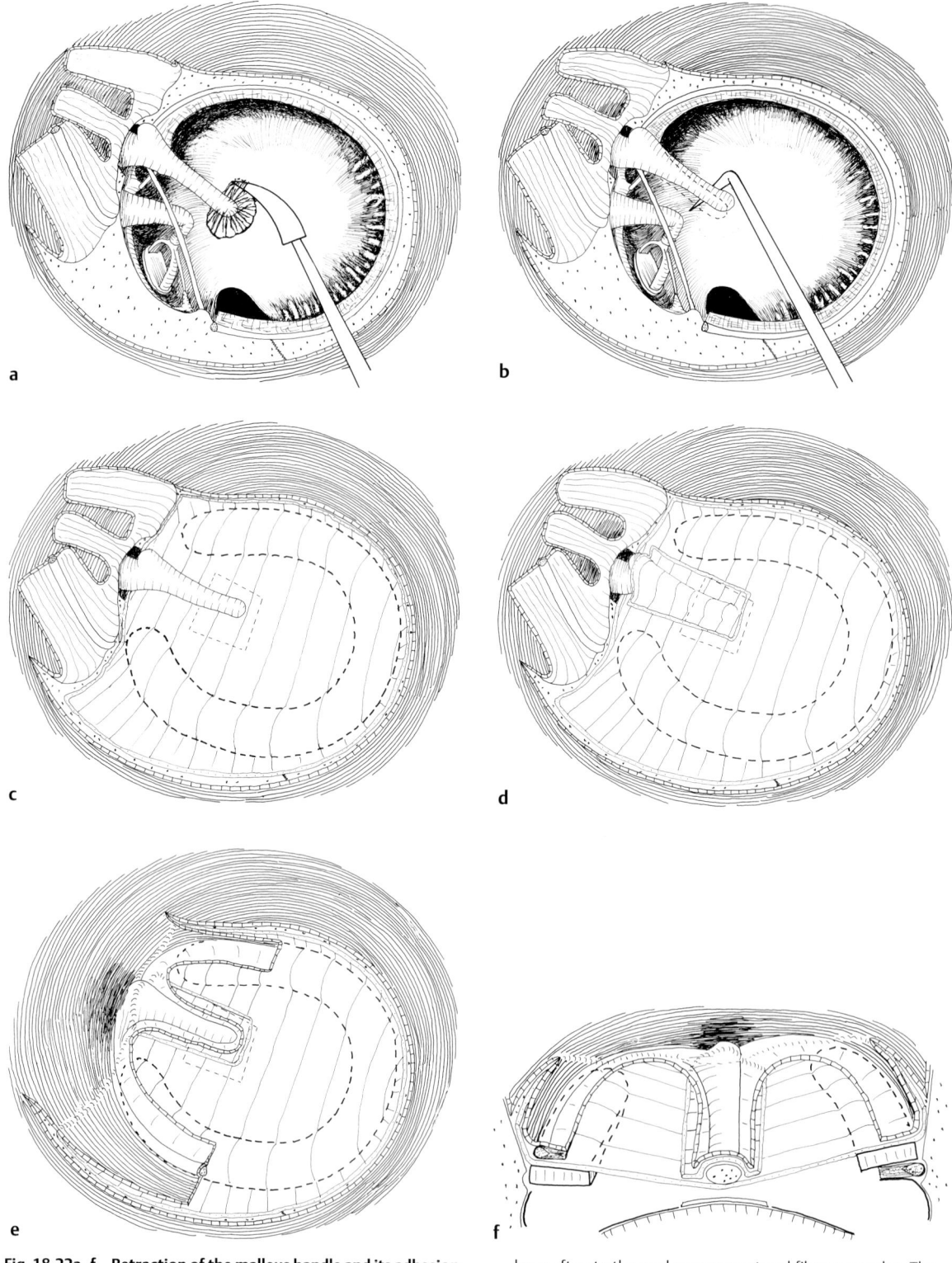

Fig. 18.22a–f Retraction of the malleus handle and its adhesion to the promontory with total perforation and annular graft.

a A circumferential incision is made and the three superior epithelial flaps are elevated. Inferiorly, the epithelium is removed. The mucosa with adhesions to the malleus is removed and the malleus handle is cleaned.

b The umbo is slightly elevated with a hook, thus allowing inspection of the movement of the incus and stapes.

c Under the umbo, the denuded area of the promontory is covered with a small piece of Silastic. The annular graft is placed as an onlay graft onto the eardrum remnant and fibrous annulus. The central perichondrium is placed under the malleus handle. The peripheral perichondrium is placed onto the bone.

d Another small piece of perichondrium is placed onto the malleus, creating a "perichondrial sandwich" (Goodhill 1967).

e The superior epithelial flaps are replaced and the perichondrium is adapted to the epithelium.

f Cross-sectional view of the retracted and adherent malleus handle and annular graft. The malleus is slightly elevated and is suspended by the perichondrium placed under the umbo.

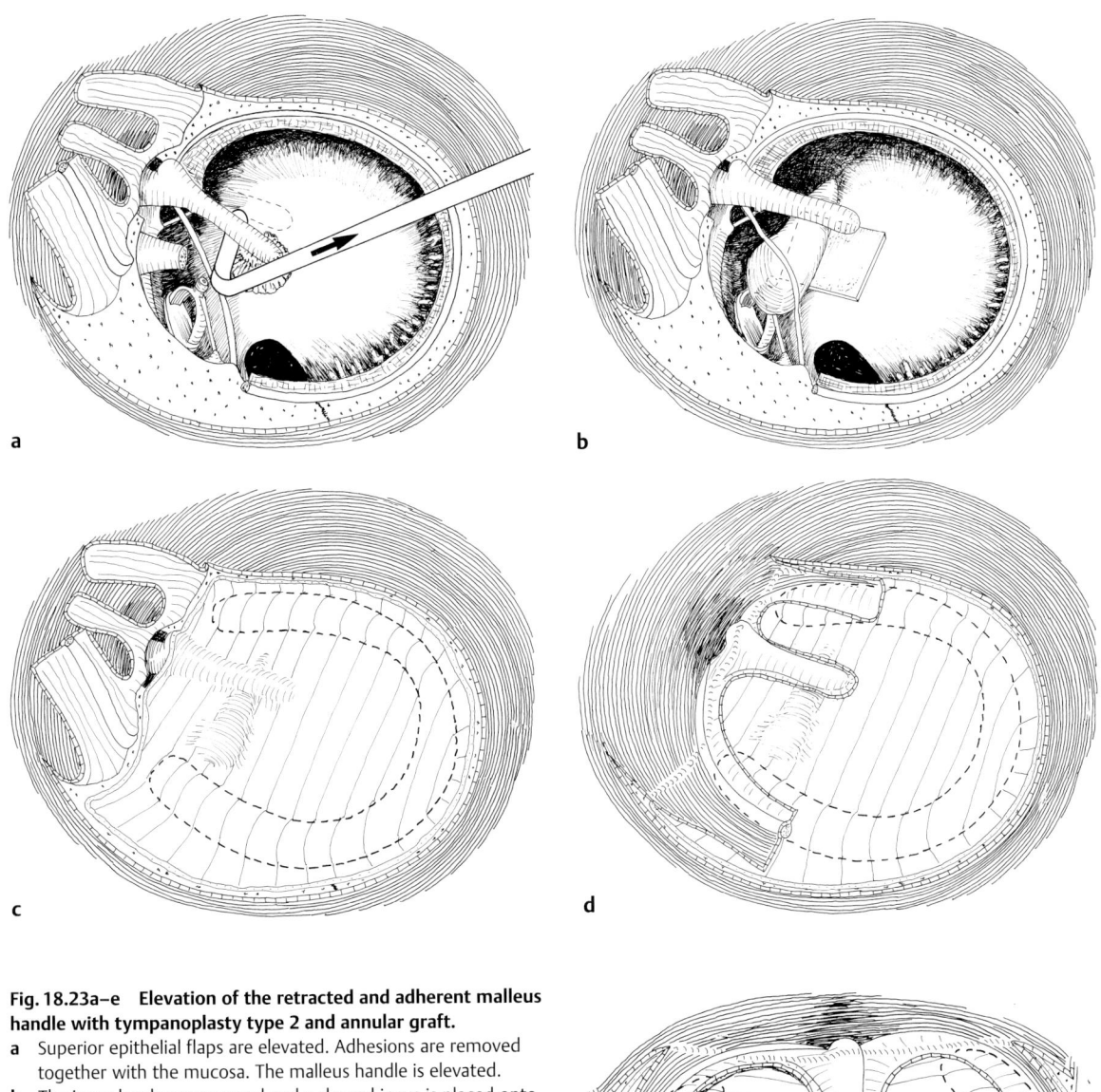

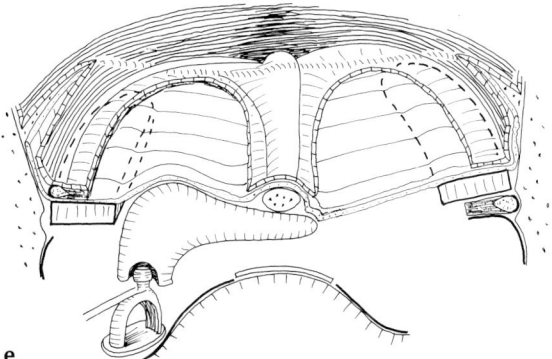

Fig. 18.23a–e Elevation of the retracted and adherent malleus handle with tympanoplasty type 2 and annular graft.
a Superior epithelial flaps are elevated. Adhesions are removed together with the mucosa. The malleus handle is elevated.
b The incus has been removed and a shaped incus is placed onto the head of the stapes,
c The annular graft is placed onto the eardrum remnant and the central perichondrium onto the elevated malleus.
d The epithelial flaps are replaced and the perichondrium is adapted to the epithelium.
e Cross-sectional view in the elevation of the malleus handle tympanoplasty type 2 with a shaped incus interposition and annular graft. A depression is made on the incus to fit onto the stapes head. The incus graft is placed under the elevated malleus handle. The central perichondrium is placed onto the malleus handle.

Missing Malleus Handle and Annular Graft

Absence of the malleus handle is caused by tensa retraction cholesteatoma, defined as the retraction of the entire pars tensa, involving the entire tympanic cavity including the posterosuperior region, hypotympanic cells, and tubal orifice. The cholesteatoma extends medial to the incus posteriorly and medial to the malleus head into the anterior attic

Incidence of Ears with Missing Malleus Handle

In an extensive analysis of ossicular defects in 1100 consecutive ears operated in Gentofte Hospital (Tos 1979, 1981), the following incidence of malleus handle defects was found in various diseases:
- Among 152 attic cholesteatomas, no ears with a missing malleus handle were found. This is logical because the bone resorption starts in the attic and continues in a superior direction.
- Among 166 ears with sinus cholesteatoma, defined as posterosuperior retraction of the pars tensa with a cholesteatomatous mass in the tympanic sinuses, no ears with a missing malleus handle only were found in the group with an intact ossicular chain, but 4% of ears had a missing malleus handle and a missing incus or missing stapes. In these advanced cases the pathology may have started with retraction of the entire pars tensa and then extended to the tympanic sinuses.
- Among 108 ears with the third type of acquired cholesteatoma—the entire tensa retraction cholesteatoma—11% of ears had a missing malleus handle only, 8% had a missing malleus handle with a missing incus, and 6% had a missing malleus handle with missing stapes. Thus 25% of ears with entire tensa retraction cholesteatoma had a missing malleus handle (Tos 1979).

Among the remaining non-cholesteatomatous diseases, the percentage of ears with a missing malleus handle was 8% (Tos 1979) and most of these ears had a total perforation. Presumably the pathological changes in these ears may have started with secretory otitis and tubal dysfunction in childhood and been followed by diffuse atrophy and retraction of the eardrum. In complete retraction around the malleus handle, retraction pockets with infection were formed, causing proliferation of squamous epithelium and bone resorption of the malleus handle. Later an acute otitis may cause necrosis of the retracted membranes with disappearance of the membranes together with the remnants of the resorbed malleus handle. The final result is a total perforation and a missing malleus handle.

Cartilage–Perichondrium Composite Graft in Missing Malleus Handle with an Intact Incudostapedial Joint and Annular Graft

There are several solutions to the problem of a missing malleus handle and an intact incudostapedial joint. Some surgeons will disrupt the incudostapedial joint and perform a type 2 tympanoplasty, but most will keep the incudostapedial joint intact and improve the connection between the incudostapedial joint and the eardrum with cartilage plates. Sheehy recommended this principle in the late 1960s (Sheehy 1972). I use this method of cartilage plates and it is illustrated in MMES_1, Figs. 944–947.

Instead of cartilage plates, a cartilage–perichondrium composite island graft can be used and adapted to the annular graft (**Fig. 18.24a, b**). The cartilage of the composite graft is placed onto the long process of the incus with the intact incudostapedial joint and onto the denuded remnant of the malleus handle. The superior free perichondrium flap covers the lateral process of the malleus and stabilizes the cartilage prosthesis to the malleus remnant. The annular graft is placed anteriorly under the eardrum remnant, and posteriorly at the level of the bony annulus (**Fig. 18.24c, d**).

Tympanoplasty Type 2 with Interposition of the Incus in Missing Malleus Handle with an Interrupted Ossicular Chain and Annular Graft

An autogenous incus is placed onto the head of the stapes with its short process close to the remnant of the malleus (**Fig. 18.25a, b**). Using a strip of perichondrium, the short process of the incus is stabilized to the malleus remnant. The posterosuperior end of the annular graft is trimmed and the graft is placed into the tympanic cavity. The perichondrium covers the incus (**Fig. 18.25c–e**).

Tympanoplasty Type 3 with Titanium Columella and Annular Graft in Missing Malleus Handle and Stapes

Using a transcanal approach, the edges of the total perforation are removed and a posterior tympanomeatal flap is elevated by an underlay swing-door technique. The titanium columella is placed onto the middle of the footplate and covered with a cartilage plate (**Fig. 18.26a, b**). The annular graft fits very well in relation to the cartilage plate (**Fig. 18.26c–e**).

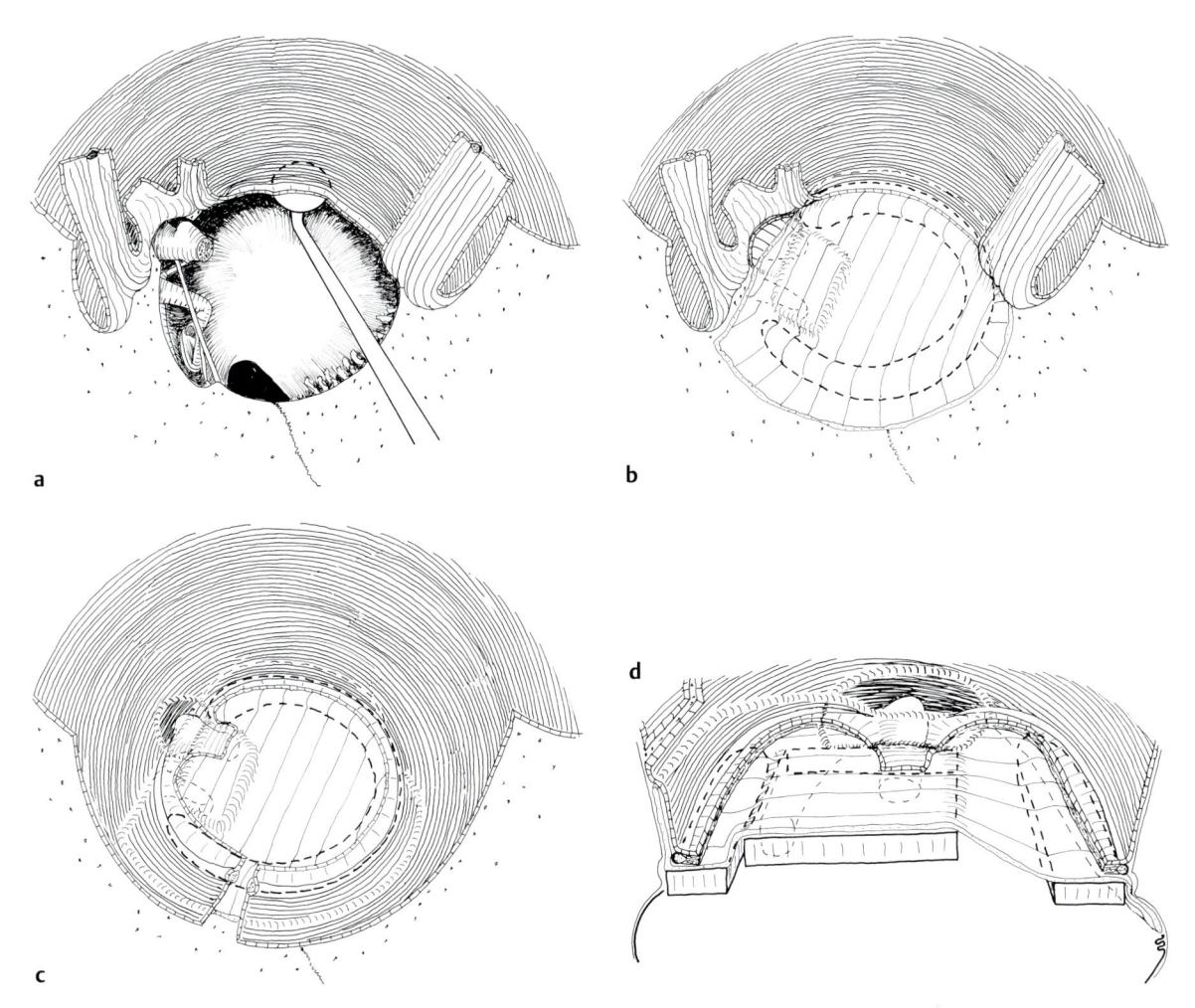

Fig. 18.24a–d Missing malleus handle and annulus graft in case of total perforation and intact ossicular chain.
a Using the retroauricular approach, the edges of the perforation are removed and a posterior tympanomeatal flap is raised by the swing-door technique. Superiorly, all epithelium is elevated, exposing the neck of the malleus. The mucosa under the anterior annulus is removed to prepare the bed for the underlay placement of the perichondrium.
b A tragal cartilage plate covered with perichondrium on the lateral side and with a small free flap is placed onto the long process of the incus and incudostapedial joint as well as onto the denuded remnant of the malleus. The free anterosuperior perichondrium flap covers the short process of the malleus. The annular graft is placed under the anterior eardrum remnant and the perichondrium is pushed under the bony annulus and toward the anterior wall of the tympanic cavity. Posteriorly, the annular graft is placed at the level of the bony annulus.
c The epithelial flaps are replaced.
d Cross-sectional view of annular graft in case of a missing malleus handle and total perforation. The cartilage plate lies on the intact incudostapedial joint and is connected with the remnant of the malleus handle and fixed with a free perichondrium flap. The annular graft lies at the level of the bony annulus. The central perichondrium covers the cartilage plate.

Circular Annular Graft in Case of Missing Entire Malleus

Sometimes the entire malleus is missing when the surgeon has removed the remnant of the malleus head, either in the case of spontaneous resorption of the malleus handle, or because of a cholesteatoma remnant, or because its removal makes easier the placement of a prosthesis and a circular annular graft (**Fig. 18.27a–d**). The head of the prosthesis placed onto the head of the stapes and the relatively large cartilage plate covering the prosthesis occupies the superior part of the tympanic cavity, with a good chance for hearing improvement. Superior to the circular cartilage ring, small cartilage palisades prevent retraction into the attic and the central perichondrium stabilizes the prosthesis (**Fig. 18.27e, f**).

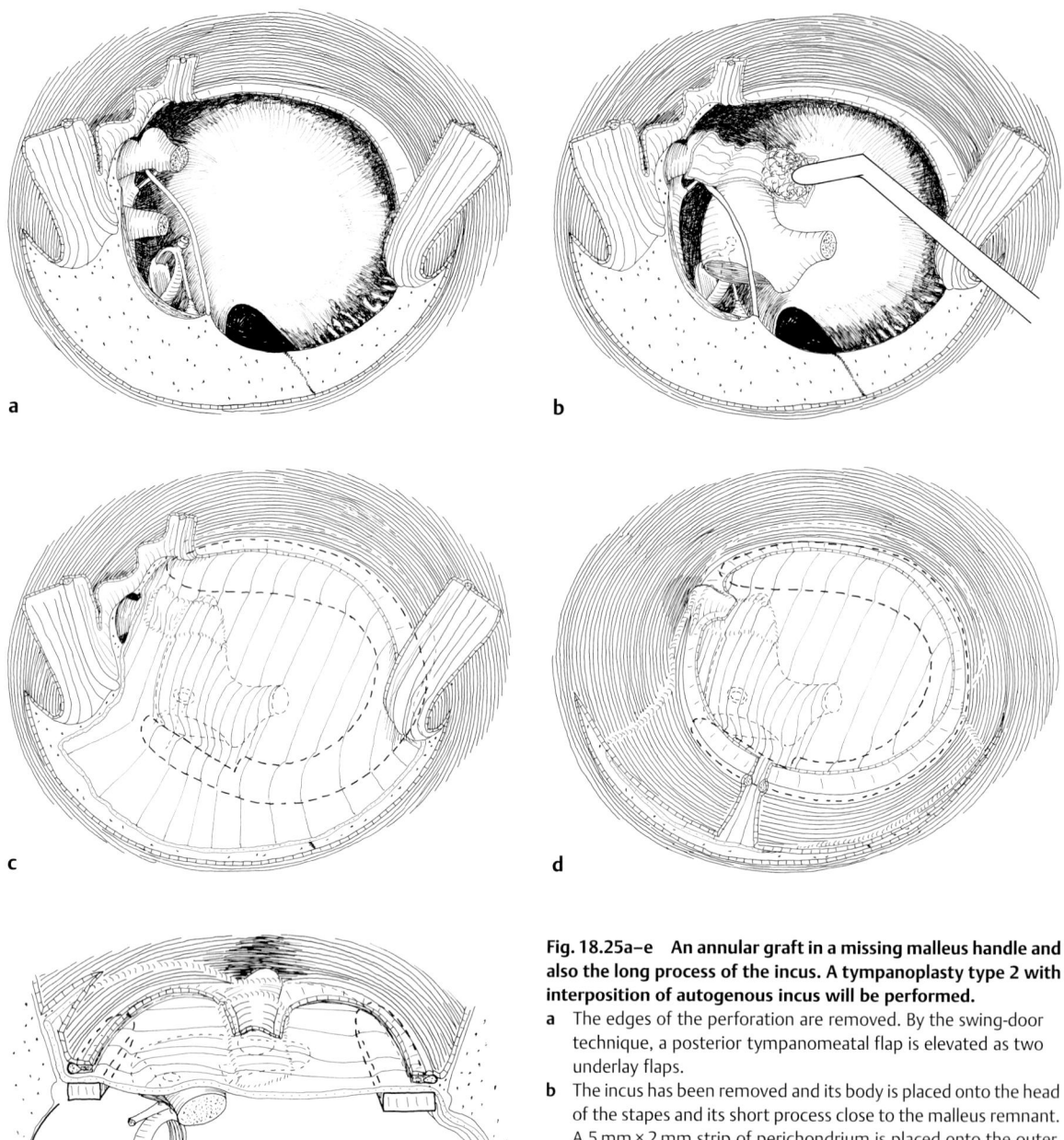

Fig. 18.25a–e An annular graft in a missing malleus handle and also the long process of the incus. A tympanoplasty type 2 with interposition of autogenous incus will be performed.

a The edges of the perforation are removed. By the swing-door technique, a posterior tympanomeatal flap is elevated as two underlay flaps.
b The incus has been removed and its body is placed onto the head of the stapes and its short process close to the malleus remnant. A 5 mm × 2 mm strip of perichondrium is placed onto the outer surface of the lateral process of the malleus and onto the short process of the incus. Then the strip of perichondrium is pushed, together with a ball of Gelfoam, around the medial site of the incus and malleus, thus fixing the incus to the malleus.
c The annular graft, slightly trimmed at the posterosuperior end is placed as an underlay graft and the perichondrium anteriorly is placed under the bony annulus.
d The epithelial flaps are replaced.
e Cross-sectional view in tympanoplasty type 2 with incus interposition and contact with the remnant of the malleus

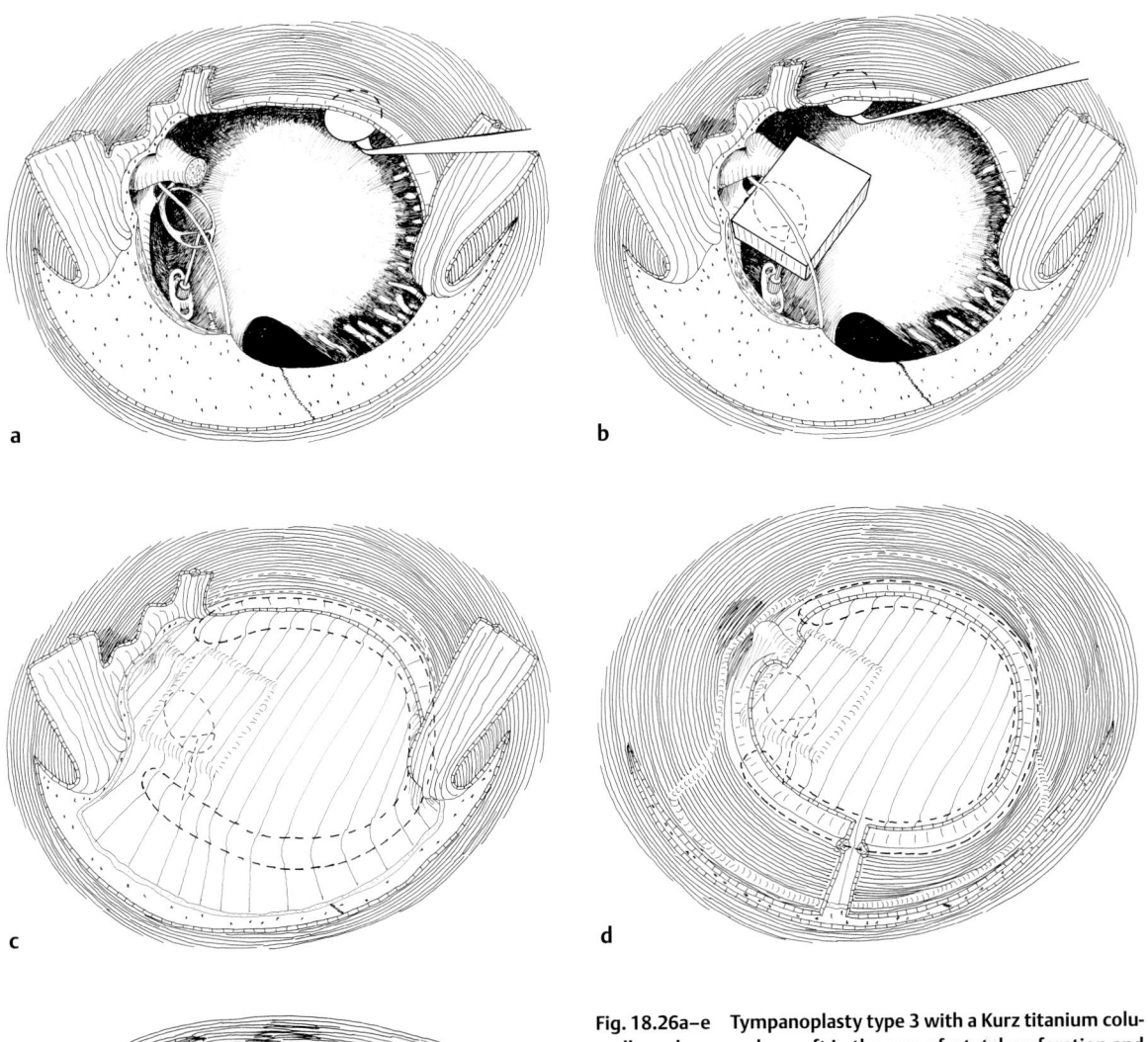

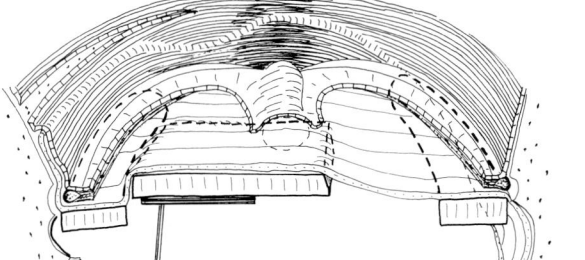

Fig. 18.26a–e Tympanoplasty type 3 with a Kurz titanium columella and an annular graft in the case of a total perforation and missing malleus handle and stapedial arch.

a By a transcanal approach, the edges of the perforation are removed, the posterior tympanomeatal flap is elevated, and the mucosa under the anterior eardrum remnant and the anterior bony annulus is removed. The columella is placed onto the central part of the footplate.

b A cartilage plate is placed onto the head of the columella, which also contacts the denuded remnant of the malleus handle.

c The annular graft is placed into the tympanic cavity at the level of the bony annulus and the anterior perichondrium is placed onto the denuded bone and under the anterior annulus. The central perichondrium covers and stabilizes the cartilage plate.

d The epithelial flaps are replaced.

e Cross-sectional view of the titanium columella covered with a cartilage plate and an underlay placement of the annular graft. The annular graft is placed more superiorly and the cartilage plate contacts the malleus remnant.

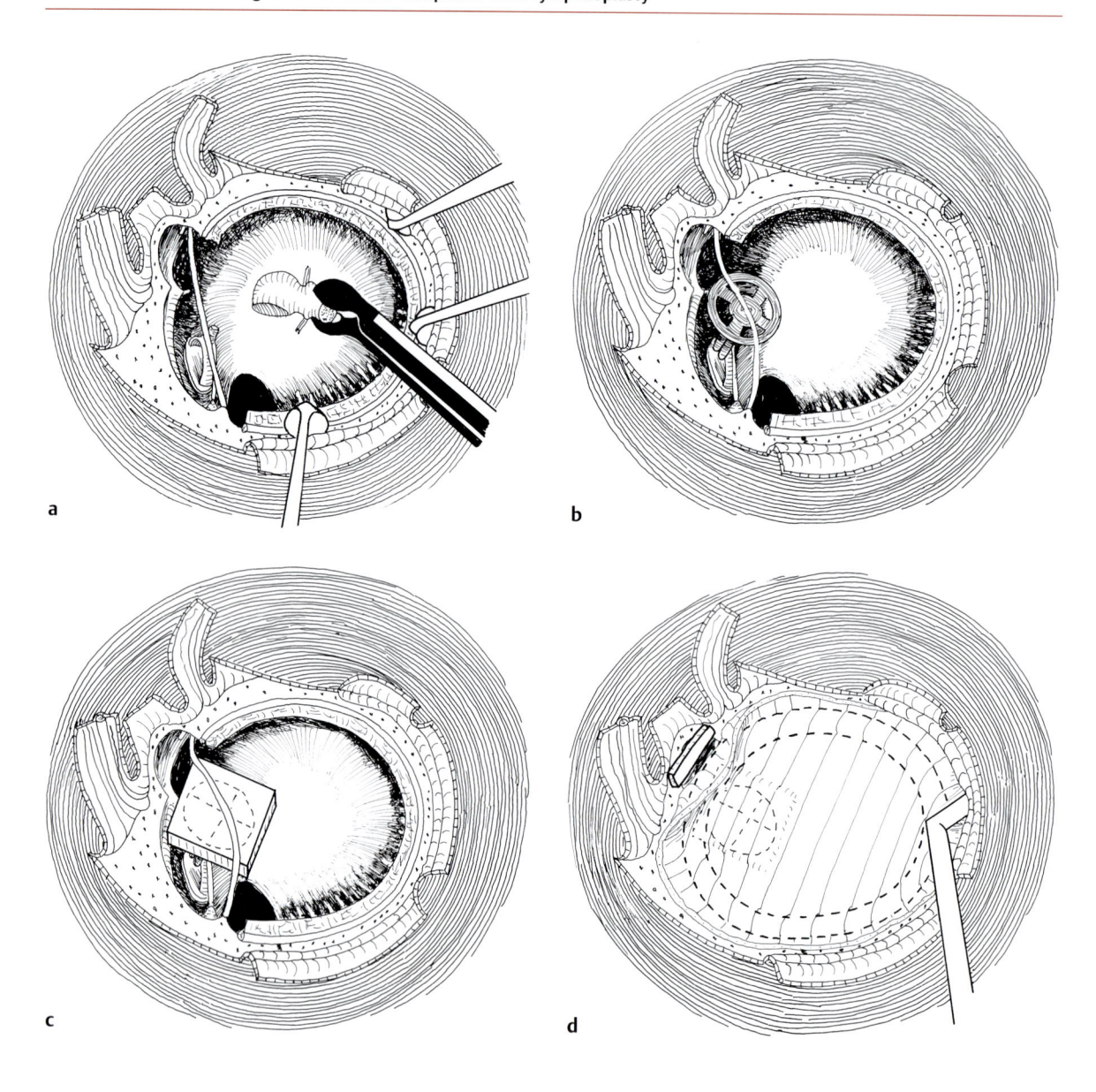

U-shaped Annular Graft in Large Inferior Perforation

In case of a large inferior perforation or a subtotal perforation, a smaller, U-shaped annular graft can be used via the transcanal, endaural, or retroauricular approaches, with an on-lay or underlay technique (**Fig. 18.28a, b**). The U-shaped graft is placed in the inferior half of the tympanic cavity at the level of the bony annulus and the peripheral perichondrium is folded out over the ear canal bone. Superiorly, the perichondrium is placed under the eardrum (**Fig. 18.28c, d**).

Annular Graft in the Reconstruction of the Tympanic Cavity after a Canal Wall Down Mastoidectomy

There are several options for the application of an annular graft in the reconstruction of the tympanic cavity after a canal wall down mastoidectomy. The attic may be open without obliteration (**Fig. 18.29a**) or partly obliterated with cartilage (**Fig. 18.29b**) or totally obliterated with cartilage plates (**Fig. 18.29c**). The peripheral perichondrium from the annular graft covers the cartilage in the attic.

The obliteration of the attic can be done with other materials, such as bone chips, bone paste and fibrous tissue (MMES_2, Figs. 687–689). The obliterated attic may also be covered with the fascia.

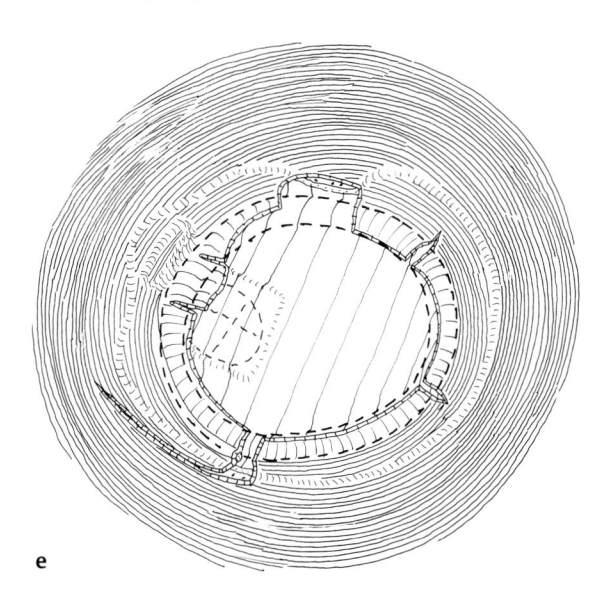

Fig. 18.27a–f Circular annular graft and tympanoplasty type 2 in a total perforation with both the entire malleus and the incus missing.

a The malleus head with the short process has been removed. A medial circumferential incision is made and the three superior epithelial flaps are elevated. Inferiorly, the eardrum epithelium is also elevated.
b A Kurz titanium prosthesis of Dresden type is placed onto the head of the stapes.
c The head of the prosthesis is covered with a cartilage plate.
d The circular annular graft is placed onto the eardrum remnant in the inferior half and in the anterosuperior part of the tympanic cavity. In the posterosuperior region and in the attic region, the circular graft is placed in the tympanic cavity. A small palisade of cartilage covers the attic region superiorly. The peripheral perichondrium covers the denuded bone.
e All the epithelial flaps are replaced.
f Cross-sectional view of the circular graft with interposition of a titanium prosthesis covered with a cartilage plate. The circular graft is placed anteriorly onto the fibrous annulus and posteriorly under the fibrous annulus.

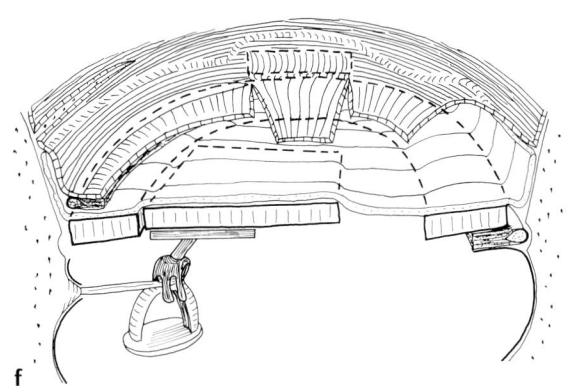

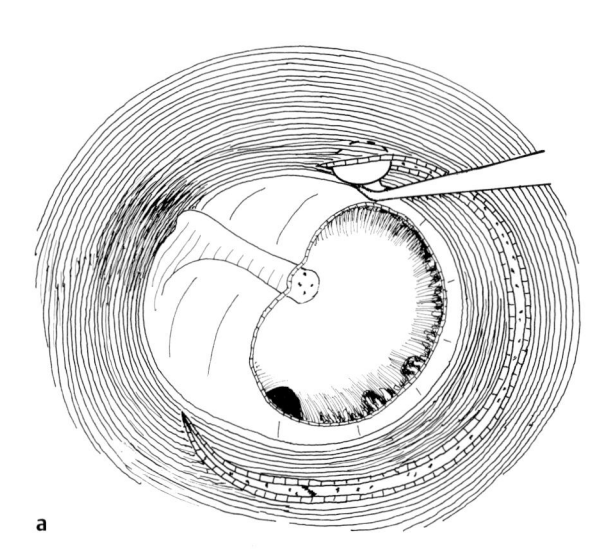

Fig. 18.28a–d Underlay myringoplasty with U-shaped annular graft in a large inferior perforation.

a The epithelium around the perforation is removed. A large inferior circumferential incision is made.
b A large inferior tympanomeatal flap is elevated and the umbo is cleaned of epithelium.

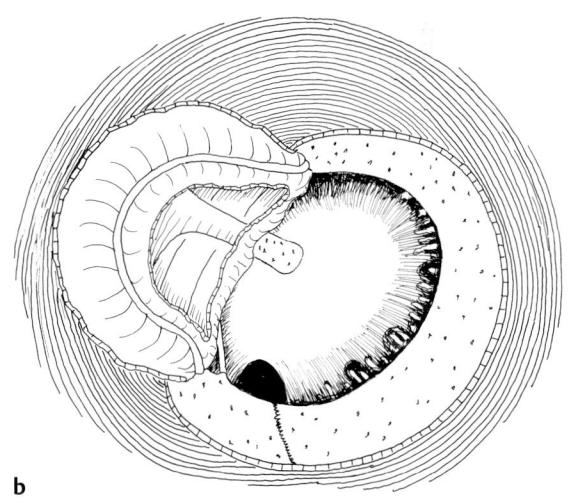

Fig. 18.28c, d ▷

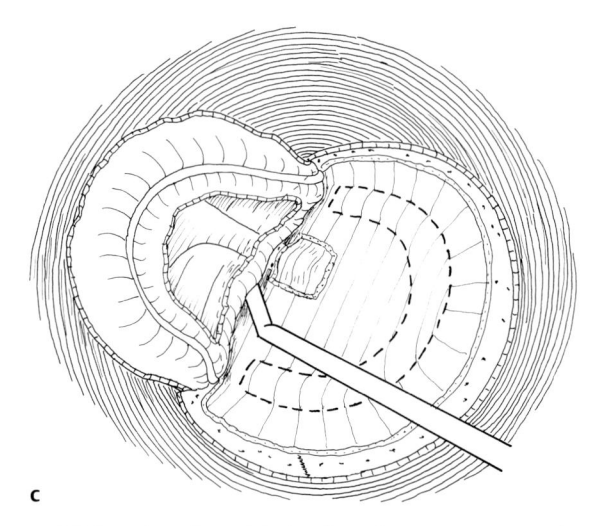

c A U-shaped annular graft is placed into the tympanic cavity at the level of the bony annulus with the central perichondrium placed under the umbu, the superior peripheral perichondrium is pushed under the eardrum, and the remaining peripheral perichondrium flap is folded out onto the denuded ear canal bone. A small piece of perichondrium covers the umbo, creating a perichondrial sandwich.

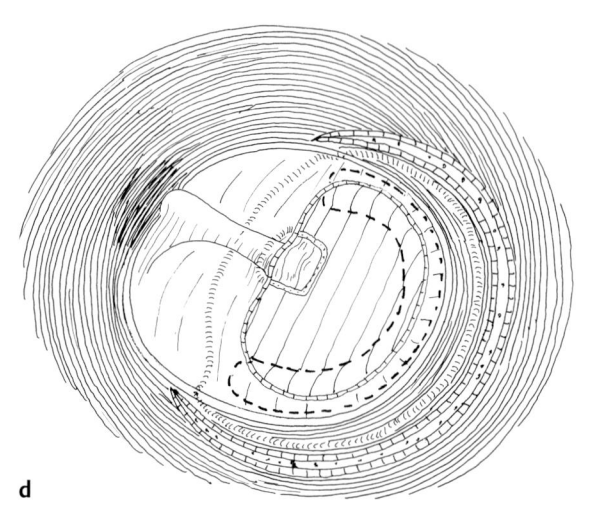

d The tympanomeatal flaps are replaced.

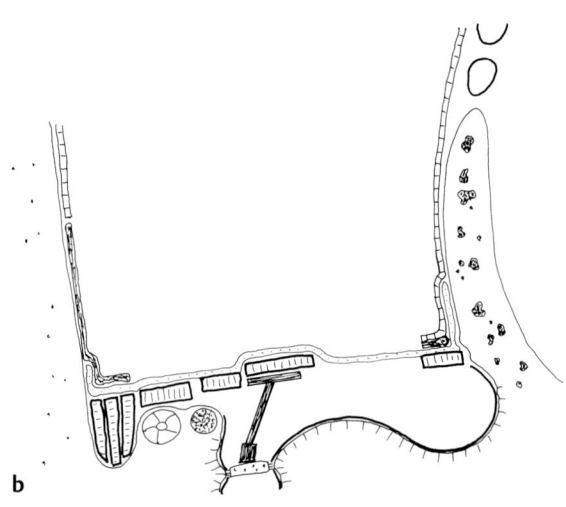

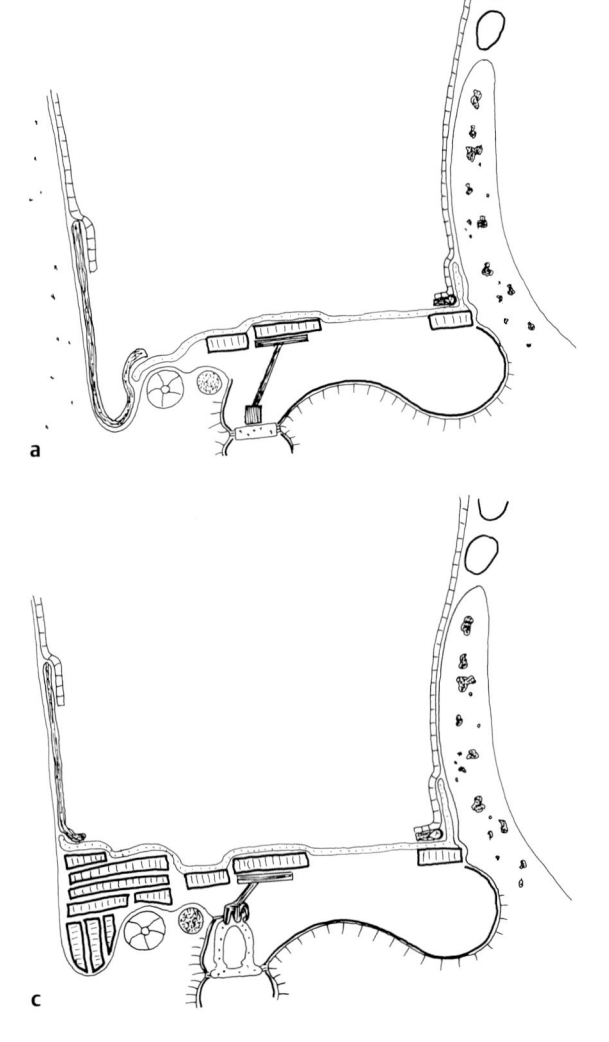

Fig. 18.29a–c Superoinferior side views of the reconstruction of tympanic cavity with circular annular graft in a situation with canal wall down mastoidectomy without or with partial or total obliteration of the attic.

a The attic is open. The annulus graft is positioned under the fibrous annulus. The titanium columella is covered with cartilage and has a solid contact with the perichondrium. The attic is covered with perichondrium.

b The attic is partly obliterated with cartilage and covered with perichondrium. The denuded superior wall of the cavity is covered with fascia.

c The attic is totally obliterated with cartilage and covered with perichondrium. The PORP titanium prosthesis is covered with a cartilage disk. The superior wall of the cavity is covered with fascia.

Annular Graft in a Total Perforation and a Floppy Malleus Handle with Remnant Stapes

After removal of an attic cholesteatoma and a totally adherent pars tensa, the result may be a total perforation of the pars tensa and a floppy malleus handle attached to the anterior malleolar ligament and the tendon of the tensor tympani muscle (**Fig. 18.30a**). After obliteration of the attic with cartilage (the remnant central cartilage from the annular graft [as in **Fig. 18.4c**] may be used), the malleus handle is included in the reconstruction of the tympanic cavity with the annular graft (**Fig. 18.30b**). After elevation of a posterior and anterior tympanomeatal flap, the incus is interposed (**Fig. 18.30c**) and the annular graft is placed close to the neck of the malleus (**Fig. 18.30d**). The superior part of the peripheral perichondrium covers the obliterated attic. After replacement of the epithelial flaps and the ear canal skin, a firm reepithelialization is likely (**Fig. 18.30e**).

Annular Graft and Tympanoplasty Type 3 in a Total Perforation without Any Ossicles

Situations without ossicles and without an eardrum are relatively common and can be seen in several circumstances:

1. Reconstruction after previous surgery, particularly after a previous radical operation in which even the fibrous annulus may have been removed.
2. Reconstruction after removal of a tensa retraction cholesteatoma with a totally atelectatic tympanic cavity with resorption of the malleus handle and stapedial arch. Such a cholesteatoma expands medially to the incus and malleus head and into the attic. In order to follow the pathology toward the antrum, the remaining ossicles are removed together with the cholesteatoma membrane. Usually a canal wall down mastoidectomy with a small cavity is performed, with a good prognosis for a dry cavity. The reason for the small pneumatization of the mastoid process is the early and chronic infection of the middle ear mucosa. In our epidemiological studies we have clearly demonstrated that diminished pneumatization is a conse-

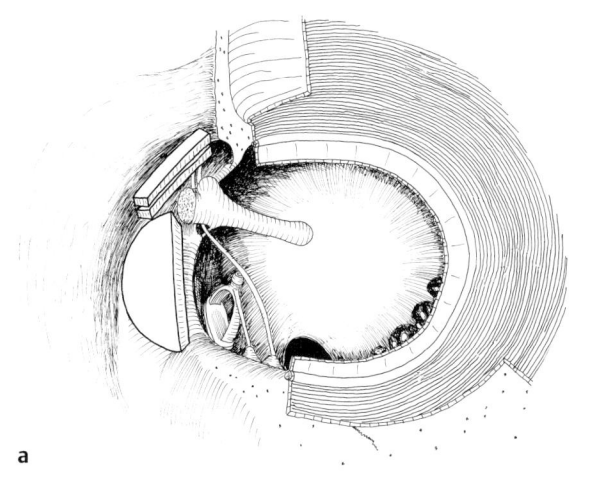

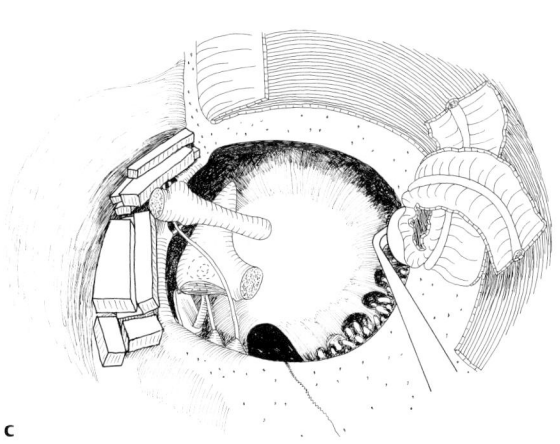

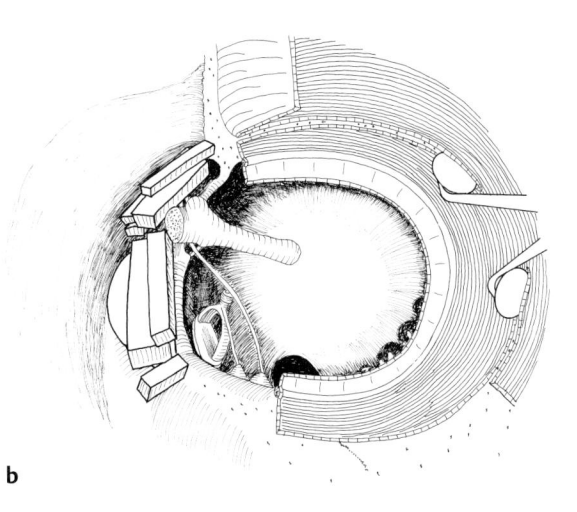

Fig. 18.30a–e Reconstruction of the eardrum and attic employing the annular graft after a canal wall down mastoidectomy with a total perforation, a floppy malleus handle, and intact, mobile stapes.

a After completion of a canal wall down mastoidectomy by a retroauricular approach, the open attic is obliterated with cartilage remnants from the annular graft preparation. First a semicircular plate cut out from the central circular cartilage remnant (see **Fig. 18.4c**) is placed. Epithelium from the border of the perforation is removed and the malleus handle is cleaned.

b The posterior circumferential incision is extended to the 6-o'clock position. The anterior circumferential incision is extended to the 5-o'clock position.

c The posterior tympanomeatal flap is elevated first, followed by the anterior tympanomeatal flap, and finally the last part of the fibrous annulus is elevated using the round knife. The autogenous incus is shaped and placed onto the head of the stapes.

Fig. 18.30d, e ▷

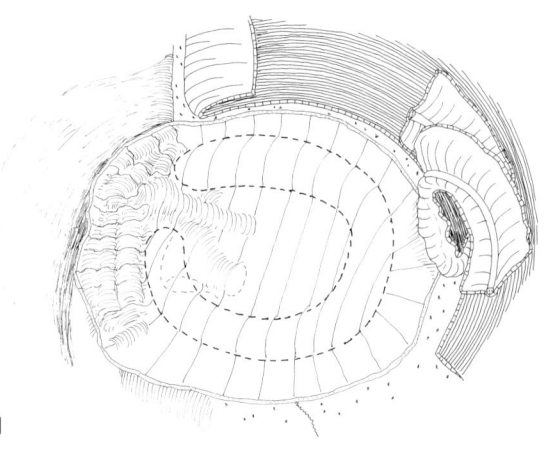

Fig. 18.30d, e
d The annular graft is placed into the tympanic cavity at the level of the bony annulus and the peripheral perichondrium is folded out over the denuded ear canal bone. Superiorly, the peripheral perichondrium covers the lateral process of the malleus and the cartilage obliterating the epitympanum. The central perichondrium covers the malleus handle and the incus body.
e The epithelial flaps are replaced. The posterior and the anterosuperior ear canal skin flaps are replaced.

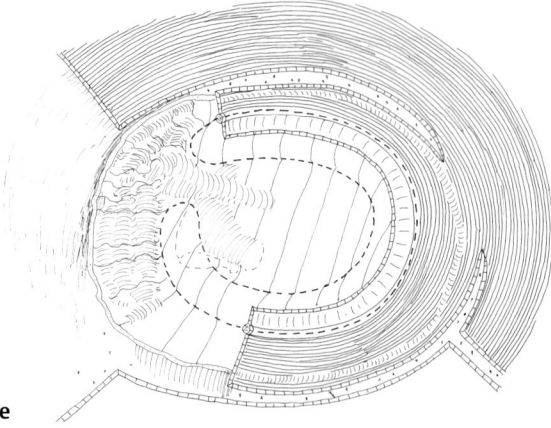

quence of the disease and not the cause of the disease (Tos and Poulsen 1979; Tos 1982; Tos and Stangerup 1984, 1985; Tos et al. 1984, 1985; Stangerup and Tos 1986, 1989; Aoki et al. 1990). Therefore, the creation of a large closed cavity does not prevent the infection or tubal dysfunction.

3. Adhesive otitis and atelectasis without an active cholesteatoma may result in a total perforation and a missing stapedial arch at surgery.

An annular graft placed onto the cartilage plates in the obliterated attic (**Fig. 18.31a, b**) provides a certain depth to the superior part of the cavity. After the elevation of the tympanomeatal flaps, a titanium Tübingen Aerial total prosthesis is placed onto the center of the stapes footplate (**Fig. 18.31c**). After the head of the prosthesis is covered with a cartilage plate (**Fig. 18.31d**), a circular annular graft is placed into the tympanic cavity. Superiorly, it is placed onto the cartilage plate in the attic. Small cartilage palisades are also placed on both sides of the graft (**Fig. 18.31e**). The peripheral perichondrium covers the palisades, the cartilage in the attic, and the denuded bone of the ear canal. After the replacement of the tympanomeatal flaps, the fascia also covers the denuded bone of the superior wall. Finally, the ear canal skin flaps are replaced (**Fig. 18.31f, g**).

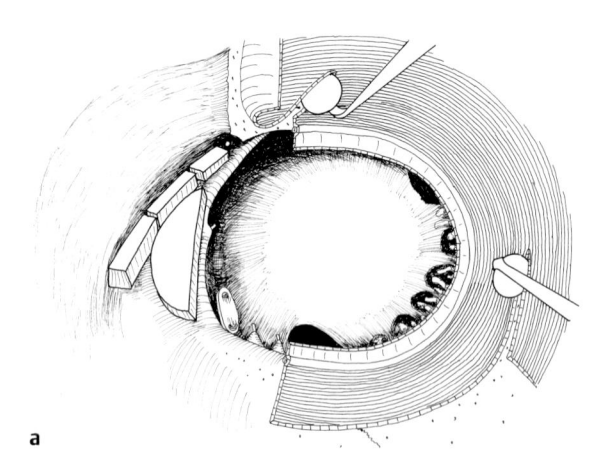

Fig. 18.31a–g Obliteration of the attic and elevation of the superior attic wall with two semicircular cartilage plates in the case with total perforation and without ossicles.
a The epithelium is removed from the edges of the perforation. Using a retroauricular approach, the posterior circumferential incision is extended in the inferior direction. Anteriorly, a small incision is performed for elevation of the anterior fibrous annulus.
b The posterior tympanomeatal flap is elevated. Anterosuperiorly, the fibrous annulus with the eardrum remnant is elevated.

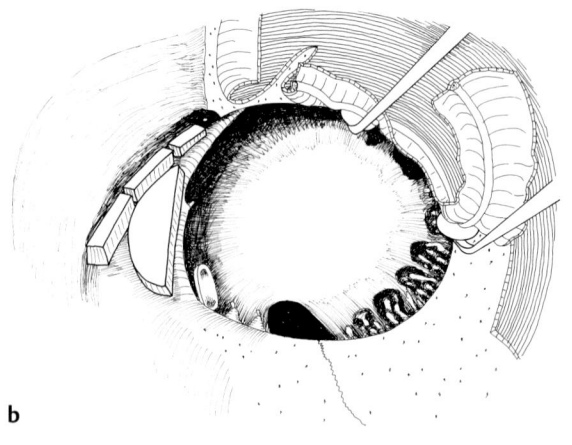

Fig. 18.31c–g

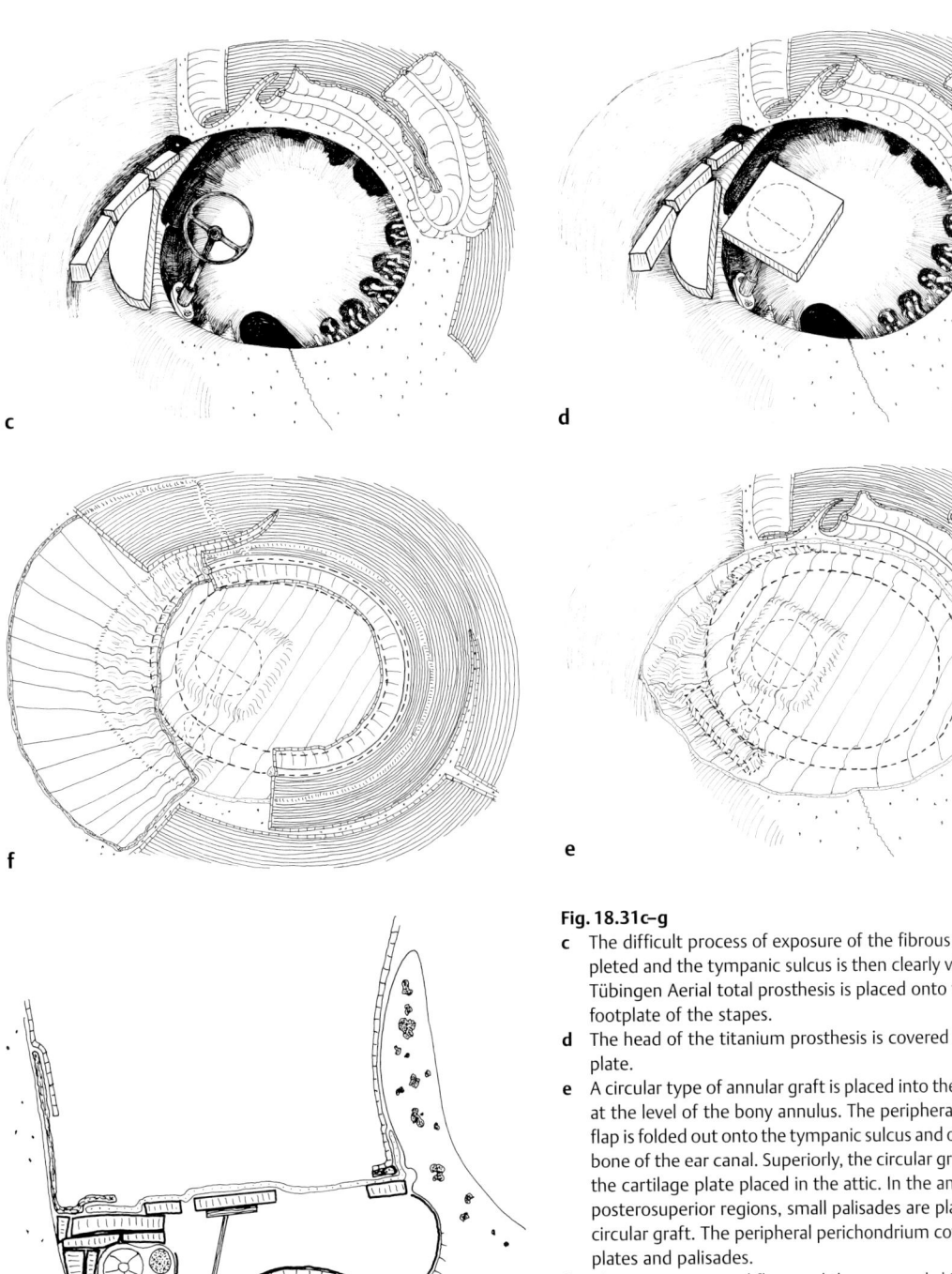

c The difficult process of exposure of the fibrous annulus is completed and the tympanic sulcus is then clearly visible. A titanium Tübingen Aerial total prosthesis is placed onto the center of the footplate of the stapes.

d The head of the titanium prosthesis is covered with a cartilage plate.

e A circular type of annular graft is placed into the tympanic cavity at the level of the bony annulus. The peripheral perichondrium flap is folded out onto the tympanic sulcus and onto the denuded bone of the ear canal. Superiorly, the circular graft is placed onto the cartilage plate placed in the attic. In the anterosuperior and posterosuperior regions, small palisades are placed along the circular graft. The peripheral perichondrium covers the cartilage plates and palisades.

f The tympanomeatal flaps and the ear canal skin flaps are replaced. The denuded bone of the cavity and the cartilage and perichondrium of the attic are all covered with fascia.

g Cross-sectional view of the tympanic cavity, attic, and antrum with the implanted circular type of annular graft and tympanoplasty type 3 with a titanium columella covered with a cartilage plate. Canal wall down mastoidectomy is performed and the attic is obliterated with cartilage plates and palisades. The annular graft is placed superiorly onto the cartilage plates and inferiorly into the tympanic cavity at the level of the bony annulus. The peripheral perichondrium is smoothed out inferiorly onto the ear canal bone and superiorly onto the cartilage plates obliterating the attic. Superiorly, fascia covers the denuded bone and laterally the fascia is covered with ear canal skin.

Results of Surgery with the Annular Graft

Only a few results of tympanoplasty with the annular graft have been published. Goodhill (1967) mentioned that his results were satisfactory, but no data on the results were published.

Klacansky et al. (1998) found that in 77 ears reconstructed with cartilage palisades, 248 ears reconstructed with total pars tensa cartilage–perichondrium island combined grafts, and 47 ears with annular grafts, that is, in a total of 372 ears operated between 1976 and 1978, peripheral defects between the cartilage and bone occurred in 25 ears (6.7%), and perforations of the perichondrium occurred in 3 ears (0.8%). In total there were only 7.5% failures and all the implanted cartilages were vital. No specific results of surgery employing the annular grafts were published. The hearing results were not presented.

Borkowski et al. (1999) used annular grafts in 21 ears with total or subtotal perforations. Some patients originally had tensa retraction cholesteatoma, which resulted in a total perforation and a missing malleus handle. In 13 ears the malleus handle was intact.

On removal of the ear dressing 3 weeks after the operation, no retractions or perforations were found. Good healing was also noted in the problematic anterior region along the anterior annulus.

The mean primary postoperative air–bone gap in 2 ears with intact ossicular chain was 10 dB and in the remaining 19 ears with a disrupted ossicular chain it was 20 dB. The late results were not published.

Author's Comments and Proposals

The annular graft appears to diminish the area of the new eardrum slightly, but the retraction of the central perichondrium of the graft apparently requires a larger negative pressure than that required by a flaccid and atrophic eardrum or large interposed fascia. Systematic postoperative tympanometry and otomicroscopy would be of great interest and may provide some new information on the mechanism of the retractions. Additionally, the adherence of the new eardrum to the edges of the cartilage ring of the annular graft is presumably less prone to retraction than the atrophic and thin eardrum or implanted fascia.

Because of the annular graft, the tympanic cavity is slightly deeper, especially in the on-lay method. The risk of adhesion of the central perichondrium to the promontory is presumably minimal, but again there are no results published with an observation time longer than 3 weeks after the operation. Further observation of the postoperative behavior of the annular graft is needed.

Contact of the interposed ossicle between the stapes and the central perichondrium of the annulus graft is good, and there is a slight pressure exerted by the central perichondrium onto the ossicle, which stabilizes the prosthesis in a tympanoplasty type 2 (**Fig. 18.10a, c**). Similarly, the central perichondrium acts as a stabilizer of the incus columella in a tympanoplasty type 3 (**Fig. 18.17b, d**). The cartilage plates covering the heads of the titanium prostheses in tympanoplasty type 2 (**Fig. 18.16c, e**) and in tympanoplasty type 3 (**Fig. 18.18c, e**) are also stabilized by the central perichondrium of the annular graft.

A disadvantage of the annular graft may be its construction and preparation, requiring the exact measurement of the diameters and the keeping of the cartilage ring intact during its preparation and during its placement in the tympanic cavity.

The three different techniques—the on-lay technique (Goodhill 1967), the underlay technique (Borkowski et al. 1999), and the technique with removal of the entire fibrous annulus and eardrum remnant (Klacansky et al. 1998)—are well described and illustrated. It is, however, necessary to compare the clinical results of the three techniques on comparable clinical series of operated patients. The technique with the removal of the entire fibrous annulus may be the fastest method, but it is not physiological to remove the fibrous annulus and the eardrum with the epithelium. The consequence is slowing of the epithelialization of the annular graft, which may explain the peripheral perforations encountered.

I recommend the application of small cartilage palisades at the sites not covered by the annular graft, such as bony defects caused by drilling along the posterosuperior bony annulus (**Figs. 18.12b, 18.13c**), in the attic region, and also on the prostheses.

The annular graft is an important graft in cartilage tympanoplasty and will become increasingly popular in the future. It can be applied in all total perforations with poor tubal function, i. e., in ears with preoperative negative Valsalva maneuver. Furthermore, it can be applied in ears with atelectasis, adhesive chronic otitis, tensa retraction cholesteatoma, or sinus cholesteatoma, and in the reconstruction of the tympanic cavity after previous surgery resulting in a radical cavity with removal of the fibrous annulus.

Need for Future Research on Clinical Series with Annular Graft

Apart from the primary results of Borkowski et al. (1999), no other studies have reported **results**. Clinical studies are therefore needed on primary results as well as on late results of the methods presented in this chapter.

The following clinical research on annular grafts needs urgent attention:
1. Evaluation of the primary results (3 months postoperatively) including hearing results of the four methods:
   a) The on–lay method of Goodhill with an intact ossicular chain (**Fig. 18.8**), with a tympanoplasty type 2 with interposition of a prosthesis onto the intact stapes and malleus handle (**Figs. 18.9–18.15**) and

again with a tympanoplasty type 3 with the placement of a columella between the footplate and the malleus handle (**Fig. 18.16**).

b) The Klacansky method with removal of the fibrous annulus and the ear drum remnants (**Fig. 18.19**) and again separately for tympanoplasty type 1 in an intact ossicular chain, type 2 with interposition of a prosthesis between intact stapes and malleus handle, and tympanoplasty type 3 with placement of a columella between the footplate and the malleus handle.

c) The Borkowski underlay method with placement of the anterior perichondrium under the bony annulus (**Fig. 18.20**) and again in tympanoplasty types 1, 2 and 3.

d) My own proposal to elevate the anterior fibrous annulus and place the perichondrium onto the ear canal bone and onto the bony annulus (**Fig. 18.21**), and again subdivided into tympanoplasty types 1, 2, and 3.

2. Evaluation of late results (2–5 years postoperatively) with the same subdivision as for the primary results.

3. Evaluation of the primary results with methods applying the annular graft to the pathology of the malleus handle: retraction, adhesion (**Figs. 18.22, 18.23**), missing malleus handle (**Figs. 18.24–18.26**), missing entire malleus (**Fig. 18.27**), and a floppy malleus handle (**Fig. 18.30**). It will be difficult to collect a large series with pathologies of the malleus, but further information is needed.

4. Comparison of the results of surgery applying the annular graft with results by other surgical methods, but with the same pathology. For example, applying the annular graft in cases of total perforation with an intact ossicular chain and positive Valsalva maneuver compared with fascia, perichondrium, small cartilage palisades, or broad cartilage palisades. Comparison of a similar series, but with negative Valsalva maneuver, should also be done.

References

Aoki K, Esaki S, Honda Y, Tos M. Effect of middle ear infection on pneumatization of the mastoid process: an experimental study in pigs. Acta Otolaryngol 1990;110:399–409.

Borkowski G, Sudhoff H, Luckhaupt H. Autologer Knorpel- Perichondrium- "Spannring" bei subtotalen oder totalen Trommelfelldefekten. Laryngorhinootologie 1999;78:68–72.

Goodhill V. Tragal perichondrium and cartilage in tympanoplasty. Arch Otolaryngol 1967;85:480–491.

Klacansky J, Kucera J, Starek I. Rekonstrukcia blanky bubienka chrupkovymi transplantati. [Reconstruction of the eardrum with cartilage transplants] Otorinolaryngologie a foniatrie 1998;47:59–63.

Sheehy JL. Surgery of chronic otitis media. In: English GM, ed. Otolaryngology. Vol. 2. Hagerstown: Harper and Row; 1972:1–86.

Stangerup SE, Tos M. Treatment of secretory otitis and pneumatization. Laryngoscope 1986;96:680–684.

Stangerup SE, Tos M. Middle ear ventilation and pneumatization. In: Tos M, Thomsen J, Peitersen E, eds. Cholesteatoma and Mastoid Surgery. Amsterdam: Kugler & Ghedini, 1989;377–381.

Steinbach E, Pusalkar A. Long-term histological fate in ossicular reconstruction. J Laryngol Otol 1981;95:1031–1039.

Steinbach E, Karger B, Hildmann H. Zur Verwendung von Knorpeltransplantaten in der Mittelohrchirurgie. Eine histologische Langzeituntersuchung von Knorpelinterponaten. Laryngorhinootologie 1992;71(1):11–14.

Tos M. Pathology of the ossicular chain in various chronic middle ear diseases. J Laryngol Otol 1979;93:769–780.

Tos M. Stability of myringoplasty based on late results. ORL J Otorhinolaryngol Relat Spec 1980;42:171–181.

Tos M. Relationship between secretory otitis in childhood and chronic otitis and its sequalae in adults. J Laryngol Otol 1981;95:1011–1022.

Tos M. Mastoid pneumatization: a critical analysis of the hereditary theory. Acta Otolaryngol 1982;94:73–80.

Tos M, Poulsen G. Changes of pars tensa after secretory otitis media. ORL 1979 1977;41:313–328.

Tos M, Stangerup SE. Mastoid pneumatization in secretory otitis: further support for the environmental theory. Acta Otolaryngol 1984;98:110–118.

Tos M, Stangerup SE. The causes of asymmetry of the mastoid air cell system. Acta Otolaryngol 1985;99:564–570.

Tos M, Stangerup SE, Hvid G. Mastoid pneumatization: evidence of the environmental theory. Arch Otolaryngol 1984;110:502–507.

Tos M, Stangerup SE, Andreasen UK. Size of the mastoid air cells and otitis media. Ann Otol Rhinol Laryngol 1985;94:386–392.

Utech H. Über diagnostischen und therapeutische Möglichkeiten der Tympanotomie bei Schalleitungsstörungen. [Tympanotomy in disorders of sound conduction; its diagnostic and therapeutic possibilities] Z Laryngol Rhinol Otol 1959;38:212–221.

Utech H. Verwendung der Knorpelgewebe bei Tympanoplastik und Stapeschirurgie. HNO 1961;9:232–233.

19 "Crown Cork" Cartilage–Perichondrium Composite Graft Tympanoplasty

Definition

In 1992 Hartwein, Leuwer, and Kehrl published a new technique for total reconstruction of the tympanic membrane with a cartilage–perichondrium composite graft, called "crown cork" tympanoplasty. The graft consists of a round piece of tragal cartilage, covered on the outer side (ear canal side) with perichondrium, which continues in a large peripheral perichondrium flap (**Fig. 19.1a**). The diameter of the cartilage is slightly smaller than the diameter of the ear canal at the level of the bony annulus (**Fig. 19.1b**). The exposed, bare inner side of the cartilage is brought into contact either with the malleus handle (**Fig. 19.1b**) or with a PORP or TORP prosthesis. The large overlapping peripheral perichondrium is radially incised, resulting in several perichondrial flaps, which, after placement and fixation on the ear canal bone, form the shape of a crown cork (**Fig. 19.1b–d**) (Hartwein and Leuwer 1992; Hartwein et al. 1992; Hartwein and Kehrl 1993).

Harvesting and Construction of the "Crown Cork" Graft

The problem of the crown cork graft is the size of the peripheral perichondrium, 3–4 mm, enlarging the diameter of the entire graft by 6–8 mm. According to Anson and Donaldson (1981), the diameter of the eardrum is 8–9 mm. Counting both measurements together, the horizontal and vertical diameters of the entire graft should be 14–17 mm. A diameter of 9 mm for the cartilage disk will be the standard.

Harvesting of Tragal Cartilage

Hartwein et al. (1992) used exclusively tragal cartilage for construction of the crown cork graft, but from their illustrations it was evident that several perichondrial flaps were considerable shorter than 3 mm. To make a crown cork graft with 3 mm perichondrium flaps and a cartilage disk of 9 mm in diameter (see **Fig. 19.1a**), a tragus graft of 15 mm × 15 mm has to be harvested. In comparison, for the annular graft (Chapter 18) an 11 mm × 11 mm tragus graft is adequate (Borkowski et al. 1999).

Hartwein et al. did not show how to harvest a 15 mm × 15 mm tragus graft. My recommendation is for a conservative technique with sufficient removal of the perichondrium and minimal removal of the cartilage.

A 15 mm long skin incision on the posterior aspect of the tragus dome 3 mm medial to the dome (**Fig. 19.2a**) allows exposure of the entire dome (**Fig. 19.2b**) and also the lateral edge of the antitragus. The perichondrium is incised along the dome. A 3 mm lateral perichondrium flap and a similar inferior flap are created (**Fig. 19.2c–e**) to allow smaller resection of the cartilage (**Fig. 19.2 f, g**).

Cutting of the cartilage disk is similar to cutting of the annular graft (Chapter 18, **Figs. 18.4–18.6**) and can be performed with a metallic tracheal cannula, ear speculum (**Fig. 19.2h**) or Klacansky chondrotome (**Figs. 18.5, 18.6**) (Klacansky et al. 1998). After removal of the superfluous cartilage (**Fig. 19.2i**), the surrounding perichondrium is radially incised, creating several flaps (**Fig. 19.2j**).

Harvesting of Conchal Cartilage

Harvesting of conchal cartilage for the crown cork graft in a normal pinna is much easier than that of tragal cartilage. However in some cases, such as congenital atresia with microtia, previous surgery with use of conchal cartilage can make it difficult to harvest a sufficient round piece of cartilage with a diameter of 15 mm.

In cases with normal concha, a postauricular incision is performed, the subcutaneous tissue is elevated, and a round area with a diameter of 16 mm is cut through all three layers: the posterior perichondrium, the cartilage, and the anterior perichondrium (**Fig. 19.3a**). The posterior perichondrium is first removed and then the cartilage along with the anterior perichondrium is elevated and removed (**Fig. 19.3b–d**). The removed graft can easily be elaborated into a crown cork graft with 3.5 mm perichondrium flaps (**Fig. 19.3e**).

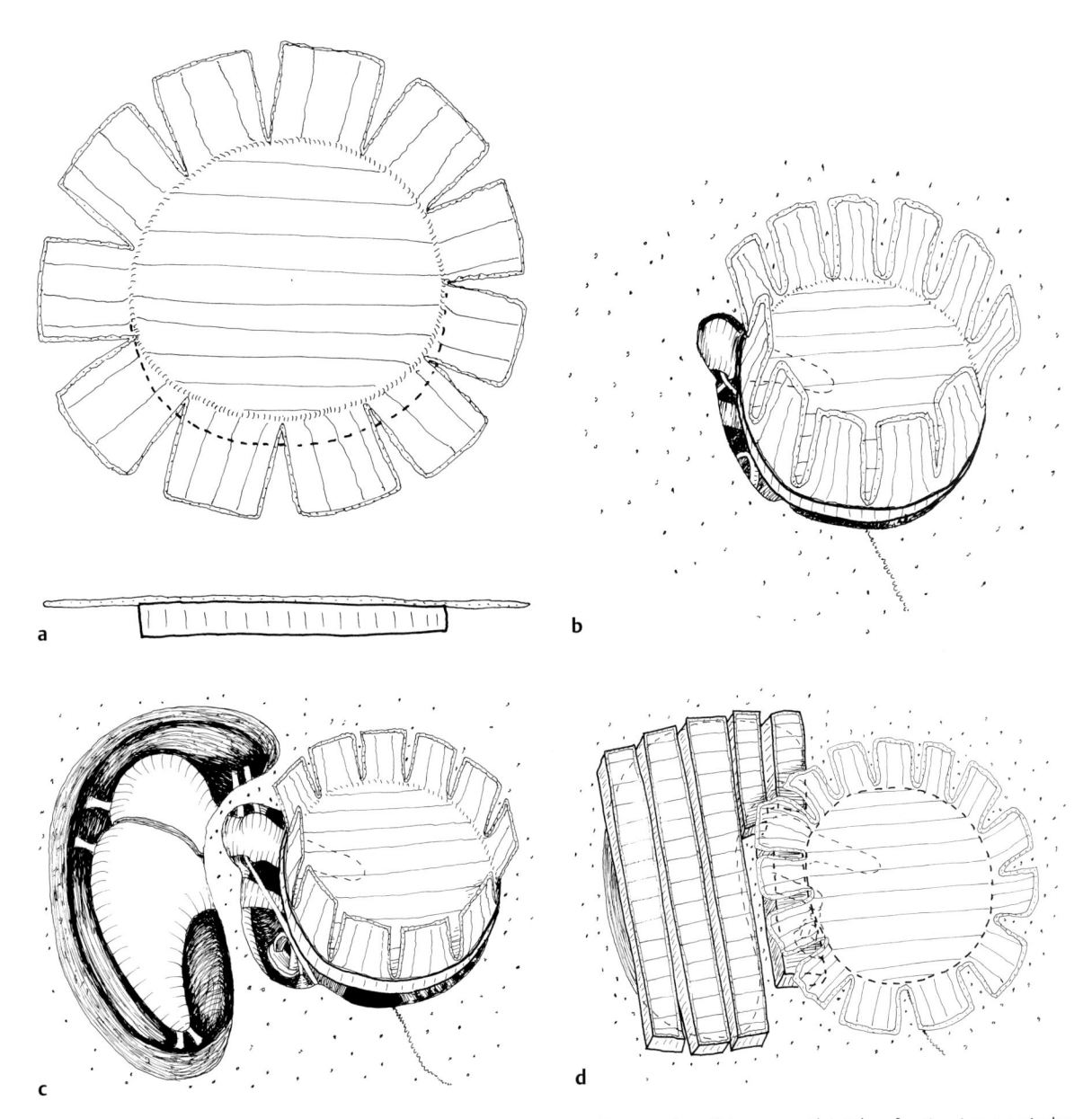

Fig. 19.1a–d The crown cork graft.
a A crown cork graft with a cartilage disk covered on the ear canal side with perichondrium with several relatively large peripheral flaps. A side view of the graft is shown below.
b Example of the crown cork graft tympanoplasty in a case of a total perforation with intact ossicular chain. The cartilage plate is placed into the tympanic cavity and is in contact with the malleus handle. The perichondrium flaps will cover the bone of the ear canal.
c Crown cork graft in a case with total perforation, intact ossicular chain and an atticotomy with preservation of the bridge. The cartilage disk is placed into the tympanic cavity.
d The atticotomy and posterosuperior bony annulus are covered with palisades placed onto the bone and the perichondrium flaps are folded out over the denuded bone and cartilage palisades.

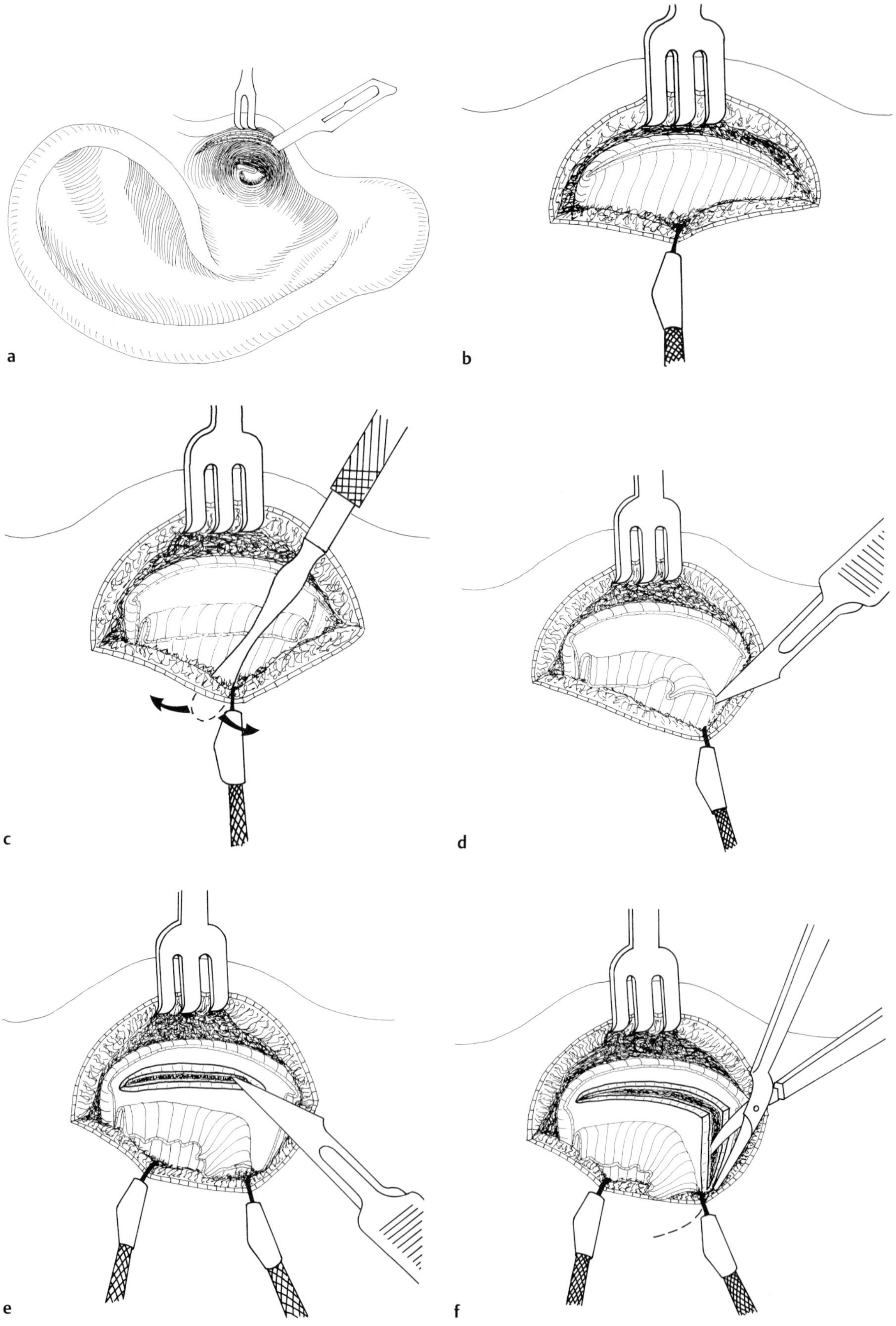
a
b
c
d
e
f

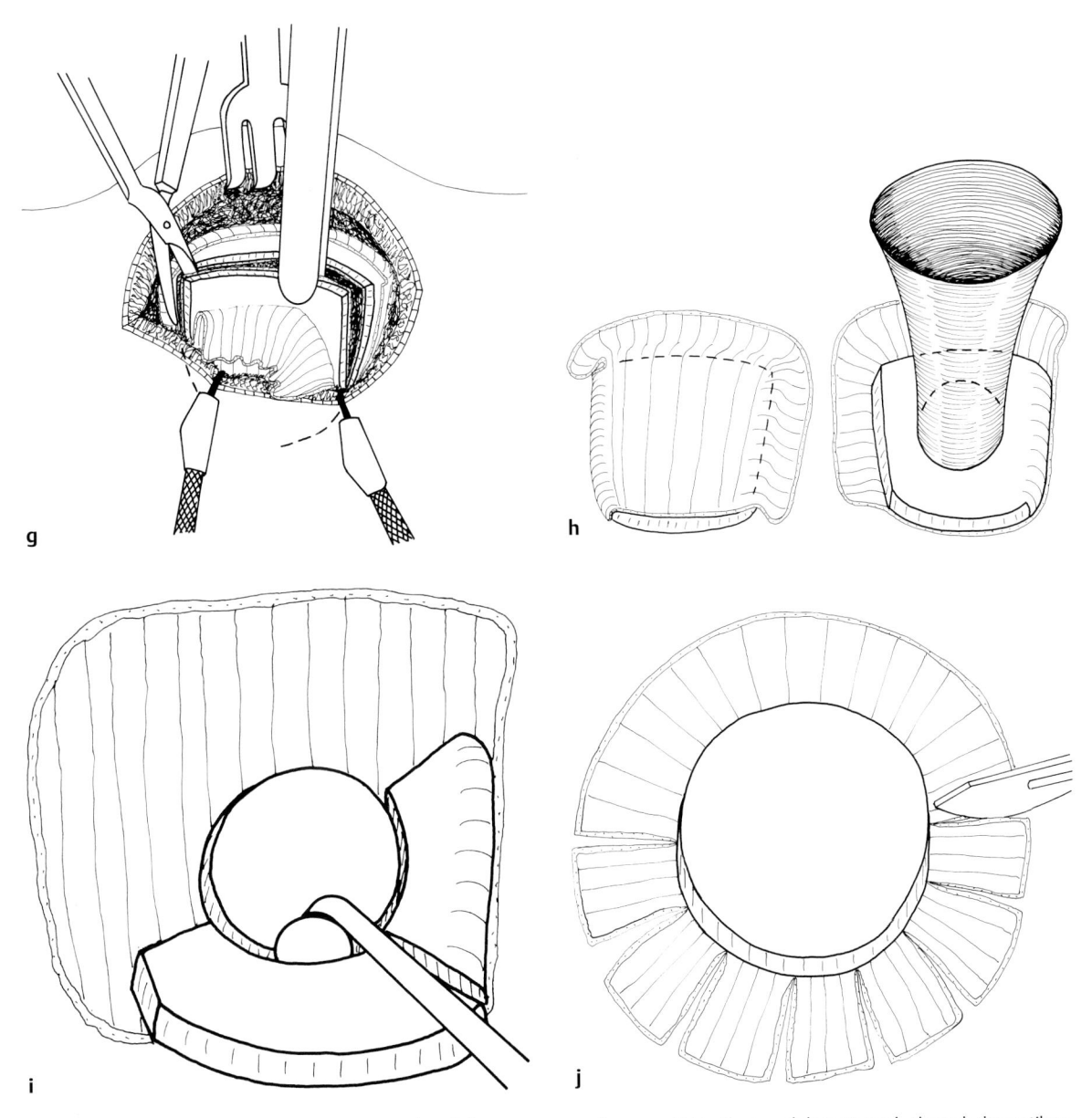

Fig. 19.2a–j Harvesting a 15 mm × 15 mm tragal graft in a case of total perforation and blunting of the ear canal.

a A 15 mm skin incision is made on the posterior side of the tragus, turning toward the inferior wall of the ear canal—the antitragus.
b The skin with the subcutaneous tissue is elevated and pulled anteriorly, exposing the entire dome of the tragus and the lateral edge of the inferior ear canal cartilage. The perichondrium is incised along the tragal dome, continuing along the lateral edge of the inferior cartilage.
c The lateral 3 mm belt of perichondrium is elevated from the dome. With a Freer's rugine, the posterior ear canal skin with subcutaneous tissue is further elevated and the entire area of the posterior perichondrium is cleaned.
d The exposed perichondrium is incised with a small knife, starting laterally and continuing medially as deep as possible.
e A 3 mm belt of the posterior perichondrium is elevated in superior direction from the inferior incision. A horizontal incision 3 mm medial to the tragal dome is made through the cartilage and the anterior perichondrium.
f With a pair of scissors, the tragal cartilage is cut inferiorly and partly medially along the stippled line.
g Finally the tragal cartilage with the perichondrium is excised superiorly and medially and a large graft is removed.
h Removed cartilage-perichondrium graft. *Left:* The cartilage graft with a superior and an inferior perichondrium flap. Perichondrium is removed from the anterior (convex) side of the graft.
Right: The graft is turned and is now placed with the cartilage up. An ear speculum cuts the 9 mm cartilage disk.
i The superfluous cartilage is removed.
j Using a scalpel with #23 blade, small wedges of perichondrium are excised all the way round the cartilage disk, creating the crown cork graft.

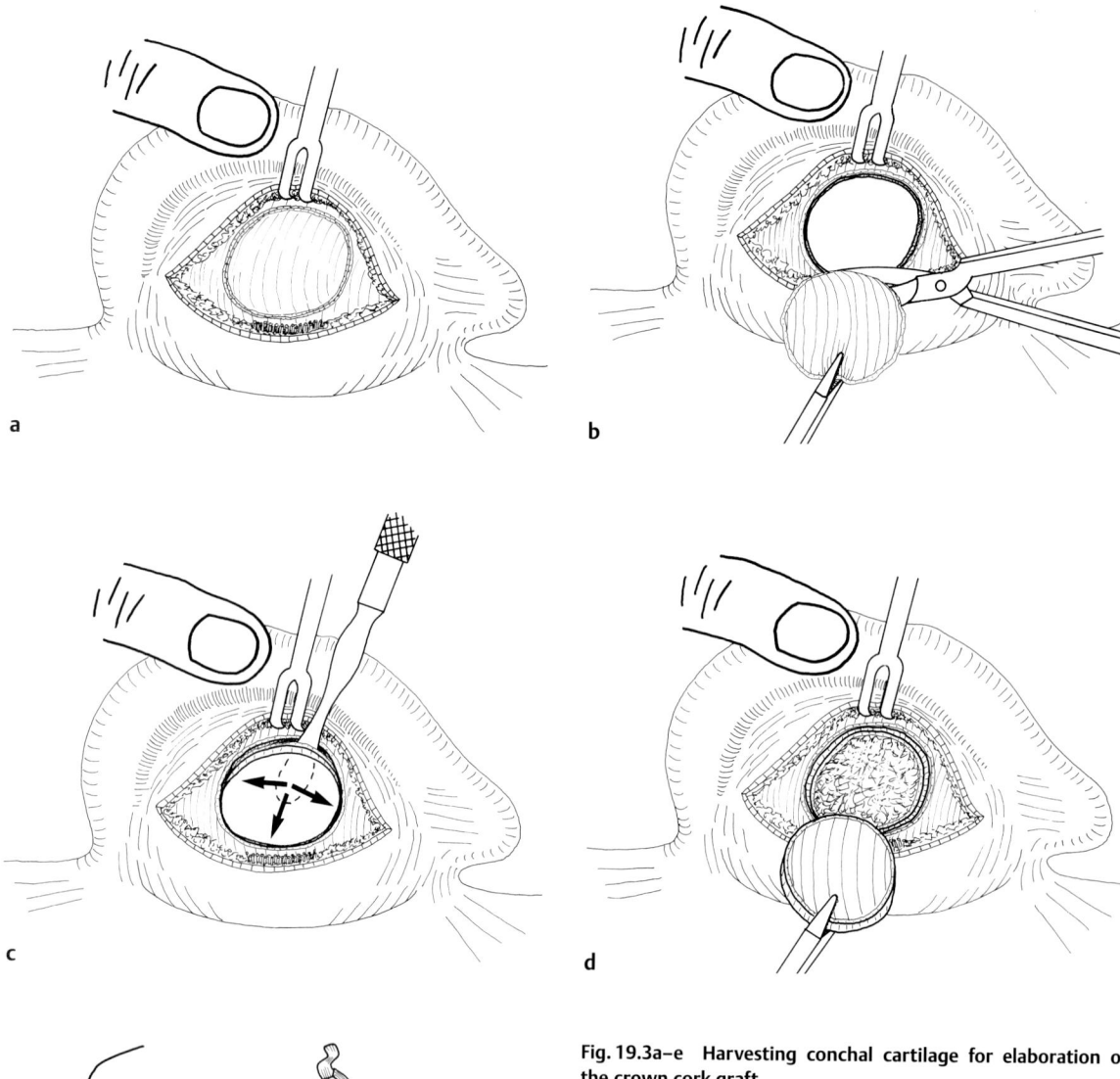

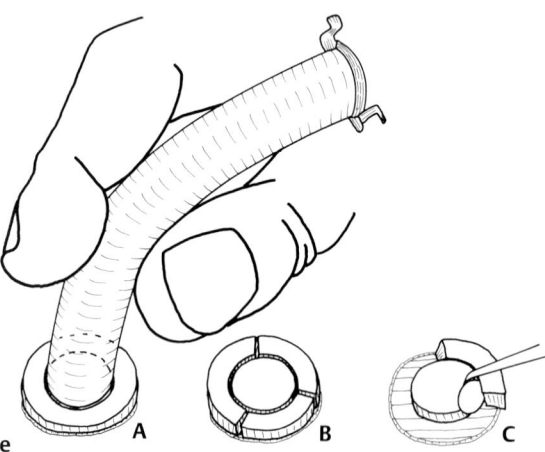

Fig. 19.3a–e Harvesting conchal cartilage for elaboration of the crown cork graft.

a A postauricular incision is made over the most prominent area. The subcutaneous tissue and posterior auricular muscle are cut and elevated, exposing the posterior perichondrium of the concha. A full circular incision is made through the posterior perichondrium, the cartilage, and the anterior perichondrium. The diameter of the round graft to be excised is 15–16 mm.
b The posterior perichondrium is elevated and removed.
c The cartilage graft with the anterior perichondrium is elevated with a Freer's rugine.
d The round graft is elevated and removed.
e The removed conchal graft, measuring 16 mm in diameter, is cut with a 9 mm tracheal cannula (**A**), allowing a 3.5 mm belt of perichondrium for the perichondrium flap. The remaining cartilage is gradually removed (**B**, **C**) to create the peripheral perichondrium flap.

Indications for "Crown Cork" Tympanoplasty

Indications for crown cork tympanoplasty are conditions with involvement of the ear canal and the tympanic cavity along with the eardrum. Some of these conditions are congenital, others are acquired.

Congenital Malformations

Following Altmann's (1949, 1951, 1955) classification, the congenital atresias are divided into three types of severity:
- An atresia of **type 1** indicates mild form with a small external ear canal, a hypoplastic tympanic bone, a small eardrum, malformed ossicles to varying degrees, and often contracted tympanic cavity. Whether the crown cork tympanoplasty should be applied, or not, in type 1 depends on the degree of hearing loss and other symptoms. A combination of hearing loss of 40 dB or less and an air–bone gap less than 30 dB, ossicular malformation, and small eardrum is an indication for surgery.
- An atresia of **type 2a** with a thick atretic plate but a small groove for the ear canal (see **Fig. 19.4**) and normal or slightly abnormal pinna is an indication for crown cork tympanoplasty. An atresia of **type 2b** (a subclassification of Cremers et al. [1984]) with absent ear canal and rudimentary pinna is an indication for crown cork tympanoplasty.
- In **type 3** atresia with an absent ear canal, hypoplastic or completely missing middle ear, and severely malformed pinna, crown cork tympanoplasty is indicated.

Among 22 patients operated with crown cork tympanoplasty, 8 patients had congenital anomalies, but the types and severity were not described (Hartwein and Kehrl 1993).

Revision surgery in congenital malformations is common and crown cork tympanoplasty may be relevant in eardrum perforation, blunting, recurrent fibrous atresia, small and immobile eardrum, and chronic granulations on the eardrum and surrounding medial ear canal wall.

Acquired Ear Canal Lesions

Postinflammatory Acquired Solid Atresia

Postinflammatory acquired solid atresia is caused either by inflammation in the tympanic cavity, extending to the ear canal, or by inflammation starting medially in the ear canal (MMES_3, Figs. 23–35). In our long-term analysis of the first 14 cases of solid fibrous atresia (Bonding and Tos 1975; Tos and Bonding 1979), half started with chronic suppurative otitis media with eardrum perforation, the other half started with external otitis with an intact eardrum. In a series of 47 patients who underwent surgery during a 27-year period at the Gentoft hospital (Becker and Tos 1998), an incidence of acquired solid postinflammatory atresia of 0.5/100 000, all of whom underwent surgery, indicates that surgery is infrequent. In the great majority of cases the atresia can be removed, leaving the fibrous annulus and the lamina propria of the eardrum intact (Tos and Balle 1986). The eardrum and the denuded ear canal are covered with split-skin grafts (MMES_3, Figs. 46–53 and 62–76).

In a few cases, especially those starting with chronic otitis media, the lamina propria may perforate, resulting in a total perforation. In such cases the crown cork graft may be indicated.

Cholesteatoma in Postinflammatory Acquired Atresia

Cholesteatoma appears in 18 % of cases with in postinflammatory acquired atresia (Tos and Balle 1986). Most cholesteatomas are localized in the ear canal and can be removed together with the atresia. Some cholesteatomas are located in the tympanic cavity and have to be removed together with the fibrous annulus and lamina propria. In such cases the crown cork tympanoplasty is indicated.

Postoperative Atresia

Postoperative atresia may occur after several types of surgical procedures where a significant loss of ear canal skin has occurred. In the medial end of the ear canal the granulations may predominate, become fibrotic, and finally be epithelialized, resulting in a 2–4 mm thick fibrous atresia (MMES_3, Figs. 105–109). After removal of atresia, a crown cork tympanoplasty is indicated.

Blunting

Blunting is an obliteration of the anterior tympanomeatal angle, making the anterior half of the eardrum thick and stiff (MMES_3, Figs. 122–129). Blunting may appear together with posterior perforation. Crown cork tympanoplasty may be a good solution for blunting. Nine of 22 patients operated with crown cork tympanoplasty had blunting phenomena after previous tympanoplasty (Hartwein and Kehrl 1993).

Total Perforation with Granulations in the Medial Ear Canal

Total perforation with granulations in the medial ear canal may also be an indication for crown cork tympanoplasty. Five out of 22 patients had a totally defective eardrum because of chronic suppurative otitis media or cholesteatoma (Hartwein and Kehrl 1993).

Surgical Techniques of "Crown Cork" Tympanoplasty

No particular surgical techniques with crown cork tympanoplasty have been described. This is understandable because the preoperative pathology includes many variations and particularly in the congenital malformations several grades of severity of atresia are included.

Hartwein et al. (1992) showed how to elaborate and place the crown cork graft. The authors indicate that the adjacent 3–4 mm of canal skin are removed in continuity with the squamous epithelium of the tympanic membrane remnants and fibrous annulus. The malleus handle is deepithelialized. At the end of the operation, the ear canal skin is realigned and the ear canal is covered with Silastic sheets for 10 days to stabilize the graft.

Because of the limited descriptions of surgical technique in the literature, I will here illustrate the application of the crown cork method on congenital atresias and blunting phenomena on the basis of my own experience in ear canal surgery (Tos 1997).

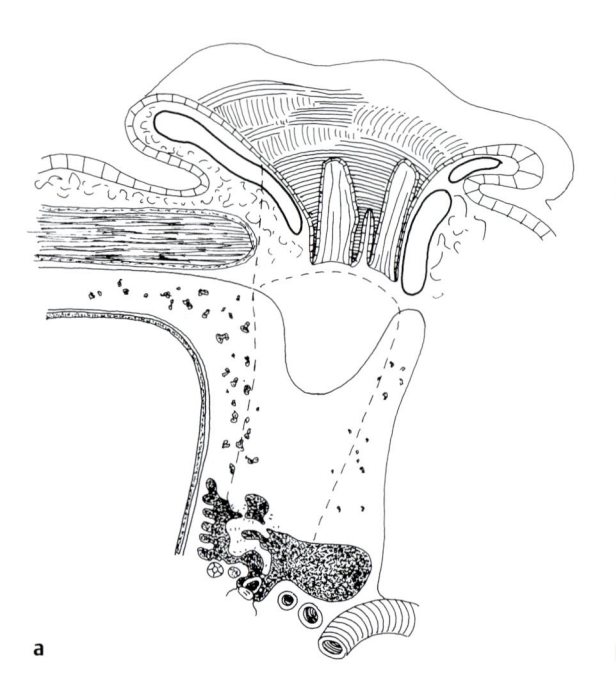

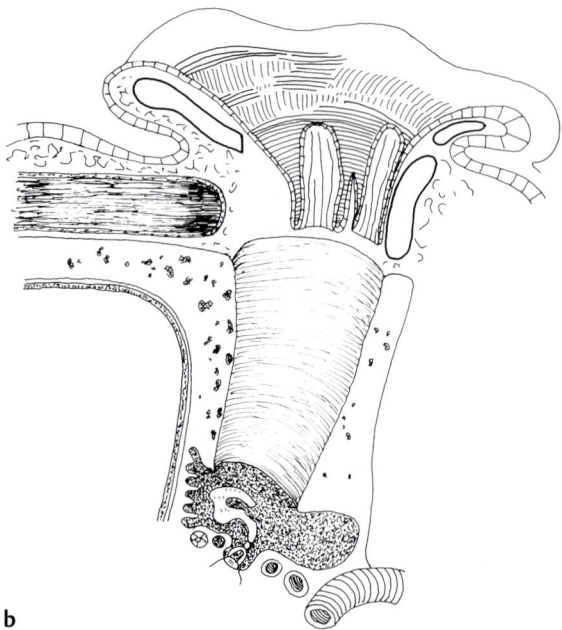

Schematic Illustration of Surgical Principle in Congenital Type 2a Atresia Reconstructed with Crown Cork Tympanoplasty

Type 2a atresia has a thick atretic plate, but the position of the ear canal is indicated by a groove, which makes initial surgery of the ear canal easier (**Fig. 19.4**). In a retroauricular approach the entrance to the ear canal is identified and the epithelial flaps are elevated (**Fig. 19.5a**). The ear canal is widened up to the attic and the tympanic cavity. A round opening of diameter 9.5 mm is made and the fixed ossicles are mobilized (**Fig. 19.5b**). The cartilage disk is placed into the round opening and onto the malleus head and incus body. The perichondrial flaps are placed in the medial end of the ear canal (**Fig. 19.5c**), A large split-skin graft covers the ear canal, some small epithelial flaps cover the new

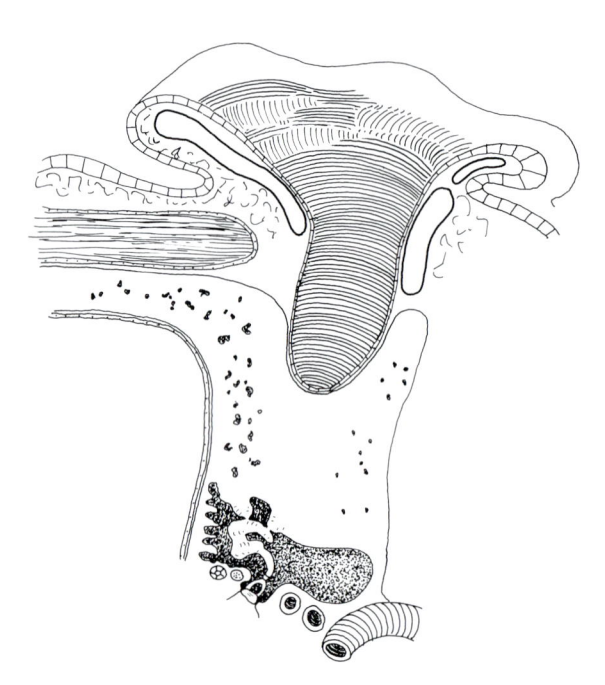

Fig. 19.4 Type 2a atresia with a groove for the ear canal and a thick atretic plate that is deformed and fused to the surrounding bone. The ossicles are malformed and fixated to the atresia plate. The pinna is only slightly malformed.

a

b

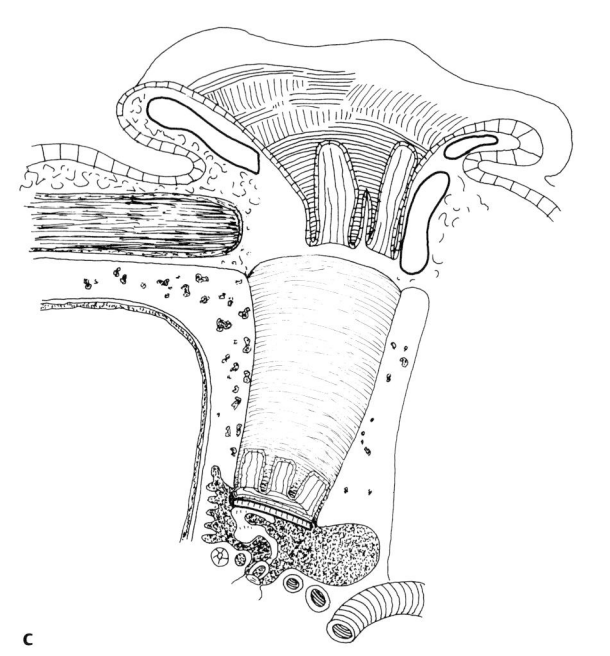

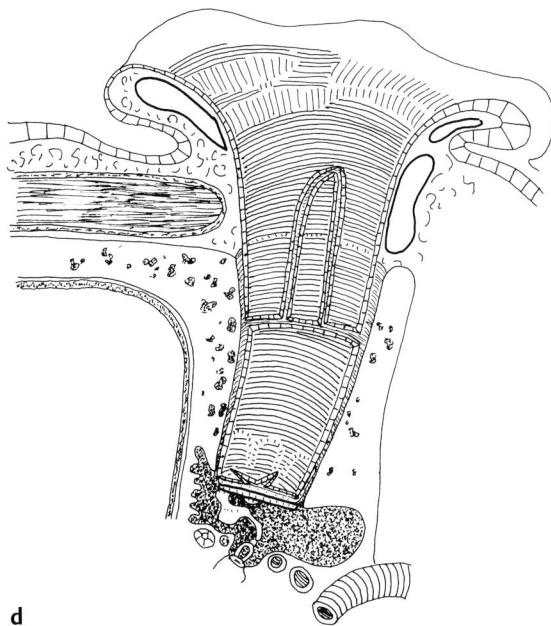

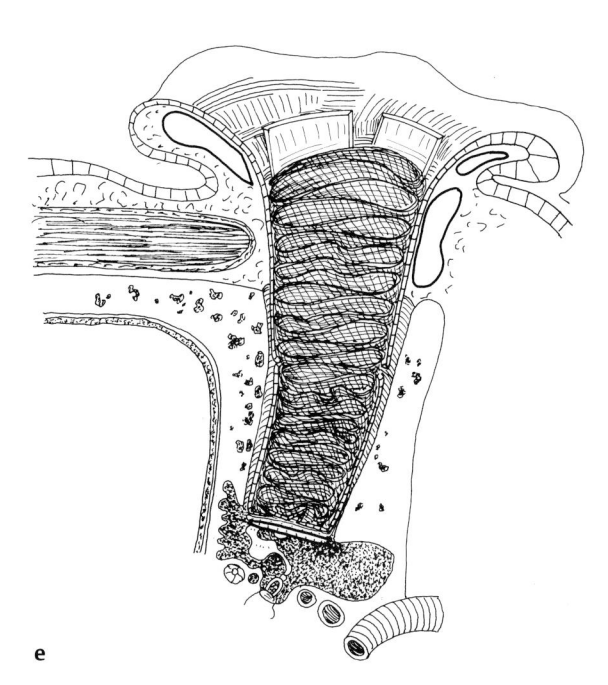

Fig. 19.5a–e Schematic illustration of surgery for type 2a congenital atresia and application of crown cork tympanoplasty.
a In a retroauricular approach, the groove of the ear canal is identified and the canal skin is cut, resulting in four elevated skin flaps. The ear canal is widened by cutting the conchal cartilage is performed. The extension of drilling of the ear canal is indicated by dotted lines.
b The ear canal is drilled out, exposing and mobilizing the ossicles in the attic. A round opening with of 9.5 mm diameter is made to enable placing of the cartilage disk. The medial end of the ear canal is smoothed to receive the crown cork graft.
c The cartilage disk of the crown cork graft is placed onto the mobile incus body and malleus head and suspended with the perichondrium flaps placed onto the medial end of the new ear canal.
d A large split-skin flap covers the wall of the new ear canal and the perichondrium flaps. The four lateral skin flaps are replaced in the bony ear canal. Additional small split-skin grafts cover the cartilage disk and the areas between the lateral skin flaps.
e The ear canal wall is covered with Silastic sheets and a moistened gauze fills the new ear canal.

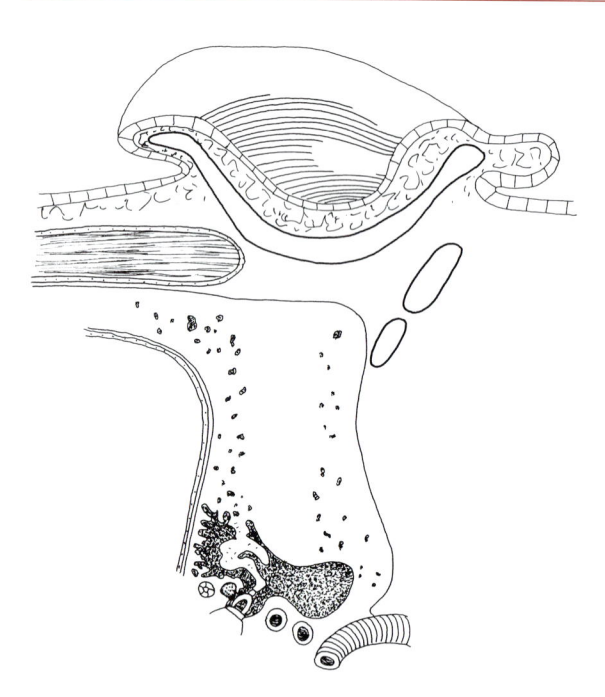

Fig. 19.6 The type 2b atresia with no indication of any ear canal, and with malformed and fixated ossicles. The pinna is severely malformed.

eardrum, and other split-skin grafts are placed between the replaced epithelial flaps (**Fig. 19.5 d**). Silastic sheets cover the entire ear canal wall, which will be filled with a gauze moistened with oxytetracycline and hydrocortisone ointment (**Fig. 19.5e**).

Surgery of Congenital Type 2b Atresia Applying Crown Cork Graft

In type 2b atresia there is no indication of an ear canal, and the pinna is small and malformed (**Fig. 19.6**).

The mastoid region is exposed in a retroauricular approach (**Fig. 19.7a**). There is no tympanic bone and the mastoid process is close to the glenoid fossa. A small supra-meatal spine indicates the place of drilling (**Fig. 19.7b, c**). The malleus head and the incus body are identified by continued drilling along the middle fossa dura (**Fig. 19.7d**). By drilling toward the tympanic cavity, a round opening of diameter of 9.5–10.0 mm is created (**Fig. 19.7e**). The cartilage disk of the crown cork graft is placed onto the malleus head and incus body as well as into the entrance of the hole (**Fig. 19.7f**). Finally, the perichondrial flaps are folded out, thus suspending and stabilizing the cartilage disk (**Fig. 19.7g**). The new ear canal and the new eardrum are covered with a large split-skin graft with five tongues cut out medially (**Fig. 19.7h**; Jahrsdoerfer 1990). The eardrum is covered with four of the tongues (**Fig. 19.7i**).

Removal of Fibrous Tissue in Blunting Phenomena When Applying Crown Cork Tympanoplasty

The goal of surgery in blunting is to preserve enough ear canal skin that the anterior tympanomeatal angle can be covered. This can be achieved according to three different principles:
1. Preservation of the ear canal skin as a flap (MMES_3, Figs. 130–137).
2. Removal of the skin together with the fibrous tissue and covering of the anterior tympanomeatal angle with split-skin grafts (MMES_3, Figs. 138–143).
3. Removal of the skin and fibrous tissue separately (MMES_3, Figs. 144–149).

In this example the principle of preservation of the ear canal skin as a flap is applied.

In a case of severe blunting and posterior perforation, a swing-door technique is employed using a retroauricular approach and elevating a large superior and inferior tympanomeatal flap (**Fig. 19.8a, b**). A malleus epithelial flap and an anterosuperior epithelial flap are also elevated, exposing the superior fibrous tissue (**Fig. 19.8c, d**). Similarly, the anteroinferior blunting tissue is exposed and the eardrum is separated from the malleus (**Fig. 19.8e**), thus allowing safe removal of the fibrous tissue and the eardrum with the fibrous annulus in one piece (**Fig. 19.8 f, g**). The cartilage disk of the crown cork graft is placed into the tympanic cavity and the perichondrial flaps are folded onto the denuded medial ear canal bone (**Fig. 19.8h**). After replacement of the elevated epithelial flaps, the epithelialization of the eardrum will occur (**Fig. 19.8i**). The eardrum and ear canal are covered with Silastic sheets, fixed with Klacansky packing (**Fig. 19.8j**) (Klacansky et al. 1998).

Results of the "Crown Cork" Tympanoplasty

In the first report (Hartwein and Leuwer 1992), 10 patients were operated with crown cork tympanoplasty; in the next paper, the series was increased to 12 patients (Hartwein et al. 1992). In the last report (Hartwein and Kehrl, 1993), in total 22 patients were included, with a postoperative observation time between 2 and 42 months. Eight patients were operated for middle ear deformation, 9 for blunting phenomena after previous surgery, and 5 for totally defective eardrum due to chronic otitis media or cholesteatoma.

Two to 42 months after operation the eardrum was intact and vital in all 22 patients. Two patients had reblunting, one patient had granulations that disappeared after conservative treatment. The remaining 19 patients had no complaints from the operated ears.

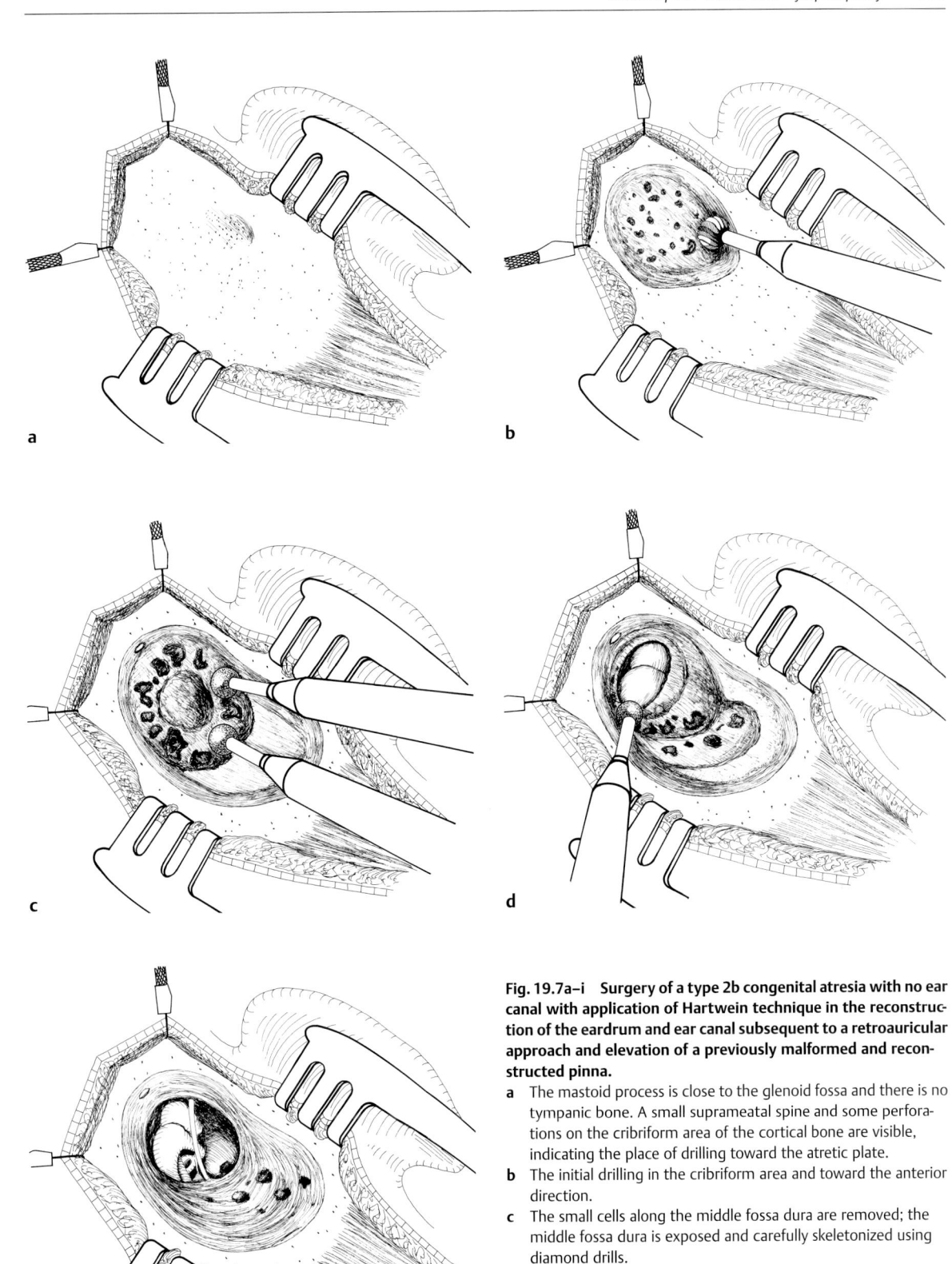

Fig. 19.7a–i Surgery of a type 2b congenital atresia with no ear canal with application of Hartwein technique in the reconstruction of the eardrum and ear canal subsequent to a retroauricular approach and elevation of a previously malformed and reconstructed pinna.

a The mastoid process is close to the glenoid fossa and there is no tympanic bone. A small suprameatal spine and some perforations on the cribriform area of the cortical bone are visible, indicating the place of drilling toward the atretic plate.
b The initial drilling in the cribriform area and toward the anterior direction.
c The small cells along the middle fossa dura are removed; the middle fossa dura is exposed and carefully skeletonized using diamond drills.
d Superiorly, the malleus head and incus body are identified.
e Removal of the bone is complete. The ossicular chain is intact and mobile and the cartilage plate will be placed onto the malleus head and incus body.

Fig. 19.7f–i ▷

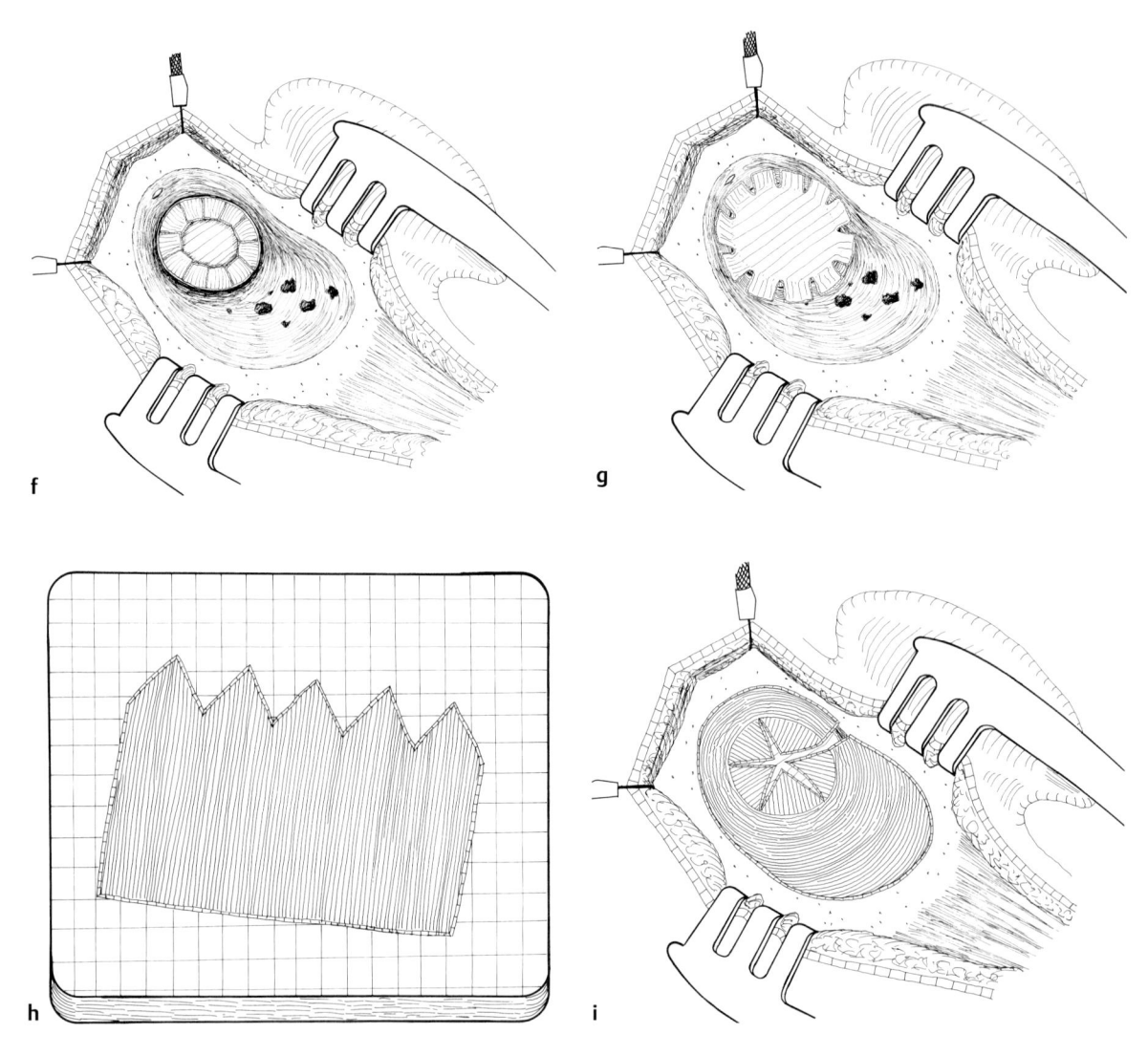

Fig. 19.7f–i

f The crown cork graft is placed into the tympanic cavity. It has good contact with the malleus and incus. The perichondrium flaps are folded inward onto the cartilage to check the relation of the cartilage plate to the new bony annulus and the free movement of the cartilage graft.

g The crown cork perichondrium flaps are placed one by one onto the bone all the way round the new ear canal.

h A large split-skin graft is harvested and cut to create five notches (Jahrsdoerfer 1990).

i The large split-skin graft covers the entire new eardrum and the new ear canal.

Fig. 19.8a–j Surgery for blunting and posterior perforation, applying a crown cork graft in retroauricular approach.

a Blunting involves the anterior half of the eardrum, the anterior tympanomeatal angle, and the anterior ear canal wall. The ossicular chain is intact. The posterior tympanomeatal flap, together with the epithelium of the eardrum remnant will be elevated and cut radially at the 9-o'clock position.

b A swing-door method is used and a superior and an inferior tympanomeatal flap are thus created. Inferiorly, some of the fibrous tissue from the blunting of the eardrum is visible (arrow).

c An epithelial flap from the malleus handle and from the blunting fibrous tissue of the superior end of the anterior part of the eardrum is elevated. Using a sickle knife, the epithelium covering the blunting fibrous tissue of the eardrum and the anterior ear canal wall is cut laterally to the normal ear canal skin.

d Epithelium from the attic region and the superior part of the blunting tissue is elevated up to the normal ear canal skin.

e The epithelium from the fibrous tissue of the inferior part of the eardrum and ear canal is elevated up to the normal skin. Using a sickle knife, the eardrum is separated from the malleus handle.

f Removal of blunting fibrous tissue together with the eardrum and the fibrous annulus. The eardrum is already separated from the malleus, so that all the tissue can be removed in one piece. Using an incudostapedial knife, all tissue—including the annulus and eardrum—is safely separated from the bone and will be removed.

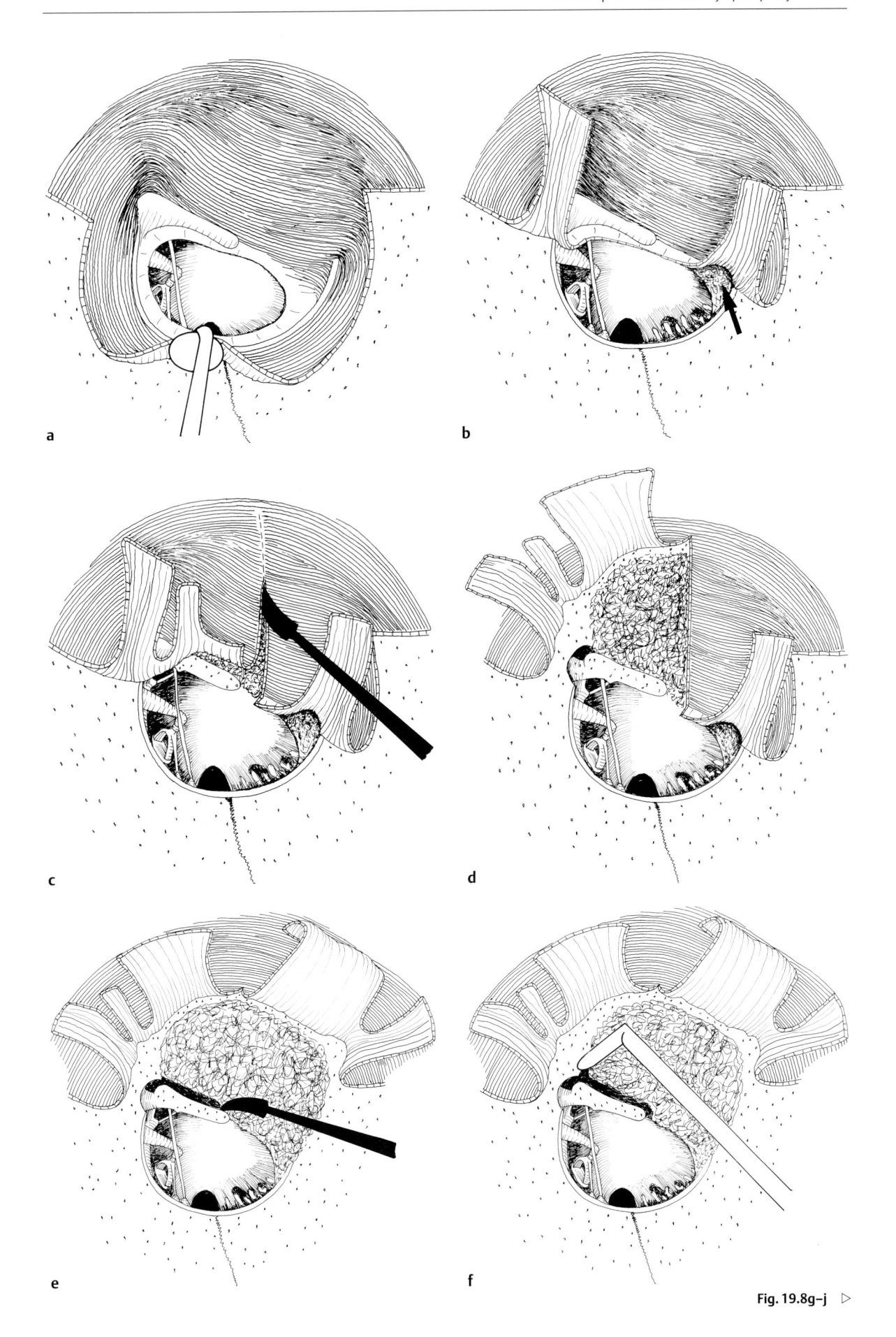

Fig. 19.8g–j ▷

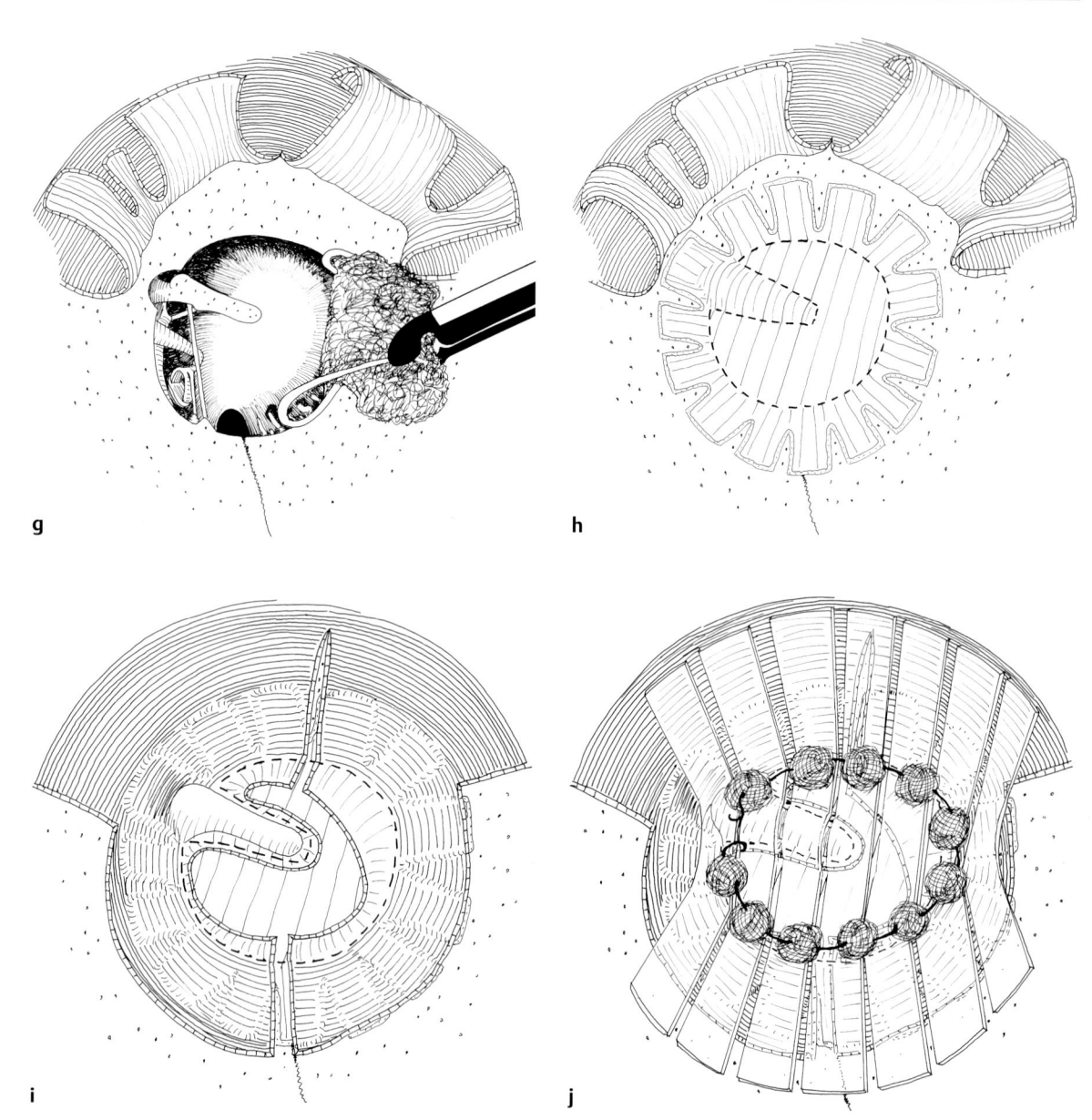

Fig. 19.8g–j

g The fibrous tissue with the anterior part of the eardrum and the fibrous annulus is pulled out in one piece.

h A wedge of the cartilage disk is removed to accommodate the handle and the short process of the malleus, but the perichondrium remains intact. The cartilage disk is placed into the tympanic cavity at the level of the bony annulus and the perichondrium flaps are individually placed onto and adapted to the denuded ear canal wall.

i The epithelial flaps are replaced and epithelialization is thus expected to be hastened. The anterior tympanomeatal angle is clearly visible.

j The ear canal is covered with Silastic sheets, fixed to the tympanomeatal angle with small balls of gauze moistened with hydrocortisone–oxytetracycline. The balls are bound together with black silk.

The average postoperative air–bone gaps at frequencies 500, 1000, 2000, and 4000 Hz were 18, 19, 17, and 11 dB, respectively.

There are no other reports on crown cork tympanoplasty.

Author's Comments and Recommendations

The crown cork graft is similar to a total pars tensa cartilage–perichondrium composite island graft, suspended on the surrounding perichondrium placed onto the denuded bone of the ear canal.

The cartilage disk of 9 mm diameter is also similar. The difference between the two grafts is the many, relatively long perichondrium flaps, cut radially or having small perichondrium strips excised, in the crown cork graft in contrast to the total pars tensa graft in which a 1–2 mm wide perichondrium belt surrounds the cartilage disk.

It may be difficult to harvest a graft of 17 mm diameter (9 + 4 + 4 mm) from the tragus or a deformed concha. However, in my experience a 2 mm perichondrium flap is sufficient posteriorly where the covering of the ear canal skin is adequate. Thus, a crown cork graft used in blunting phenomena may have posterior and superior perichondrium flaps of 2 mm, and a graft of 15 mm diameter (9 + 2 + 4 mm) may be large enough.

The results of surgery with crown cork tympanoplasty are satisfactory, without any eardrum perforation 2–42 months after surgery. However, in very different pathological categories, such as a blunting group of 9 patients, a middle ear malformation group of 8 patients, and a chronic otitis group with 5 patients, the preoperative and postoperative hearing should be reported for each group separately. We may hope that the authors will publish late results of the crown cork method.

Apart from the late results of this series and some reports on new series with crown cork tympanoplasty from the same group, we cannot expect new research on crown cork tympanoplasty. The severe ear canal atresias with total perforation are relatively rare, and new techniques of surgery for congenital atresia are becoming popular (Siegert 2004; Teufert and De la Cruz 2004).

References

Altmann F. Problem of so-called congenital atresia of the ear. Arch Otolaryngol 1949;50:759–788.

Altmann F. Malformation of the auricle and the external auditory meatus. Arch Otolaryngol 1951;54:115–135.

Altmann F. Congenital atresia in the ear in man and animals. Ann Otol Rhinol Laryngol 1955;64:824–858.

Anson BJ, Donaldson JJ. Surgical Anatomy of the Temporal Bone. 3rd ed. Philadelphia: WB Saunders; 1981.

Becker BC, Tos M. Postinflammatory acquired atresia of the external auditory canal. Treatment and results of surgery over 27 years. Laryngoscope 1998;108:903–907.

Bonding P, Tos M. Postinflammatory acquired atresia of the external auditory canal. Acta Otolaryngol 1975;79:115–123.

Borkowski G, Sudhoff H, Luckhaupt H. Autologer Knorpel- Perichondrium- "Spannring" bei subtotalen oder totalen Trommelfelldefekten. Laryngorhinootologie 1999;78:68–72.

Cremers CWRJ, Oudenhoven JMTM, Marres EHMA. Congenital aural atresia: a new subclassification and surgical management. Clin Otolaryngol 1984;9:119–127.

Hartwein J, Kehrl W. "Crowncork tympanoplasty": a technique for total reconstruction of the tympanic membrane. In: Nakano Y, ed. Cholesteatoma and Mastoid Surgery. Amsterdam: Kugler; 1993: 607–609.

Hartwein J, Leuwer R. Die "Kronenkorkentympanoplastik"— eine Methode zur Trommelfelltotalrekonstruktion. Laryngorhinootologie 1992;71:102–105.

Hartwein J, Leuwer RM, Kehrl W. The total reconstruction of the tympanic membrane by the "crowncork" technique. Am J Otolaryngol 1992;13:172–175.

Jahrsdoerfer RA. Surgical correction of congenital malformations of the sound-conducting mechanism. In: Glasscock ME, Shambough GE, eds. Surgery of the Ear. 4th ed. Philadelphia: WB Saunders; 1990:321–333.

Klacansky J, Kucera J, Starek I. Rekonstrukcija blanky bubieka chrupkovymi transplantanti [Reconstruction of the eardrum with cartilage transplants] Otorinolaryngologie a foniatrie 1998; 47:59–63.

Siegert R. [New surgical techniques for the treatment of auricular atresia]. [In German] HNO 2004;52(3):275–286.

Teufert KB, De la Cruz A. Advances in congenital aural atresia surgery: effects on outcome. Otolaryngol Head Neck Surg 2004;131(3): 263–270.

Tos M. Manual of Middle Ear Surgery. Vol. 3. Surgery of the External Auditory Canal. New York, Stuttgart: Thieme; 1997..

Tos M, Balle V. Postinflammatory acquired atresia of the external auditory canal: late results of surgery. Am J Otol 1986;7:365–370.

Tos M, Bonding P. Treatment o postinflammatory acquired atresia of the external auditory canal. ORL J Otorhinolaryngol Relat Spec 1979;41:85–90.

20 Cartilage Shield T-Tube Tympanoplasty

Definition

In 1990 Larry Hall first introduced the long-term ventilation of the middle ear with a T-tube placed in a hole made in the tragus cartilage–perichondrium composite island graft. After a tympanotomy with elevation of the posterior tympanomeatal flap with the intact eardrum, the cartilage–perichondrium graft with the T-tube is placed into the posteroinferior part of the tympanic cavity and the small perichondrium flap onto the posteroinferior part of the ear canal (**Fig. 20.1**). Thus the goal of placement of the permanent tube is to prevent repeated insertions of ventilating tubes, especially in children with severe and chronic secretory otitis media. The series published by Hall did not have eardrum perforations (Hall 1990).

Duckert, Müller, Makielski, and Helms (1995) from the University of Washington and the University of Würzburg have developed an interesting cartilage T-tube device to ventilate the tympanic cavity long-term in cases with perforation of the eardrum and chronically severe poor tubal function. A hole is made in a relatively large round or oval cartilage–perichondrium composite island graft and a T-tube is placed through the hole (**Fig. 20.2**). The cartilage graft with the T-tube is placed under the eardrum remnant and is suspended by the surrounding perichondrium flap placed onto the ear canal bone.

Danner and Dornhoffer (2001) applied primary intubation in cartilage tympanoplasty by making a hole in the anterior part of the total tensa cartilage–perichondrium composite graft and placing a T-tube into the hole. This graft is placed as an underlay graft under the eardrum remnant. The two cartilage half-disks are suspended by the perichondrium flap placed onto the bone of the ear canal. The relatively short flaps of the T-tube are folded out, either in posteroanterior or in superoinferior direction (**Fig. 20.3**)

Fig. 20.1 The Larry Hall cartilage–perichondrium graft. The T-tube graft is placed, after a tympanotomy, in the posterosuperior part of the tympanic cavity and is suspended by a small perichondrium flap.

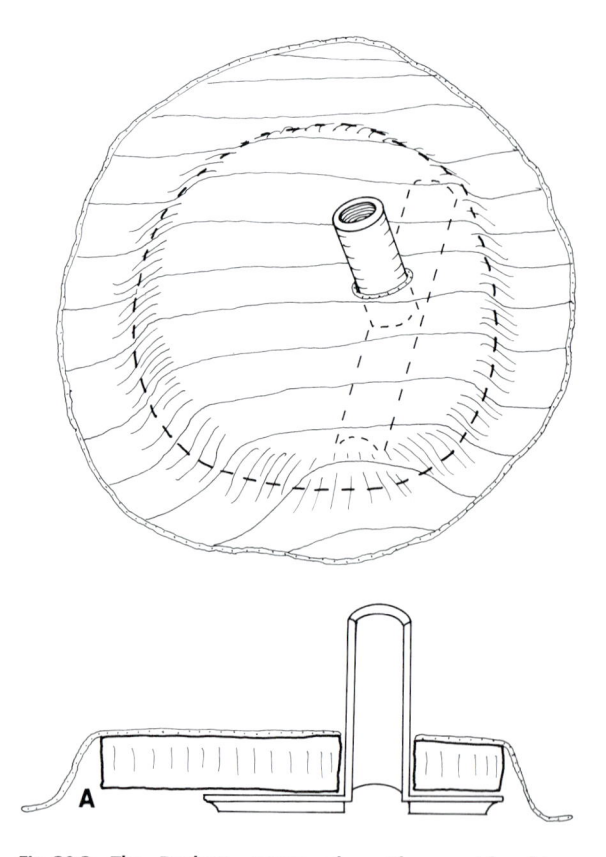

Fig. 20.2 The Duckert compound cartilage–perichondrium graft with a T-tube with long flanges placed in the inferior part of the cartilage. The surrounding perichondrium will be placed onto the bony ear canal wall as an underlay graft. The cartilage will be suspended by the perichondrium flap.

Recently Elsheikh et al. (2006) published an interesting prospective, randomized study, comparing results in 23 patients with intact ossicular chain and various grades of atelectasis. After removal of the retracted part of the eardrum, a cartilage–perichondrium graft, with a ventilating tube inserted, was placed in the tympanic cavity as an underlay graft. In another group of 23 patients with similar pathology, a similar surgical procedure was performed but without insertion of the ventilating tube in the cartilage graft. The shape of the graft and the surgical method differ from those of the other grafts.

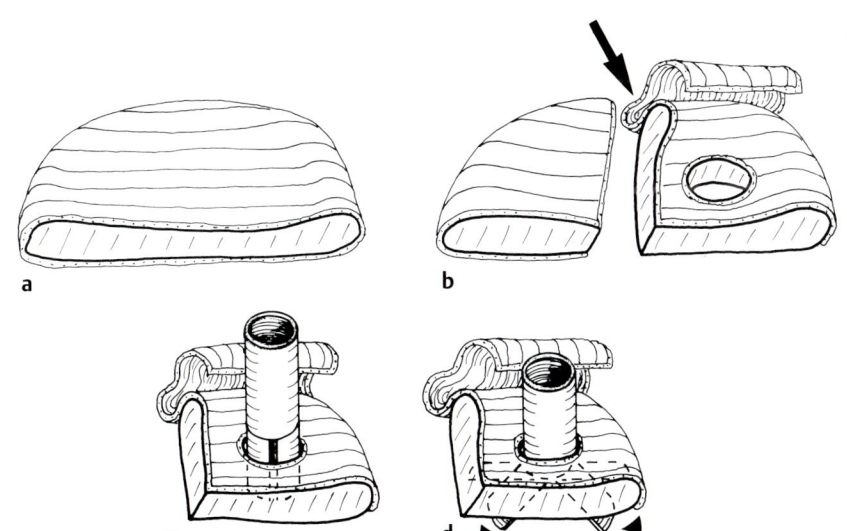

Harvesting and Construction of the Cartilage Shield T-Tube Grafts

The four different methods use different grafts and construct them in a different ways. The harvesting and construction of the grafts will be described separately for each method.

Construction of the Hall Cartilage Shield T-Tube Graft in Intact Eardrum

Under general anesthesia, a skin incision is made posterior to the tragus dome and the skin with the subcutis is elevated on both sites of the tragus dome. A 5 mm × 5 mm piece of the tragus, including the dome, is removed (**Fig. 20.4a**). This cartilage is divided into two pieces (as shown in **Fig. 20.4b**). The perichondrium is elevated from the anterior side of the cartilage and it is trimmed into a small perichondrium graft (**Fig. 20.4b**). On the posterior side the perichondrium is not removed as it will be in contact with the undersurface of the eardrum. A hole is made in the middle of the graft using a 1.8 ID Treace Gelfoam punch or a round knife. A 1.14 mm C-flex Treace T-tube is inserted through the hole (**Fig. 20.4c, d**) (Hall 1990).

Construction of the Duckert Cartilage Shield T-Tube Graft

The round cartilage shield T-tube graft is harvested from the concha via a retroauricular approach (**Fig. 20.5a**). The diameter of the cartilage disk is usually 9 mm and the surrounding perichondrium should measure at least 2 mm. Thus the diameter of the entire graft is 13 mm (2 + 9 + 2 mm). The perichondrium is removed from the convex side of the cartilage (**Fig. 20.5b**) and this side will face the middle ear. The round cartilage graft is isolated together with the perichondrium on its concave side (**Fig. 20.5c–e**).

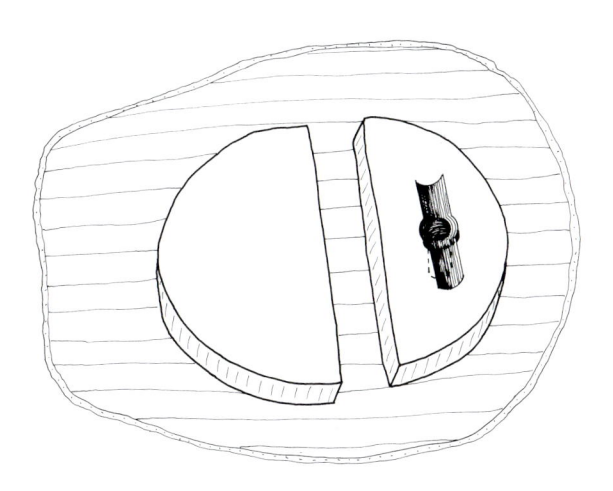

Fig. 20.3 The Dornhoffer total pars tensa graft with a T-tube placed in the anterior cartilage disk. The flanges of the T-tube are short and are directed superoinferiorly.

Fig. 20.4a–d Construction of the cartilage shield T-tube graft by Hall.
a A 5 mm piece of tragal cartilage with the dome is harvested.
b The cartilage is cut sagittally into two pieces. The anterior perichondrium is elevated up to the dome and trimmed to a flap (arrow). A hole is made with a 1.8 ID Treace Gelfoam punch, or with a small round knife.
c A 1.14 mm C-flex Treace T-tube is placed through the hole.
d The flanges of the T-tube are opened.

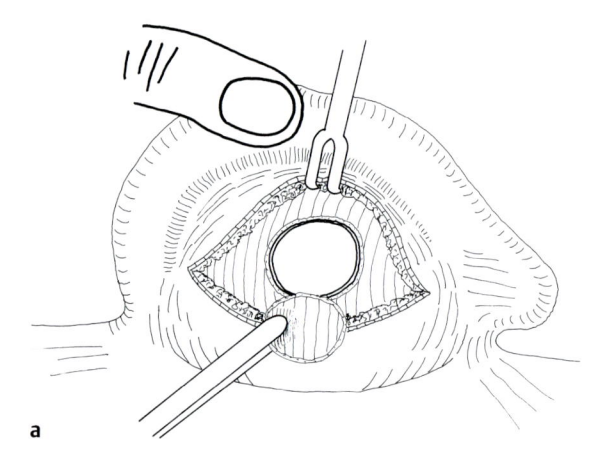

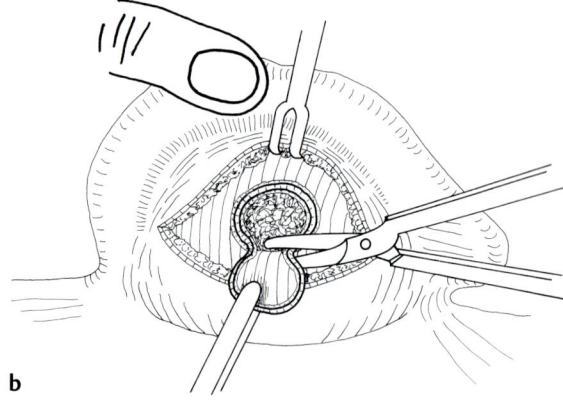

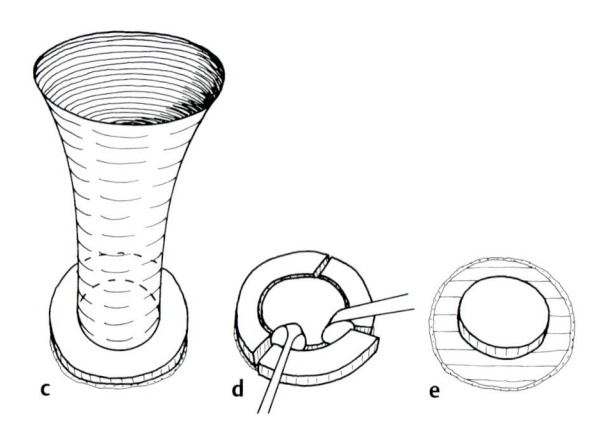

Fig. 20.5a–e Harvesting of a 13 mm round concha cartilage–perichondrium disk.
a A postauricular incision is made at the most prominent area of the concha and the subcutaneous tissue is elevated. A round incision is made though all three layers: the posterior perichondrium, the cartilage, and the anterior perichondrium. The posterior perichondrium is elevated and removed.
b The 13 mm cartilage with the anterior perichondrium is carefully elevated from the anterior subcutaneous tissue and removed.
c–e Trimming the cartilage graft. The graft is placed with the perichondrium on the undersurface. Using a 9 mm ear speculum, the cartilage disk is mapped and cut, leaving a 2 mm belt for the perichondrium flap (**c**). The cartilage is elevated and removed from the peripheral belt (**d**). The round cartilage disk of 9 mm will be placed into the tympanic cavity and the perichondrium onto the ear canal (**e**).

The size and the round shape of the ring are easily marked with a 9 mm ear speculum (Klacansky et al. 1998) (see **Fig. 19.2h**). The cartilage within the marked ring is removed, creating a round hole for the T-tube.

The size and shape of the cartilage graft are adapted to the conditions in the tympanic cavity, especially the ossicular chain, or as needed in an ossiculoplasty. In the presence of the malleus handle, the cartilage is notched or a specially shaped graft is made to fit the malleus handle (**Fig. 20.6**). Duckert et al. (1995, 2003) use a 1.5 mm punch to trephine a hole through the cartilage and the perichondrium in the inferior half of the graft. A Richards modified T-tube, 1.32 mm in diameter and 4.8 mm long, is passed through the hole to create the shield unit (**Figs. 20.2** and **20.6**).

Construction of the Dornhoffer Cartilage Shield T-Tube Graft

The cartilage is harvested from the tragus (Dornhoffer 1997). Danner and Dornhoffer (2001) used a total pars tensa cartilage–perichondrium composite island graft divided into a posterior and an anterior island. The cartilage is surrounded by a belt of perichondrium. In the anterior island graft, a hole is made in the cartilage for the T-tube using a round knife (**Fig. 20.7**). Then a straight pick is used to create and enlarge the hole in the perichondrium (**Fig. 20.8**) to allow easier tube placement. Using small surgical scissors, the T-tube is remodeled by trimming the flanges to 3–4 mm. Finally, the T-tube is placed into the cartilage window and brought out through the perichondrium surface (**Fig. 20.9**). The graft is now ready to be placed into the tympanic cavity.

The Elsheikh U-shaped Cartilage–Perichondrium T-Tube Graft

The graft is harvested from the tragus in the way shown by Dornhoffer (1997). A U-shaped cartilage–perichondrium total pars tensa graft with a horizontal diameter of 9–10 mm is cut. Superiorly, a rectangular wedge of cartilage is cut, to accommodate the graft to the malleus handle. A hole is made through the cartilage–perichondrium graft and a tube without flanges is pushed through the hole (**Fig. 20.10a, b**). The perichondrium is attached on the ear canal side and not on the tympanic side. There is no peripheral perichondrium flap as found in the grafts of Hall, of Duckert, and of Dornhoffer.

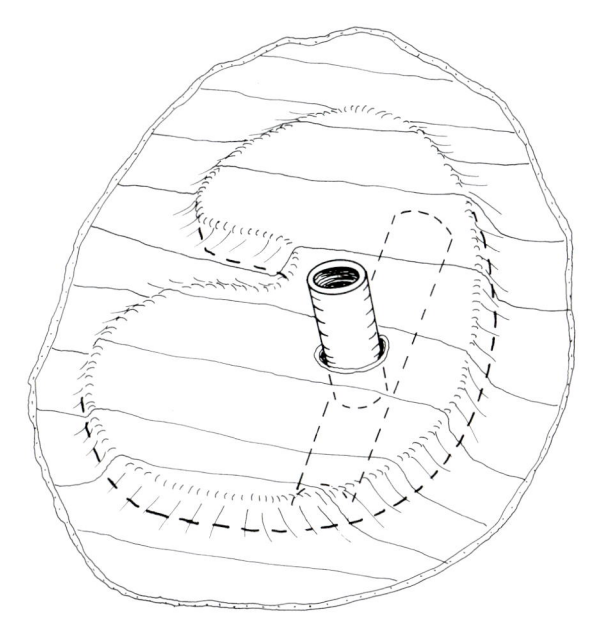

Fig. 20.6 The Duckert graft with the T-tube. The graft is shaped to fit the malleus handle exactly.

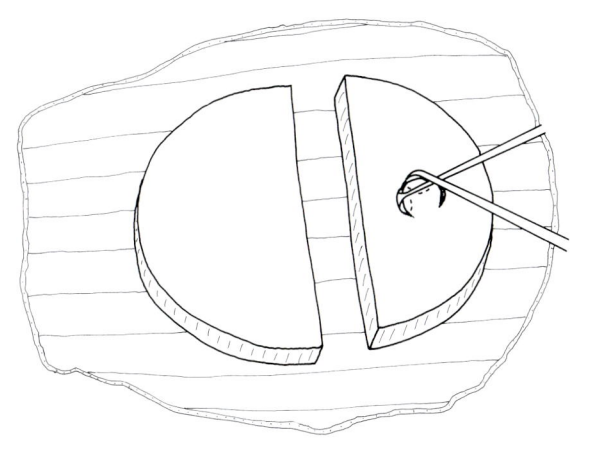

Fig. 20.7 The Dornhoffer total pars tensa compound cartilage–perichondrium island graft. A hole is made in the anterior island using a round knife. (See also **Figs. 20.8** and **20.9**.)

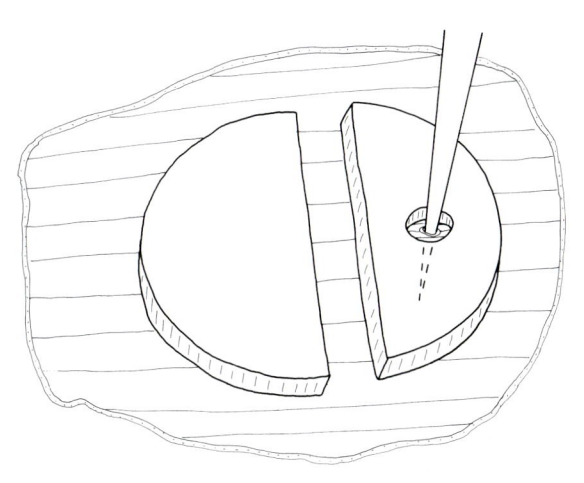

Fig. 20.8 (Cont.) A straight pick dilates a hole in the perichondrium.

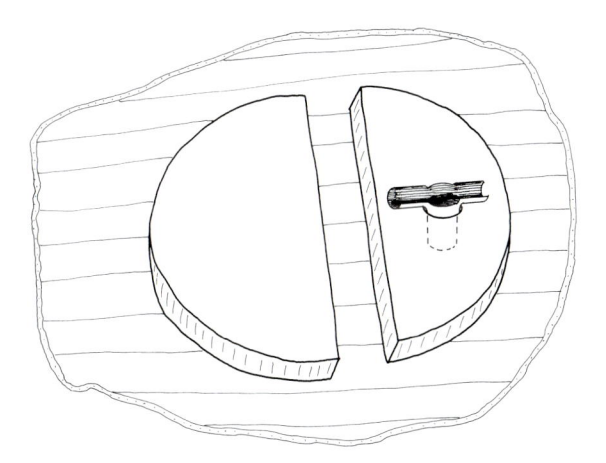

Fig. 20.9 (Cont.) A T-tube is placed in the hole and the graft is ready to be placed in the tympanic cavity.

Indication for Cartilage Shield T-Tube Tympanoplasty

Chronic severe eustachian tube dysfunction is the main indication for cartilage shield T-tube tympanoplasty. Such a situation is most often present in:
- Craniofacial abnormalities, Down syndrome.
- Nasopharyngeal adenoid cystic carcinoma.
- Previous head and neck cancer involving the nasopharynx.
- Patients with recurrences of chronic otitis media and a history of multiple surgeries, with demonstrated eustachian tube dysfunction. However, in the published reports it is not mentioned which tubal function tests are used or should be used.
- Recurrent long-term middle ear effusion and atelectasis.

These indications of Danner and Dornhoffer (2001) explain why the cartilage shield T-tube tympanoplasty is relatively seldom used by them. During a period of 6 years from 1994 to 2000, Danner and Dornhoffer (2001) performed 25 primary cartilage shield T-tube intubations in a total of 694 cartilage tympanoplasties.

Duckert et al. (1995) performed cartilage-shield T-tube tympanoplasty on 294 ears (290 patients) between 1990 and 1992—a high number. The indications for surgery were different:
- Total absence of tympanic membrane in a nondraining ear, which means a total perforation involving more than 90 % of the eardrum.

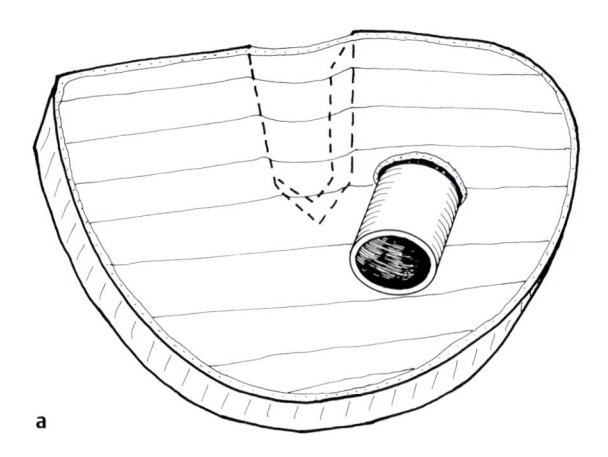

Fig. 20.10a, b The Elsheikh U cartilage–perichondrium graft with a tube without flanges, placed in a hole at the anterior part of the graft.
a Perichondrium covers the ear canal side, but the graft has no free flaps and is not suspended on the ear canal wall. A wedge in the upper part of the cartilage is cut to accommodate the inferior half of the malleus handle.
b The tympanic side of the same Elsheikh cartilage graft. The tympanic side of the graft is not covered with perichondrium.

- Chronic otitis media "characterized by recurrent drainage and long-standing tympanic membrane perforation over a number of years."

In a later series of 40 patients (12 children and 28 adults) operated from 1994 the indications were: atelectasis with chronic effusion (13 ears); chronic otitis media with perforation (8 ears); adhesive otitis media with effusion (7 ears); cholesteatoma (10 ears); and cholesterol granuloma (2 ears) (Duckert et al. 2003).

In the randomized study of Elsheikh et al. (2006), 46 adult patients with a mean age of 28 years had atelectasis of the following severity, according to Sade's classification (Sade 1979):
- Thirty-one patients had grade 2 with posterosuperior atrophy and retraction down to the incudostapedial joint without resorption of the lenticular process or down to the stapes with resorption of the lenticular process and eventually the head of the stapes.
- Fifteen patients had atelectasis of grade 3 with atrophy and retraction of the entire pars tensa to the incudostapedial joint and down to the promontory, but without adhesion to the promontory.

Ears with atelectasis of grade 4 and adhesion to the promontory, called adhesive otitis, are not included.

The indication of Hall for his technique was "cartilage shield T-tube after two trans-tympanic grommet insertions." Hall does not insert trans-tympanic tubes more than twice and believes that "continuing to place tubes is most often like beating a dead horse."

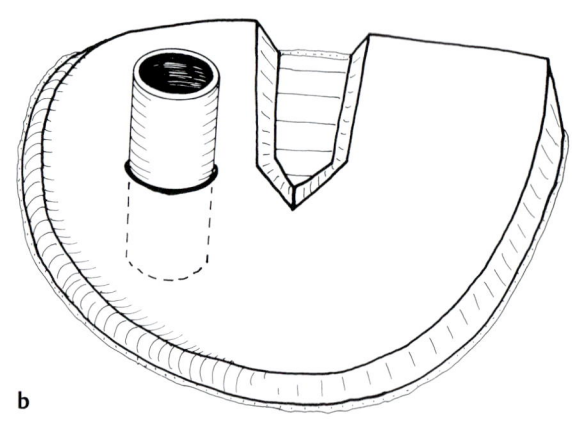

Surgical Techniques

Only the three surgical teams mentioned have published their techniques and results. The differences in construction of T-tube shield grafts have already been described. Since the island grafts differ between the three teams, there are also some differences between the surgical techniques employed.

The Hall Technique

The Hall series comprised selected children with severe eardrum changes.

With a sickle knife, a small incision of the eardrum is made at the 8-o'clock position and another circumferential incision on the posterior canal wall (**Fig. 20.11a**). The incision of the atrophic eardrum is continued 3 mm in the inferoanterior direction. Posteriorly, the ear canal wall skin flap is divided (**Fig. 20.11b**). The two tympanomeatal flaps are elevated and the cartilage–perichondrium graft with the T-tube is placed into the inferoposterior part of the tympanic cavity at the level of the bony annulus. The perichondrium flap is placed onto the ear canal bone, suspending the graft (**Fig. 20.11c**). The tympanomeatal flaps are replaced and the eardrum epithelium is adapted to the ventilation tube (**Fig. 20.11d**). Closure of the eardrum is quicker because the outer surface of the cartilage graft is covered with perichondrium.

To illustrate the high incidence and severity of eardrum pathology, one of our first **unselected** series of chronic secretory otitis with several previous grommet insertions will be briefly mentioned (Tos et al. 1989). In our oldest series of 278 children (527 ears) with secretory otitis,

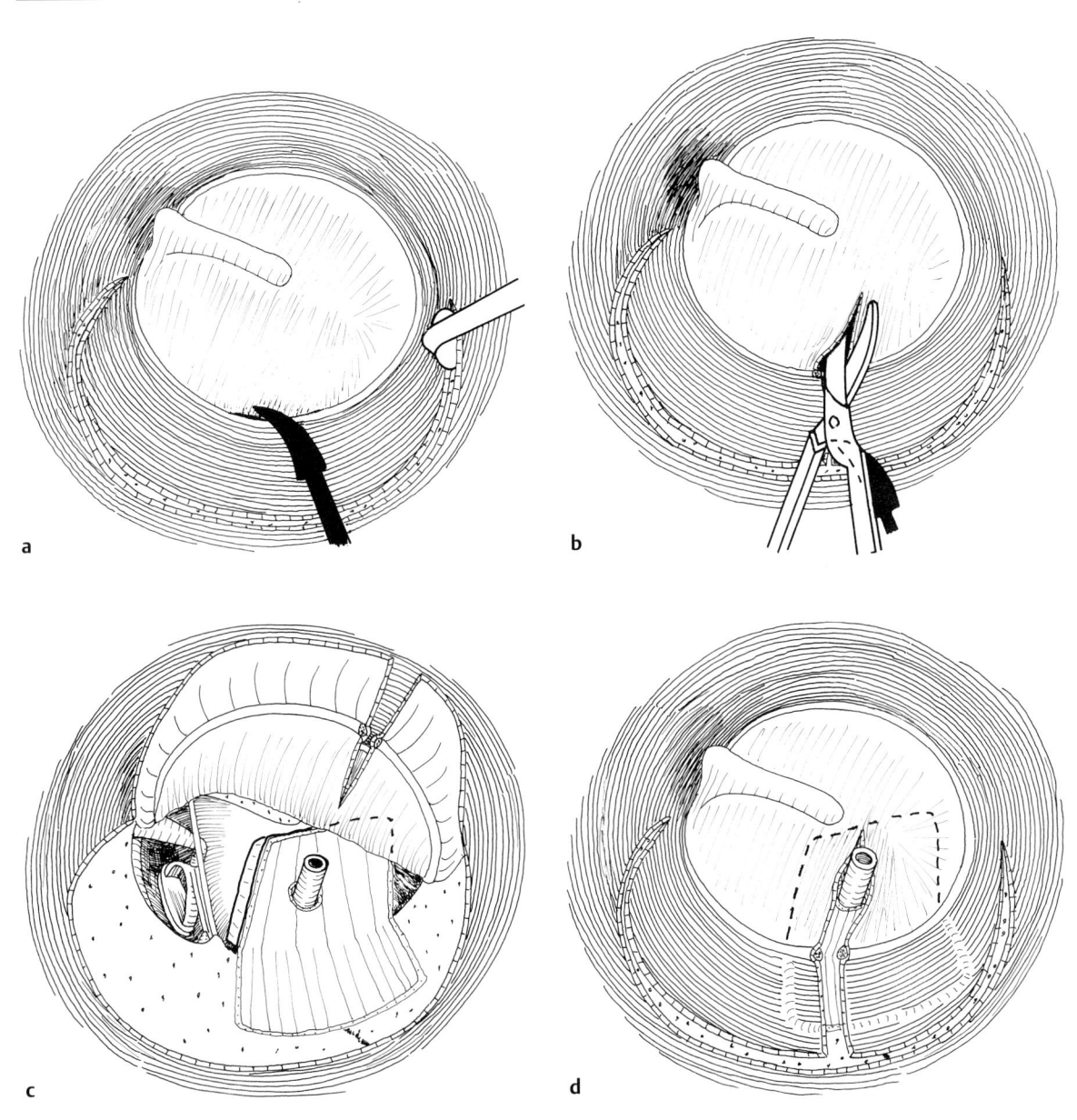

Fig. 20.11a–d The Hall technique of prolonged middle ear ventilation using the cartilage shield T-tube tympanoplasty in a case of chronic secretory otitis media with atrophic but intact eardrum.

- **a** Using a transcanal approach with a fixed ear speculum, a circumferential incision is made. Using a sickle knife, a small perforation of the eardrum is made at the 8-o'clock position and just anterior to the fibrous annulus. A circumferential incision is made between the 11-o'clock and 6-o'clock positions.
- **b** Using a pair of scissors, the incision in the eardrum is continued 3 mm in the inferoanterior direction. The radial skin incision of the ear canal skin is continued outward using a sickle knife.
- **c** The tympanomeatal flap is elevated and the cartilage–perichondrium flap with the T-tube is placed in the posteroinferior part of the tympanic cavity at the level of the bony annulus. The perichondrium flap is placed onto the bony wall of the ear canal.
- **d** The tympanomeatal flaps are replaced and the incision on the eardrum is adapted to the tube. The mucosa of the eardrum is in contact with the perichondrium of the graft.

treated during the period 1970–1975 with adenoidectomy and grommet insertion, the following changes of the pars tensa were found 10–16 years after treatment: myringosclerosis 25.7 %; myringosclerosis and atrophy 10.8 %; atrophy 14.4 %; atrophy and adherence to incudostapedial joint 4.7 %; adhesive otitis 2.2 %; sinus cholesteatoma 0.3 %; perforation 0 (two patients had a successful myringoplasty). In total, 58.1 % of ears had abnormal pars tensa. In addition 27 % of ears had attic retractions, including 7.5 % of ears with advanced retractions of types 3 and 4 and one ear with an attic cholesteatoma (Tos et al. 1989).

This unselected clinical series indicates that the selected series of Hall may have had more, possibly much more, severe eardrum pathology than our series. The surgery of such cases with advanced atrophy of the pars tensa is accordingly a delicate procedure and may sometimes end with a perforation.

The Duckert Technique

Initially Duckert et al. (1995) used the retroauricular approach but later they used the transcanal approach, raising a large tympanomeatal flap (Duckert et al. 2003) (**Fig. 20.12a, b**). It is important to elevate the anterior fibrous annulus together with the eardrum remnant and anterior ear canal skin to be able to place the perichondrium flap onto the exposed bony annulus and ear canal wall (**Fig. 20.12c, d**). The T-tube shield graft is placed under the malleus and gently pulled toward the anterior bony annulus (**Fig. 20.12e**). The cartilage disk is positioned onto the intact long process of the incus and under, but close to, the malleus handle. It lies at the level of the bony annulus but without touching it (**Fig. 20.12f**). The perichondrium is pushed onto the anterior bony annulus and bony ear canal wall, allowing the cartilage to be suspended from the perichondrium. Inferiorly and posteriorly, it is much easier to fold out a large perichondrium flap (**Fig. 20.12f**). Superiorly, only a small perichondrium flap can be used. All epithelial flaps, including the elevated fibrous annulus, are replaced onto the graft and tympanomeatal flaps are also replaced (**Fig. 20.12g–i**). The patency of the T-tube is tested using a pick or a probe.

Instead of placing the cartilage plate under the malleus handle, the cartilage may be shaped to fit the contours of the malleus handle (**Fig. 20.6**). The cartilage plate can also be placed more laterally, thus enlarging the tympanic cavity. Another option is to place the perichondrium as an on-lay graft along the malleus handle and the anterosuperior part of the eardrum remnant. After the endaural incision (**Fig. 20.13a**), the tympanomeatal flap with the fibrous annulus is elevated all the way around the perforation (**Fig. 20.13b**). The epithelium from the malleus handle and the anterosuperior part of the eardrum is elevated as one flap, allowing the in-lay grafting in this part. After placement of the cartilage T-tube graft (**Fig. 20.13c**), the on-lay perichondrium flap covers the malleus handle and the lamina propria (**Fig. 20.13d**). The elevated epithelial flap is replaced, covering the malleus handle and the anterosuperior part of the eardrum (**Fig. 20.13e**). The tympanomeatal flap with the fibrous annulus is next replaced (**Fig. 20.13f, g**).

Contouring of the Anterior Annular Sulcus

In some patients with a total perforation, the anterior fibrous annulus is atrophic or missing and the annular bony sulcus is flat or nonexistent (Duckert et al. 1995, 2003). Duckert recommends contouring and enlarging the anterior sulcus and the anterior bony ear canal wall. In the retroauricular approach this can be achieved by elevation of the anterior eardrum remnant with the fibrous annulus and anterior ear canal skin. Duckert even used two medial radial incisions—at 2-o'clock and 5-o'clock positions—to elevate an anterior skin flap and widened the ear canal by drilling to better accommodate the perichondrium flap.

Widening of the Anterior Annular Sulcus without Anterior Radial Skin Incisions

In the retroauricular approach, widening can be performed with elevation of the anterior fibrous annulus and the gradual drilling of a groove in the ear canal bone along the bony annulus (**Fig. 20.14a, b**). After placement of the cartilage shield T-tube graft, the anterior perichondrium flap can be accommodated in the groove of the enlarged anterior tympanic sulcus (**Fig. 20.14c, d**). Fibrous tissue around the perichondrium will fixate the flap and gradually fill out the groove (**Fig. 20.14e**).

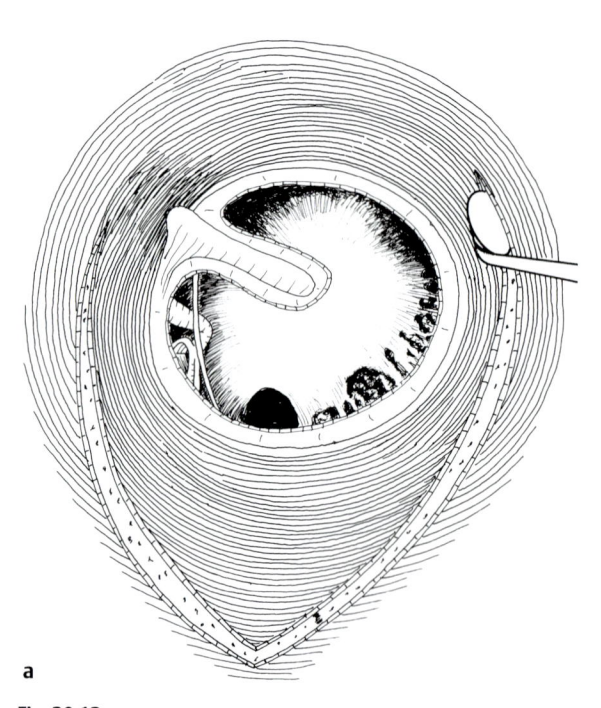

Fig. 20.12a

Surgical Techniques 303

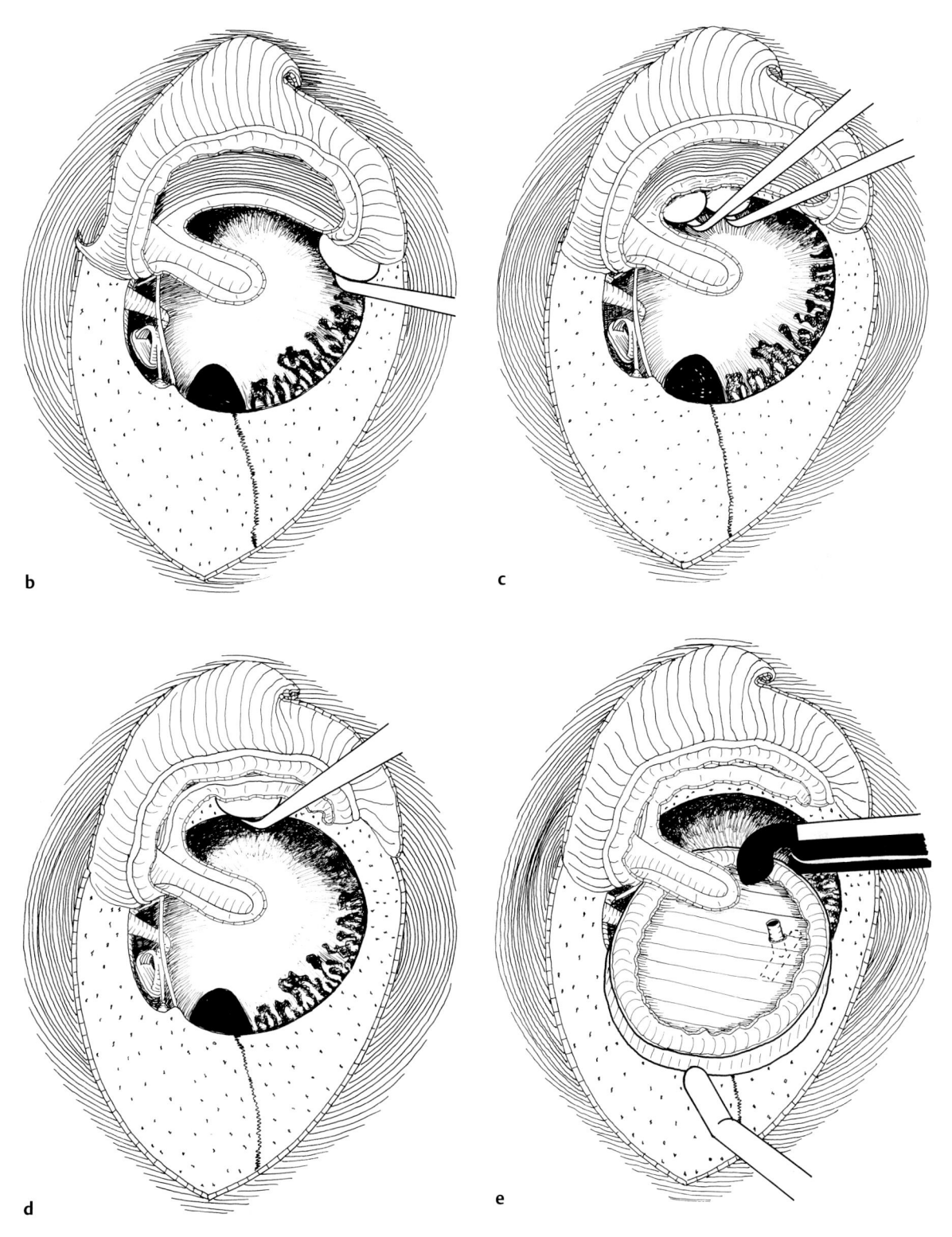

Fig. 20.12b–i The Duckert cartilage shield T-tube tympanoplasty in a case with chronic tubal dysfunction, total perforation, and an intact ossicular chain.

a The edges of the perforation are removed all the way around and along the malleus handle. A large canal skin incision is made, continuing far anteriorly to the anterior canal.

b A large tympanomeatal flap with the fibrous annulus and the eardrum remnants is elevated. Using a round knife, the anterior fibrous annulus is also elevated, exposing and visualizing the anterior bony annulus.

c The anterior fibrous annulus is elevated further.

d The anterior bony annulus is now clearly visible.

e The cartilage T-tube graft is placed under the malleus handle and will then be pushed toward the bony annulus.

Fig. 20.12f–i ▷

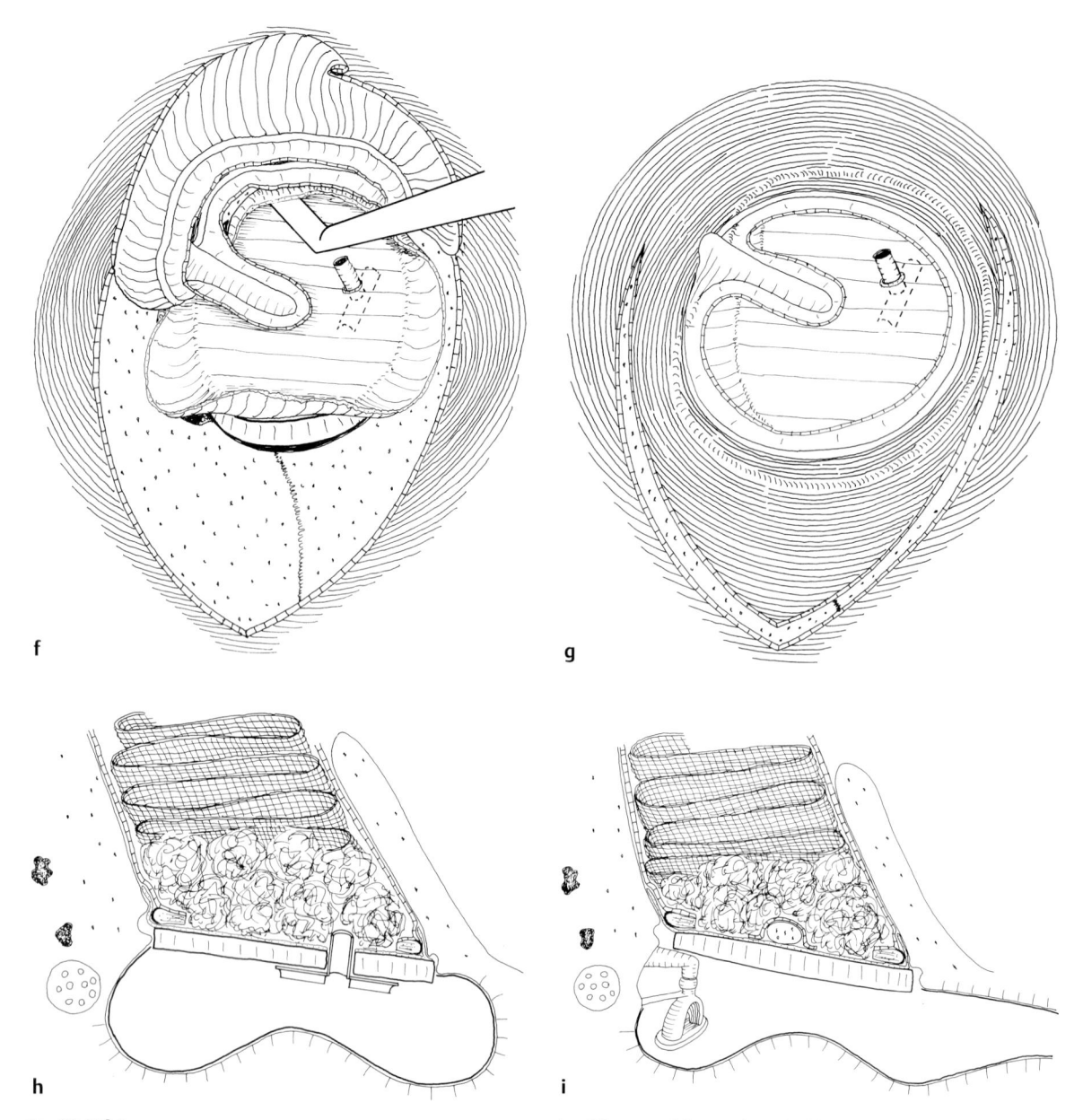

Fig. 20.12f–i

f The cartilage T-tube graft is now placed close to the bony annulus and is fixed by placing the perichondrium onto the denuded bony annulus and ear canal wall as well as onto the inferior and superior bony ear canal wall. The hole for the T-tube is in the anteroinferior part of the cartilage disk.

g The graft with the T-tube is in place, the anterior and the inferior fibrous annulus is pulled back together with the remnants of the eardrum. Superiorly, the perichondrium flap is placed under the malleus and superior part of the eardrum. Posteriorly, the large perichondrium flap covers the bone. The tympanomeatal flap is replaced.

h Side view of the cartilage shield T-tube tympanoplasty at the level of the position of the T-tube. The cartilage plate with the T-tube is placed at the level of the bony annulus. Its lateral surface is covered by the perichondrium, which continues as a flap on the anterior and posterior ear canal walls. The cartilage with the T-tube is thus hanging from the perichondrium.

i Side view of the same tympanoplasty at the level of the lenticular process. The cartilage plate is almost touching the distal part of the long process of the incus. The cartilage plate is in contact with the malleus handle, providing a fair chance for good hearing.

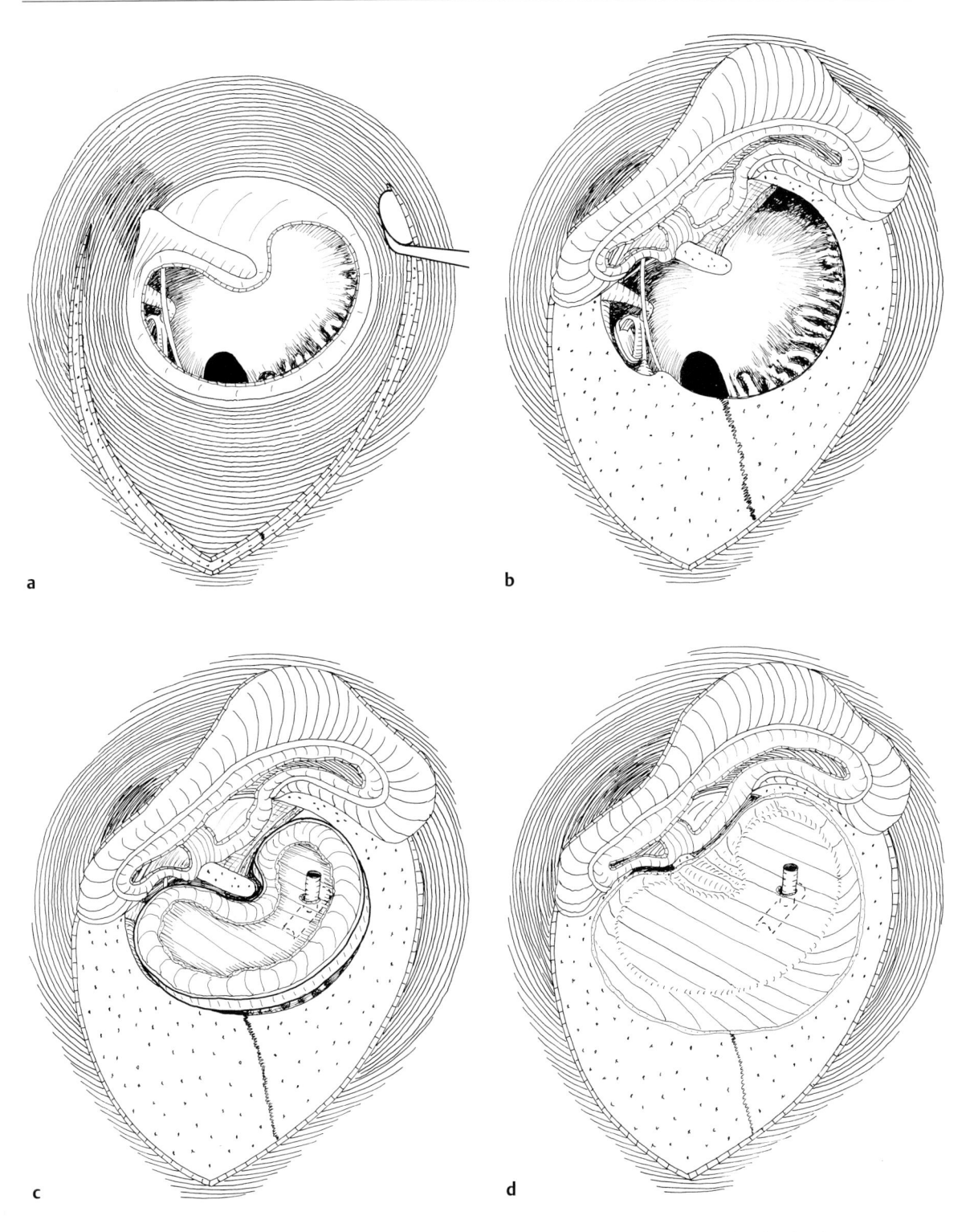

Fig. 20.13 a–g Cartilage shield T-tube tympanoplasty with a cartilage plate adapted to the malleus handle in a subtotal perforation and an intact ossicular chain.

a Epithelium is removed from the edges of the perforation. A large endaural incision extending to the anterior ear canal wall is made.
b The tympanomeatal flap with the fibrous annulus and the eardrum remnant is elevated. The anterior bony annulus is visible. The epithelium from the malleus handle and the anterosuperior part of the eardrum is elevated as one flap.
c The cartilage shield T-tube graft is placed in the tympanic cavity. It is adapted well to the malleus handle and it is positioned at the level of the malleus. The perichondrium flaps will be folded out.
d Superiorly, the perichondrium is folded out over the malleus handle and over the lamina propria of the anterosuperior part of the eardrum. Anteriorly, inferiorly, and posteriorly, the perichondrium is placed onto the bony annulus and the ear canal bone.

Fig. 20.13 e–g ▷

Fig. 20.13e–g

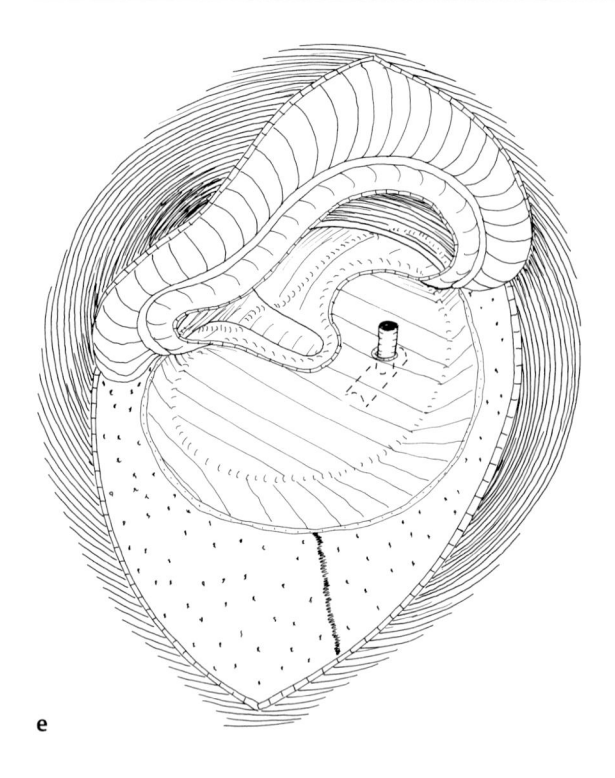

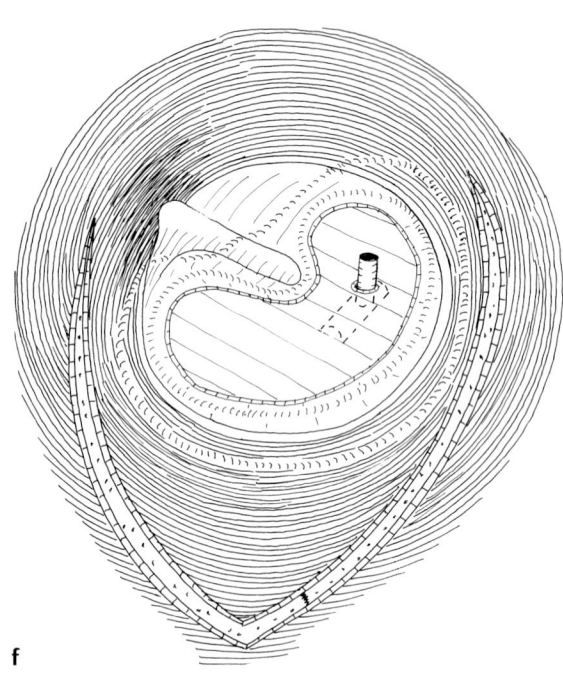

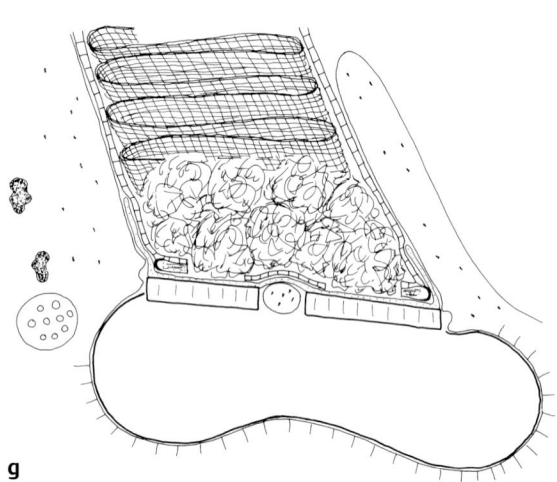

e The epithelial flap of the malleus handle and the anterosuperior eardrum remnant are replaced as on-lay grafts.

f The tympanomeatal flap and the fibrous annulus and the eardrum remnants are replaced, stabilizing the cartilage–perichondrium T-tube compound graft.

g Side view of the graft at the level of the malleus handle. The graft is hanging from the perichondrium at the level of the bony annulus and the malleus handle. The perichondrium covers the malleus.

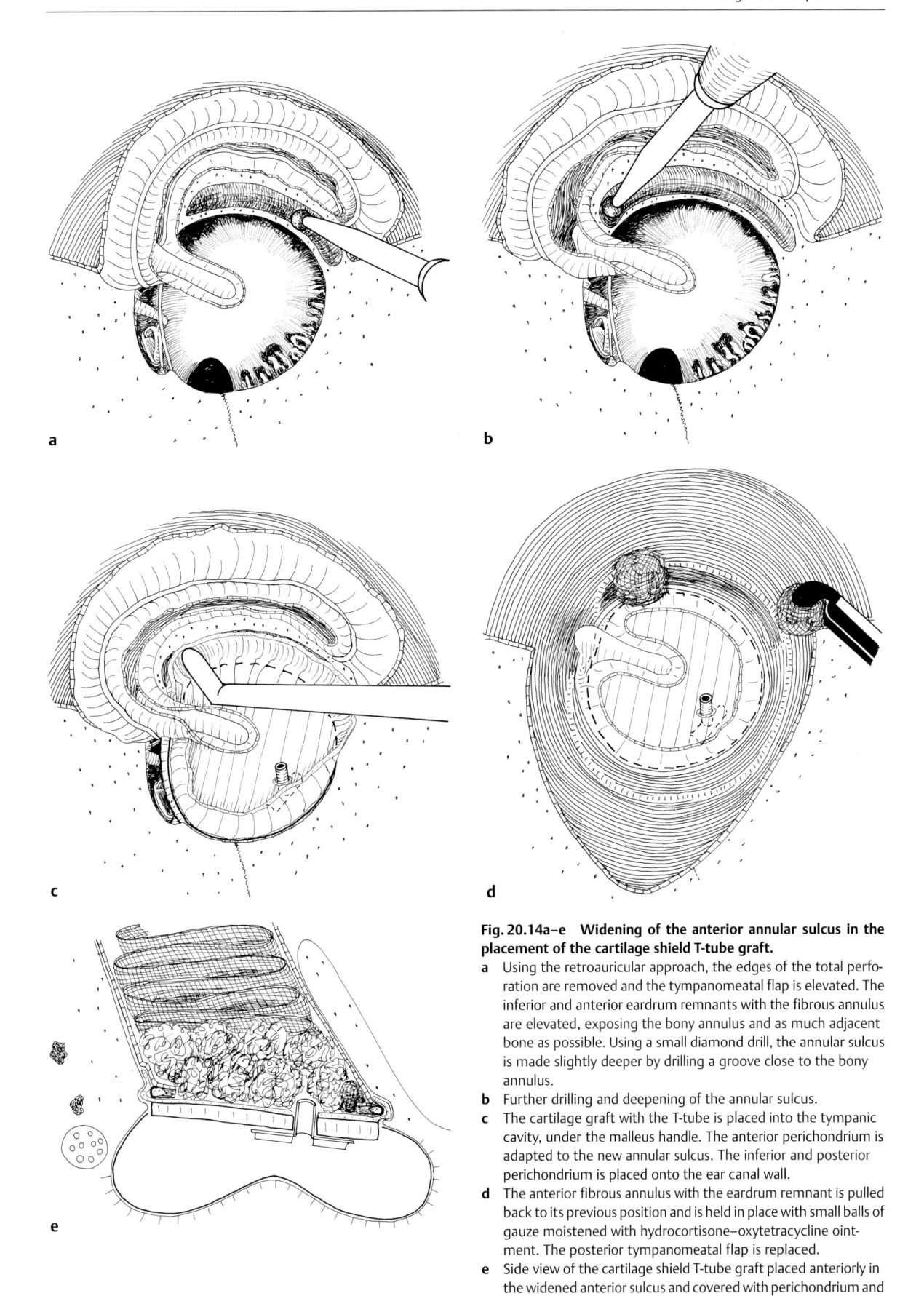

Surgical Techniques 307

Fig. 20.14a–e Widening of the anterior annular sulcus in the placement of the cartilage shield T-tube graft.

a Using the retroauricular approach, the edges of the total perforation are removed and the tympanomeatal flap is elevated. The inferior and anterior eardrum remnants with the fibrous annulus are elevated, exposing the bony annulus and as much adjacent bone as possible. Using a small diamond drill, the annular sulcus is made slightly deeper by drilling a groove close to the bony annulus.

b Further drilling and deepening of the annular sulcus.

c The cartilage graft with the T-tube is placed into the tympanic cavity, under the malleus handle. The anterior perichondrium is adapted to the new annular sulcus. The inferior and posterior perichondrium is placed onto the ear canal wall.

d The anterior fibrous annulus with the eardrum remnant is pulled back to its previous position and is held in place with small balls of gauze moistened with hydrocortisone–oxytetracycline ointment. The posterior tympanomeatal flap is replaced.

e Side view of the cartilage shield T-tube graft placed anteriorly in the widened anterior sulcus and covered with perichondrium and epithelium. The anterior tympanomeatal angle is filled with small balls of gauze and the ear canal with Gelfoam and gauze moistened with hydrocortisone–oxytetracycline ointment.

Widening of the Anterior Annular Sulcus with Anterior Radial Skin Incisions

When conditions are narrow along the anterior annulus with new bone formation, more drastic drilling is needed to widen the anterior sulcus and accommodate the anterior perichondrium flap. Duckert et al. (1995, 2003) recommend two radial incisions via a retroauricular approach, at the 2-o'clock and 5-o'clock positions and the elevation of an anterior tympanomeatal flap (**Fig. 20.15a, b**). Along the anterior bony annulus a groove is drilled with a diamond drill (**Fig. 20.15c**). After placement of the cartilage shield T-tube graft, the anterior perichondrium flap is accommodated in the groove, thus providing a solid fixation of the graft (**Figs. 20.15d–f**).

Placement of the Anterior Perichondrium Flap into the Tympanic Cavity

Duckert et al. (1995) proposed placement of the anterior perichondrium flap into the tympanic cavity by drilling bone along the bony annulus. This can be done by drilling a deep groove anterior to the bony annulus directly through the bone and ending in the tympanic cavity. Optimally such a groove can be made between the 1-o'clock and 5-o'clock positions with preservation of the bony annulus (**Fig. 20.16a**). After placement of the cartilage disk, the anterior perichondrium flap can be pushed into the groove and into the tympanic cavity (**Fig. 20.16b**). After the replacement of the anterior annulus, the eardrum remnant covers the perichondrium (**Fig. 20.16c**). The cartilage disk is safely suspended on the bony annulus (**Fig. 20.16d**).

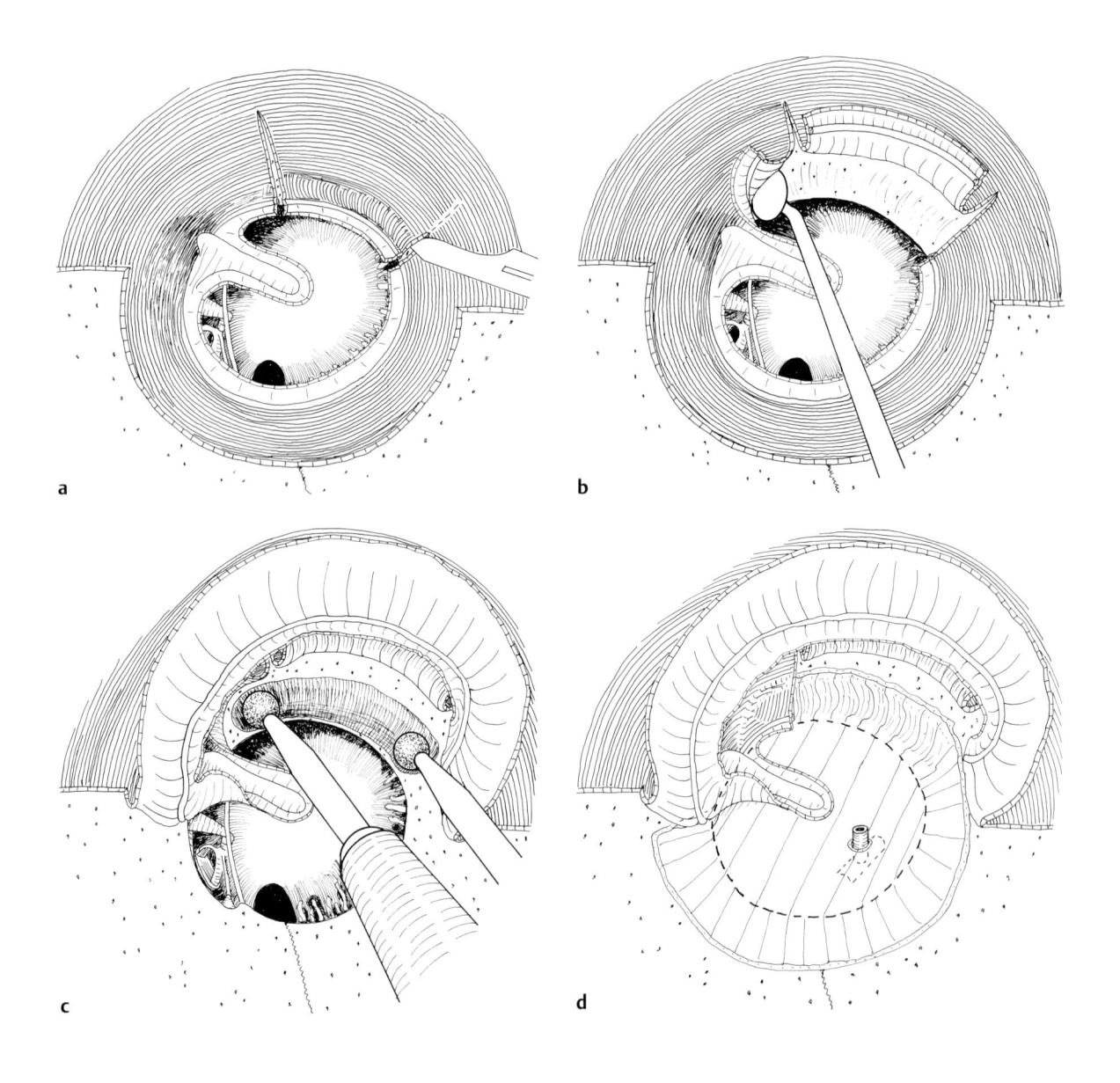

a

b

c

d

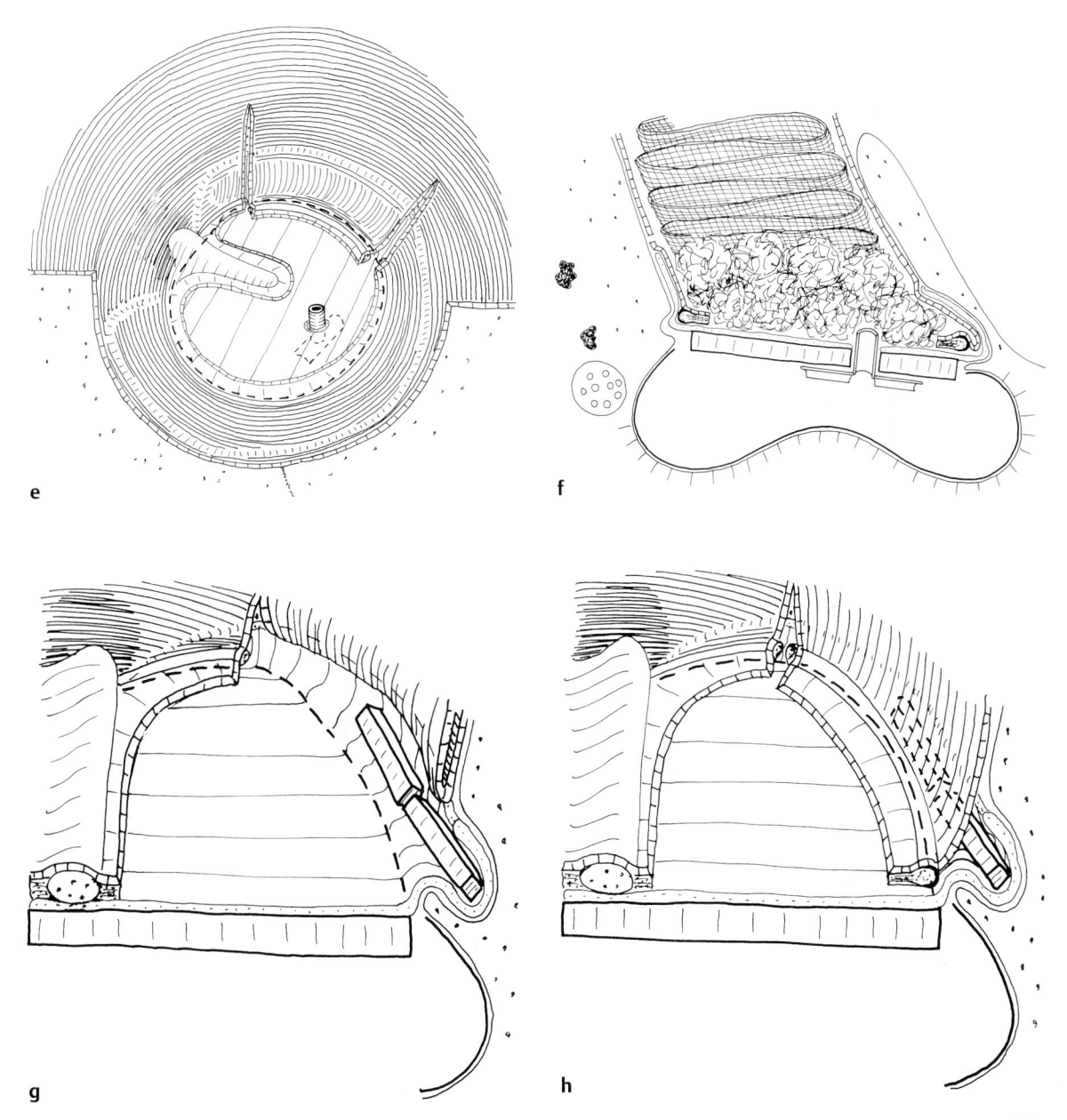

Fig. 20.15a–h Widening of the anterior sulcus and the ear canal with elevation of an anterior skin flap to accommodate the perichondrium flap of the cartilage shield T-tube graft in a case with total perforation and bone formation in the anterior tympanomeatal angle.

a Using a retroauricular approach, a posterior circumferential incision is made and the posterior canal skin is elevated. The edges of the total perforation are removed. Anteriorly, two radial skin incisions are made at the 2-o'clock and 5-o'clock positions, to include the eardrum remnant with mucosa and fibrous annulus. Some bony protrusion is visible in the anterior tympanomeatal angle.

b The anterior flap is elevated, exposing the bone in the anterior tympanomeatal angle, which will be removed. An anterosuperior flap is elevated using a round knife.

c The posterior tympanomeatal flap is elevated. The bone along the bony annulus is gradually removed starting anterosuperiorly with a diamond drill, resulting in a groove.

d The cartilage disk, together with the T-tube and the surrounding perichondrium is placed in the tympanic cavity at the level of the bony annulus and under the malleus handle. The anterior perichondrium flap covers the groove. Anterosuperiorly, a small flap is replaced over the perichondrium.

e The anterior tympanomeatal flap is replaced to cover the ear canal and the anterior perichondrium. Finally, the posterior tympanomeatal flap is replaced.

f Side view of the cartilage shield T-tube tympanoplasty with a groove in the anterior tympanomeatal angle to accommodate the placement of the anterior perichondrial flap. The groove is covered by the perichondrium and the skin of the ear canal. The ear canal is packed with Gelfoam balls and gauze moistened with hydrocortisone–oxytetracycline ointment.

g Placement of small cartilage palisades onto the anterior perichondrium flap to fixate the flap and to fill out the sulcus that has been created. A side view with some perspective of the anterior half of the reconstructed eardrum with cartilage shield T-tube graft. The cartilage palisade presses the perichondrium flap both anteriorly to the bone of the ear canal and posteriorly to the bony annulus.

h The skin flap and the eardrum remnant with the annulus are replaced without dehiscence of the new anterior sulcus.

Fixation of the Anterior Perichondrium Flap by Placing Small Cartilage Palisades into the Deep Anterior Sulcus

In the case of a deep new anterior sulcus, after placement of the anterior perichondrium flap (**Fig. 20.15f**), I recommend small cartilage palisades to be placed onto the perichondrium flap, thus fixating the flap and filling the empty place in the groove (**Fig. 20.15g**). After replacement of the epithelium there will be no dehiscence (**Fig. 20.15h**).

Any connection from the anterior sulcus to the tympanic cavity (**Fig. 20.16d**) can be closed similarly and the anterior perichondrium flap is further fixated by placing some small cartilage palisades into the anterior sulcus (**Fig. 20.16e, f**).

Application of Anterior Sulcus Methods in Other Cartilage Tympanoplasty Techniques

The procedures of contouring and widening of the anterior sulcus for safe placement of the anterior perichondrium flap (**Figs. 20.14a, b** and **20.15c, d**) as well as the placement of the anterior perichondrium flap into the tympanic cavity (**Fig. 20.16a–f**) have been illustrated in detail. These methods enhance the safer placement of the anterior perichondrium flap. They can also be applied in other tympanoplasty methods with cartilage–perichondrium island flaps, such as the total pars tensa island graft (Chapter 17), the annular cartilage–perichondrium graft (Chapter 18), and the crown cork cartilage–perichondrium graft (Chapter 19), as well as in the classic tympanoplasty with fascia or perichondrium alone. The most difficult and delicate procedures are the elevation of the anterior eardrum remnants and the firm placement of the anterior perichondrium flap. Surgical failures arise most often from insufficient anterior fixation of the cartilage disk. By pulling the anterior perichondrium flap through the anterior sulcus into the tympanic cavity, the disk is firmly fixated.

Notched Cartilage Disk

A notched cartilage disk is applied in any situation where the malleus disturbs a satisfactory placement of the round cartilage disk, especially when the distal half of the malleus handle is missing, or in case of a grossly retracted malleus handle with adhesions to the promontory. The notch may be of various lengths depending on the particular need.

In the case of a retracted malleus (**Fig. 20.17a**), the short process is dominant and the notch should be wide superiorly. First the edges of the total perforation are removed and cleaned of epithelium. The adhesions between the umbo and the promontory are also removed and the malleus is slightly elevated. The mucosa under the umbo is removed and the denuded bone is covered with a small piece of thin Silastic. A malleus flap is elevated (**Fig. 20.17b**). A tympanomeatal flap with the eardrum remnants and the fibrous annulus is elevated (**Fig. 20.17c**). The notched cartilage shield T-tube graft with the surrounding perichondrium is placed into the tympanic cavity. The perichondrium of the notch covers the superior half of the malleus handle and the short process of the malleus (**Fig. 20.17d**). The surrounding perichondrium is placed onto the denuded bone of the ear canal (**Fig. 20.17e**). The tympanomeatal flap and malleus flap are replaced (**Fig. 20.17f**).

Cartilage Shield T-Tube Tympanoplasty Type 2 with PORP

In Duckert's first series of 294 ears with cartilage shield T-tube tympanoplasty, 24% of ears had an intact ossicular

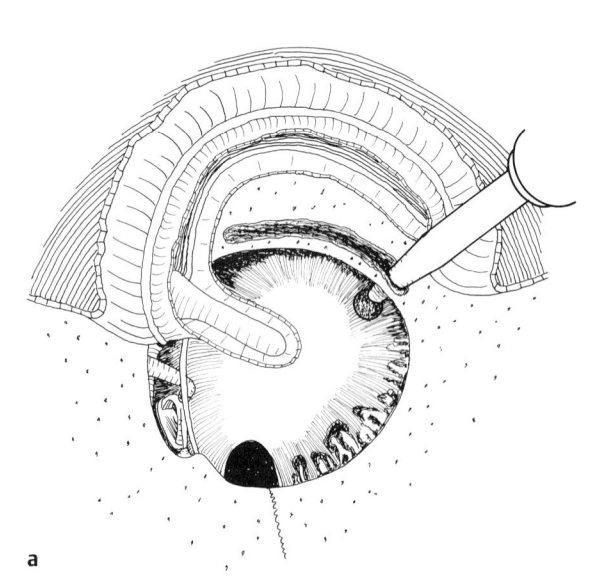

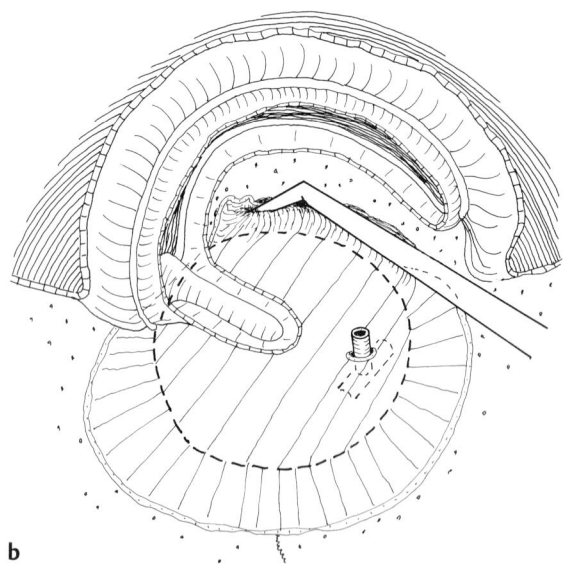

a

b

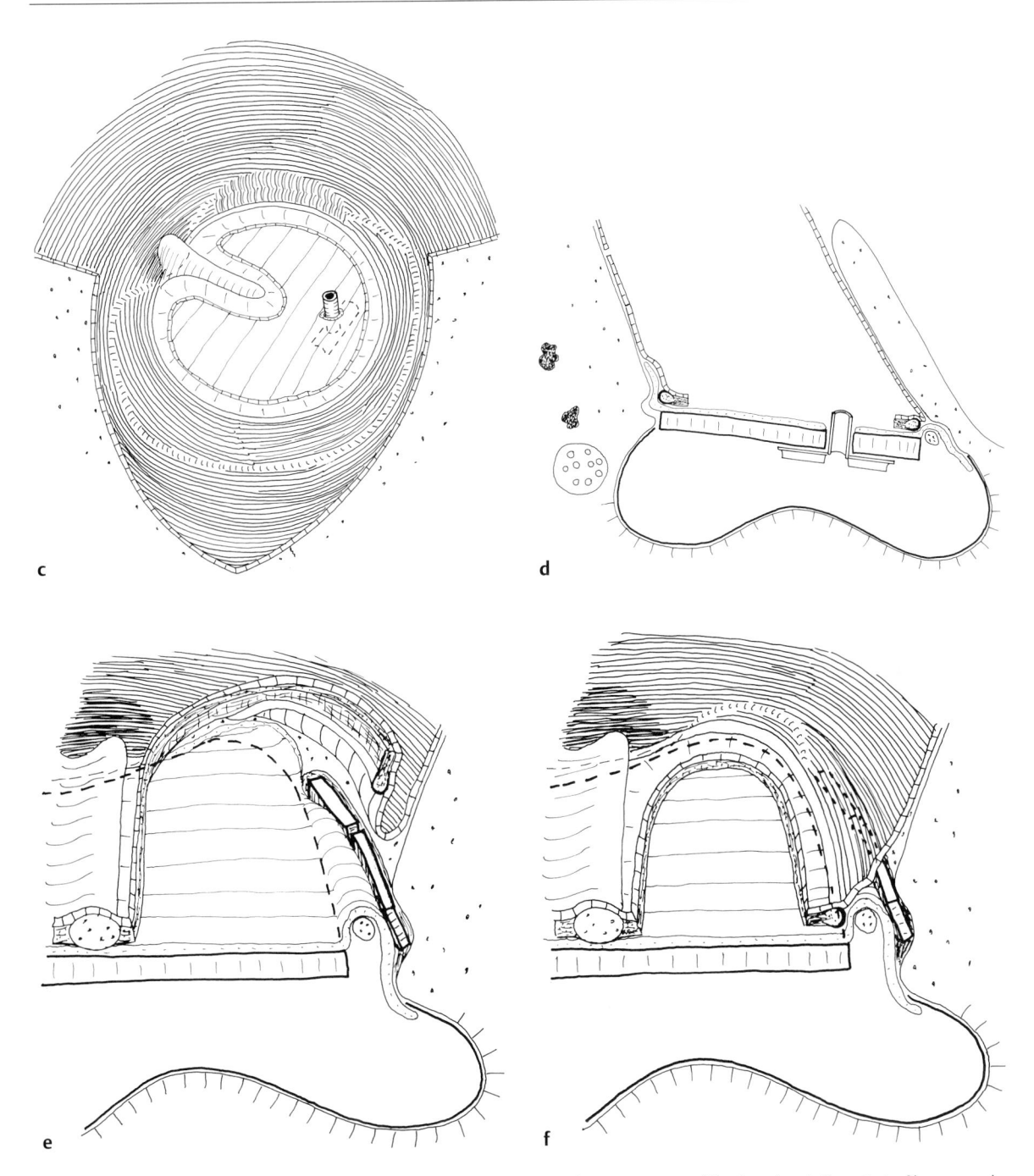

Fig. 20.16a–f Placement of the anterior perichondrium flap into the tympanic cavity in a cartilage shield T-tube tympanoplasty, in a case with total perforation and an intact ossicular chain.

a Using a retroauricular approach, the epithelium from the edges of the perforation is removed. The posterior tympanomeatal flap is elevated and the epithelial remnant with the anterior fibrous annulus is elevated, exposing the bony annulus. Using diamond drills of 3–4 mm diameter, a deep groove is drilled anterior to the bony annulus. With careful drilling toward the tympanic cavity, the head of the drill penetrates the bone of the tympanic cavity. Further drilling is easier and the groove can be extended to the 5-o'clock position.

b The cartilage shield T-tube graft is placed under the malleus handle in the tympanic cavity at the level of the bony annulus and the anterior graft is pushed into the tympanic cavity by using a pick or a hook. The posterior and inferior segments of the flap are placed onto the bony ear canal.

c The tympanomeatal flap is replaced. The anterior fibrous annulus and eardrum remnant are pulled back to cover the perichondrium.

d Side view of placement of the anterior perichondrium flap into the tympanic cavity. The flap is suspending the cartilage shield T-tube graft. It lies onto the anterior bony annulus and into the anterior wall of the tympanic cavity. Posteriorly, the perichondrium flap is placed onto the ear canal wall.

e Side view of placement of small cartilage palisades into the drilled opening connecting the anterior sulcus and the tympanic cavity in a cartilage shield T-tube tympanoplasty. The thin palisade is placed between the anterior perichondrium flap and the ear canal bone. The palisades fix the flap and close the drilled opening into the tympanic cavity.

f The ear canal skin and the eardrum remnants with the fibrous annulus are replaced.

20 Cartilage Shield T-Tube Tympanoplasty

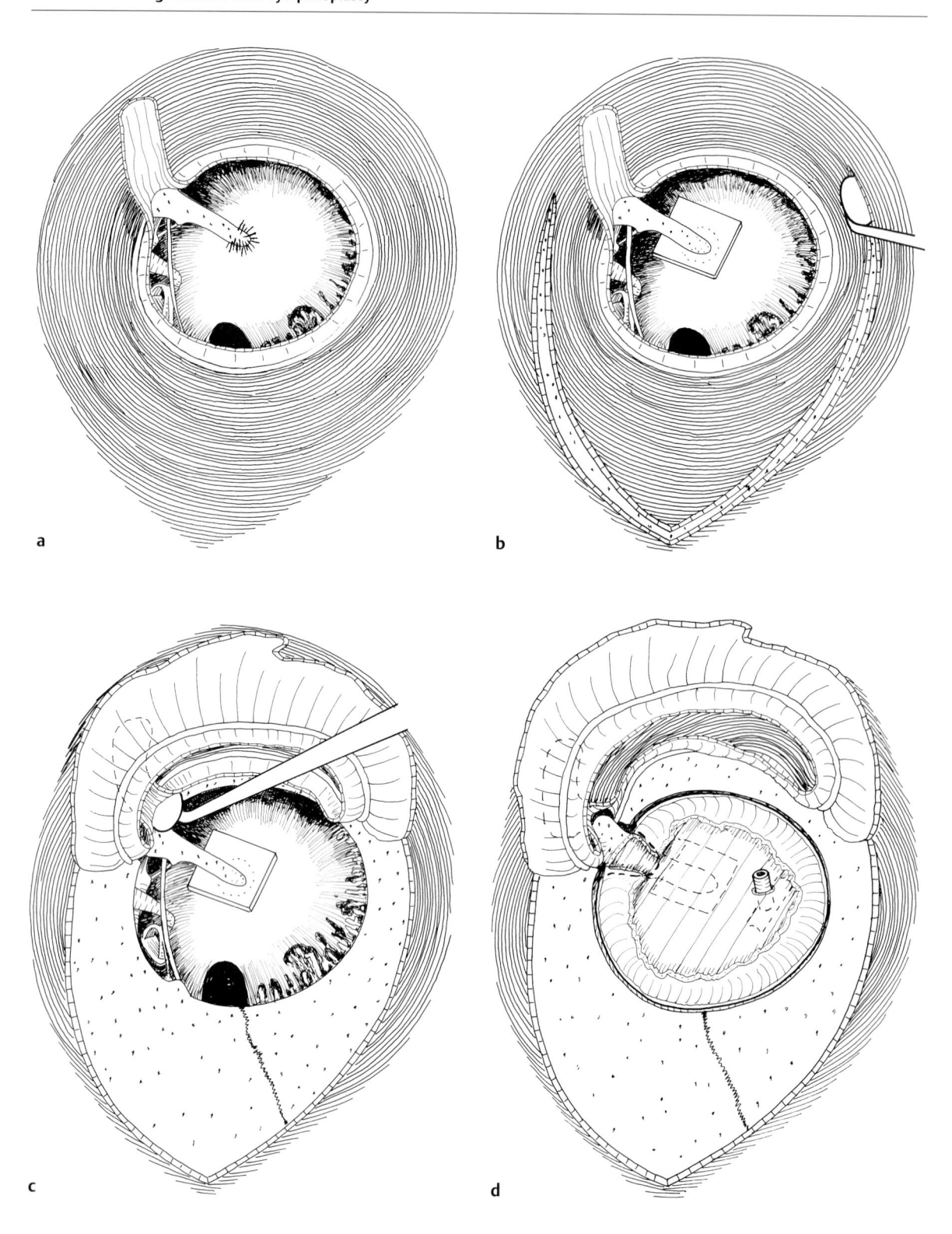

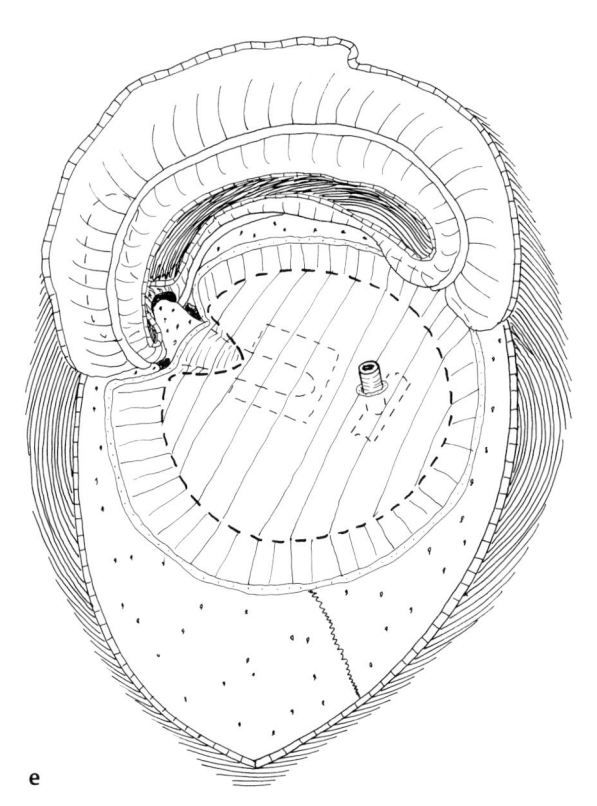

Fig. 20.17a–f Cartilage shielded T-tube graft in a case with chronic poor tubal function, total perforation with a retracted and adherent malleus handle, but otherwise intact ossicular chain.

a The malleus handle is cleaned, the malleus flap elevated, and the adhesions to the malleus handle are to be removed.
b The mucosa of the promontory with adhesions under the malleus handle is removed and the small mucosal defect is covered with Silastic. A large circumferential incision of the ear canal skin is made.
c A large tympanomeatal flap with the eardrum remnant and the fibrous annulus is elevated. In particular, the epithelium is removed from the short process of the malleus.
d The notched cartilage disk with the T-tube and the surrounding perichondrium is placed into the tympanic cavity at the level of the bony annulus. The upper part of the notched cartilage disk is placed onto the malleus handle.
e The perichondrium flap is folded out onto the denuded ear canal bone and under the anterior fibrous annulus.
f The tympanomeatal flap with the eardrum remnants is replaced and also the malleus flap.

chain. In these ears, a tympanoplasty type 1 was performed. In 51% the long process of the incus was resorbed but the stapes was intact. In these cases a tympanoplasty type 2 was performed with interposition of a PORP prosthesis. In 25% of ears the stapes was resorbed and a tympanoplasty type 3 with a columella was performed. Only allografts were used in both tympanoplasty type 2 and type 3 and over 90% were of a glass-ionomer cement-based material (Duckert et al. 1995). This material has today more or less been abandoned and replaced by prostheses made of titanium.

In tympanoplasty type 2, a short titanium PORP prosthesis of Dresden type is placed onto the stapes head (**Fig. 20.18a**). It is important to measure the distance from the head of the stapes to the undersurface of the cartilage disk.

The cartilage shield T-tube graft is placed under the malleus (**Fig. 20.18b**) If the prosthesis is too long, the umbo can be elevated or the posterior part of the cartilage disk can be slightly elevated (**Fig. 20.18c, d**).

Cartilage Shield T-tube Tympanoplasty Type 3 with TORP

In the case of a missing stapes, a titanium columella with a large head is placed between the footplate and the cartilage graft (**Fig. 20.19a–c**). In the side view, the titanium columella and mobile cartilage disk appear stable (**Fig. 20.19d**).

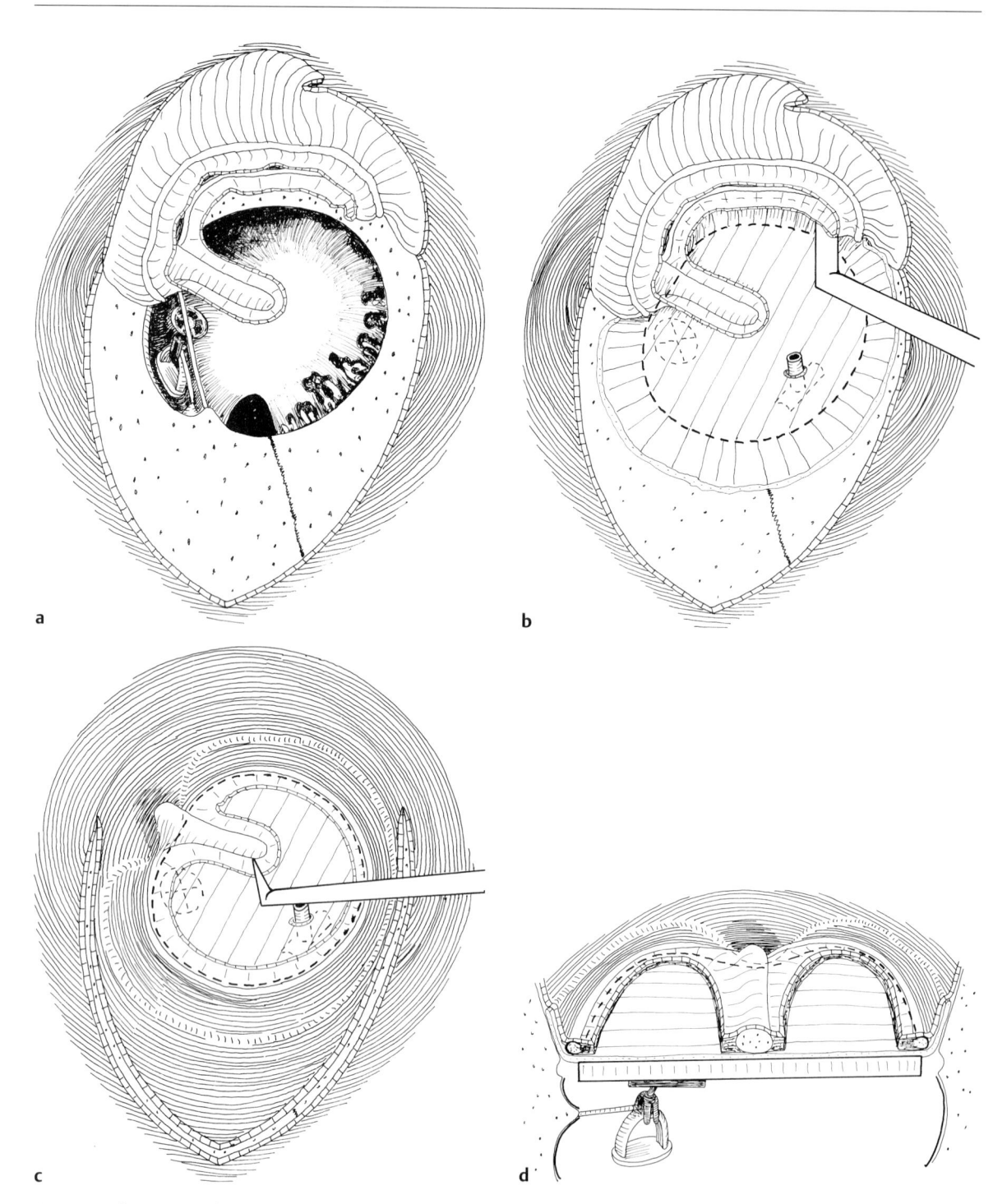

Fig. 20.18a–d Tympanoplasty type 2 with a titanium PORP Kurz prosthesis of Dresden type placed onto the intact stapes before the placement of the cartilage shield T-tube graft.

a The edges of the total perforation are removed and the tympanomeatal flap and the anterior fibrous annulus and the eardrum remnant are elevated, exposing the anterior bony annulus. The head of the stapes is scarified and the distance from the head to the undersurface of the cartilage graft is measured. The relatively short prosthesis is placed onto the stapes head.

b The cartilage shield T-tube graft is placed in the tympanic cavity, under the malleus handle and onto the head of the stapes. The anterior perichondrium flap is placed onto the denuded bone or pushed up under the fibrous annulus and eardrum remnant.

c In the case of too long a PORP prosthesis, the malleus handle can be gently prized out to accommodate the prostheses. The tympanomeatal flaps are replaced.

d Side view of tympanoplasty type 2 with interposition of a titanium prosthesis between the stapes and the cartilage shield T-tube graft. The T-tube is positioned in the lower part of the graft, suspended by the perichondrium flaps.

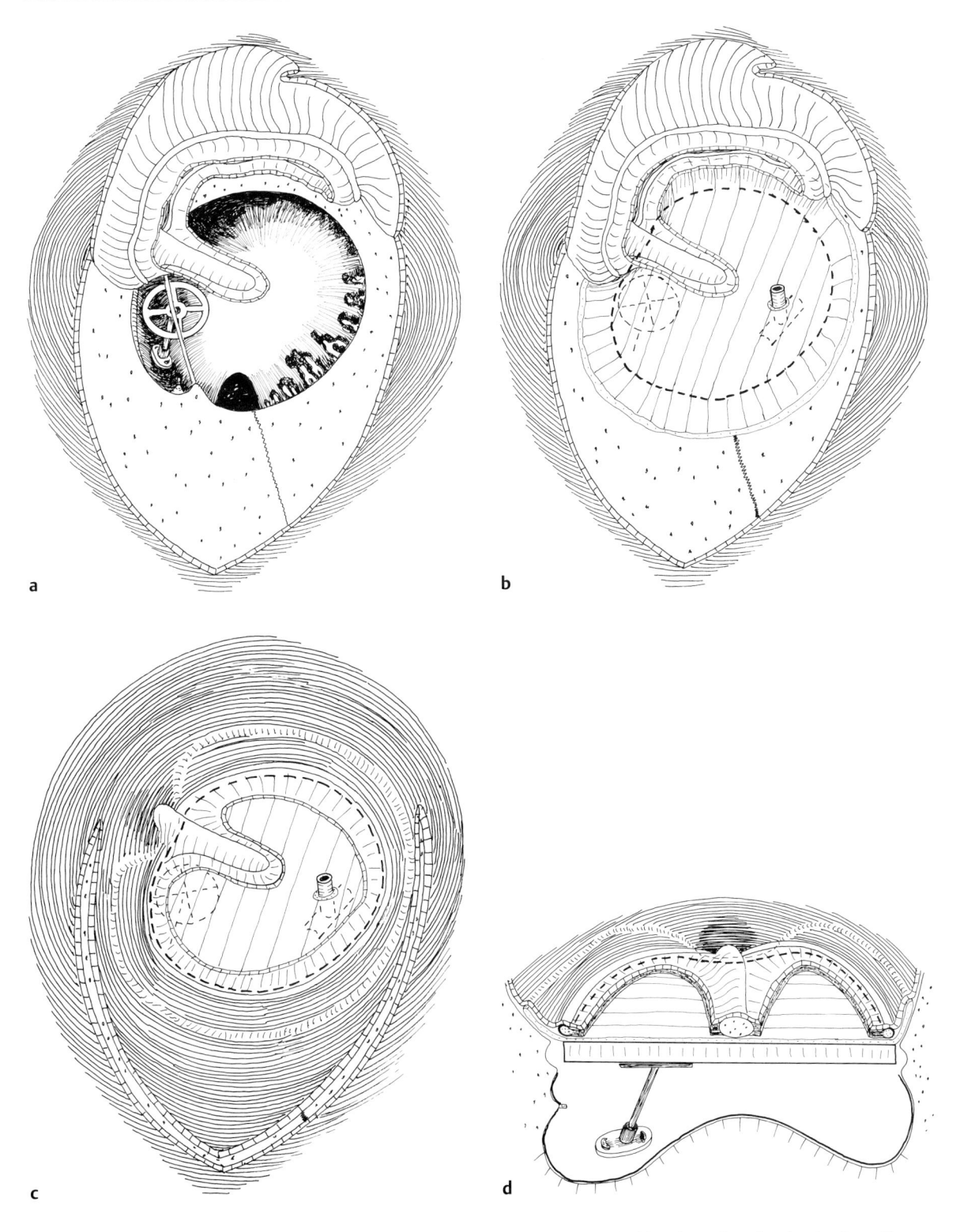

Fig. 20.19a–d Tympanoplasty type 3 with a titanium TORP columella placed onto the footplate and under the cartilage shield T-tube graft.

a The edges of the total perforation are removed, and the posterior tympanomeatal flap and the anterior fibrous annulus with the eardrum remnant are elevated. After measurement of the length of the prosthesis, it is placed onto the center of the footplate. The prosthesis may be supported with Gelfoam balls.

b The cartilage shield T-tube graft is placed under the malleus handle and onto the head of the prosthesis. It is suspended by the perichondrium placed onto the denuded bone.

c The tympanomeatal flaps are replaced.

d Side view with some perspective of tympanoplasty type 3 with a titanium columella placed between the footplate and the undersurface of the cartilage shield T-tube graft. The cartilage disk is suspended by the perichondrium flap.

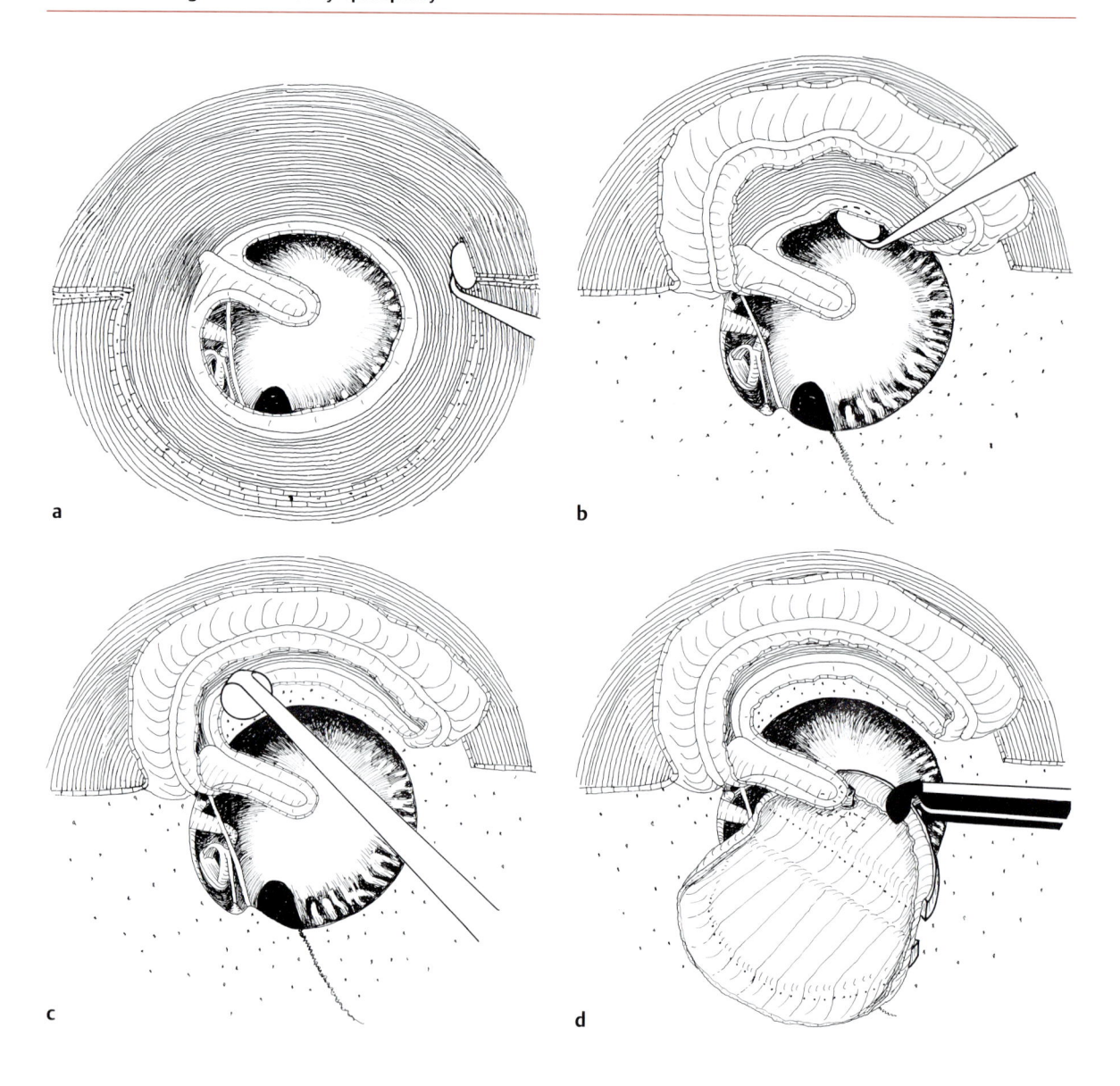

The Dornhoffer Technique

Danner and Dornhoffer (2001) use the retroauricular approach (**Fig. 20.20a**) with the removal of the epithelium from the edges of the perforation and elevation of a large posterior tympanomeatal flap, and continuing with the elevation of the inferior and the anterior parts of the eardrum remnants and the fibrous annulus (**Fig. 20.20b, c**). After exposure of the anterior bony annulus and medial end of the ear canal, the Dornhoffer cartilage shield T-tube graft is placed under the malleus into the tympanic cavity (**Fig. 20.20d**). First, the anterior half of the graft with the T-tube is angled under the manubrium with a small alligator forceps. Finally, the graft is adapted to the anterior and posterior bony annulus as well as to the malleus handle (**Fig. 20.20e**). Because the Dornhoffer graft consists of two semicircular cartilage pieces connected with perichondrium, it is relatively easily moved under the malleus handle and adapted to the bony annulus, to be suspended by the perichondrium flap. It is important to push the anterior perichondrium flap under the ear canal skin, and under the fibrous annulus (**Fig. 20.20f**). With a cup forceps, the anterior eardrum remnant is gently pulled onto the perichondrium of the cartilage (**Fig. 20.20g**), allowing rapid epithelialization of the anterior part of the eardrum.

The T-tube is usually placed in the anterior disk, either superiorly (**Fig. 20.20g, h**) or inferiorly.

If the malleus is absent, the graft–tube complex is slid directly into its final position.

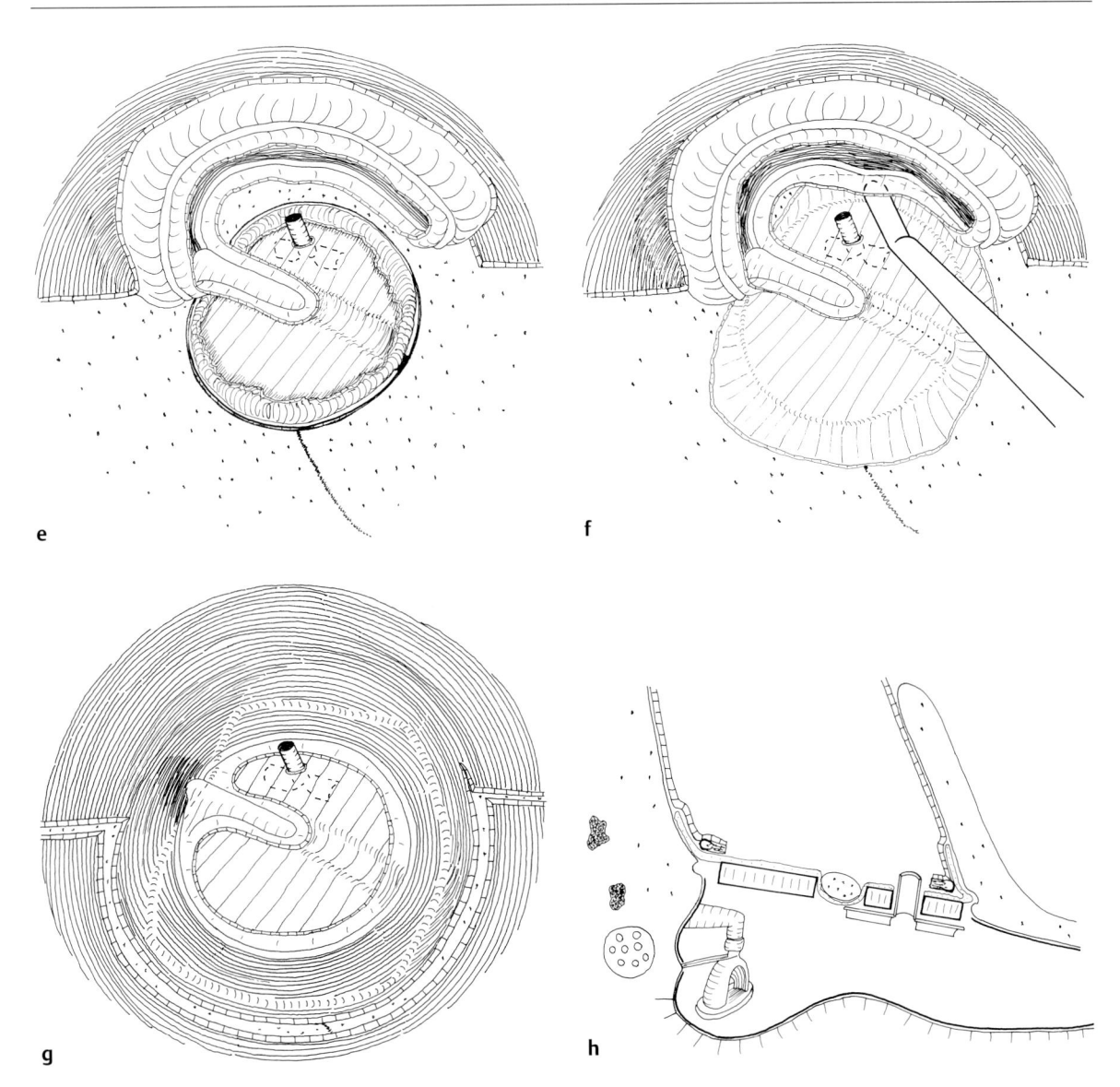

Fig. 20.20a–h The Dornhoffer technique of cartilage shield T-tube tympanoplasty in a case with total perforation and intact ossicular chain.

- **a** Using the retroauricular approach, a circumferential incision is performed allowing the elevation of a large tympanomeatal flap. The epithelium from the edges of the perforation is removed.
- **b** A large posterior and inferior tympanomeatal skin flap together with the fibrous annulus and the eardrum remnants are elevated, allowing a good view of the anterior annulus and ear canal wall.
- **c** Using a round knife, the anterior annulus with the eardrum remnant and the attached ear canal skin are elevated, thus exposing the anterior bony annulus and the ear canal bone and allowing sufficient space to place the anterior perichondrium flap.
- **d** The anterior cartilage of the Dornhoffer T-tube complex is positioned under the malleus handle. Half of the posterior cartilage disk is still in the ear canal.
- **e** The entire Dornhoffer T-tube cartilage shield graft is placed in the tympanic cavity.
- **f** The perichondrium is pushed anteriorly under the ear canal skin and under the fibrous annulus. Inferiorly and posteriorly, the perichondrium is folded out onto the denuded bone.
- **g** The tympanomeatal flap with the fibrous annulus and eardrum remnants is replaced. The posterior ear canal flap is replaced next.
- **h** Side view of the Dornhoffer method of cartilage shield T-tube tympanoplasty in a case with total perforation and intact ossicular chain. The Dornhoffer graft with the two semicircular cartilage disks connected by perichondrium is placed in the tympanic cavity at the level of the malleus handle. A T-tube is inserted through a hole in the anterior disk at the level of the Eustachian tube with the flanges turned in the superoinferior direction. The graft is suspended by the perichondrium flap placed onto the denuded bone of the medial part of the ear canal.

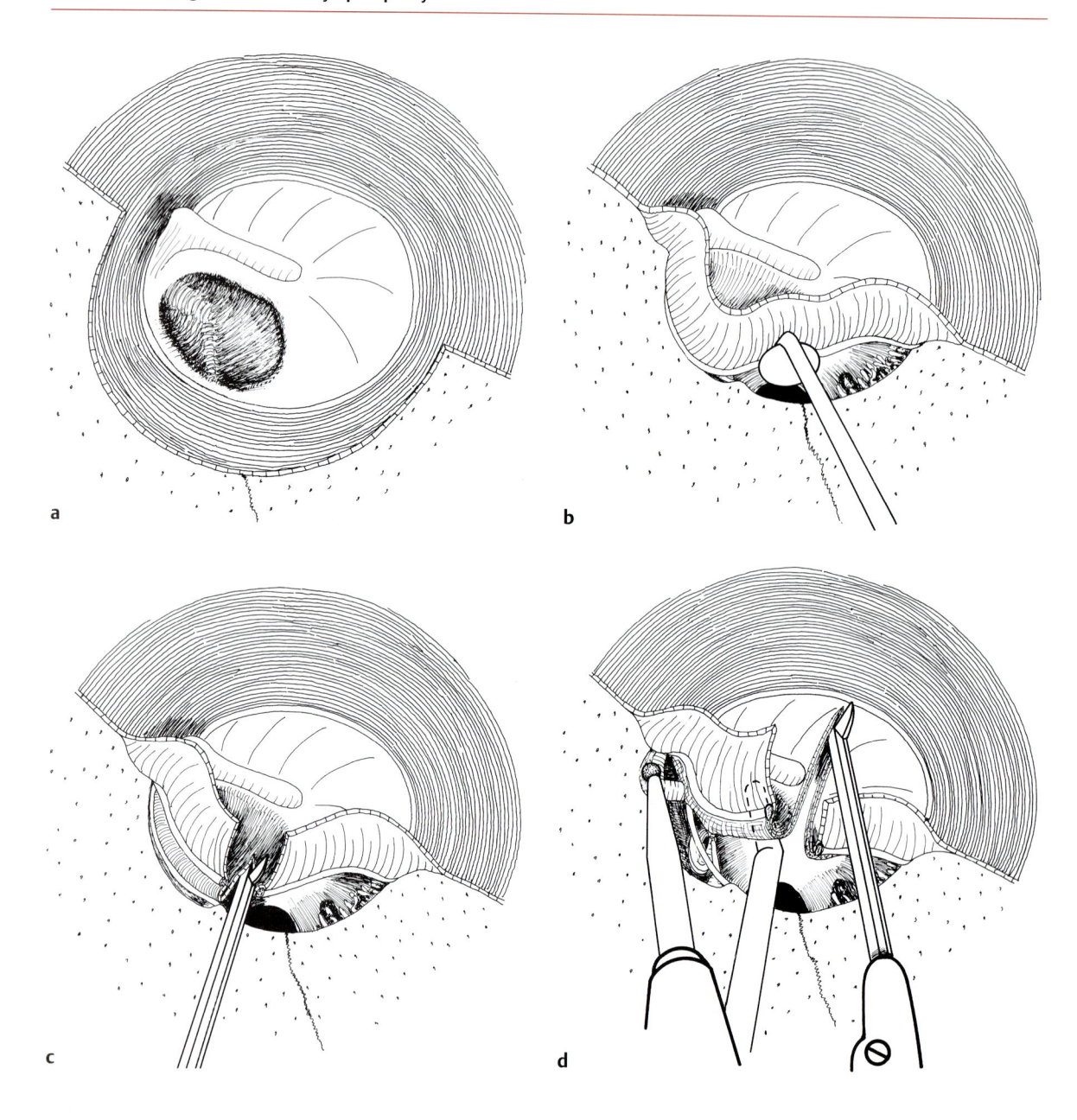

Application of the Elsheikh Graft

Via a retroauricular approach, Elsheikh et al. (2006) applied a U-shaped perichondrium–cartilage graft in grade 2 and grade 3 atelectasis. Because they did not describe their own tympanoplasty procedure, I will here illustrate methods that may be applied in these conditions to place the U-shaped cartilage–perichondrium ventilating tube graft. The principle of the methods is to preserve as much of the epithelium as possible without leaving hidden residual epithelium.

Tympanoplasty with U-Graft in Grade 2 Atelectasis

In the grade 2 tympanoplasty of Sade (1979), a posterosuperior atrophy and retraction is fixed to the incudostapedial joint with or without resorption of the lenticular process or the stapes head. The anterior half of the eardrum is not atrophic and is not retracted (**Fig. 20.21a**) and the anterior half of the tympanic cavity is ventilated. Because of infection within the retraction, a sinus cholesteatoma involving the tympanic sinuses may appear despite the ventilation of the anterior part of the tympanic cavity. After removal of the retraction, a posterosuperior perforation has to be closed in such a way that a recurrent retraction does not occur.

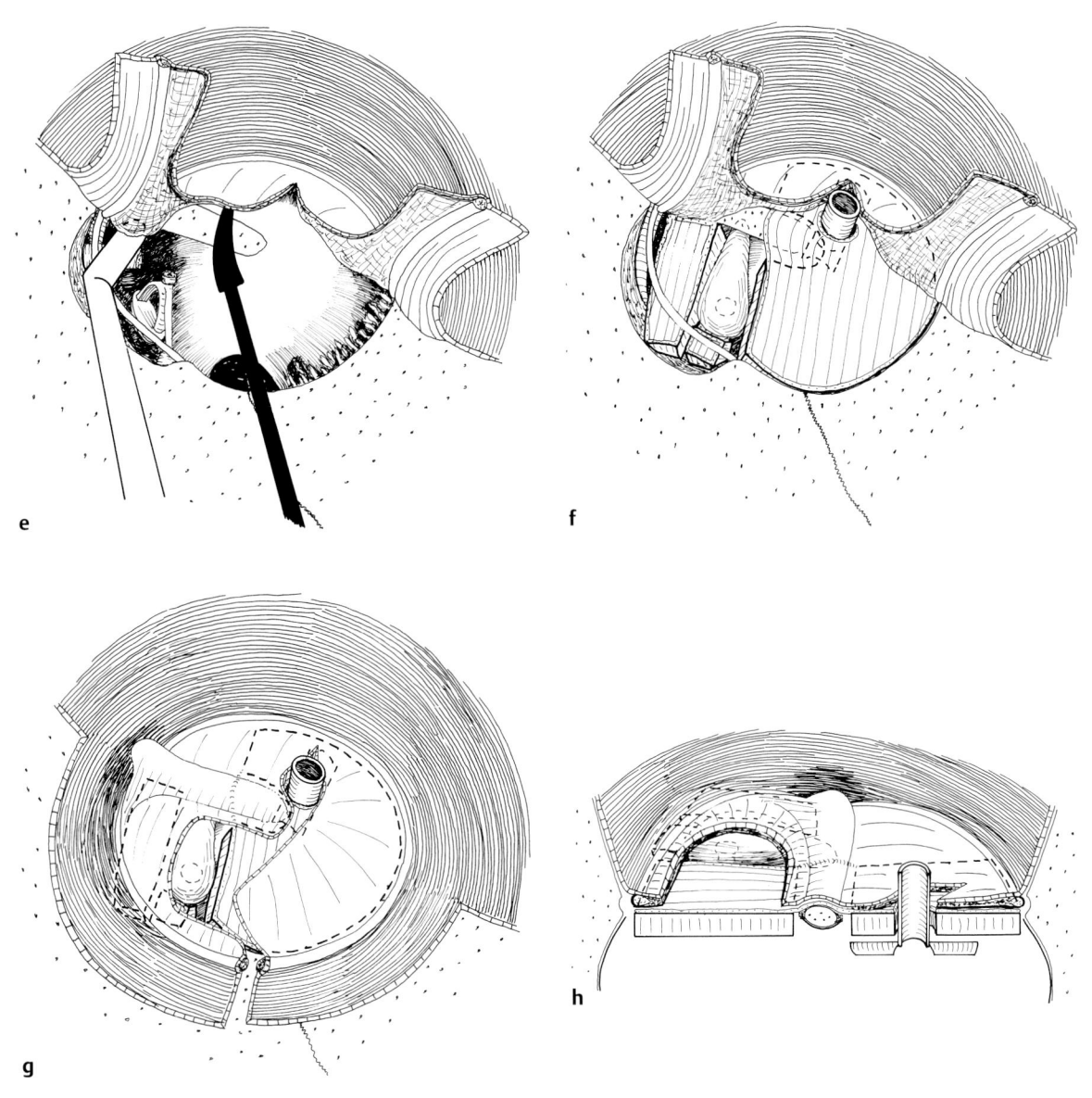

Fig. 20.21a–h The retroauricular approach in a posterosuperior retraction with resorption of the lenticular process.

a The retracted and atrophic eardrum is fixed to the long process of the incus and to the stapes, but the anterior part of the tympanic cavity is ventilated

b The tympanomeatal flap is partly elevated and the tympanic cavity is entered inferiorly to the retraction. Using the round knife, the fibrous annulus is further elevated in superior direction, localizing the bottom of the retraction and pushing it as an intact sac forward and upward.

c The annulus is further elevated and the inferior part of the retraction is exposed and elevated. To create more space for the U-graft with the T-tube, the tympanomeatal flap with the fibrous annulus and the inferior part of the retraction membrane is cut.

d The incision is carried forward to the anterior part of the eardrum. Posterosuperiorly, the retraction extends under the bony annulus, which is gradually removed by drilling. The inferior and anterior parts of the retraction are elevated and gradually removed. The stapes and the long process of the incus are thus cleaned.

e The posterosuperior fibrous annulus is maximally elevated and the posterior and superior parts of the retraction are also elevated from the defective long process of the incus and the stapes head. Using a sickle knife, the tympanic membrane is separated from the malleus handle.

f The incus without the lenticular process is removed and cleaned of epithelium, shaped by making a groove for the stapes head, and next placed onto the stapes head. The short process is placed under the malleus handle. The U-shaped cartilage–perichondrium tube graft is placed under the anterior tympanic membrane with the perichondrium section over the malleus handle. Two pieces of cartilage covered with perichondrium have been placed superior to the interposed incus.

g The anterior part of the eardrum and the remnants of the posterior part of the eardrum with the attached remnants of the retraction are replaced.

h Side view with some perspective of a tympanoplasty type 2 and placement of a U-shaped cartilage–perichondrium graft with a ventilating tube, after removal of a posterosuperior retraction. The graft is not suspended by the perichondrium flap. It is partly suspended by the perichondrium covering the malleus handle.

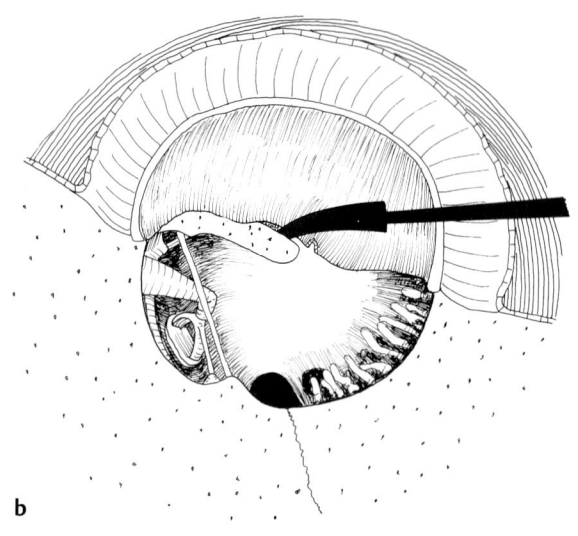

Fig. 20.22a–c

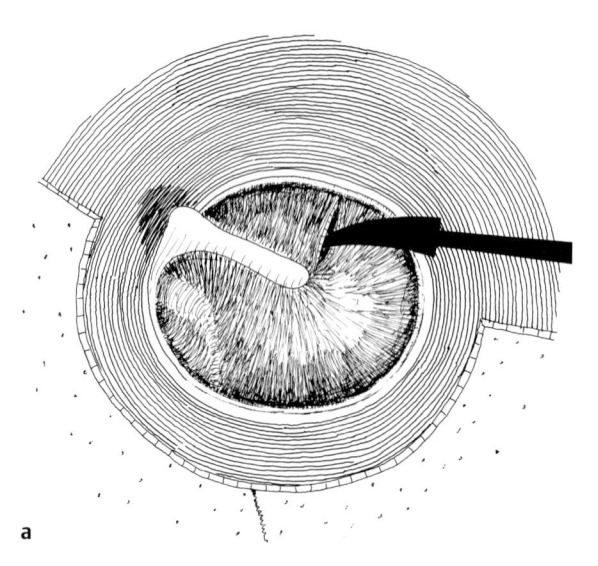

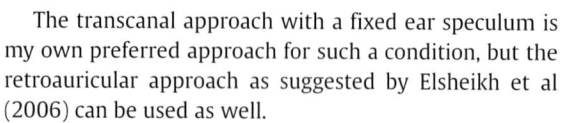

The transcanal approach with a fixed ear speculum is my own preferred approach for such a condition, but the retroauricular approach as suggested by Elsheikh et al (2006) can be used as well.

The tympanomeatal flap is partly elevated and the tympanic cavity is entered inferior to the retraction (**Fig. 20.21b**). A horizontal incision of the elevated skin flap, the fibrous annulus, and the atrophic eardrum is made at the 8-o'clock position (**Fig. 20.21c**), allowing elevation of the inferior part of the eardrum (**Fig. 20.21 d**) and the superior part of the eardrum together with the retraction, which is partly removed. After total exposure of the posterosuperior part of the tympanic cavity and the removal of the bone, the entire retraction is exposed, elevated, and removed (**Fig. 20.21e**). The incus with the defective long process is removed as well. To create space for the U-graft, the eardrum is separated from the malleus handle and further elevated. The incus is shaped and a groove for the head of the stapes is drilled. The incus body is placed onto the head of the stapes and the short process is placed under the malleus handle (**Fig. 20.21 f**). The U-graft with the ventilating tube is placed into the tympanic cavity at the level of the bony annulus. The notch of the cartilage is adapted to the inferior part of the malleus, which is thus covered by the perichondrium. Superior to the U-graft, a small piece of the cartilage is placed to prevent a future retraction. Another piece of cartilage is placed superior to the interposed incus. The eardrum is replaced, covering most of the U-graft (**Fig. 20.21 g, h**).

Tympanoplasty with U-Graft in Atelectasis of Grade 3

The entire pars tensa is atrophic and retracted but it is not adherent to the promontory (**Fig. 20.22a**). The malleus handle may be retracted. Posterosuperiorly the changes are the same as in atelectasis grade 2. Using a retroauricular approach, a perforation is created on the eardrum for the site of the T-tube, and then a tympanomeatal flap is elevated to include the retraction around the intact incudostapedial joint and the malleus handle, which is separated from the eardrum (**Fig. 20.22b, c**). The U-graft with the T-tube and a large notch for the malleus handle is gradually placed into the tympanic cavity (**Fig. 20.22 d, e**) and adapted to the malleus handle. Two small pieces of cartilage, with perichondrium, are placed superior to the U-graft, and the nearly intact eardrum is replaced (**Fig. 20.22 f, g**).

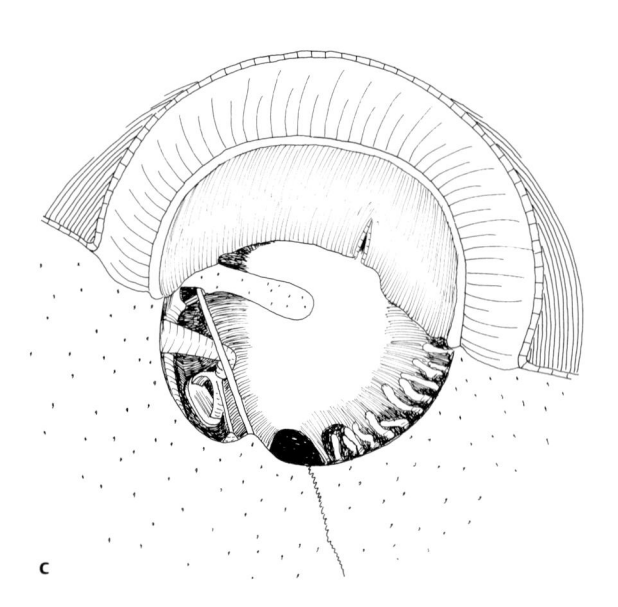

In a severe retraction of the entire pars tensa of a grade 3 atelectasis type with deep posterosuperior retraction and resorption of the stapes, a perforation is made in the region of the retraction (**Fig. 20.23a**) and then the tympanomeatal flap is elevated and separated from the malleus handle (**Fig. 20.23b, c**). If the stapes is totally resorbed, the remnant retraction is now removed and the footplate is cleaned. Finally, the anterior half of the eardrum is further

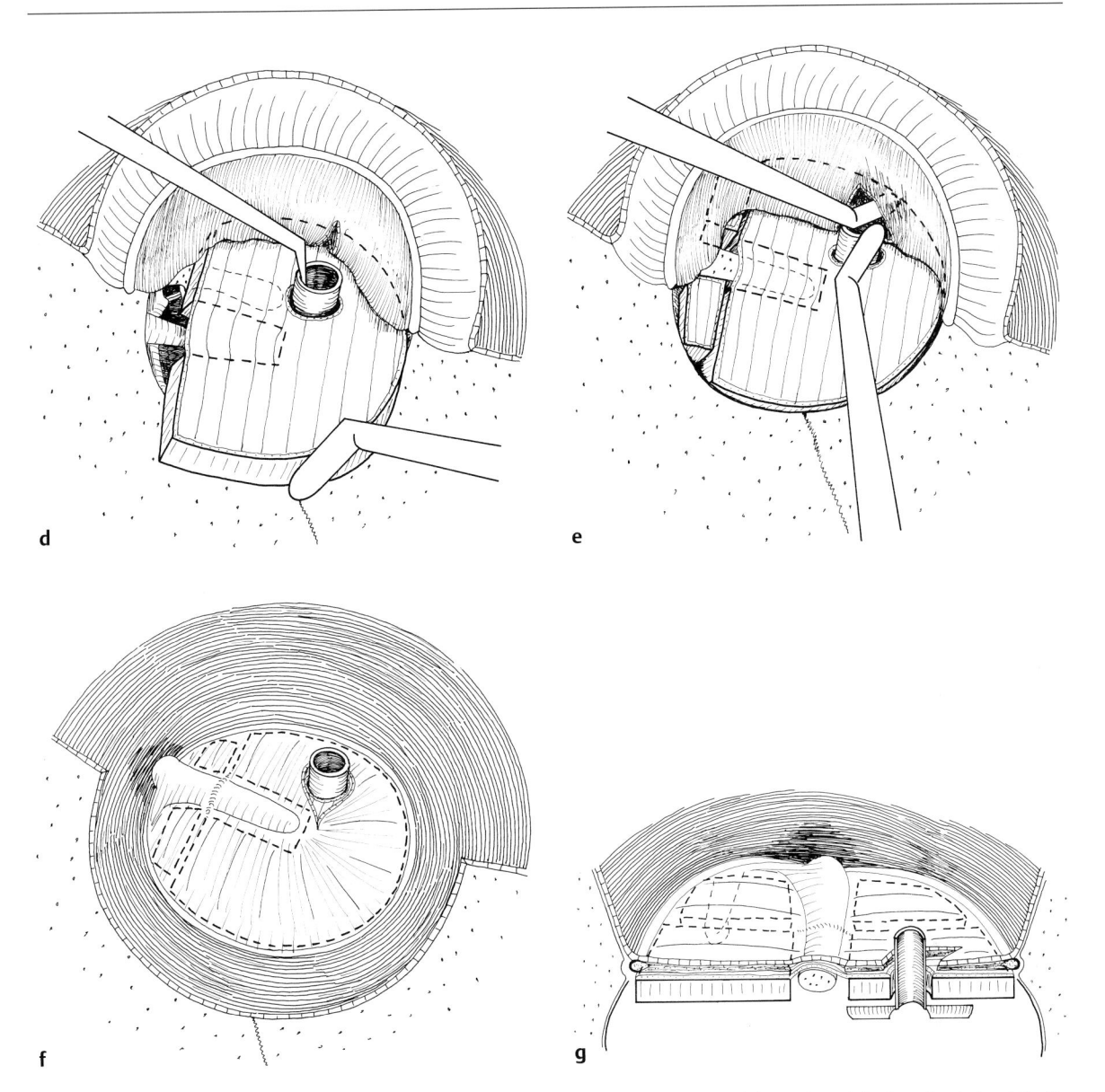

Fig. 20.22a–g Tympanoplasty using a U-shaped cartilage–perichondrium graft with T-tube in a case with atelectasis grade 3 with atrophy and retraction of the entire pars tensa and with attachment of the retraction to the incudostapedial joint, but without adhesion of the retraction to the promontory.

a The adhesion of the atrophic membrane to the long process of the incus is evident. A perforation of the anterior atrophic tympanic membrane at the level of the umbo is made to accommodate and allow placement of the ventilating tube.
b The tympanomeatal flap with the eardrum is elevated in a retroauricular approach. Using a sickle knife, the eardrum is separated from the malleus handle and the umbo.
c The eardrum is further elevated, to allow placement of the U-graft.
d The U-graft with the tube is pushed toward the anterior part of the tympanic cavity between the elevated atrophic eardrum and the lateral surface of the malleus handle.
e The anterior part of the eardrum is further elevated and the U-graft with the tube is pushed toward the anterior bony annulus. The tube is pushed through the tympanic perforation created. The graft is adapted to the malleus handle, which is covered with the perichondrium. The graft is touching the bony annulus and is suspended by the perichondrium covering the malleus handle. Two small pieces of cartilage with perichondrium are placed superior to the graft to prevent a new retraction.
f The atrophic tympanic membrane is replaced together with the ear canal flap.
g Side view with some perspective of tympanoplasty type 1 in a case of total retraction of the entire pars tensa in atelectasis grade 3 using a U-shaped cartilage graft with perichondrium. The T-tube is placed in the anterior part of the eardrum at the level of the umbo. The cartilage graft is placed in the tympanic cavity at the level of the bony annulus.

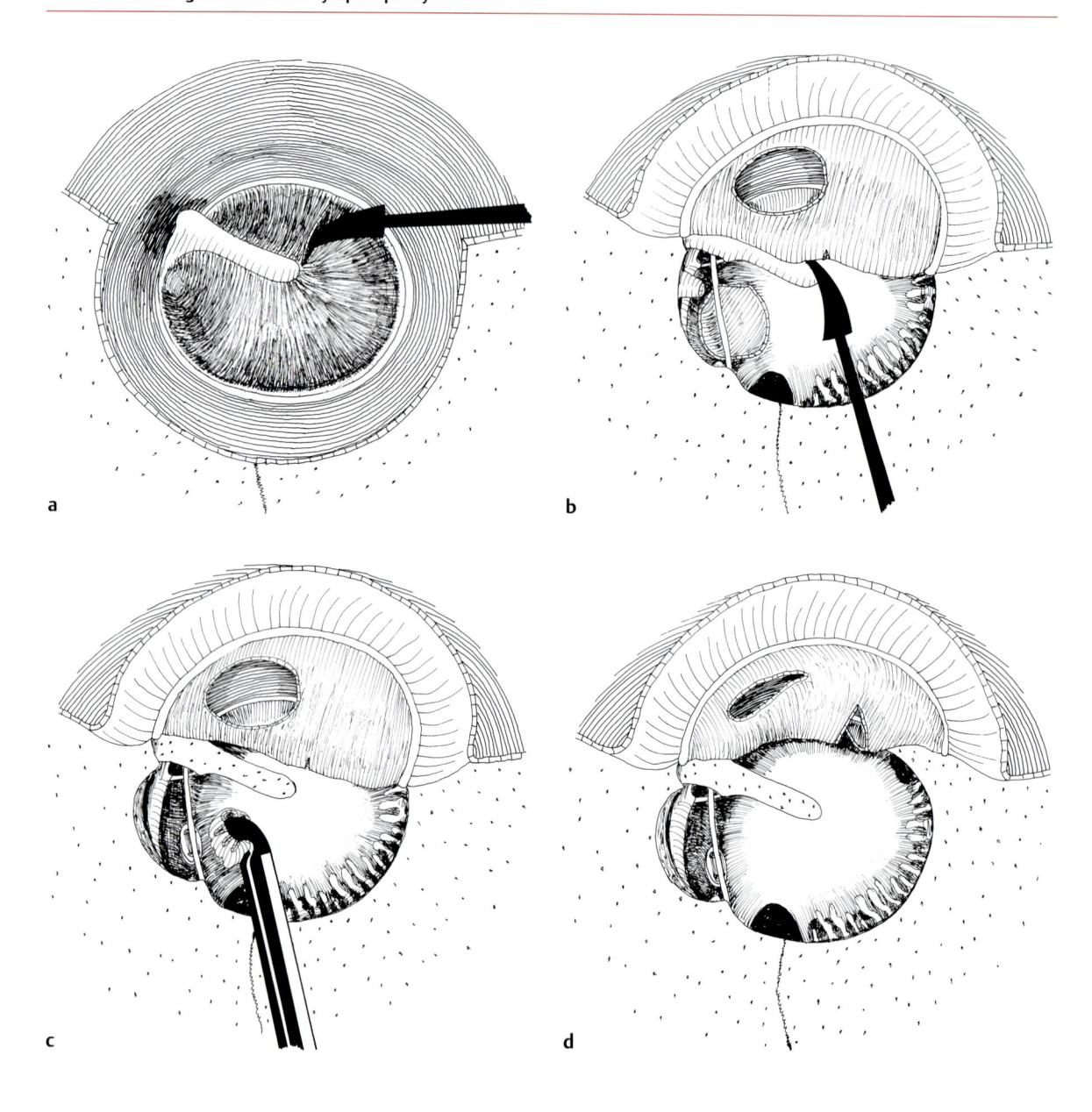

elevated, allowing placement of the U-graft with the T-tube (**Fig. 20.23d, e**). The U-shaped cartilage–perichondrium graft with the tube is suspended by the perichondrium covering the malleus handle. A titanium Kurz columella is placed onto the center of the footplate. The head of the prosthesis is covered with cartilage. The tympanomeatal flap is replaced (**Fig. 20.23f**).

Postoperative Care and Problems

It is expected and hoped that the T-tube stays in place in the cartilage graft and remains open without any further problems. This is not always the case, however, and patients will need long-term postoperative monitoring and care of the ear. The following events and complications may occur.

Accidental or Intentional Removal of the Tube

In the series of Danner and Dornhoffer (2001) of 25 patients, two patients had the tube inadvertently removed while cerumen was being cleaned. Another patient had an immune dysfunction with cartilage necrosis around the tube and subsequent extrusion of the tube. The perforation closes rapidly with a thin membrane, but the hole in the cartilage remains open, facilitating reinsertion of the T-tube in the same hole.

Duckert et al. (2003) have not found any extrusion of the tubes among 40 patients of their latest series.

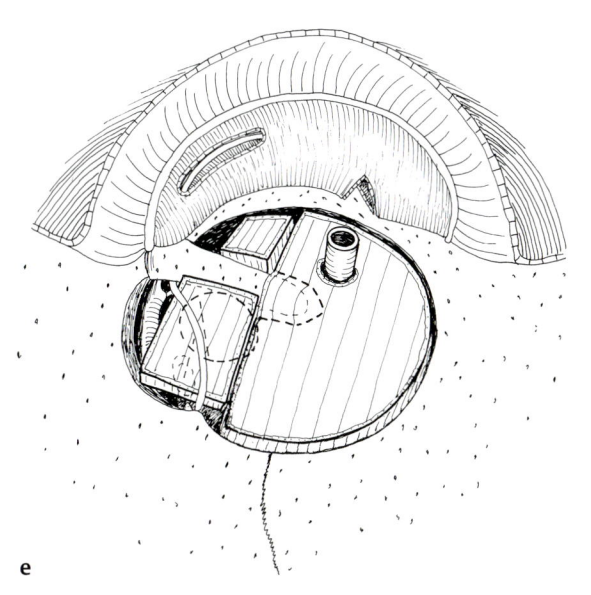

Fig. 20.23a–f Tympanoplasty type 3 with a titanium Kurz columella prosthesis of Tübingen type in an atelectasis grade 3 with atrophy and retraction of the entire pars tensa and resorption of the stapes.

a An incision in the anterior part of the thin and retracted eardrum is performed at the level of the umbo in a retroauricular approach.
b A tympanomeatal flap with most of the retracted and atrophic eardrum is elevated, leaving behind that in the region of the footplate. Using a sickle knife, the eardrum is separated from the malleus handle.
c Using various hooks, the adherent epithelial membrane from the posterosuperior part of the tympanic cavity is gradually removed and the footplate is cleaned of epithelium. The incus is removed as well.
d The anterior part of the atrophic and retracted eardrum is elevated.
e A U-shaped cartilage graft with T-tube is inserted into the tympanic cavity. The upper part of the U-graft is suspended by the perichondrium that covers the lower part of the malleus handle. A titanium columella of Tübingen type is placed onto the center of the footplate with its head touching the malleus handle anteriorly. The inferior edge of the head of the prosthesis is placed under the upper edge of the U-graft. Finally, a small rectangular piece of cartilage is placed onto the head of the titanium columella.
f The tympanomeatal flap is replaced. The atrophic eardrum covers most of the cartilage.

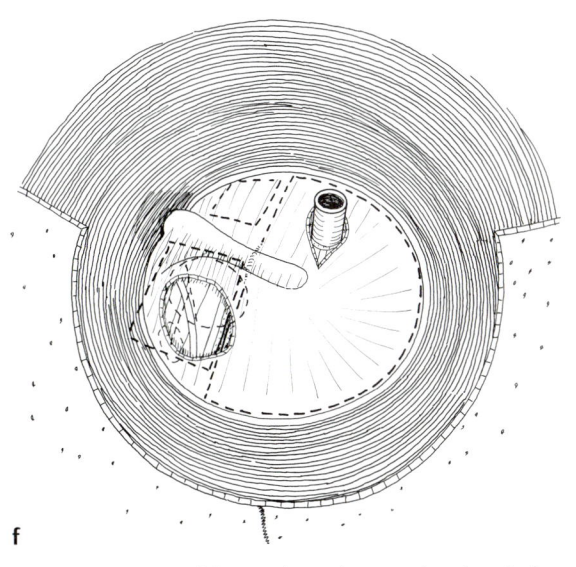

Reinsertion of the T-Tube in a Cartilage Shield Graft

The membrane covering the previous hole in the cartilage is elevated (**Fig. 20.24a**). The new T-tube is grasped with a small alligator forceps and pushed with the flanges through the previous hole into the tympanic cavity. The flanges will open out after the tube is pulled slightly outward (**Fig. 20.24b**). Because of the increased rigidity of the eardrum, secondary tube insertion is relatively easy without any risk of medialization of the eardrum during pushing of the tube through the hole.

Furthermore, the reinsertion is well tolerated because the previously implanted cartilage–perichondrium graft remains insensate after healing.

Malfunction of the T-Tube due to Plugged Cerumen

Closure of the T-tube by cerumen is the most common, but harmless, event and can easily be treated at regular follow-up for cleaning by placing a straight pick through the tube into tympanic cavity and by suction.

Formation of Granulation Tissue at the Tube–Perichondrium Interface

Granulation tissue forms in 10–20% of cases (Danner and Dornhoffer 2001), but it has responded well to steroid-containing drops and has never prompted tube removal in the series of Danner and Dornhoffer. Duckert et al. (2003) found obstruction of the tube by granulation tissue and hyperplastic mucosa, with or without infection, to be relatively common (6 adults and 3 children). Usually these patients were treated by tube reinsertion.

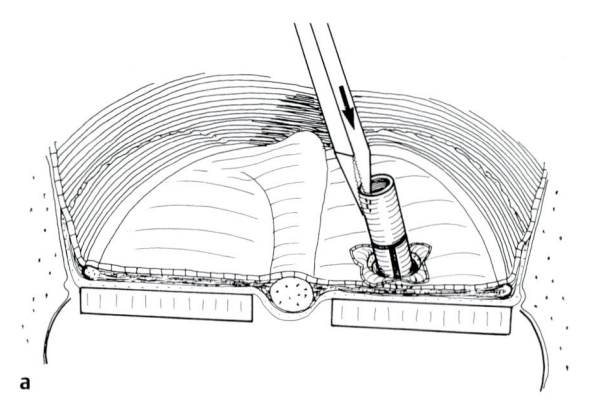

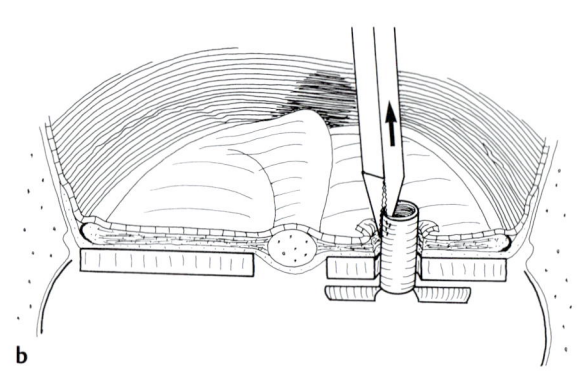

Fig. 20.24a, b Side view with some perspective of reinsertion of a new T-tube through the same hole in the cartilage graft.
a The thin epithelial membrane covering the previous hole in the cartilage is elevated. With an alligator forceps the tube and its flanges are pushed through the hole.
b The flanges of the tube are folded out and the tube is slightly pulled out.

Infection and Otorrhea

In Duckert's series of 28 adults and 12 children, 4 adults and 3 children had recurrent otorrhea. The drainage from infection did not respond well to systemic or local antibiotics. Temporary resolution was followed by recurrent drainage once therapy was stopped, but was eliminated once the colonized T-tube was removed.

Medialization of the Cartilage Graft

In the Danner and Dornhoffer series, medialization or retraction have not been a problem. Four patients have had an insignificant retraction around the periphery of the cartilage graft. They were followed for several years without progression and the retractions have been classified as nonsignificant.

Duckert et al. (2003) found recurrent atelectasis in 5 children.

Results of Cartilage Shield T-Tube Tympanoplasty

Hall's Series of Children

Hall (1990) presented a series of 19 children (24 ears) with long-term middle ear ventilation problems, applying his technique of T-tube with tragus cartilage–perichondrium graft. Median age at surgery was 8.6 years. At the time of evaluation the tubes had been in place for an average of 24.2 months and none of the tubes had extruded. Average hearing was 31 dB preoperatively and 9.2 dB postoperatively. Postoperative drainage appeared in 2 patients within 6 weeks and started after 6 weeks in 3 patients.

In another 6 patients, the cartilage T-tube was placed together with tympanomastoid surgery. The results were slightly poorer, with 33% infections.

No other paper has been published on this series and there is no report on the final outcome of this method.

The First Series of Duckert and Co-workers

In the first series of Duckert et al. (1995) of 294 ears (290 patients) the follow-up was for only 6 months. At 6 months, persistent or recurrent perforation was found in 9 ears, yielding a successful closure in 97%. Residual perforations appeared within one month, most often in the anterior quadrants where the support from the perichondrium flap was the weakest. The best hearing results were found in tympanoplasty type 1 measured at 6 months as frequency-specific mean air–bone gap: 5.3 dB at 500 Hz, 5.1 dB at 1000 Hz, and 4.0 dB at 2000 Hz.

In tympanoplasty type 2 with intact stapes and a PORP prosthesis made of glass-ionomer cement (Ionos), the mean air–bone gap was 10.0 dB at 500 Hz, 9.5 dB at 1000 Hz, and 6.7 dB at 2000 Hz.

In tympanoplasty type 3 without stapes, a TORP columella of the same material was used. The mean air–bone gap was 14.0 dB at 500 Hz, 14.0 at 1000 Hz, and 8.6 dB at 2000 Hz. Thus the postoperative hearing was good.

Calculating the mean air–bone gap for all 294 ears for frequencies 500, 1000, and 2000 Hz, a range of 0–10 dB was achieved in 66%, 11–20 dB in 14%, and 21–30 dB in 13% of all patients.

The Later Series of Duckert and Co-workers

Duckert et al. (2003) reported on **a later series** of 40 patients (12 children, 28 adults,) operated since 1994, in which 62.5% patients had retained functional tubes in a 6-year observation period (minimum of 4 years). The average time of tube retention was 38 months (range 3–96 months).

Graft failure, extrusion, epithelial in-growth, or residual perforation occurred in none of the ears. The most common cause of tube failure leading to removal was otorrhea and/or obstruction.

The average conductive hearing loss at 0.5, 1, 2, and 4 kHz was 0–10 dB in 30%, 11–25 dB in 52%, and > 25 dB in 18%.

Duckert et al. (2003) concluded that the cartilage-shielded T-tube unit can effectively reverse atelectasis, reconstruct the tympanic membrane, and eliminate effusion in at least 65% of adult patients for a minimum of 4 years. In children the results are less predictable and less often favorable. Undoubtedly, some of these tubes may remain in position longer, but Duckert et al. "cannot promote this method of intubation as permanent or indefinitive [sic]." The authors believe that the method offers an attractive alternative to the more temporary methods of middle ear intubation in a selected group of patients.

The Series of Danner and Dornhoffer

Since 1994 Danner and Dornhoffer (2001) have operated over a 6-year period on 25 patients and have had only 3 failures, which have already been described in this chapter: accidental removal of tube in two ears and necrosis of the cartilage around the tube followed by extrusion in one ear. The remaining 22 tubes have functioned well since their insertion with only minor complications, such as granulations and medialization.

No data on postoperative hearing are presented but no evident difference in hearing results between the intubated and nonintubated ears was found.

The Randomized Prospective Study of Elsheikh and Co-workers

In their randomized prospective study, Elsheikh et al. (2006) did not find any statistically significant difference between the two groups of 23 adults with a tube inserted in the U-graft compared with 23 adults without the ventilating tube in the U-graft.

Preoperatively, both groups were almost identical: mean age 27/29 years; men 15/14; women 8/9; middle ear risk index 1.72/1.76; atelectasis of grade 2, 15 (65%) / 16 (70%); atelectasis of grade 3, 8 (35%) / 7 (30%).

Testing of tubal function: Elsheikh and co-workers (2006) carried out extensive testing of tubal function:

Tympanometry of patients showed negative values of peak tympanometric pressure in both groups. No statistically significant differences were present in tubal patency or tubal function between the two groups.

The mean tubal opening pressure under static conditions in the first group was 324 ± 145 mmH$_2$O and in the second group was 319 ± 150 mmH$_2$O.

The mean tubal closing pressure in the first group was 106 ± 61 mmH$_2$O and in the second group was 103 ± 64 mmH$_2$O

Tubal opening test under dynamic conditions after swallowing—the deflation test of equalizing the positive pressure: At a positive pressure of + 200 mmH$_2$O in the ear canal, 56% in the first group and 52% of patients in the second group could successfully equalize the positive pressure after 10 swallows.

Tubal opening test under dynamic conditions after swallowing—the aspiration test of equalizing the negative pressure: A negative pressure of –200 mmH$_2$O in the ear canal could be equalized after 10 swallows in 34% cases in the first group and in 30% in the second group.

The Valsalva maneuver was positive preoperatively in 48% in the first group and in 52% in the second group.

Elsheikh and co-workers concluded that the extent of test–retest variability in both groups was consistent with the finding that middle ear pressure is not constantly negative but fluctuates over time in atelectatic middle ears.

Postoperatively, in both groups there were no complications, no graft failure, and no sensorineural hearing loss. After the surgery, three patients from the second group had conductive hearing loss. Two patients developed middle ear effusion and required a secondary insertion of the ventilating tube through the cartilage. In the first group, two patients had recurrent conductive hearing loss. In one patient this was caused by middle ear effusion as a result of occlusion of the ventilating tube, which was replaced.

In both groups, **hearing results** one year after surgery (**Table 20.1**) were significantly better than before surgery ($p < 0.001$, chi-squared test). However, they were no better in the first group with ventilation tubes than in the second group without the ventilating tube ($p > 0.05$).

The conclusion of the excellent study by Elsheikh and co-workers was that the primary insertion of the ventilation tube into the cartilage–perichondrium graft is not necessary for the reconstruction of the atelectatic eardrum.

Table 20.1 Hearing results after tympanoplasty for atelectasis in group 1 with ventilation tube inserted in the U-shaped cartilage graft compared with group 2 without insertion of ventilating tube in the U-shaped cartilage graft (Elsheikh et al. 2006)

	Hearing (0.5, 1, 2, 3 kHz average)			
	Group 1 (23 patients)		Group 2 (23 patients)	
	Preoperative	Postoperative	Preoperative	Postoperative
Pure-tone average (dB)	36.0	23.9	34.5	21.7
Air–bone gap (dB)	24.6	12.2	22.7	10.9
WDS (%)	97.6	98.2	97.2	97.8

WDS, word discrimination score.

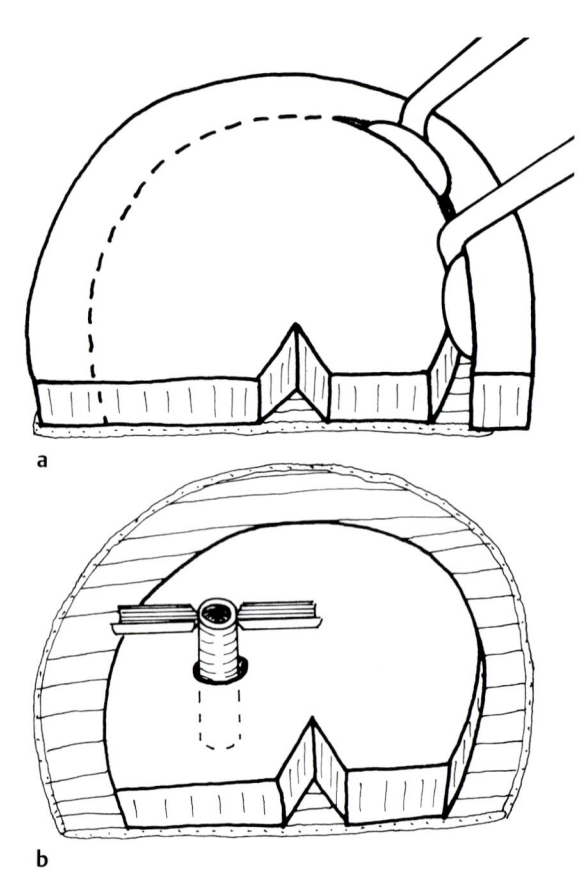

Fig. 20.25a, b Trimming of the tragal cartilage to convert to an inferior cartilage shield T-tube compound graft.
a The perichondrium is removed from the posterior side of the tragal cartilage. The notch for the umbo is made. The dotted line indicates the removal of the peripheral cartilage.
b The T-tube is inserted and the perichondrium flap is trimmed.

Author's Comments and Recommendations

Proposal of an Inferior Cartilage Shield T-Tube Graft

The cartilage graft of Hall (1990) is rather small and is suspended by the perichondrium flap only on the posteroinferior part of the ear canal bone.

My own impression is that a larger semicircular cartilage disk with surrounding perichondrium will provide a better fixation of the cartilage to the ear canal bone. I propose that an inferior cartilage shield T-tube composite graft be placed under the inferior half of the eardrum and suspended by a large perichondrium flap placed on the inferior half of the ear canal wall.

Such a graft can be applied in children with secretory otitis with an intact eardrum, relatively good hearing, and a chance for improvement or normalization of tubal function during the teenage period.

The graft can be harvested from the tragus (**Fig. 20.25a**) or from the concha. It is trimmed to a maximal diameter of 9 mm. A notch is cut for the umbo and a T-tube is placed in the posteroinferior part of the cartilage disk (**Fig. 20.25b**).

A large inferior circumferential incision with elevation of the inferior half of the eardrum is made and the umbo is exposed (**Fig. 20.26a**). The graft with the notch for the umbo and incorporating the T-tube is placed into the tympanic cavity at the level of the bony annulus (**Fig. 20.26b**). The perichondrium flap is folded out (**Fig. 20.26c**) and a hole for the T-tube is made in the eardrum (**Fig. 20.26d**) and the tympanomeatal flap is replaced (**Fig. 20.26e**). The edges of the eardrum are adapted around the tube.

Comments on Tubal Function

I agree with the conclusion of Elsheikh and co-workers (2006) in their series. A cartilage–perichondrium graft alone without the primary insertion of a ventilating tube is a sufficient treatment for the following reasons:

1. The series was dominated by cases with grade 2 atelectasis with posterosuperior retractions where the anterior and inferior parts of the tympanic cavity are ventilated. The series did not include any atelectasis grade 4 cases.
2. There have apparently been no cholesteatomas and active chronic infection in the series.
3. The measured tubal function was apparently not particularly poor:
   The tympanometry showed peaks of negative pressure, but no tympanograms of type B.
   - The mean opening pressure in static condition was similar to a normal series of 33 normal ears with traumatic perforation (Honjo 1988) and other normal series (Yuasa and Takakura 1971; Bylander

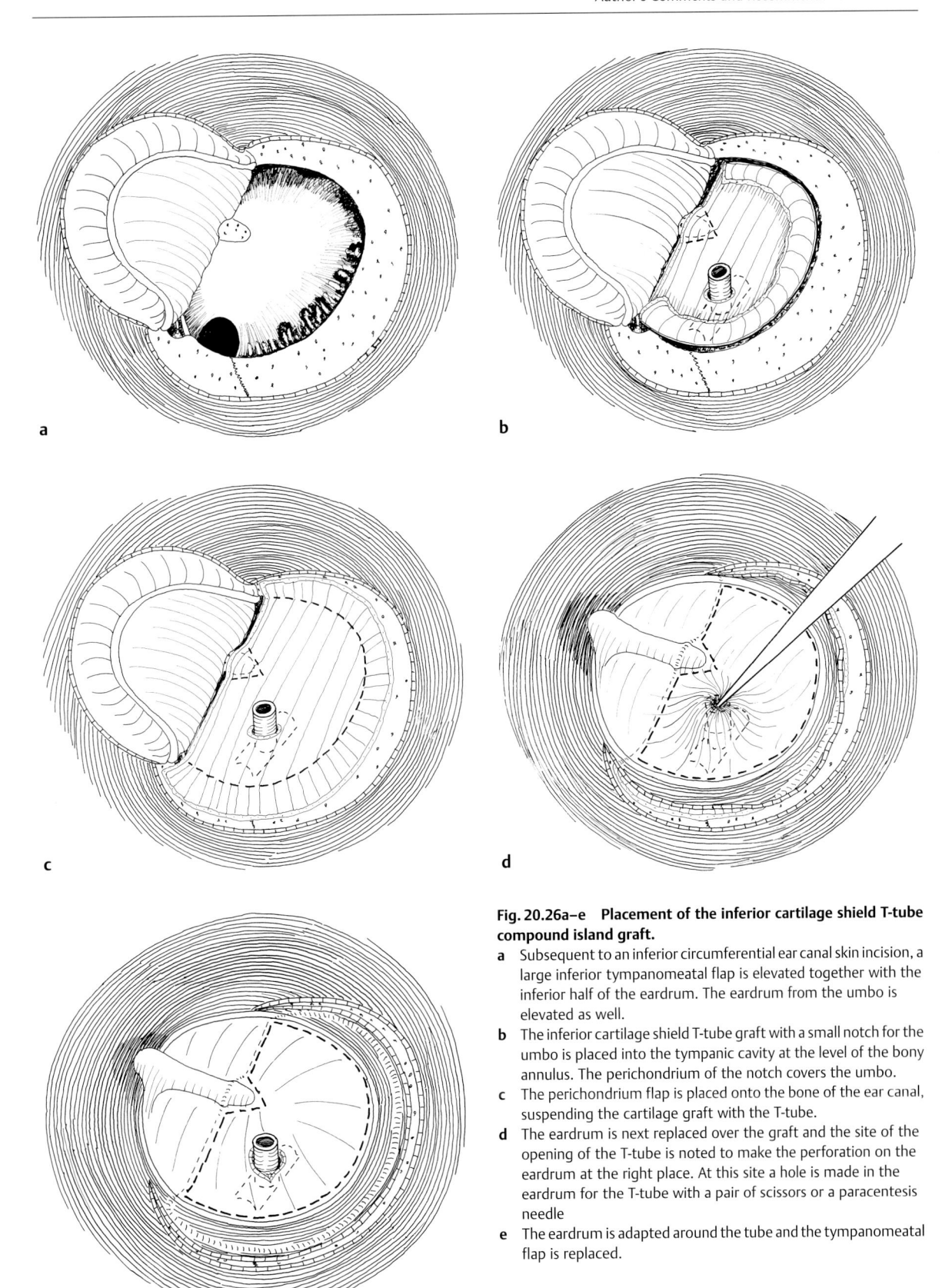

Fig. 20.26a–e Placement of the inferior cartilage shield T-tube compound island graft.

a Subsequent to an inferior circumferential ear canal skin incision, a large inferior tympanomeatal flap is elevated together with the inferior half of the eardrum. The eardrum from the umbo is elevated as well.

b The inferior cartilage shield T-tube graft with a small notch for the umbo is placed into the tympanic cavity at the level of the bony annulus. The perichondrium of the notch covers the umbo.

c The perichondrium flap is placed onto the bone of the ear canal, suspending the cartilage graft with the T-tube.

d The eardrum is next replaced over the graft and the site of the opening of the T-tube is noted to make the perforation on the eardrum at the right place. At this site a hole is made in the eardrum for the T-tube with a pair of scissors or a paracentesis needle

e The eardrum is adapted around the tube and the tympanomeatal flap is replaced.

1980; Bluestone and Cantekin 1981). In the normal series of Honjo (1998), the normal range of tubal opening pressure was 545–165 mmH$_2$O with a mean pressure of 355 H$_2$O (±2SD). Honjo judged the tube to have stenosis or obstruction when it did not open at a pressure of 800 mmH$_2$O.
- The deflation test indicating successful equalization of positive pressure of +100 decapascals in 56 % in the first group and in 52 % in the second group. The percentages of equalization of negative pressure of −100 decapascals in the aspiration test were 34 % and 30 %. In 33 normal ears, Honjo found 73 % in the deflation test and 61 % in aspiration test. This means that performance in the deflation and aspiration tests was not especially poor.
- Preoperative Valsalva was positive in 48 % and 52 % cases respectively in the two groups. In one of our series (Tos 1974a) of 171 dry ears with a diagnosis of sequelae to chronic otitis media and having a tympanoplasty only, the preoperative Valsalva was positive in 64 % of patients. In 128 ears with cholesteatoma (63 %) and active chronic granulating otitis (37 %) being operated with mastoidectomy and tympanoplasty, the preoperative Valsalva was positive in 48 % of the ears, i. e., a similar percentage to the series of Elsheikh et al.

4. The series of Danner and Dornhoffer (2001) were clinically much more severe even though the tubal function tests or tubal patency tests were not performed. This is presumably also the case with the later series of Duckert et al. (2003). It will be of great interest to see the late results of both studies.

Need for Testing of Tubal Function

This chapter deals with special surgery in patients with poor tubal function, but the testing of tubal function was not mentioned at all in the first three surgical papers. There is no documentation to support the suggestion that the 290 patients from the first series of Duckert et al. (1995), all receiving cartilage shield T-tube graft at the time of surgery, in fact had severe tubal dysfunction. A simple test, such as the Valsalva maneuver, would be able to split such series into a group with positive Valsalva, indicating patent eustachian tube, and a group with negative Valsalva, indicating no patent eustachian tube. In measurements of the static opening pressure test, more than a half of the patients with negative Valsalva will presumably be able to open the eustachian tube with a pressure of 800 mmH$_2$O in the ear canal. Measurement of the tubal function with deflation test and aspiration test will further improve the quality of tubal function testing.

In the paper of Elsheikh et al. (2006) all the tubal tests were done, allowing a comparison of their own series with other normal or other abnormal surgical series. This brings greater scientific rigor to cartilage tympanoplasty papers. When we argue that this method or any other cartilage tympanoplasty methods have to be performed because of poor tubal function, then we must document the tubal function.

Cartilage Shield T-Tube Tympanoplasty Provides Ideal Opportunities for Long-Term Research on Tubal Function

Tubal function and tubal patency can change: it can deteriorate and it can improve. Such changes can be followed postoperatively by the deflation test and the aspiration test. Patients with a T-tube have to be followed clinically for a long time after surgery. By including systematic testing of tubal function through the open T-tube, long-term postoperative studies of tubal function can be carried out. It can be expected that tubal function in ears with preoperative active infection or inflammation of middle ear mucosa may be improved by permanent ventilation of the middle ear. Middle ear mucosa and tubal mucosa may gradually improve and become less edematous, allowing better passage of air and better conditions for mucocilliary clearance. In addition, mucus production by the mucosa can be reduced and even normalized.

There is good documentation of the very common changes in tubal function during childhood (Fiellau-Nikolajsen et al. 1977; Poulsen and Tos 1978; Tos et al. 1978), as shown in epidemiological and etiological studies on prevalence and incidence of secretory otitis media in cohorts of otherwise healthy children. It is caused mainly by upper respiratory tract infections; 90 % of otherwise healthy Danish children (80 % of ears) have had at least one episode of secretory otitis media with initial deterioration and then spontaneous improvement, which is documented by repetitive tympanometry (Tos 1980; Holm-Jensen et al. 1981; Tos 1983, 1988; Thomsen and Tos 1981). Fifteen percent of ears have had one short episode of 1–3 months' duration, 25 % have had recurrent short episodes, 15 % have had long-lasting (3–9 months) episodes, 15 % have had long-lasting recurrent episodes, and 10 % have had very long-lasting (1–4 years) episodes (Tos 1984). Among the children of the three cohorts, at age 5 years 23.7 % and at age 10 years 32.8 % had eardrum pathology. The most common changes were atrophy in 8.1 %, atrophy with fixated retraction in 2.3 %, atrophy with tympanosclerosis in 2.3 %, and tympanosclerosis in only 5.1 % The remaining 15 % had attic retractions and only 5 % had grade 3 or grade 4 (Tos et al. 1990).

Influence of the Tubal Mucosa on the Tubal Function

The constant deterioration and improvement of tubal function as documented by repeated tympanometry during childhood can only be explained by the changes of the middle ear mucosa and the tubal mucosa.

During the late 1960s and 1970s our quantitative histopathological studies on goblet cells of temporal bones showed that the density of the goblet cells in the tympanic part of the eustachian tube and tympanic cavity is increased in ears previously exposed to infection. In ears with subacute and acute pathological reactions, the density of goblet cells was considerably increased (Tos and Bak-Pedersen 1976, 1977). We have demonstrated that mucous glands form during acute and chronic infection of the middle ear (Bak-Pedersen and Tos 1971; Tos and Bak-Pedersen 1972, 1973; Tos 1974b). The newly formed glands are active and produce mucus during the period of active disease. The glands do not disappear during the period of improvement, but they do degenerate and become inactive. We found degenerated glands in 90% of normal temporal bones and concluded (10 years before the epidemiological studies) that the glands were sequelae of previous disease (Tos 1985a; Tos and Cayé-Thomasen 2002). The most severe cases have thick tubal mucosa that could influence tubal function.

The density of goblet cells in the tubal mucosa was increased during and up to 6 months after acute otitis media in animal models of acute otitis media caused by *Streptococcus pneumoniae* (Cayé-Thomasen and Tos 2003). In another similar study, the volume of eustachian tube glands increased during and up to at least 3 months after acute otitis media, primarily because of hypertrophy of the mucous gland components. This may compromise tubal ventilatory and drainage function (Cayé-Thomasen and Tos 2004a). In a third study, four different types of bacteria were inoculated into various bullae of rats: *Streptococcus pneumoniae*, non-typable *Haemophilus influenzae*, *Haemophilus influenzae* type b, and *Moraxella catarrhalis*. All four bacteria caused increase of goblet cells and mucous glands in the eustachian tube. The non-typable *Haemophilus* strain induced the highest increase of goblet cells and mucous gland volume (Cayé-Thomasen and Tos 2004b). Excessive mucus secretion up to 6 months after acute otitis media contributes to the deteriorated tubal function after acute otitis media and thus predisposes, sustains or aggravates middle ear disease.

Chronic Hyperplasia of the Eustachian Tube Mucosa

On the basis of histopathological studies of the middle ear mucosa and tubal mucosa on human temporal bones and also surgical biopsies, in 1985 I introduced the term "chronic mucosal hyperplasia of the eustachian tube" (Tos 1985b). This includes hyperplasia of the epithelium, the basal membrane, and the lamina propria in which the fibrous, vascular, and glandular elements are all increased as found in our human studies. In the case of adults, with sequelae of chronic otitis with eardrum perforation, active chronic otitis, and chronic secretory otitis, the mucosa was thickened to varying degrees and there was an increased number of round cells and fibrous elements in the lamina propria (Tos 1974b). The recent experimental studies on the eustachian tube mentioned above support the findings in humans.

Such hyperplasia of the mucosa hampers the ventilation of the middle ear, but this may improve in long-term ventilation and therefore the measurement of tubal patency and tubal function through the T-tube is important for a considerable time after surgery.

References

Bak-Pedersen K, Tos M. The mucous glands in chronic secretory otitis media. Acta Otolaryngol 1971;72:14–27.

Bluestone CD, Cantekin EI. Panel on experiences with testing eustachian tube function. Current clinical methods, indications and interpretation of eustachian tube function tests. Ann Otol Rhinol Laryngol 1981;90:552–562.

Bylander A. Comparison of Eustachian tube function in children and adults with normal ear. Ann Otol Rhinol Laryngol Suppl 1980;89(3 Pt 2):20–24.

Cayé-Thomasen P, Tos M. Eustachian tube goblet cell density during and after otitis media caused by streptococcus pneumoniae: a morphometric analysis. Otol Neurotol 2003;24:365–370.

Cayé-Thomasen P, Tos M. Eustachian tube gland changes in acute otitis media. Otol Neurotol 2004a;25:14–18.

Cayé Thomasen P, Tos M. Eustachian tube gland tissue changes are related to bacterial species in acute otitis media. Int J Pediatr Otorhinolaryngol 2004b;68:101–110.

Danner CJ, Dornhoffer JL. Primary intubation of cartilage tympanoplasties. Laryngoscope 2001;111:177–180.

Dornhoffer JL. Hearing results with cartilage tympanoplasty. Laryngoscope 1997;107:1094–1097.

Duckert LG, Müller J, Makielski KH, Helms J. Composite autograft "shield" reconstruction of remnant tympanic membranes. Am J Otol 1995;16:21–26.

Duckert LG, Makielski KH, Helms J. Prolonged middle ear ventilation with the cartilage shield T- tube tympanoplasties. Otol Neurotol 2003;24:153–157.

Elsheikh MN, Elsherief HS, Elsherief SG. Cartilage tympanoplasty for management of tympanic membrane atelectasis: is ventilatory tube necessary? Otol Neurotol 2006;27:859–864.

Fiellau-Nikolajsen M, Lous J, Vang Pedersen S, Schousboe HH. Tympanometry in three-year-old children. Scand Audiol 1977;6:199–204.

Hall LJ. T-tube with tragus cartilage flange in long- term middle ear ventilation. Am J Otol 1990;11:454–457.

Holm-Jensen S, Sørensen HC, Tos M. Repetitive screenings in 4-year-old children. Seasonal influence on secretory otitis and tubal dysfunction. ORL J Otorhinolaryngol Relat Spec 1981;43:164–174.

Honjo I. Eustachian Tube and Middle Ear Diseases. Tokyo: Springer-Verlag; 1988:25–29.

Klacansky J, Kucera J, Starek I. Rekonstrukcija blanky bubienka chrupkovymi transplantati. [Reconstruction of the eardrum with cartilage transplants.] Otorinolaringologie a Fonietrie 1998;47:59–63.

Poulsen G, Tos M. Screening tympanometry in newborn infants and during the first six months of life. Scand Audiol 1978;7:159–166.

Sade J. The atelectatic ear. In: Sade J, ed. Secretory Otitis Media and Its Sequelae. New York: Churchill Livingstone; 1979:64–88.

Thomsen J, Tos M. Spontaneous improvement of secretory otitis. A long-term study. Acta Otolaryngol 1981;92:493–499.

Tos M. Tubal function and tympanoplasty. J Laryngol Otol 1974a;88:1113–1124.

Tos M. Production of mucus in the middle ear and Eustachian tube. Embryology, anatomy, and pathology of the mucous glands and goblet cells in the Eustachian tube and middle ear. Ann Otol Rhinol Laryngol 1974b;83(Suppl. 11):44–58.

Tos M. Spontaneous improvement of secretory otitis and impedance screening. Arch Otolaryngol 1980;106:345–349.

Tos M. Epidemiology and spontaneous improvement of secretory otitis. Acta Otorhinolaryngol Belg 1983;37:31–43.

Tos M. Epidemiology and natural history of secretory otitis. Am J Otol 1984;5:459–462.

Tos M. Normalization of the middle ear mucosa. Auris Nasus Larynx 1985a;12(suppl 1):S30–S32.

Tos M. Pathology of the Eustachian tube. Ann Otol Rhinol Laryngol 1985b;94(Suppl. 120):17–18.

Tos M. Etiologic factors in secretory otitis. Adv Otorhinolaryngol 1988;40:57–64.

Tos M, Bak-Pedersen K. The pathogenesis of chronic secretory otitis media. Arch Otolaryngol 1972;95:511–521.

Tos M, Bak-Pedersen K. Density of mucous glands in a biopsy material of chronic secretory otitis media. Acta Otolaryngol 1973;75:55–60.

Tos M, Bak-Pedersen K. Goblet cell population in the normal middle ear and Eustachian tube of children and adults. Ann Otol Rhinol Laryngol 1976;85(2 Suppl. 25 Pt 2):44–50.

Tos M, Bak-Pedersen K. Goblet cell population in the pathological middle ear and the Eustachian tube in children and adults. Ann Otol Rhinol Laryngol 1977;86:209–218.

Tos M, Cayé-Thomasen P. Mucous glands in the middle ear—what is known and what is not. ORL J Otorhinolaryngol Relat Spec 2002;64:86–94.

Tos M, Poulsen G, Borch J. Tympanometry in 2-year-old children. ORL J Otorhinolaryngol Relat Spec 1978;40:77–85.

Tos M, Stangerup S-E, Larsen P, Siim S, Hvid G, Andreassen UK. The relationship between secretory otitis and cholesteatoma. In: Tos M, Thomsen J, Peitersen E, eds. Cholesteatoma and Mastoid Surgery. Amsterdam: Kugler & Ghedini Publications; 1989;325–330.

Tos M, Hvid G, Stangerup S-E, Andreassen UK. Prevalence and progression of sequelae following secretory otitis. In: Bluestone CD Casselbrandt ML, eds. Workshop on otitis media. Ann Otol Rhinol Laryngol 1990; 99(Suppl. 149):36–38.

Yuasa R, Takakura M. Analysis of physical properties of the Eustachian tube. J Otolarynol Jpn 1971;749:53.

21 Underlay Tympanoplasty Techniques with Cartilage–Perichondrium Composite Island Graft

Definition

Two typical and well-known underlay composite island grafts are the posterior island graft for posterior retraction or perforation and the total pars tensa island graft for the total perforation or total atelectasis of the eardrum. The posterior island graft, described in Chapter 15, is exclusively an underlay graft. The total island graft, described in Chapter 17, is mostly used as an underlay graft but it can also be used as an on-lay graft. The methods and results of the posterior and total graft are well described in the literature

In this chapter, underlay grafting with cartilage island grafts of anterior, inferior, and subtotal perforations or retractions will be illustrated. The cartilage–perichondrium composite island graft is occasionally used for anterior and inferior perforations, but there are no publications on techniques and results. The drawings of techniques presented here have been made exclusively for this chapter.

The cartilage–perichondrium composite island graft is defined as a piece of tragus or concha cartilage, covered on at least one side with perichondrium, which surrounds the cartilage as a flap (**Fig. 21.1**).

The **size of the cartilage** is slightly larger than the size of the perforation. The **shape of the cartilage** follows the shape of the perforation. It is desirable that the perichondrium flap reach at least the bony annulus. The **thickness of the cartilage** may vary and may depend on the cause and the size of the perforation. In large perforation, retraction, poor tubal function, and recurrent surgery, a full-thickness cartilage disk will be used. In small anterior and inferior perforations, grafts of half-thickness or even less will be used.

Harvesting and Shaping of the Island Graft

The graft is harvested from the tragus (see **Figs. 3.21–3.23**) or concha cartilage (see **Figs. 3.26, 3.27**), as described in Chapter 3 The perichondrium is removed on the convex side. The reduction of the thickness is accomplished using the Kurz Precise Cartilage Knife Set illustrated in Chapter 3 (see **Fig. 3.36**). Finally, the thinned graft is trimmed to the appropriate size and shape (**Fig. 21.2**).

Indication for Application of the Underlay Island Graft

In principle, there is no contraindication to the use of the cartilage island graft for closure of anterior, inferior, and subtotal perforation, especially when using a half-thickness graft or an even thinner graft. However, there are no publications on comparison of island grafts of various thickness, and no comparison between the fascia or the perichondrium with the island graft in anterior or inferior perforation.

Clear individual indications for application of the island graft are poor tubal function with negative preoperative Valsalva maneuver, cholesteatoma, retraction, infection, and recurrent surgery.

Surgical Techniques

Anterior Perforation

Even if symptoms from the anterior perforation are few, the closure of the perforation is sometimes difficult, with a high rate of recurrence. Several methods employing fascia or perichondrium are described and illustrated in Volume 1 of *Manual of Middle Ear Surgery* (Tos 1993), and new

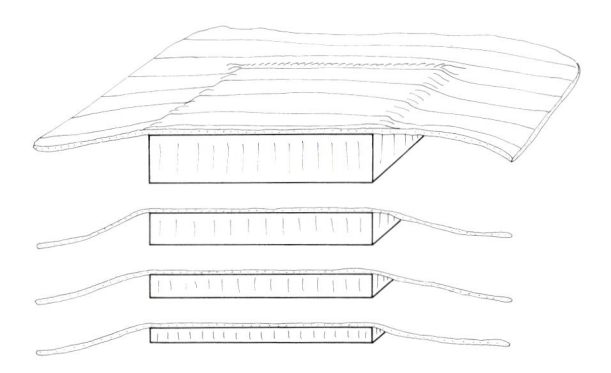

Fig. 21.1 Cartilage–perichondrium composite island grafts of various thicknesses. Full thickness, two-thirds or three-quarters, half, and one-third thickness of the cartilage. Perichondrium covers the eardrum side of the cartilage and surrounds the cartilage as a flap.

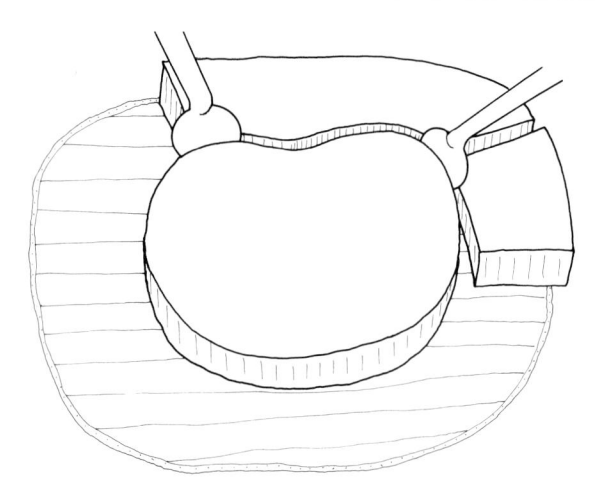

Fig. 21.2 Trimming of a three-quarters thickness island graft. The cartilage disk is made slightly larger than the inferior perforation.

methods have subsequently been published (Potsic et al. 1996; Schraff et al. 2005; Jung and Park 2005).

Transcanal Technique without Flaps

In transcanal approach with fixed ear speculum (Chapter 3), the edges of the perforation are cleaned and the mucosa under the eardrum remnant is scarified and partly removed (**Fig. 21.3a**). The anterosuperior part of the tympanic cavity is filled with Gelfoam to support the perichondrium flap, which stays in place through surface tension (**Fig. 21.3b**). A half-thickness cartilage island graft is placed under the edges of the perforation and the perichondrium is folded out under the denuded mucosa. The perforation is covered with Gelfoam balls (**Fig. 21.3c–f**).

Fixation of the Anterior Perichondrium Flap

It can sometimes be desirable to fixate the perichondrium flap in underlay techniques and to use Gerlach technique (MMES_1, Figs. 421–424), pushing or pulling the fascia through the holes created in the eardrum remnant (Gerlach 1972, 1975). Gerlach's idea has been used by Primrose and Kerr (1986) in fascia grafting of marginal anterior perforations. The authors cut a small tag on the anterosuperior part of a large fascia graft and pull the tag through the hole under the anterior fibrous annulus.

I use a similar method, with some modifications, in closure of anterior perforations by underlay cartilage island graft. First a hole is made through the anterior ear canal skin Then a curved elevator is pushed under the anterior fibrous annulus at the same location as the previous perforation of the skin, creating a small channel (**Fig. 21.4a**). The island graft is placed into the perforation (**Fig. 21.4b**), the anterior perichondrium is pushed though the newly formed hole with the curved elevator, and the perichondrium is further pulled with a hook into the ear canal. Finally, the cartilage disk is positioned under the eardrum and the remaining perichondrium is folded out (**Fig. 21.4c**).

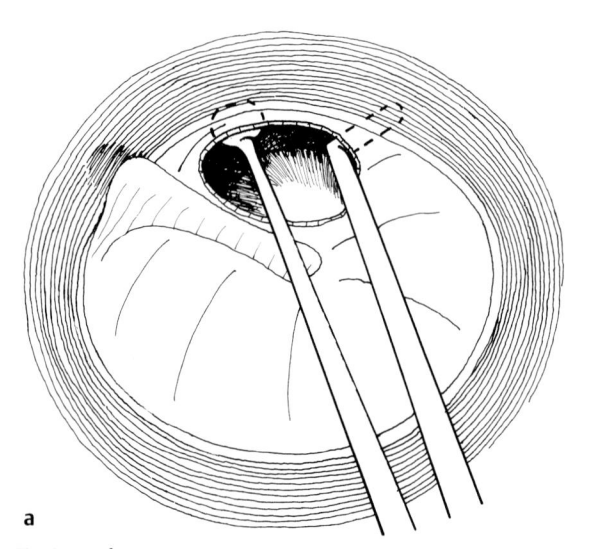

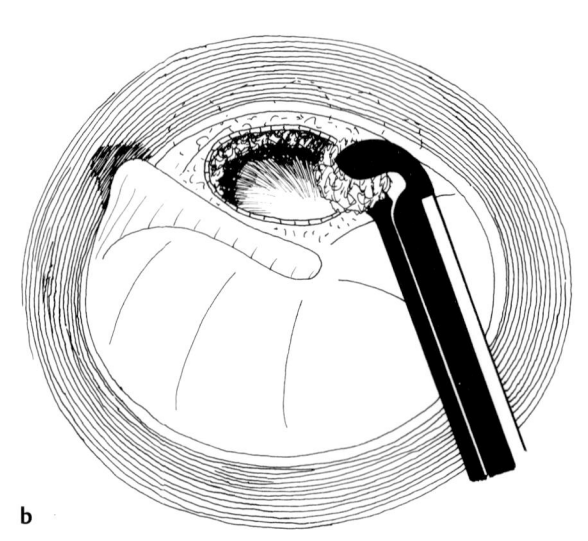

a b

Fig. 21.3a, b

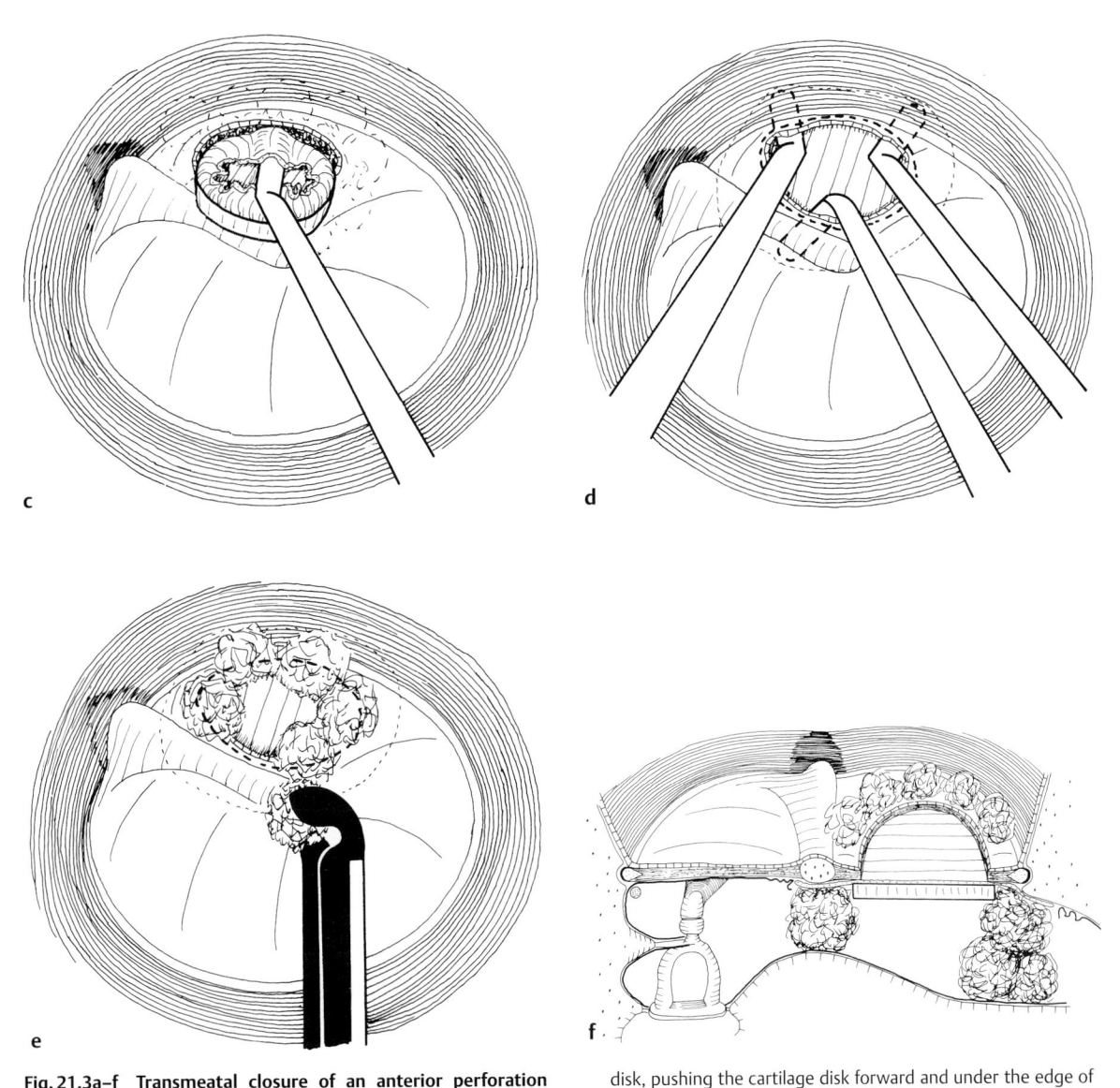

Fig. 21.3a–f Transmeatal closure of an anterior perforation with underlay application of an island graft.

a The edge of the perforation is cleaned and the epithelium is removed. Using a round knife or incudostapedial knife, the mucosa of the undersurface of the eardrum is scarified all the way around the perforation, and that of the medial side of the malleus handle and the bony annulus.

b The anterosuperior part of the tympanic cavity is firmly packed with slightly moist Gelfoam balls.

c The island graft with a three-quarters thickness cartilage disk is placed onto the perforation with the perichondrium folded back onto the cartilage disk. A curved incudostapedial knife is placed under the anterior perichondrium flap and onto the cartilage disk, pushing the cartilage disk forward and under the edge of the perforation.

d Using a curved incudostapedial knife the perichondrium is folded out under the denuded eardrum remnant all the way around the perforation.

e Slightly moist Gelfoam balls are placed around the edge of the perforation, fixing the cartilage graft.

f Side view of the transmeatal closure of the anterior perforation with an underlay three-quarters thickness cartilage island graft. The mucosa of the eardrum and malleus handle is scarified, the cartilage island graft is supported and stabilized with Gelfoam, and the perichondrium flaps stay in place due to the surface tension with the eardrum remnant.

The Large Anterior Tympanomeatal Flap Technique

Anterior perforations can be closed by all three approaches, but the transcanal approach with fixed ear speculum is less invasive than the retroauricular and endaural approaches, especially in cases with disturbing bony prominences of the anterior ear canal wall.

A large anterior incision and elevation of the large ear canal skin flap allows extensive drilling of the bony prominence and a subsequent anterior tympanotomy (**Fig. 21.5a**). Placement of the cartilage island underlay graft is easy, especially that of the anterior perichondrium flap, which is placed onto the anterior ear canal bone (**Fig. 21.5b, c**).

Posterior Perichondrium Flap Attached to the Malleus Handle

To avoid poor attachment of the posterior perichondrium flap, I recommend placement of the posterior perichondrium flap onto the denuded malleus handle. The epithelium is further elevated from the lateral and posterior sides of the malleus handle (**Fig. 21.6a**), creating a fissure between the malleus handle and the lamina propria, where the posterior perichondrium, covering the malleus handle, continues under the posterior part of the eardrum (**Fig. 21.6b**). At the umbo region the lamina propria is not disconnected from the malleus handle. After replacement of the tympanomeatal flap, the healing will be rapid and the grafting effective (**Fig. 21.6c, d**).

Instead of placing the entire posterior perichondrium flap and elevating the lamina propria from the malleus handle, two small fissures are made along the anterior border of the malleus handle (**Fig. 21.6e**). After placement of the island graft with the perichondrium, two strips of the posterior perichondrium flap are cut at the level of the corresponding fissures (**Fig. 21.6f**). Using forceps, each strip is pulled though the channel and over the malleus handle into the tympanic cavity (**Fig. 21.6g**). The remaining perichondrium is placed under the malleus handle and the tympanomeatal flap is replaced (**Fig. 21.6h**).

Anterior Perforation Closed through Posterior Tympanotomy

In cases with more severe hearing loss than expected in an anterior perforation, it will be desirable to perform a posterior tympanotomy and inspect the incudostapedial joint. Additionally, an elevation of the eardrum from the malleus handle, to place the posterior perichondrium flap, can be used to suspend the cartilage graft.

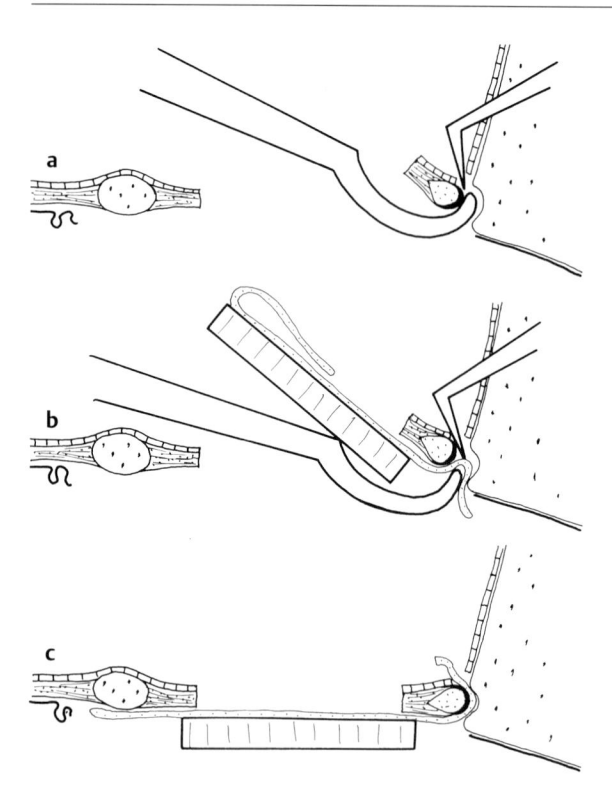

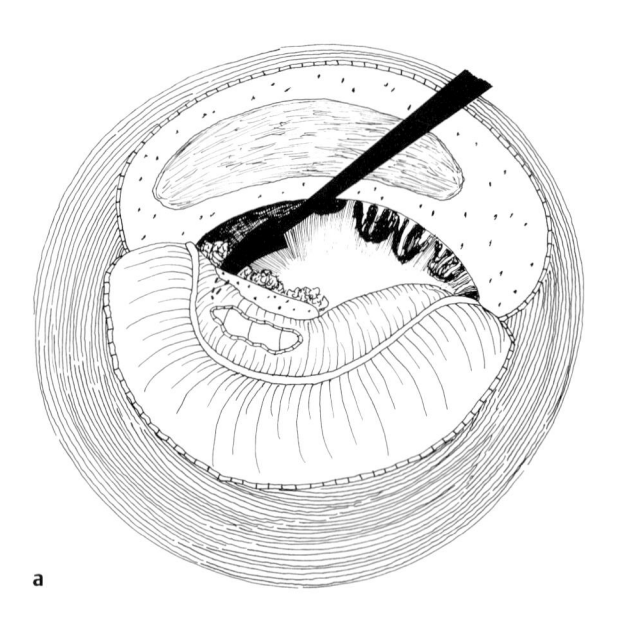

Fig. 21.4a–c Fixation of the anterior perichondrium flap.
a Using a hook, an incision lateral to the anterior fibrous annulus is made and the annulus is loosened, making a hole toward the tympanic cavity. A curved elevator further subluxates the fibrous annulus, creating a small channel reaching to the hook.
b The anterior edge of the island graft is placed into the perforation and, with the curved elevator, the anterior perichondrium flap is pushed into the channel. Using the hook, the edge of the perichondrium is pulled slightly into the ear canal.
c The half-thickness cartilage disk and the surrounding perichondrium are placed under the eardrum remnant.

Fig. 21.5a–c The large anterior tympanomeatal flap technique, removing the bony protrusion of the ear canal and closing an anterior perforation with an island graft.
a First the edges of the perforation are cleansed, then a large anterior skin flap is gradually elevated and the bony protrusion is gradually removed by the diamond drill. Finally, an anterior tympanotomy is performed and a large tympanomeatal flap, including the perforation is elevated. Using a sickle knife, the underside of the malleus handle and the eardrum mucosa are scarified.
b Gelfoam is placed under the malleus handle and into the anterior tympanic cavity and the cartilage half-thickness island graft with the surrounding perichondrium flaps is placed under the eardrum remnant and onto the anterior ear canal bone.
c The tympanomeatal flap is replaced, covering the perichondrium flaps.

a

Surgical Techniques

Fig. 21.5b, c

Fig. 21.6a–h Placement of the posterior perichondrium flap onto the malleus handle.

a In a situation with anterior perforation and elevation of a large anterior tympanomeatal flap together with the eardrum remnant with the perforation, the epithelium of the malleus handle is elevated and the lamina propria is loosened from the posterior side of the malleus handle. This creates a fissure for the posterior perichondrium.

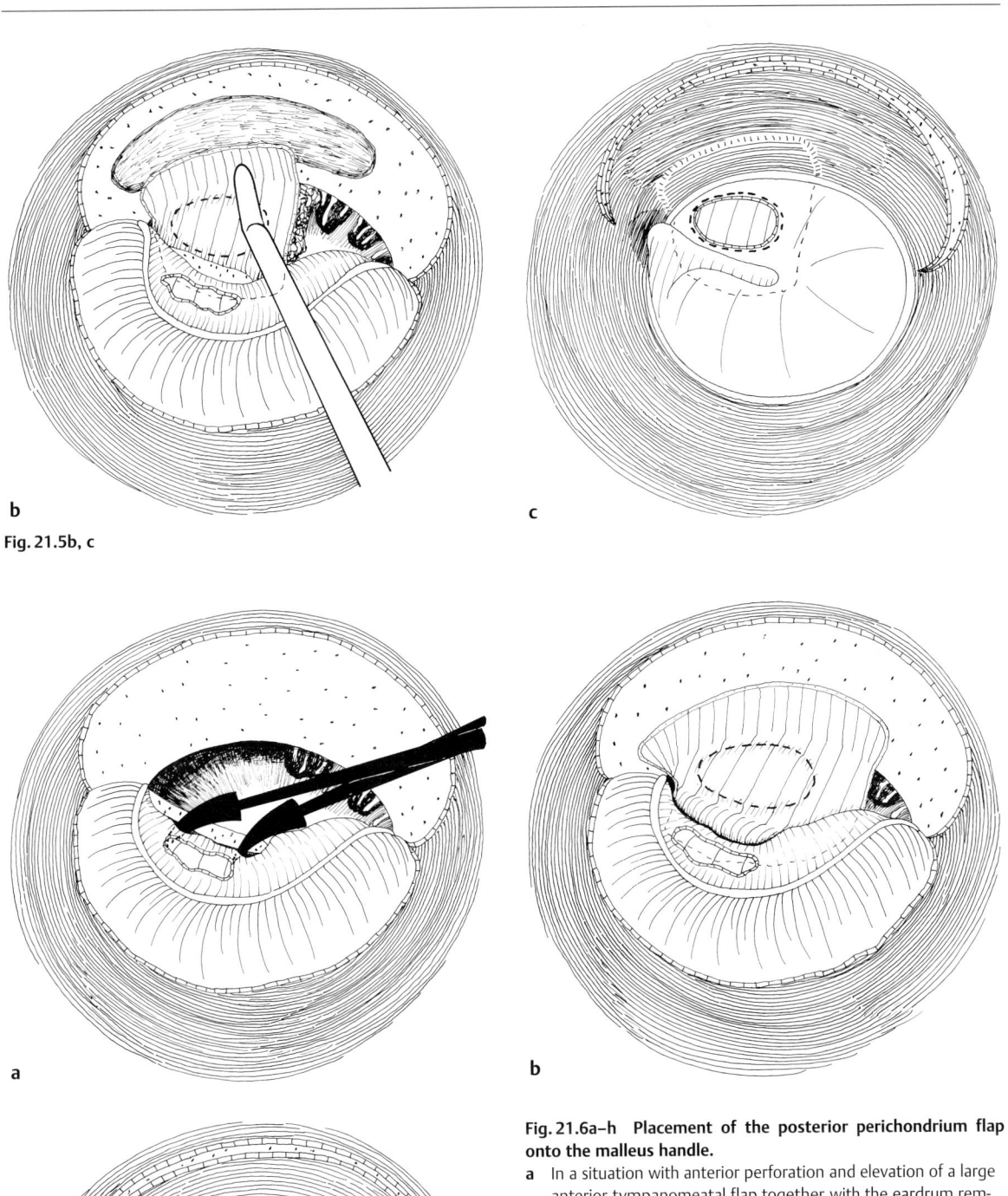

b The half-thickness cartilage island graft is placed as an underlay graft, with the anterior perichondrium flap onto the anterior bony ear canal wall and the posterior flap onto the denuded malleus handle to continue under the lamina propria. The superior and inferior perichondrium flaps are also folded out.

c The tympanomeatal flap is replaced and the elevated epithelium covers the perichondrium at the malleus handle.

Fig. 21.6d–h ▷

Fig. 21.6d–h

d Side view of the anterior perforation closed with the half-thickness cartilage island graft, and the posterior perichondrium flap, covering the malleus handle. The anterior flap is placed onto the bony annulus.

e Placement of two perichondrium strips over the malleus handle in an anterior perforation covered with underlay cartilage island graft. A large anterior tympanomeatal flap including the anterior half of the eardrum with the anterior perforation is elevated, exposing the malleus handle. Two openings to the tympanic cavity are made by elevating the eardrum from the malleus handle in two places.

f The half-thickness cartilage island graft is placed into the anterior tympanic cavity and the perichondrium flaps are folded out. Posteriorly, two strips of perichondrium are cut, to be pushed over the malleus handle through the two openings into the posterior tympanum.

g Two perichondrium strips are pushed through the two openings into the tympanic cavity. The anterior flap and most of the superior perichondrium flap are placed onto the anterior bony ear canal.

h The tympanomeatal flap is replaced.

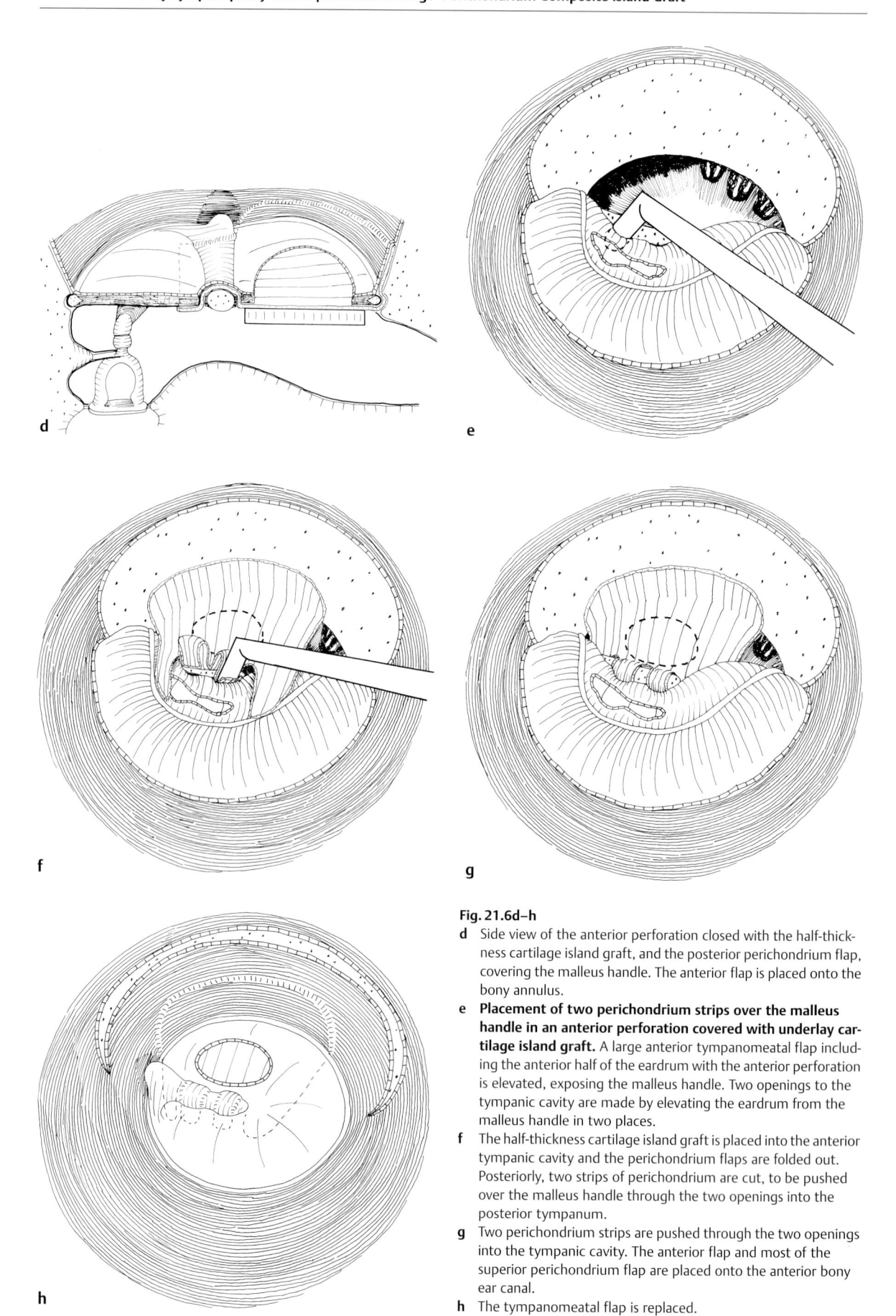

First, the edges of the perforation are cleaned, the mucosa from the eardrum remnant is scarified or removed, and then a small hole is made anterior to the fibrous annulus (**Fig. 21.7a**). After elevation of the posterior tympanomeatal flap, the periosteum with the eardrum is elevated from the malleus handle (**Fig. 21.7b**), but the connection of the eardrum to the umbo remains intact. The island graft is placed in the anterior tympanum and pushed under the eardrum remnant. The posterior tympanomeatal flap is replaced and the anterior perichondrium flap is pushed through the anterior hole previously prepared anterior to the fibrous annulus (**Fig. 21.7c**). The island graft is accommodated in relation to the perforation and the perichondrium flap is folded out (**Fig. 21.7d**). Finally, the posterior tympanomeatal flap is again elevated, the posterior perichondrium flap is pulled onto the denuded malleus handle, and the perichondrium flaps are folded out from the inner side of the eardrum using a curved elevator (**Fig. 21.7e, f**).

In the grafting of an anterior perforation with fascia in the retroauricular approach, Potsic et al. (1996) performed a posterior tympanotomy, elevated the periosteum and the eardrum from the malleus handle, and then elevated the anterior annulus with the anterior ear canal skin; finally, they positioned a long fascia from the anterior ear canal wall to the posterior ear canal wall.

Inferior Perforation

Inferior perforation of various sizes can easily be closed with an underlay cartilage island graft, either without or with tympanotomy. Several techniques have been used in grafting with fascia or perichondrium; most can also be used in grafting with the underlay cartilage island graft.

Transmeatal Closure of the Inferior Perforation with Underlay Cartilage Island Graft without Tympanotomy

A fixed ear speculum with ability to tilt to all sides provides the best conditions for transmeatal surgery (Chapter 3).

Epithelium is cleaned away along the edge of the perforation. The mucosa under the eardrum remnant is scarified (**Fig. 21.8a**) or removed. The half-thickness cartilage island graft is manipulated and pushed under the edge of the perforation (**Fig. 21.8b**) and the perichondrium flaps are folded out. The inferior half of the tympanic cavity and the lateral side of the eardrum are filled with Gelfoam (**Fig. 21.8c**).

Transmeatal Gerlach Suspension of the Underlay Cartilage Island Graft

The Gerlach suspension of the fascia graft (Gerlach 1972, 1975) is thoroughly illustrated in MMES_1 (Figs. 414–424). The method is easily adapted to any underlay method with cartilage–perichondrium island graft. Suspension of the graft by pulling the perichondrium flaps into the holes obviates the need for any further support with Gelfoam.

After cleaning of the edge of the perforation, five incisions are made with the sickle knife through the eardrum, 0.5–0.75 mm from the edge. After positioning of the cartilage under the border of the perforation, the edge of the perichondrium flap is pulled into the five holes with a small hook (**Fig. 21.9**).

Swing-Door Technique with Underlay Cartilage Island Graft

Swing-door technique is a very popular opening of the tympanic cavity, performed in transmeatal, endaural, and retroauricular approaches.

In transmeatal approach with fixed ear speculum, the edges of the perforation are cleaned, then a circumferential incision and a vertical incision at 8-o'clock are made and superior and inferior tympanomeatal flaps are elevated, providing a good view into the tympanic cavity (**Fig. 21.10a**). The mucosa under the eardrum is scarified. The anterior fibrous annulus can be slightly elevated, just enough to allow an edge of the perichondrium flap to be pushed between the bony annulus and the fibrous annulus (**Fig. 21.10b**). The inferior and posterior perichondrium flaps are placed onto the bone of the ear canal (**Fig. 21.10c**).

Large Tympanomeatal Flap Techniques with Underlay Cartilage Island Graft

Large tympanomeatal flap technique can be applied in all three approaches. A large tympanomeatal flap is elevated in the inferosuperior direction together with the fibrous annulus. Because the medial ear canal bone with the bony annulus is exposed, the method is recommended for cartilage–perichondrium composite island grafts. The perichondrium flaps can be large and are placed onto the ear canal bone.

For a large inferior perforation, a circumferential incision is made between the 2-o'clock and 10-o'clock positions and one large tympanomeatal flap with the remnants of the eardrum is elevated, including the periosteum from the umbo (**Fig. 21.11a**). The half-thickness cartilage island graft is placed into the tympanic cavity at the level of the bony annulus. The perichondrium flaps are mainly placed onto the bony ear canal wall (**Fig. 21.11b**). The superior flap is placed onto the denuded malleus handle and under the scarified eardrum. After replacement of the eardrum remnant with the tympanomeatal flap, the suspension of the graft is firm and safe (**Fig. 21.11c**).

Subtotal Perforation

Subtotal perforation involves all four quadrants, but the upper halves of the superoposterior and the superoanterior quadrants are not involved. The inferoposterior and inferoanterior quadrants are always involved and the subtotal perforation extends to the superior quadrants. Thus, a large inferior perforation extending 1–2 mm superior to the umbo may be called a subtotal perforation.

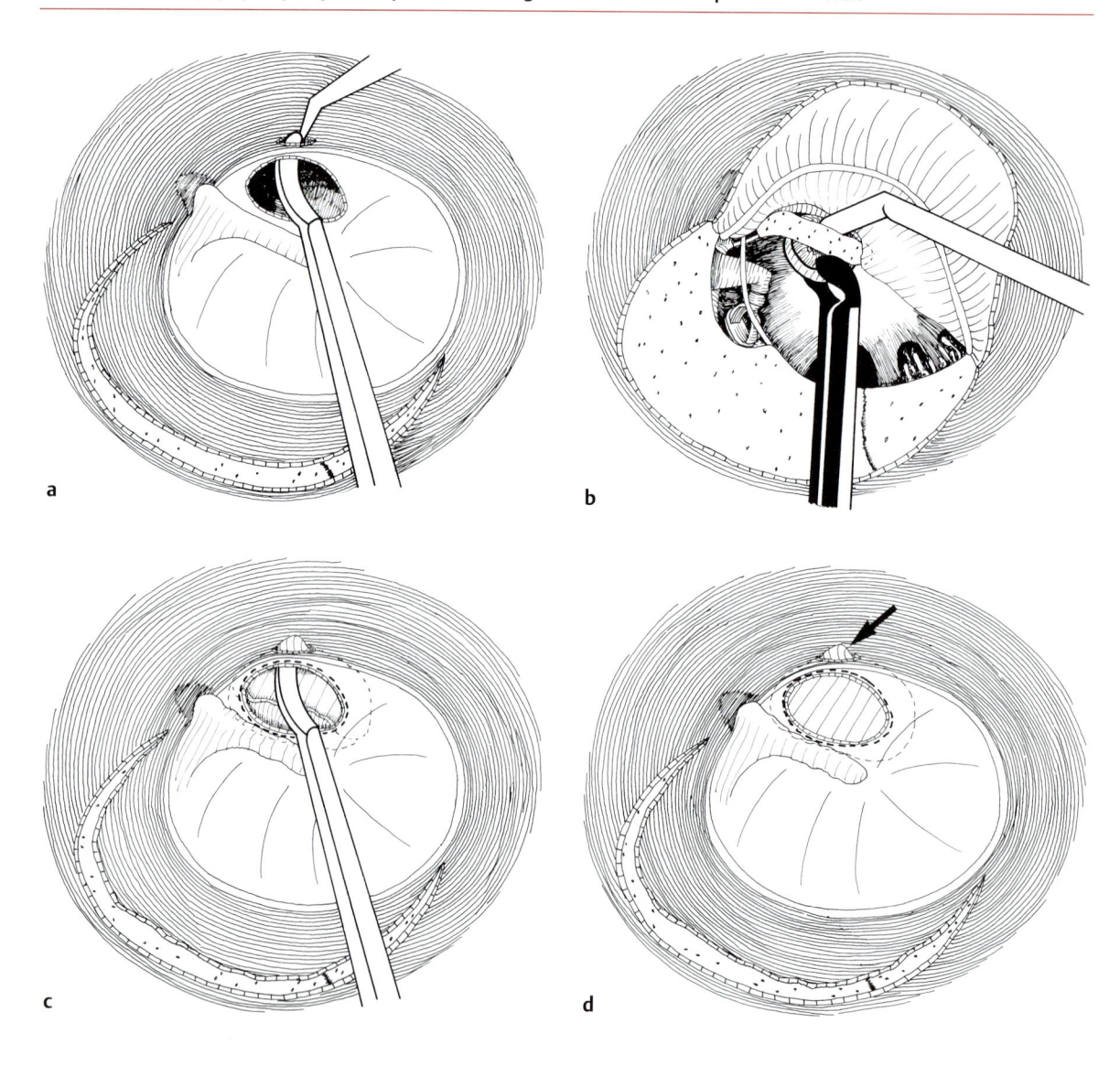

The methods for closure of the total and subtotal perforation with total cartilage island graft are thoroughly described and illustrated in Chapter 17; in this chapter, therefore, only one example of reconstruction of subtotal or total perforation will be shown.

The edges of the perforation are cleaned, a large circumferential incision is made, and a large tympanomeatal flap is elevated (**Fig. 21.12a, b**). A large malleus flap is elevated as well. The cartilage island graft of three-quarters thickness is placed into the tympanic cavity and is suspended by the perichondrium flaps, placed mostly onto the ear canal bone (**Fig. 21.12b–d**).

Cartilage Graft in Type 1 Tympanoplasty— A Modification without Perichondrium Flaps

Recently Ben Gamra et al. (2008) published a modification of the technique described here, placing a tragal or conchal full-thickness graft under the eardrum. The cartilage was covered with the perichondrium on the outer side, in contact with the undersurface of the eardrum. The graft is larger than the size of the perforation, but it does not have a perichondrium flap. The authors used this method in 90 patients for closure of posterior (49 ears), central (14 ears), inferior (10 ears), and anterior (10 ears) perforations, and 7 subtotal perforations. The cartilage–perichondrium graft is placed under the malleus handle and immediately adjacent to the incus to reconstruct the entire tympanic membrane. To achieve the closure of the perforation, fragments of perichondrium are placed on the graft to fill the space between the perforation borders and the cartilage—a kind of small free flap.

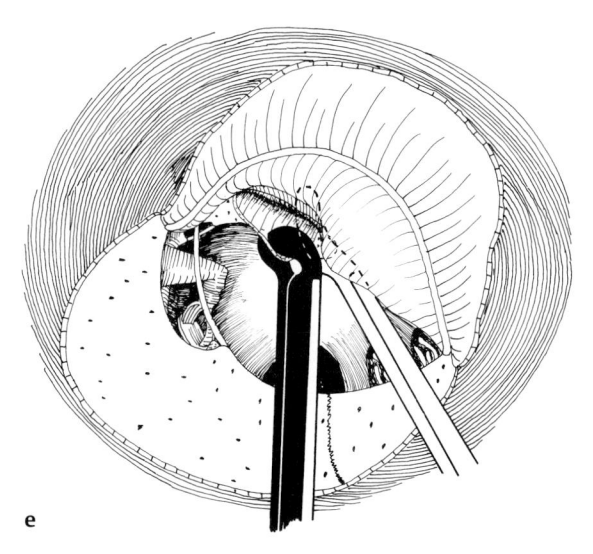

Fig. 21.7a–f Closure of an anterior perforation with underlay cartilage island graft by posterior tympanotomy.

a The edge of the anterior perforation is cleaned and mucosa is removed from the undersurface of the eardrum remnant. With a hook, a perforation is made anterior to the fibrous annulus. Through the anterior perforation, the anterior fibrous annulus is subluxated and a connection is made to the ear canal. An incision is made for posterior tympanotomy.

b The posterior tympanomeatal flap is elevated and the epithelium with the attached lamina propria on both sides of the malleus handle is elevated. The connection of the eardrum to the umbo is untouched. The cartilage island graft is placed into the anterior part of the tympanic cavity.

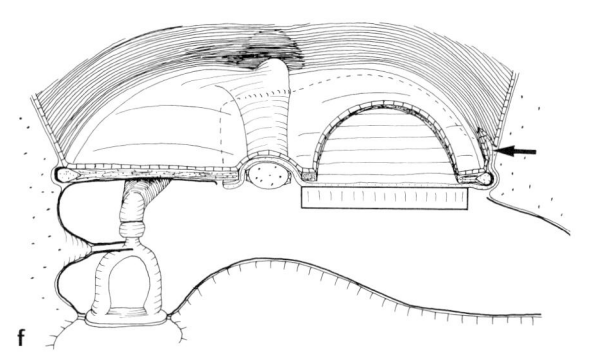

c Using a curved elevator, the anterior perichondrium flap is pushed though the hole into the ear canal, effectively suspending the cartilage disk.

d The half-thickness cartilage island graft is adapted to the perforation. The remaining perichondrium is folded out under the eardrum.

e The posterior perichondrium flap is pulled over the malleus handle. The tympanomeatal flap will be replaced.

f Side view of grafting of the anterior perforation with underlay cartilage island graft. The anterior perichondrium flap is pulled into the ear canal (arrow), the posterior flap is placed onto the malleus handle, both suspending the cartilage disk.

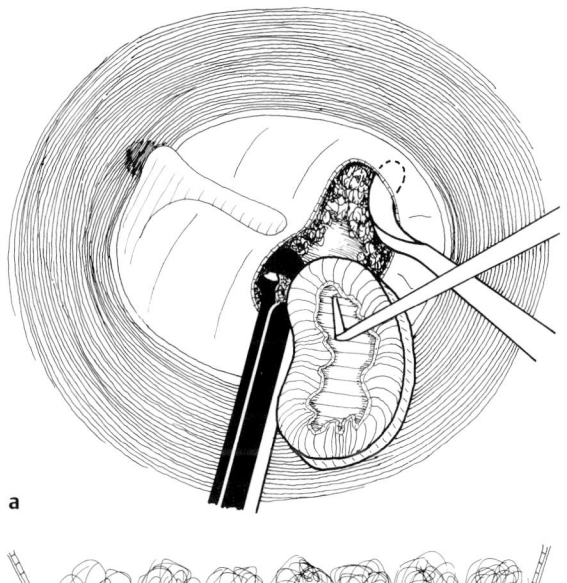

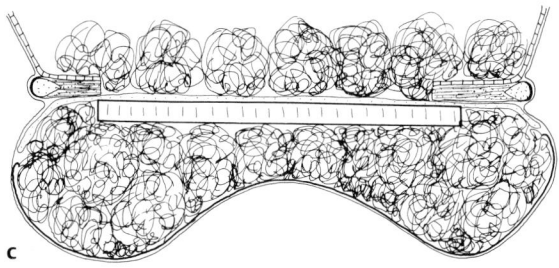

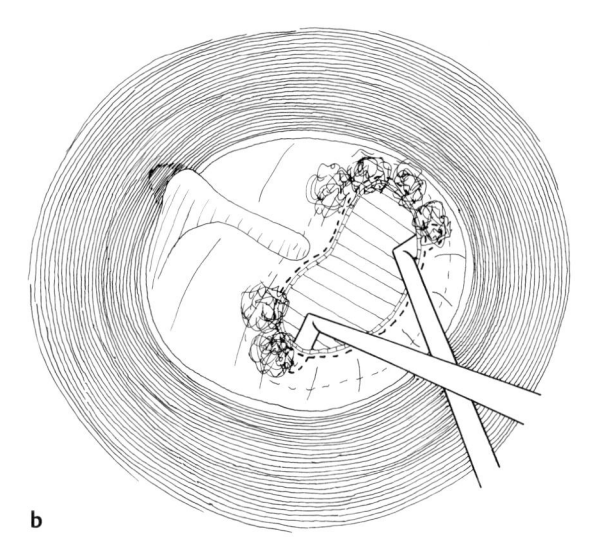

Fig. 21.8a–c Transmeatal closure of inferior perforation with underlay cartilage island graft without tympanotomy.

a The edges of the perforation are cleaned. The mucosa under the eardrum remnant is elevated or scarified and partly removed, using a curved elevator and curved cup forceps. The inferior half of the tympanic cavity is then filled with Gelfoam balls and the half-thickness cartilage island graft is ready to be positioned under the edge of the perforation.

b The slightly larger cartilage disk is positioned under the edges of the perforation and the perichondrium flaps are folded out. The edges of the perforation are covered with Gelfoam balls, fixing the graft.

c Side view of the inferior perforation closed with the underlay half-thickness cartilage island graft. Gelfoam balls support the graft on both sides.

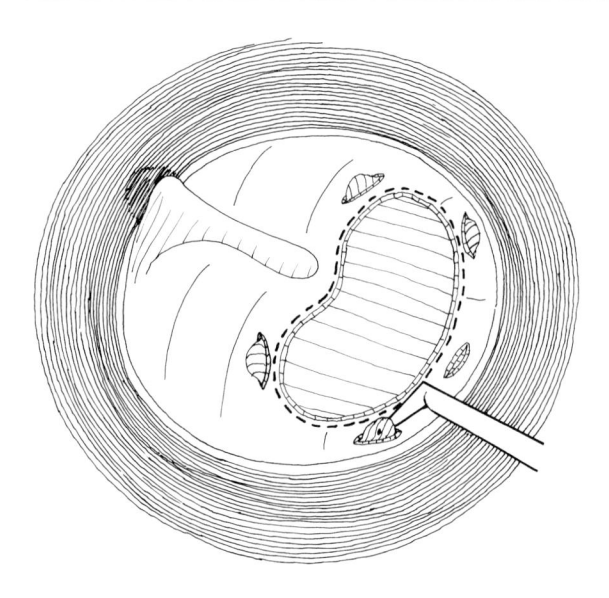

Fig. 21.9 Fixation of the underlay cartilage island graft with Gerlach technique in transmeatal closure of an inferior perforation. Epithelium is removed from the edge of the perforation. Using a sickle knife, five holes are made through the eardrum remnant 0.5 mm peripherally to the edge of the perforation. After positioning of the cartilage disk, the edges of the perichondrium flap are pulled into the holes using a small hook, suspending the half-thickness cartilage disk.

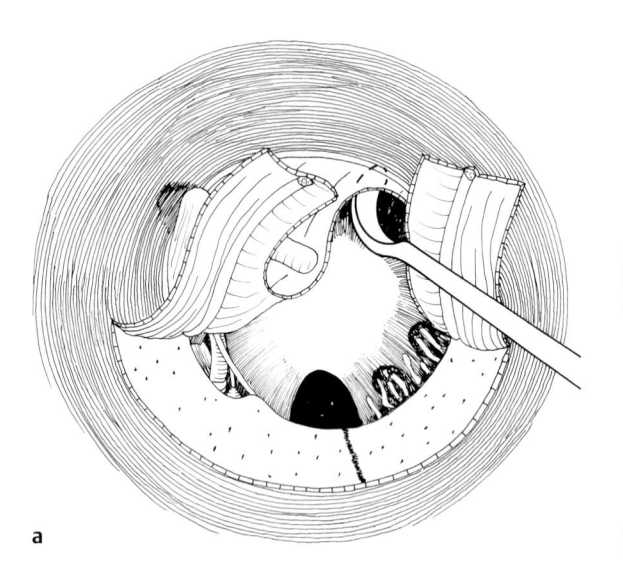

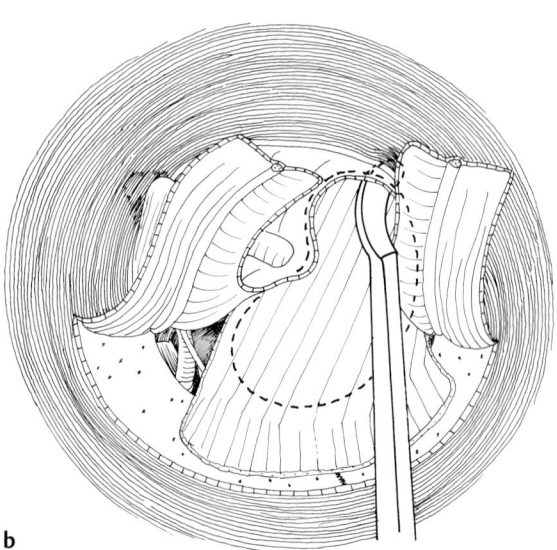

Fig. 21.10a–c Swing-door technique in grafting of an inferior perforation with underlay cartilage island graft.
a After cleaning of the edges of the perforation and scarification of the mucosa around the perforation, a circumferential incision is made between the 11-o'clock and 6-o'clock positions and a radial incision at the 8-o'clock position is made, and two tympanomeatal flaps are elevated.
b The half-thickness cartilage island graft is positioned under the edge of the perforation and the perichondrium flaps are folded out. The inferior and posterior perichondrium flaps are folded out onto the bone of the ear canal. The anterior fibrous annulus may be slightly elevated and the edge of the anterior perichondrium pushed between the bony annulus and the fibrous annulus.
c The tympanomeatal flaps are replaced. The perichondrium flaps safely suspend the cartilage graft. A small perichondrium flap is pushed under the slightly elevated anterior fibrous annulus (arrow).

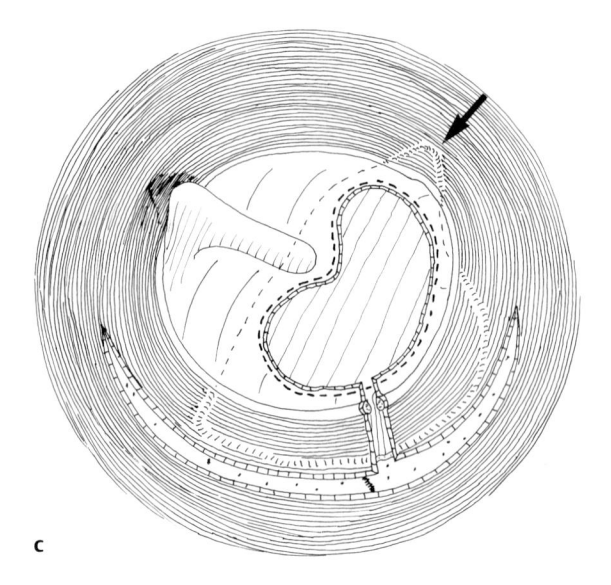

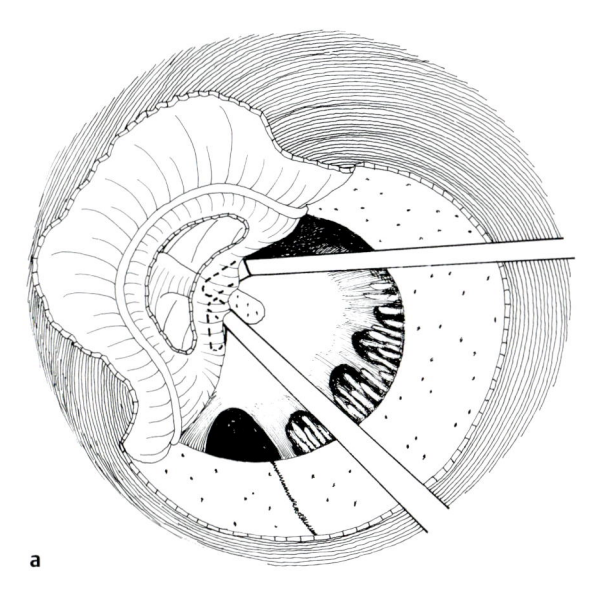

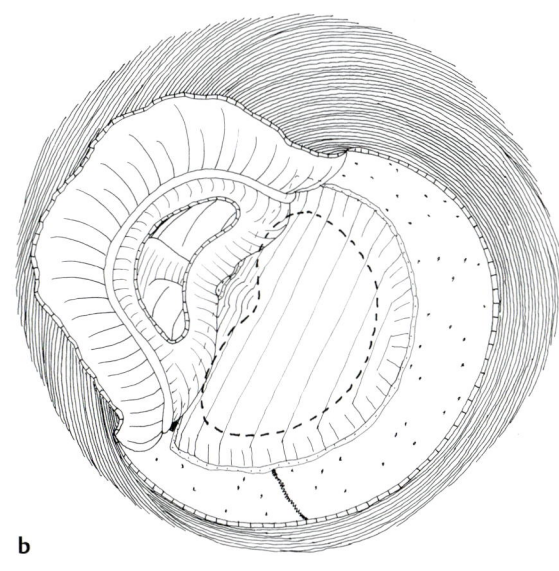

Fig. 21.11a–c Large tympanomeatal flap technique with application of cartilage island graft in a large inferior perforation.
a After cleaning of the edges of the perforation and scarification of the mucosa under the perforation, a circumferential incision is made and elevation of the tympanomeatal flap is performed. The umbo is also denuded.
b The half-thickness cartilage island graft is placed into the tympanic cavity and the perichondrium flap is folded out onto the ear canal bone, onto the umbo, and under the superior eardrum.
c The tympanomeatal flap is replaced.

Results of Surgery with the Island Graft

El-Hennawi (2001) reported on a pediatric series of 30 children with closure of 6 subtotal, 8 anterior, 10 central (inferior), and 6 posterior perforations. All children were treated with the Dornhoffer cartilage island graft (Chapter 17) via the retroauricular approach and elevation of the posterior ear canal skin and of the eardrum. The same graft is placed as an underlay graft, unrelated to the size and location of the perforation. The graft is supported with Gelfoam.

At the one-year follow-up, the take rate was 86.6%, regardless of the site and type of perforation and regardless of the status of the operated ear. Improvement of the air conduction at the one-year follow-up of more than 10 dB was found in 90% of children.

At the mean follow up of 2 years (range 3 months–6 years), Ben Gamra et al. (2008) achieved good **anatomical results** in 88 ears out of 90 (97.7%), compared with 281 ears (out of 290) with fascia (96.9%), ($p > 0.05$).

Hearing results. Mean air conduction gain was 21 ± 11 dB in the cartilage group, and 20 ± 11 dB in the fascia group.

Postoperative average air–bone gap was 16 ± 10 dB in the cartilage group, and 18 ± 7 dB in the fascia group.

Closure of the air–bone gap was 48.8% in cartilage, and 16.2% in fascia.

The **anatomical and functional** results were slightly better than in the fascia group.

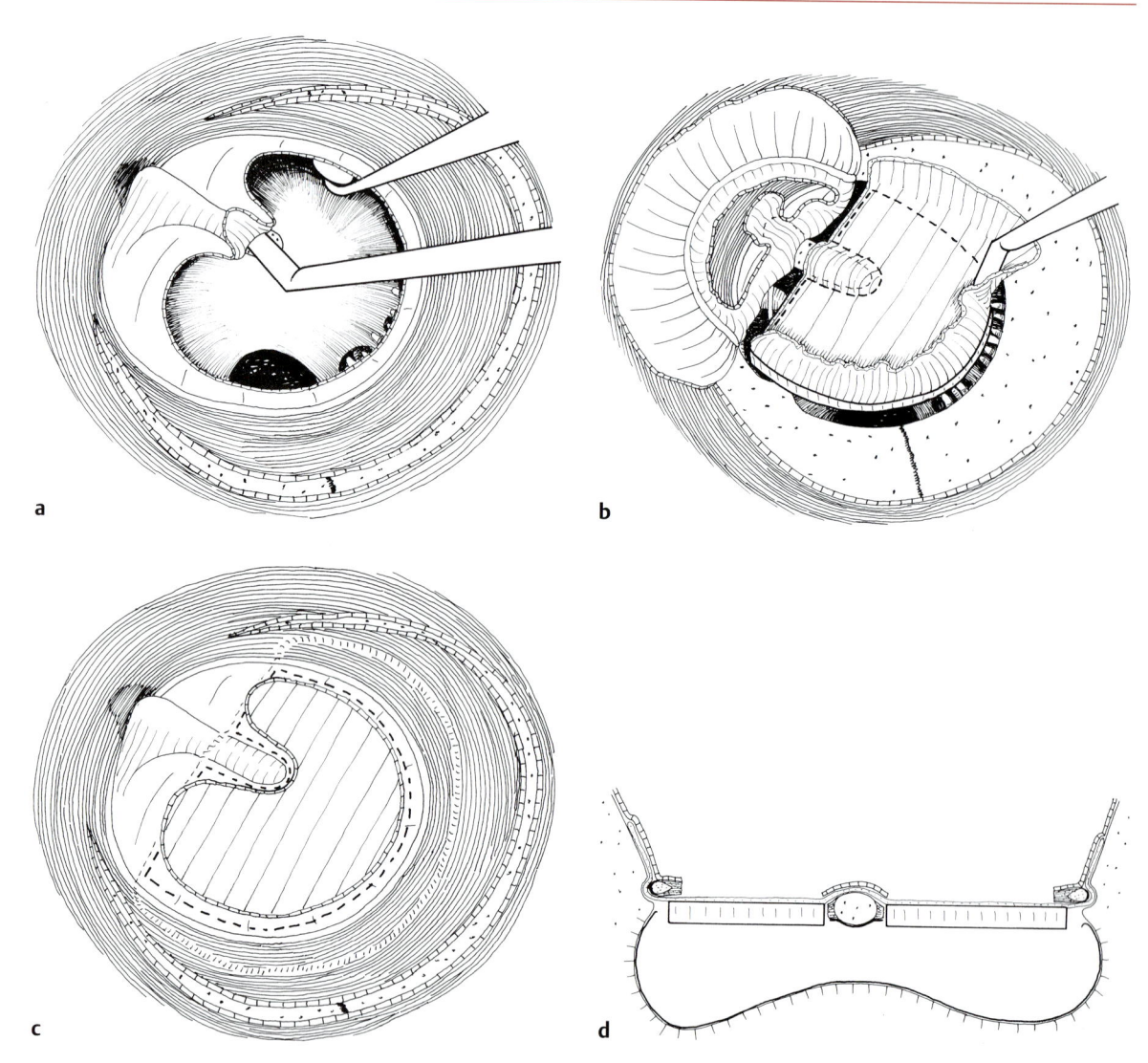

Fig. 21.12a–d Underlay cartilage island graft in a subtotal perforation with intact ossicular chain.

a The edges of the perforation are cleaned, the mucosa from the under surface eardrum remnant is scarified, a large circumferential incision between the 11-o'clock and 1-o'clock positions is made, and the umbo is cleaned by elevating a small flap.

b The tympanomeatal flap and the malleus flap are elevated. A U-shaped cut-out is made in the cartilage disk to accommodate the inferior half of the malleus handle. The cartilage island graft is positioned into the tympanic cavity. The perichondrium from the wedge covers the malleus handle; the superior perichondrium flap is placed under the eardrum, the anterior flap onto the bone.

c The posterior perichondrium flap is placed onto the ear canal bone and the malleus flap and the tympanomeatal flap are replaced.

d Side view of the underlay cartilage island graft at the level of the umbo. The perichondrium covers the malleus handle and the ear canal bone all the way around.

Comparison with Fascia

Sapci et al. (2006), in 25 patients, closed dry inferior or dry subtotal perforations with an underlay cartilage–perichondrium composite island graft tympanoplasty. In the other, identical group of 25 patients the perforations were closed with underlay, temporalis fascia graft. In both groups the ossicular chain was intact. The mean age was 30 years, range 11–63 years. At the end of the first year of observation, graft survival was 92% in the cartilage group and 85% in the fascia group, which is not significant because of the small number of patients. In comparison with a steady increase of hearing in the cartilage group, hearing levels remained unchanged after the 6 months in the fascia group. However, the two methods did not differ significantly in terms of hearing improvement.

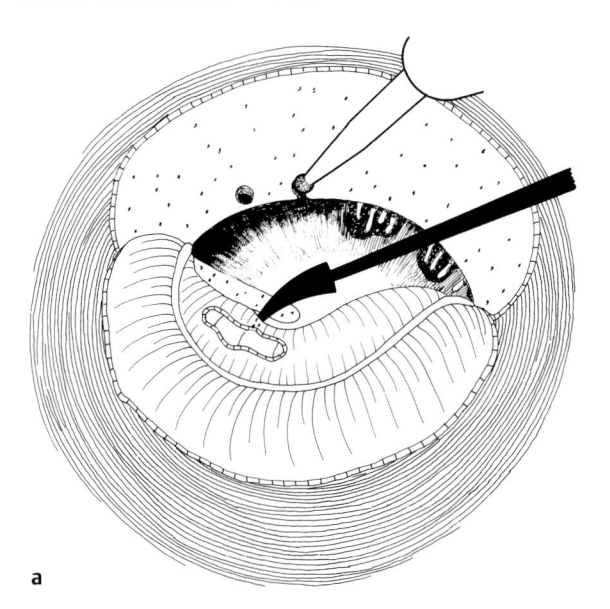

Fig. 21.13a, b Drilling a hole or a groove into the bony annulus to suspend the perichondrium flap in an anterior perforation.
a An anterior tympanomeatal flap is elevated together with the anterior half of the eardrum and the anterior perforation. The epithelium of the malleus handle is elevated and partly separated from the malleus handle, making a fissure for the posterior perichondrium flap. Using a small diamond drill, a hole is drilled through the bony annulus and a groove is made in the bony annulus.

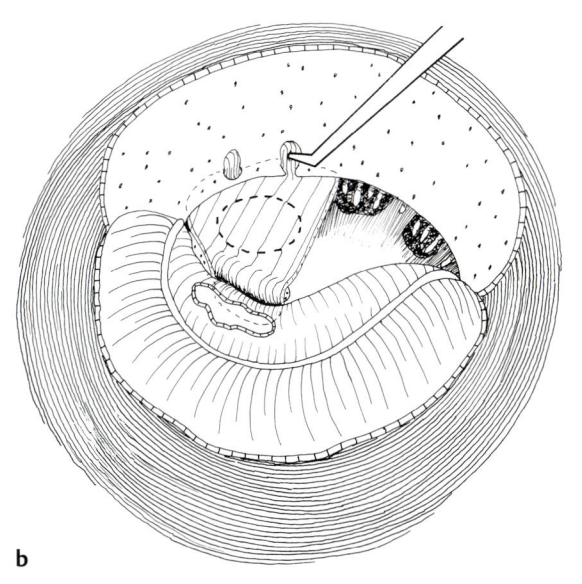

b The island cartilage graft is placed in the tympanic cavity with the anterior perichondrium flap under the bony annulus. The posterior perichondrium flap is placed onto the malleus handle and pushed through the fissure into the tympanic cavity. Using a small hook, the edge of the perichondrium is pulled thought the superior hole and into the inferior groove.

Author's Comments and Recommendations

No results and no particular methods for closure of the anterior and inferior perforations with cartilage island graft have yet been published, but several surgeons using underlay technique with fascia and/or perichondrium will also use cartilage–perichondrium composite island grafts if they feel it necessary.

On the basis of the methods used for fascia and perichondrium, and of my own experience with cartilage tympanoplasty, I have elaborated the methods illustrated and propose their use for the underlay cartilage–perichondrium composite island graft.

It is to be hoped that the methods will be used and the results compared with those of comparable series treated with fascia or perichondrium grafting. Comparison of hearing in comparable series of subtotal or smaller perforations, closed with either a half-thickness graft or a full thickness cartilage island graft, is also necessary.

Drilling a Hole or a Groove into the Bony Annulus

Underlay technique is popular, but still the fixation of the perichondrium to the undersurface of the eardrum remnant or under the bony annulus may not always be easy or effective. Some surgeons remove the mucous membrane, some scarify it, some use the Gerlach technique (**Fig. 21.9**) or its modification by Primrose and Kerr (1986) (**Fig. 21.7a–d**).

Some surgeons use Gelfoam to support the flap, others do not use Gelfoam in the tympanic cavity at all. Most surgeons just place the perichondrium (or the fascia) under the eardrum remnant.

In some special situations in closure of the anterior perforation I have drilled a hole or a small groove and with a small hook pulled the edge of the perichondrium through the hole or into the groove (**Fig. 21.13a, b**), with convincing fixation of the perichondrium to the undersurface of the eardrum and bony annulus.

The same technique can be used in the inferior perforation and in the total perforation as well.

Modifications of the Techniques

We must expect that in the future more modifications of the techniques may appear, especially with regard to the size and thickness of the graft in relation to the size of the perforation, but also in the use of a cartilage disk with the perichondrium on one side or on both sides, or of a "naked " cartilage disk without perichondrium. Additionally, a small or large perichondrium flap or no flap may be used, as found in the graft of Ben Gamra et al (2008). In this technique the grafts were larger than the perforations, but without a perichondrium flap. The advantage of the perichondrium flap is the complete closure along the edge of the perforation and the edge of the cartilage graft. Ben Gamra placed small pieces of perichondrium to fill the space between the perforation borders and cartilage. However the anatomical and functional results were good.

References

El-Hennawi DM. Cartilage perichondrium composite graft (CPCG) in paediatric tympanoplasty. Int J Pediatr Otorhinolaryngol 2001; 59:1–5.

Gamra OB, Mbarek C, Khammassi K, . Cartilage graft in type I tympanoplasty: audiological and otological outcome. Eur Arch Otorhinolaryngol 2008;265:739–742.

Gerlach H. Die Stepp-Plastik zur Erhaltung der Trommelfellebene. [Stepp method for the conservation of the tympanic membrane level] Arch Klin Exp Ohren Nasen Kehlkopfheilkd 1972;202: 662–666.

Gerlach H. Unsere Erfahrungen mit der Stepp-Plastik bei tympanoplastischen Operationen. [Experience with the quilt-plasty in tympanoplastic operations (author's transl.)] Laryngol Rhinol Otol 1975;54:196–197.

Jung TTK, Park SK. Mediolateral graft tympanoplasty for anterior or subtotal tympanic membrane perforation. Otolaryngol Head Neck Surg 2005;132:532–536.

Potsic WP, Winawer MR, Marsch RR. Tympanoplasty for the anterior-superior perforation in children. Am J Otol 1996;17:115–118.

Primrose WJ, Kerr AG. The anterior marginal perforation. Clin Otolaryngol 1986;11:175–176.

Sapci T, Almac S, Usta C, Karavus A, Mercangoz E, Evcimik MF. Comparison between tympanoplasties with cartilage-perichondrium composite graft and temporal fascia graft in terms of hearing levels and healing. [In Turkish] Kulak Burun Bogaz Ihtis Derg 2006;16:255–260.

Schraff S, Dash N, Strasnick B. "Window shade" tympanoplasty for anterior marginal perforations. Laryngoscope 2005;115: 1655–1659.

Tos M. Manual of Middle Ear Surgery. Vol. 1. Approaches, Myringoplasty, Ossiculoplasty and Typanoplasty. New York, Stuttgart: Thieme; 1993

22 In-lay Underlay Tympanoplasty Techniques with Cartilage–Perichondrium Composite Island Graft

Definition

The in-lay underlay composite graft consists of a cartilage disk and a relatively large perichondrium flap (**Fig. 22.1**). The cartilage disk is placed into the perforation and the perichondrium flap is placed under the eardrum remnant (**Fig. 22.2**).

The difference from the in-lay on-lay graft (Chapter 24) is the position of the perichondrium flap: in the in-lay on-lay method the perichondrium is placed onto the denuded eardrum remnant; in the in-lay underlay technique the graft is positioned under the eardrum remnant.

The size and shape of the cartilage disk are determined by the size and shape of the perforation. This is the case in both techniques, but the perichondrium flap is larger in the in-lay underlay technique than in the in-lay on-lay technique.

Comparing the in-lay underlay technique with the underlay technique (Chapter 21), the cartilage disk is larger than the perforation in the underlay technique and is placed on the inner side (tympanic side) of the perichondrium (see **Figs. 21.6 d, 21.7 f, 21.12 d**). In the in-lay underlay technique the cartilage disk is placed into the perforation, and protrudes into the ear canal. The size and the shape of the cartilage disk are the same as those of the perforation.

The thickness of the graft may vary from the full-thickness graft to the one-third thickness graft, similarly to the underlay composite grafts (see **Fig. 21.1**). In the in-lay underlay techniques the most appropriate thickness of the cartilage disk is that of a half-thickness graft, in particular for minor and middle-sized perforations. For large perforations with poor tubal function the three-quarters and full-thickness grafts are appropriate.

The purpose of placing an in-lay underlay graft is to fixate and stabilize the graft by means of the lamina propria from the border of the perforation. The firm fixation of the cartilage disk within the perforation is an advantage over the underlay graft, which sometimes may fall into the tympanic cavity

There are no publications on the methods or on the results of in-lay underlay techniques. The drawings presented here are my own, made exclusively for this chapter.

Harvesting and Shaping of the Graft

The graft is taken from the tragus (see **Fig. 3.21**), or from the concha (see **Fig. 3.26**). The perichondrium is removed from the convex side of the graft. The perichondrium from the concave side is cleaned and acts as a perichondrium flap. A crucial step in in-lay technique is accurate measurement of the dimensions of the perforation.

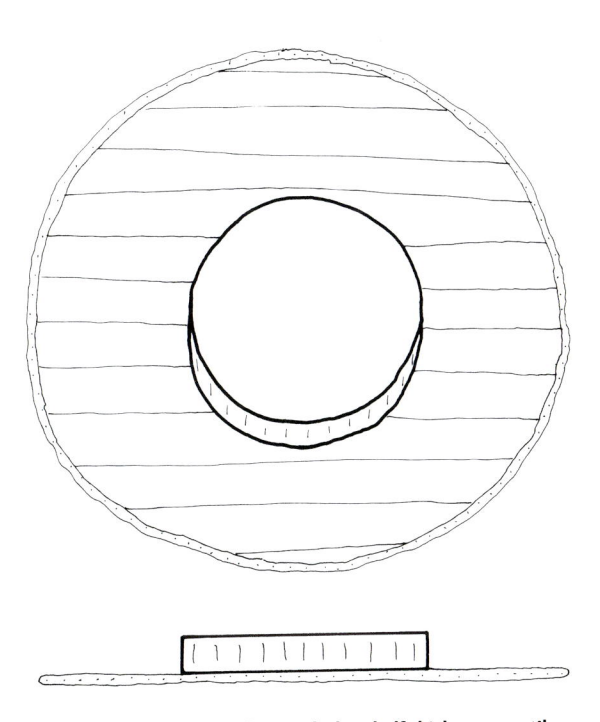

Fig. 22.1 The round in-lay underlay half-thickness cartilage perichondrium composite graft with a relatively large perichondrium flap.

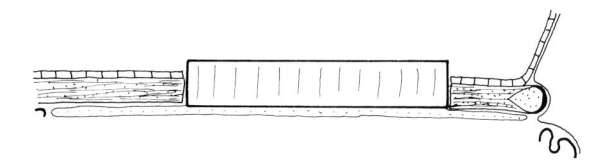

Fig. 22.2 In-lay underlay composite island graft as positioned in the eardrum perforation. The cartilage disk lies within the edges of the perforation, and the perichondrium lies under the eardrum remnant.

Indications for In-lay Underlay Technique

The technique I present here is new and there are no previous publications on the method itself or on the results. This method differs from the classic underlay technique in the placement of the cartilage disk from the tympanic cavity up and into the perforation, even with some protrusion of the cartilage disk into the ear canal.

In principle, the in-lay underlay technique could be used in the same indications as the underlay technique with cartilage–perichondrium composite graft. Clear indications are all ears with poor tubal function or negative preoperative Valsalva maneuver. Additionally, retractions, adhesive otitis media, atelectasis, recurrent surgery, cholesteatoma, and thick moist tympanic mucous membrane are conditions with a clear indication for cartilage–perichondrium composite graft and for the in-lay underlay technique, especially in minor and middle-sized perforations,

I consider that there are indications for use of this method with half-thickness or even thinner cartilage grafts for small and medium-sized perforations as sequelae of noncholesteatomatous disease and normal tubal function.

Although there are no published results for in-lay underlay island technique, other methods, such as cartilage tympanoplasty using palisades, have shown significantly better anatomical and functional results than fascia in pediatric cholesteatoma (Andersen et al. 2004). Kazikdas et al. (2007) found a clear tendency, but not statistical significance, to better results in cartilage tympanoplasty with cartilage strips than with fascia (Chapter 7) and advocate more liberal application of cartilage methods in less severe cases.

The In-lay Underlay Techniques

The in-lay underlay technique can be used in anterior, inferior, posterior, subtotal, and even total perforations. The cartilage disk may be of full thickness, of three-quarters thickness, of half thickness, or of quarter thickness. In small perforations, half or one-third thickness is enough; in large perforations and poor tubal function, the full-thickness graft is used.

Anterior Perforation

As mentioned in Chapter 21 and Chapter 24, the anterior perforation can be closed by various methods of elevation of the surrounding epithelium or by elevation of various tympanomeatal flaps.

Technique without Elevation of Tympanomeatal Flaps

After removal of the edges of the perforation and after scarification of the undersurface of the eardrum remnant (**Fig. 22.3a**), the anterior part of the tympanic cavity is filled with Gelfoam (**Fig. 22.3b**). The cartilage–perichondrium composite island graft is trimmed to the correct size and shape and placed onto the anterior perforation with the perichondrium flap folded out. The anterior part of the perichondrium graft is pushed under the eardrum remnant (**Fig. 22.3a**) Then the inferior and the superior parts of the perichondrium flap are pushed under the eardrum remnant (**Fig. 22.3b**) and finally the posterior flap is pushed under the malleus handle (**Fig. 22.3c**) There is a good chance for a rapid epithelialization and the cartilage disk may be solidly fixated.

Elevation of the Anterior Tympanomeatal Flap

The half-thickness island graft is trimmed and shaped. The anterior tympanomeatal flap is elevated together with the eardrum surrounding the anterior perforation. The undersurface of the eardrum and the malleus handle are scarified. A cartilage–perichondrium composite graft is placed under the eardrum remnant, under the posterior edge of the malleus handle and onto the bone of the ear canal (**Fig. 22.4a**). The tympanomeatal flap is replaced, exposing the protruding cartilage disk surrounded by the epithelium of the eardrum (**Fig. 22.4b**).

After the elevation of the tympanomeatal flap and the anterior eardrum remnant together with the perforation, the eardrum is separated and partly elevated from the malleus handle (**Fig. 22.4c**). The umbo remains connected to the eardrum. The cartilage–perichondrium graft covers the anterior part of the tympanic cavity. The posterior perichondrium flap is placed onto the ear canal bone and the anterior flap is pushed over the malleus handle into the posterior part of the tympanic cavity (**Fig. 22.4d**). The tympanomeatal flap is replaced (**Fig. 22.4e**), then a half-thickness cartilage disk is placed in the perforation. As shown in **Fig. 22.4f**, the posterior flap can be placed either under the malleus handle (1) or onto the malleus handle (2) after elevating the eardrum from the malleus handle.

Inferior Perforation

There are several ways to place an in-lay underlay cartilage–perichondrium composite graft and close an inferior perforation.

Transmeatal Closure without Tympanotomy

The edges of the perforation are cleaned of squamous epithelium and the undersurface of the eardrum around the perforation is scarified. The inferior part of the tympanic cavity is filled with Gelfoam balls and the shaped island graft with the perichondrium is placed onto the

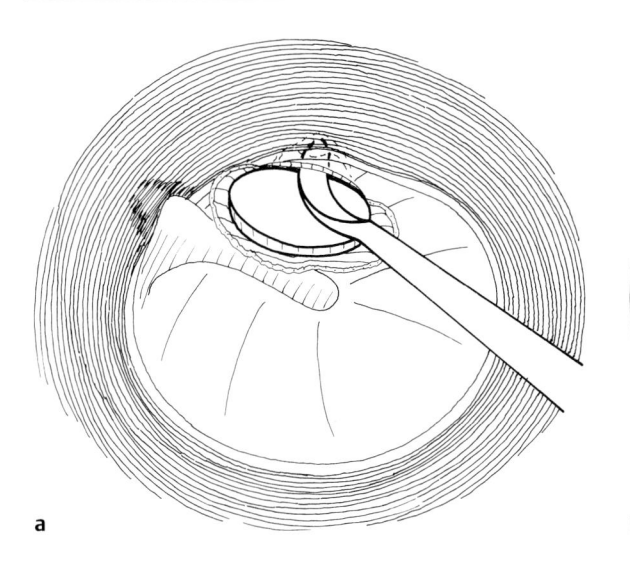

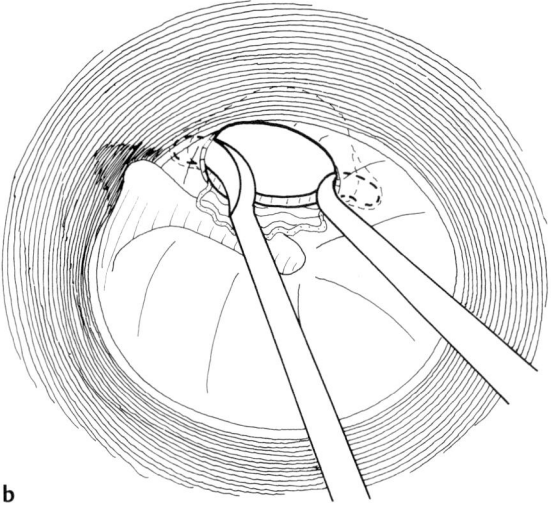

Fig. 22.3a–c Closure of an anterior perforation with the in-lay underlay technique, without elevation of tympanomeatal flaps.

a The edge of the perforation is removed. The anterior part of the tympanic cavity is filled with Gelfoam. The half-thickness composite graft with the perichondrium folded out is placed onto the perforation. The anterior perichondrium is pushed under the anterior eardrum remnant, using a curved rugine.

b The inferior and the superior parts of the perichondrium flap are pushed under the eardrum remnant.

c The last posterior part of the flap is pushed under the malleus handle. The cartilage disk is positioned in the perforation and the perichondrium flaps under the eardrum remnant.

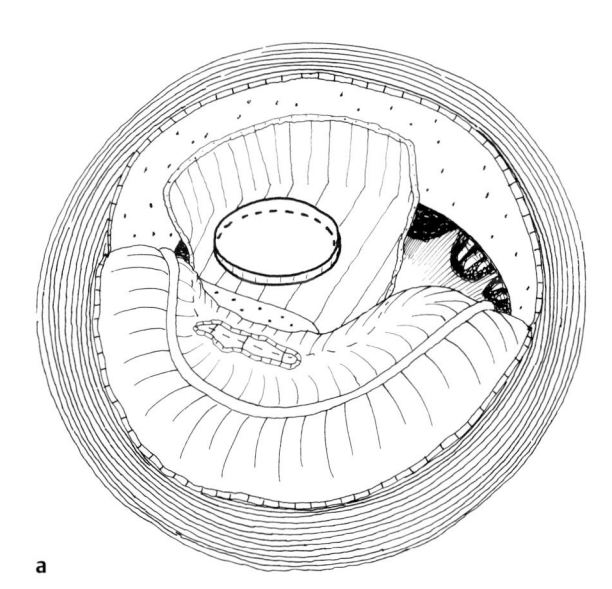

Fig. 22.4a–f Elevation of the tympanomeatal flap and the placement of the cartilage–perichondrium composite graft to cover an anterior perforation.

a The posterior perichondrium flap is placed onto the ear canal bone, and the anterior flap is placed under the malleus handle. Gelfoam balls support the graft.

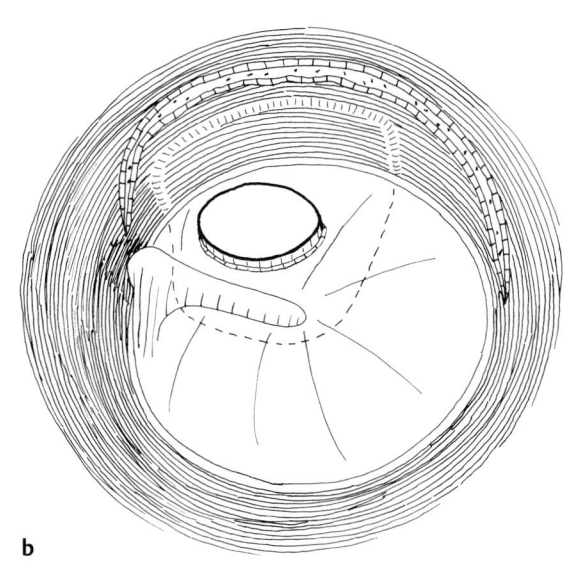

b The tympanomeatal flap is replaced; the edges of the perforation with the epithelium surround the cartilage disk.

Fig. 22.4c–f ▷

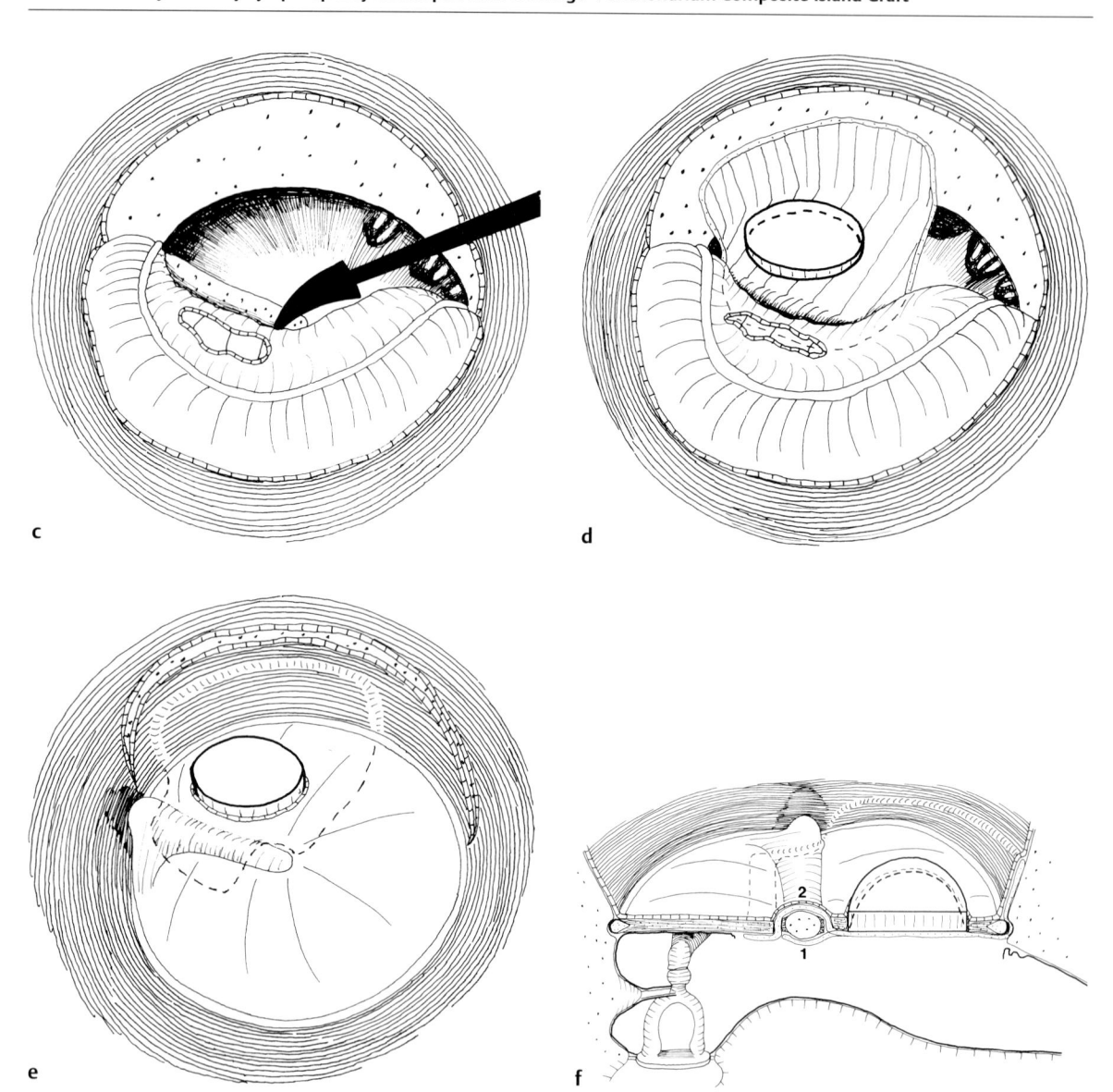

Fig. 22.4c–f

c Placement of the perichondrium flap onto the malleus handle. After elevation of the tympanomeatal flap, the eardrum is elevated from the malleus handle.

d The island graft is first placed into the anterior part of the tympanic cavity. The anterior perichondrium flap is placed onto the malleus handle and then pushed under the posterior eardrum.

e The tympanomeatal flap is replaced and the epithelium surrounds the cartilage disk.

f Side view with some perspective of two alternative placements of the posterior perichondrium flap. (1). The posterior perichondrium flap is placed under the malleus handle. (2). The posterior perichondrium flap is placed onto the malleus handle and under the posterior part of the eardrum.

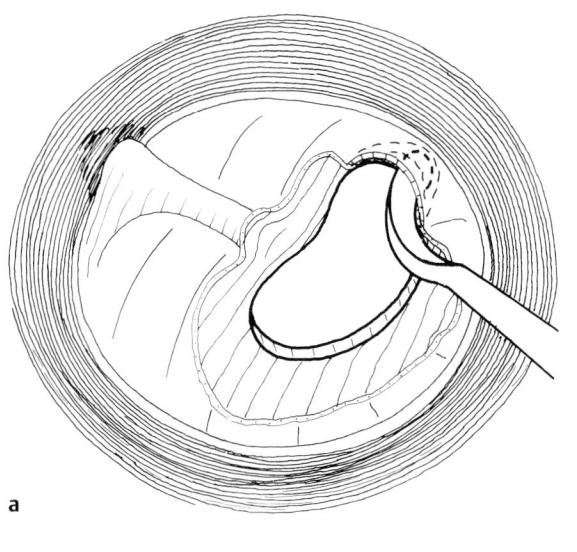

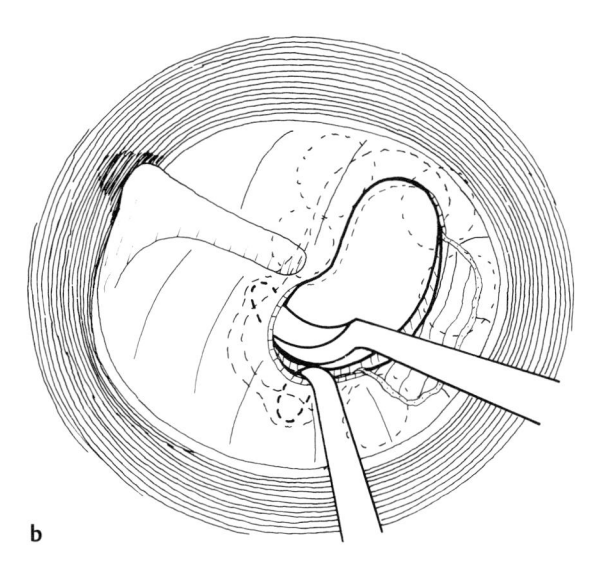

Fig. 22.5a–c In-lay underlay placement of the island graft to close an inferior perforation without tympanotomy.

a The edges of the perforation are cleaned and the mucosa under the eardrum is scarified. The inferior half of the tympanic cavity is filled with Gelfoam. The trimmed and shaped in-lay underlay cartilage–perichondrium graft is placed onto the perforation and the anterior part of the perichondrium flap is pushed under the eardrum remnant.
b The superior and posterior parts of the perichondrium flap are pushed under the eardrum remnant.
c All perichondrium flaps are under the eardrum and the cartilage disk is protruding out of the perforation and is surrounding by the epithelium of the eardrum remnant.

eardrum. Using a curved rugine, the anterior part of the perichondrium flap is pushed under the eardrum remnant (**Fig. 22.5a**). The superior and the posterior parts of the perichondrium flap are pushed under the eardrum (**Fig. 22.5b**) and finally all perichondrium is placed and folded out under the eardrum (**Fig. 22.5c**). The half-thickness cartilage disk is surrounded by the epithelium and the lamina propria of the edge of the perforation.

Swing-Door Technique with In-lay Underlay Graft

After removal of the edge of the inferior perforation and after scarification of the undersurface of the eardrum remnant, a circumferential incision and a radial incision are made at the 5-o'clock position and two tympanomeatal flaps are elevated, exposing the inferior part of the tympanic cavity. Gelfoam balls are placed into the inferior part of the cavity and then the cartilage–perichondrium composite graft is placed into the tympanic cavity. The anterior perichondrium flap (**Fig. 22.6a**) and then the entire flap are folded out. After replacement of the tympanomeatal flap, the eardrum epithelium surrounds the half-thickness cartilage disk, which protrudes slightly through the perforation (**Fig. 22.6b**).

Closure of the Inferior Perforation with the In-lay Underlay Composite Graft

A large tympanomeatal flap is elevated together with a short malleus handle flap. The edges of the perforation are scarified. The composite graft is placed into the tympanic cavity and the perichondrium flap is folded out over the bone of the ear canal. Superiorly, the flap is placed onto the malleus handle (**Fig. 22.7a**). After replacement of the tympanomeatal flap (**Fig. 22.7b**), the half-thickness cartilage disk is surrounded by the epithelium and protrudes slightly above the perforation.

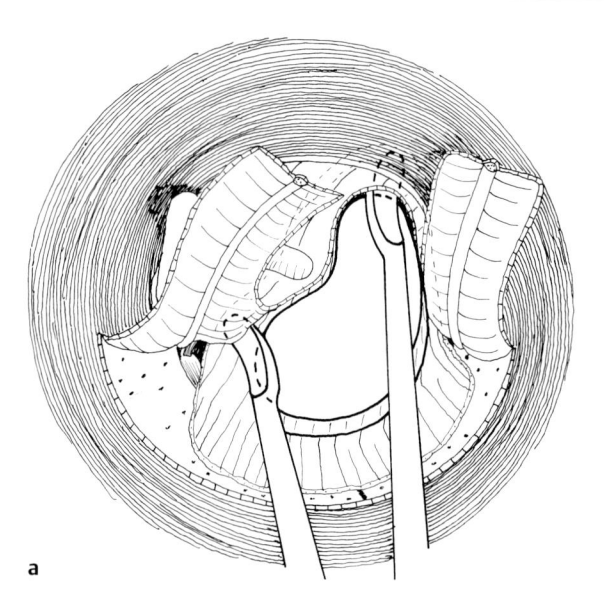

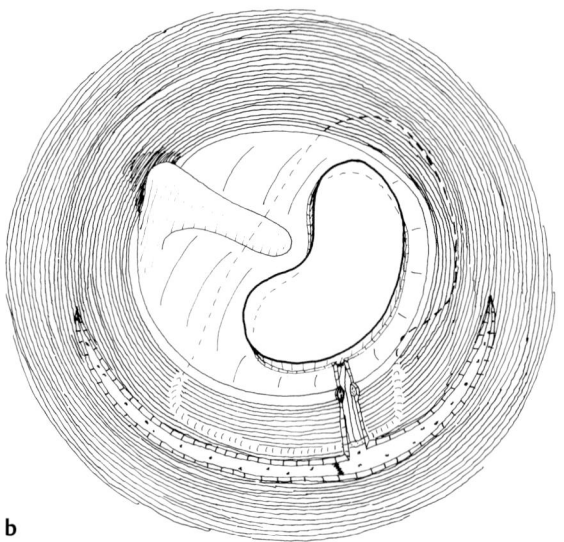

Fig. 22.6a, b Swing-door technique in closure of an inferior perforation with in-lay underlay technique.

a The edges of the perforation are cleaned and the undersurface of the eardrum is scarified. A circumferential and a radial incision are made and two tympanomeatal flaps are elevated. The tympanic cavity is filled with Gelfoam and the cartilage–perichondrium composite graft is placed into the tympanic cavity. The perichondrium flaps are folded out using a curved rugine.

b The tympanomeatal flaps are replaced and the eardrum epithelium surrounds the half-thickness cartilage disk, which protrudes slightly out of the perforation.

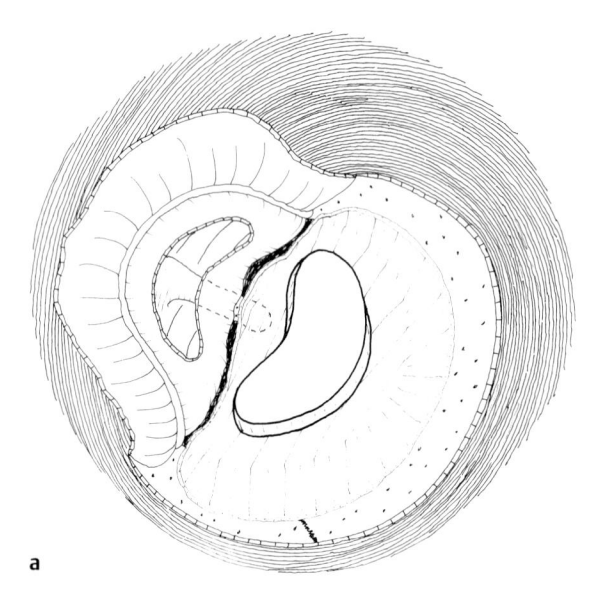

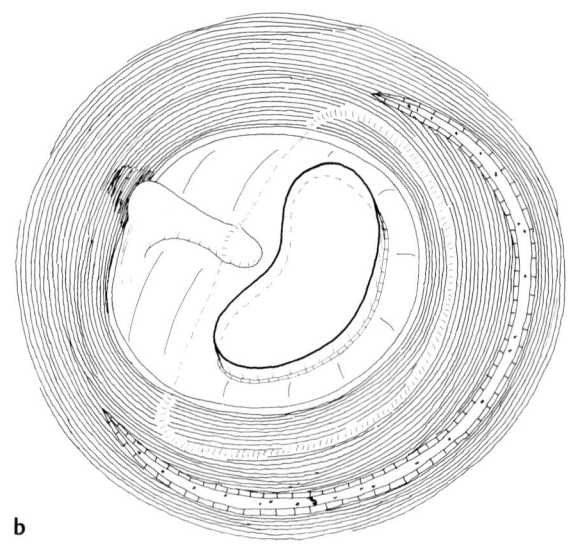

Fig. 22.7a, b Elevation of a large tympanomeatal flap to close a large inferior perforation with in-lay underlay composite graft.

a After cleaning of the edges of the perforation and scarification of the undersurface of the eardrum, a large tympanomeatal flap is elevated. Gelfoam balls are placed into the tympanic cavity. The island graft is placed into the cavity and the perichondrium flaps are folded out.

b The tympanomeatal flaps are replaced and the epithelium surrounds the half-thickness cartilage disk, which protrudes slightly out of the perforation.

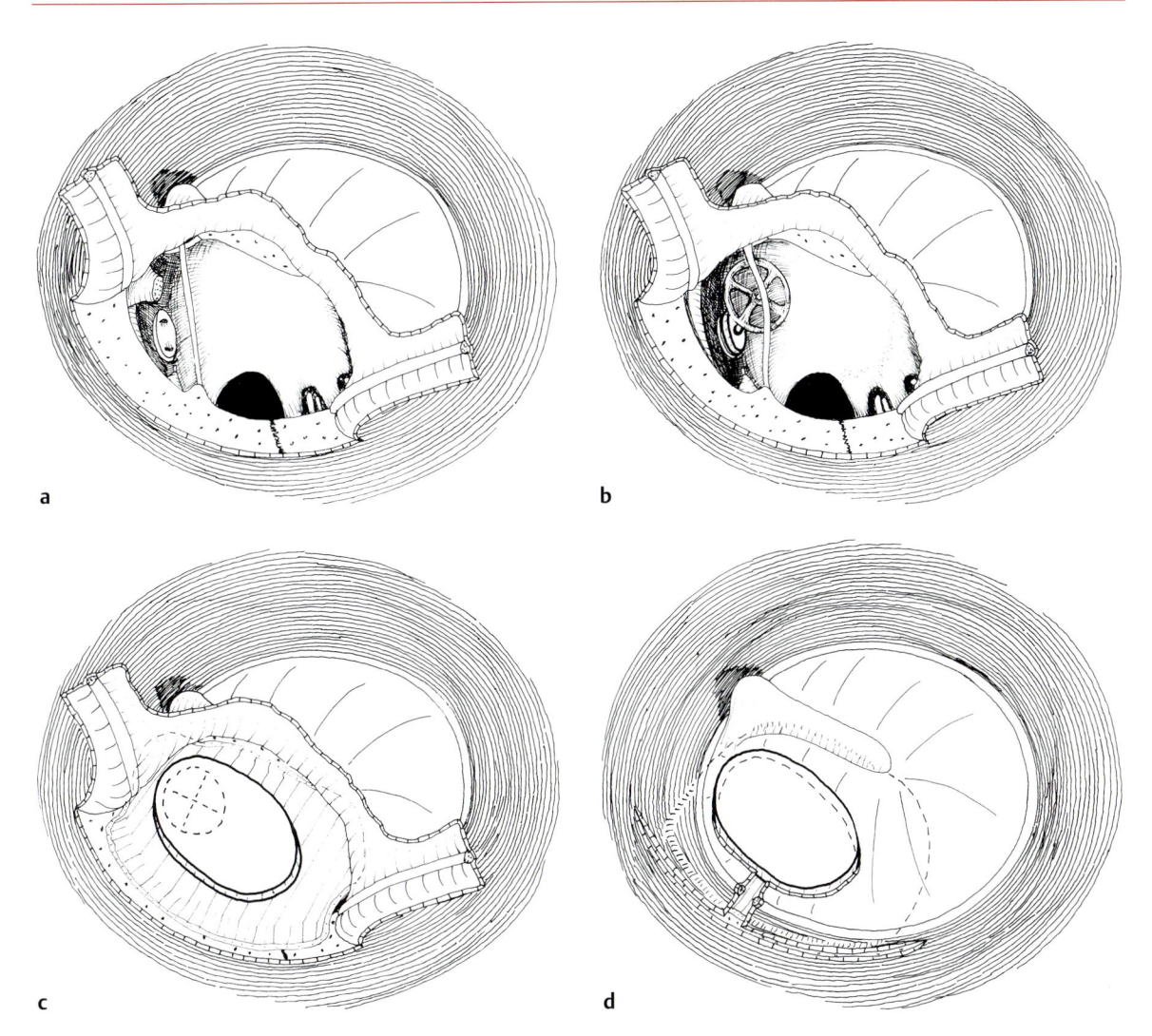

Fig. 22.8a–d In-lay underlay cartilage island graft in closure of a posterior perforation and tympanoplasty type 3.
a The swing-door technique is used and the defective incus will be removed.
b A Kurz titanium TORP is placed through a cartilage guide onto the footplate.
c The half-thickness composite graft is placed onto the head of the prosthesis and the perichondrium flap is folded out, onto the posterior border of the malleus handle and onto the posterior ear canal wall.
d The tympanomeatal flaps are replaced and the cartilage disk protrudes slightly out of the perforation.

Posterior Perforation

Although the underlay cartilage perichondrium graft, described in Chapter 15, usually functions well, the in-lay underlay grafting of a posterior perforation might be useful. After cleaning of the edges of the perforation and after scarification of the undersurface of the eardrum remnant, a swing-door incision is made and two tympanomeatal flaps are elevated (**Fig. 22.8a–d**). A defective incus is removed and a cartilage guide is made and placed onto the footplate. The Kurz titanium TORP is placed through the hole of the guide, onto the footplate (**Fig. 22.8b**). The composite island graft is placed onto the head of the prosthesis (**Fig. 22.8c**) and the perichondrium flap is folded out under the eardrum remnant and under the malleus handle. The tympanomeatal flaps are replaced and the half-thickness cartilage disk protrudes slightly out of the perforation. The epithelium surrounds the cartilage disk (**Fig. 22.8d**).

Subtotal Perforation

A large tympanomeatal flap is elevated together with the malleus flap. A cartilage–perichondrium graft is trimmed to the size of the perforation and a notch is made to accommodate the malleus handle. The graft is placed into the tympanic cavity and the perichondrium flaps are folded out over the bone of the ear canal (**Fig. 22.9a**). The

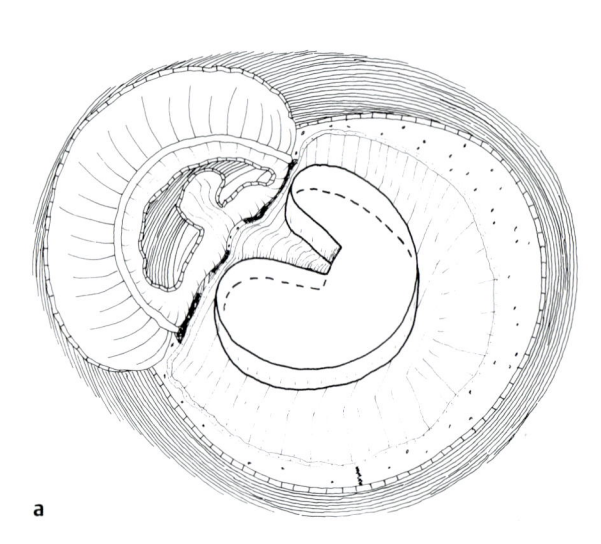

Fig. 22.9a, b Closing of the subtotal perforation with an in-lay underlay cartilage–perichondrium composite graft.
a A large tympanomeatal flap is elevated together with a malleus flap. The full-thickness graft with perichondrium is placed into the tympanic cavity. The perichondrium flaps are easily folded out onto the bone. A notch of cartilage is excised to accommodate the distal half of the malleus handle.
b The tympanomeatal flap is replaced. The epithelium is placed around the cartilage disk. The malleus flap is also replaced.

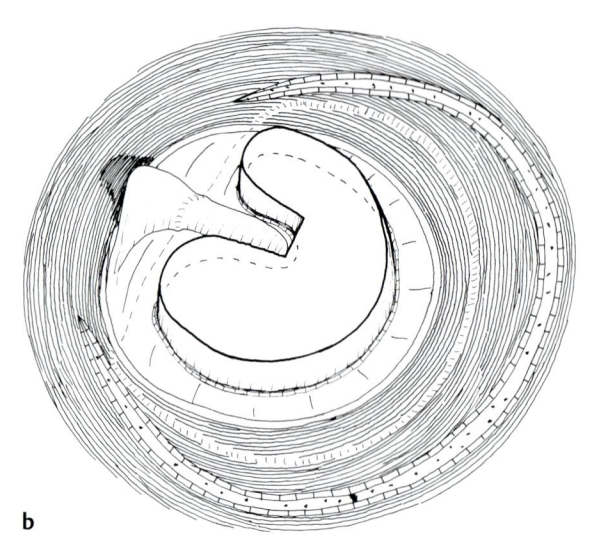

superior perichondrium flaps are placed under the superior eardrum remnant. The tympanomeatal flaps are replaced and the full-thickness cartilage disk will be epithelialized (**Fig. 22.9b**).

Results of Surgery

Since the method has not been published previously, there are no published results of the in-lay underlay method.

Author's Comments and Recommendations

In optimal cases, with exact trimming and shaping, the placement of the cartilage disk into the perforation may look like closure of a bottle with a cork.

A disk that is slightly too large may be pushed into the perforation; an evidently too large cartilage disk can be reduced, or used as an underlay island graft, placed with the perichondrium flap under the scarified mucous membrane.

A slightly too small disk will occupy almost as much of the area of the perforation as possible, but will have a slightly longer time for epithelialization than will an absolutely correctly sized disk. Fibrous tissue from the lamina may grow along the perichondrium to the cartilage disk and fill out the structural defect.

The advantage of the in-lay underlay graft is the expected firm fixation of the cartilage disk to the edges of the perforations and of the perichondrium flap to the undersurface of the eardrum remnant.

It is my hope that surgeons will use this method and compare it with the traditional underlay cartilage–perichondrium composite graft method and with fascia grafting.

References

Andersen J, Cayé-Thomasen P, Tos M. A comparison of cartilage palisades and fascia in tympanoplasty after surgery for sinus or tensa retraction cholesteatoma in children. Otol Neurotol 2004;25:856–863.

Kazikdas KC, Onal K, Boyraz I, Karabulut E. Palisade cartilage tympanoplasty for management of subtotal perforations: a comparison with the temporalis fascia technique. Eur Arch Otorhinolaryngol 2007;264:985–989.

23 On-lay Tympanoplasty Techniques with Cartilage–Perichondrium Composite Island Graft

Definition

The on-lay composite cartilage–perichondrium composite graft has a cartilage disk slightly larger than the perforation. The disk is covered on the convex side with the perichondrium, which continues as a perichondrium flap. After elevation or removal of the epithelium around the perforation, the graft can be placed onto the denuded lamina propria in two ways:

1. The first option may be called the "cartilage–perichondrium on-lay method." The graft is placed onto the denuded edge of the perforation, with the **cartilage** side turned onto the denuded lamina propria. The perichondrium covers the ear canal side of the disk, the edge of the cartilage disk, and the lamina propria. The replaced epithelium will cover all the perichondrium, up to the edge of the cartilage disk (**Fig. 23.1**).
2. The second option may be called the "perichondrium–cartilage on-lay method." The graft is placed with the **perichondrium** side turned onto the denuded lamina propria, in such a way that the cartilage disk is positioned onto the edge of the perforation. The side of the cartilage disk turned to the ear canal is not covered by the perichondrium, and the edges of the disk are not covered by the perichondrium. The replaced epithelium covers the perichondrium but not the cartilage (**Fig. 23.2**).

Desarda and Bhisegaonkar (2005) reported the results of surgery on 600 patients older than 14 years with various chronic middle ear diseases. The patients were treated during 1980–2000 with cartilage–perichondrium composite grafts at the K.E.M. Hospital, Pune, India. The surgical series were divided into 300 myringoplasties, 110 ossiculoplasties, 120 "osseous plasties" and 70 mastoid cavity obliterations.

In 300 treated myringoplasties, on-lay grafting was done in 172 patients and underlay grafting in 128 patients. The details of the method used were not described and the pathology was not further specified.

Apart from the cases of Desarda and Bhisegaonkar, there are no other publications on the on-lay cartilage tympanoplasty methods or results. It is therefore not possible to determine which of the two methods shown in **Figs. 23.1** and **23.2** is the better.

The cartilage–perichondrium on-lay method seems to be physiologically better, because all exposed cartilage is covered by the perichondrium and the epithelialization of the perichondrium may be faster than that of the naked cartilage (**Fig. 23.1**). The cartilage disk, turned to the perforation, will be covered by middle ear mucosa. This method requires exact measurement of the size of the cartilage disk, which should be slightly larger than the perforation. It is better to have too large than too small a

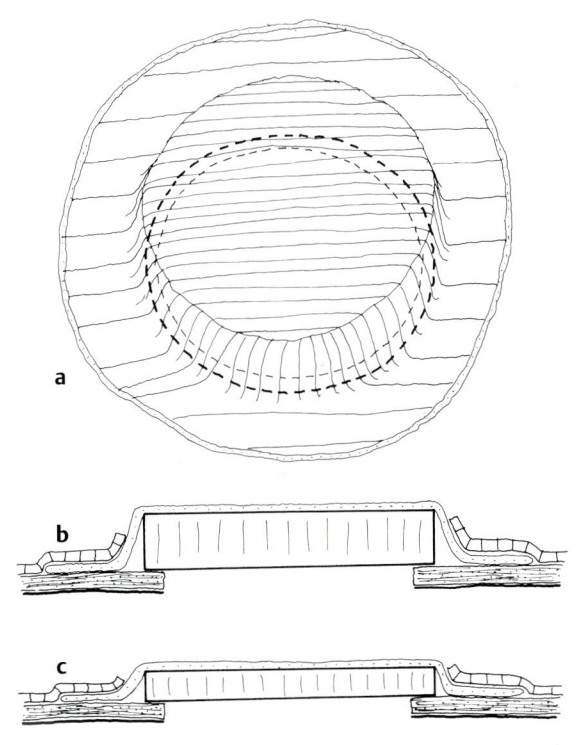

Fig. 23.1a–c The "cartilage–perichondrium on-lay method." The combined cartilage–perichondrium island graft is placed onto a perforation.
a The full-thickness cartilage disk (thick dotted circle) is placed onto the edge of the perforation (thin dotted circle). The perichondrium covers the cartilage disk and, as a flap, the edge of the disk and the denuded lamina propria.
b Side view of the reconstructed eardrum with full-thickness cartilage graft. The cartilage disk closes the perforation and is covered by the perichondrium. The replaced epithelial flaps cover the perichondrium up to the edge of the cartilage disk.
c The same as **b** with a half-thickness cartilage–perichondrium island graft.

Harvesting and Elaboration of the On-lay Island Graft

Because the on-lay techniques will most often be performed with the transcanal approach with fixed ear speculum (see **Figs. 3.1–3.4**), tragal cartilage will often be used. It is best to save the dome of the tragus and in one sweep to make a horizontal incision 2 mm medial to the tragus dome (see **Fig. 3.21a–d**) through the skin, tragal cartilage, and the perichondrium.

Harvesting of cartilage from the concha (see **Figs. 3.26** and **20.5a, b**), cymba, and scapha is also possible (see **Figs. 3.27–3.28**).

It is advisable to postpone further trimming until after final measurement of the size and the shape of the perforation.

Thinning, Trimming, and Shaping of On-lay Island Grafts

In on-lay techniques for closure of small and middle-sized perforations, the full-thickness composite grafts are not needed. The full-thickness cartilage graft with perichondrium can be thinned to half-thickness using the Kurz Precise Cartilage Knife (see **Fig. 3.36**) or the Hildmann cartilage clamp (see **Fig. 3.35**).

The thinned cartilage graft, covered with perichondrium on one side, is further trimmed to adapt the graft to the appropriate size and shape of the perforation. In small and middle-sized perforations, the size of the cartilage disk is measured with thin, angulated instruments such as a large hook or an incudostapedial knife. Small holes on the cartilage graft mark the border for trimming (**Fig. 23.3a**) and the superfluous cartilage is removed using a round knife. The extent of the perichondrium flap may also be trimmed.

To avoid possible curling of a thinned cartilage disk covered with the perichondrium, four gentle incisions are made in the perichondrium with a scalpel (**Fig. 23.3b**). It seems that curling will not occur in a composite graft because the perichondrium flap fixates the cartilage disk, but knowledge of this phenomenon is very inadequate.

Indications for Surgery

Closure of small and middle-sized anterior, posterior, and inferior perforations with half-thickness or even with one-third-thickness island grafts may give the same hearing results as obtained by closure with fascia and perichondrium grafting. If this is the case, the indications for cartilage–perichondrium island grafting are wide, even in cases with normal tubal function. This very solid and compact

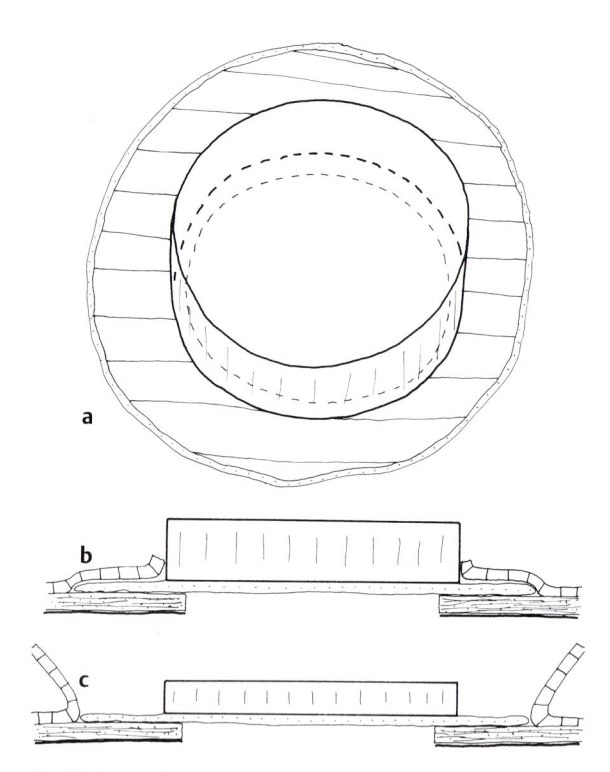

Fig. 23.2a–c The "perichondrium-cartilage on-lay method."
a The perichondrium with the full-thickness cartilage disk (thick dotted circle) is placed onto the perforation (thin dotted circle) and its surrounding flap onto the denuded lamina propria. The outer side of the cartilage disk is not covered with the perichondrium.
b Side view of the reconstructed eardrum with the perichondrium and full-thickness cartilage graft covering the perforation and the surrounding lamina propria. The epithelial flaps cover the perichondrium.
c The same as b with a half thickness perichondrium–cartilage island flap. The epithelial flaps have not yet been replaced.

cartilage disk. Too small a disk will fall through the perforation and will became an in-lay on-lay graft as described in Chapter 24.

The perichondrium–cartilage on-lay method, due to the good contact with the lamina propria, provides a good chance for early vascularization of the perichondrium from the denuded lamina propria and from the middle ear mucosa (**Fig. 23.2**). The epithelialization of the uncovered cartilage disk may be delayed, but the exact size of the cartilage disk is less important in this method. In case of too small a disk, the graft is fixed adequately by the underlying perichondrium and will not protrude into the tympanic cavity. With too small a disk, the perichondrium–cartilage on-lay method necessarily has to be used.

Thus, both methods can be used and the future will reveal which is better.

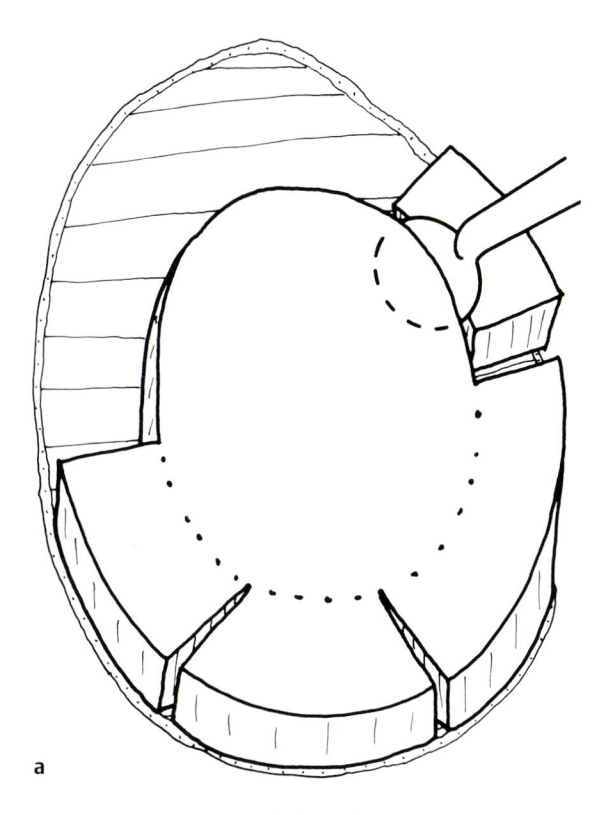

Fig. 23.3a, b Preparation of the graft.
a Trimming of a half-thickness island graft to adapt it to an oval perforation. Superfluous cartilage is gradually removed with a round knife.

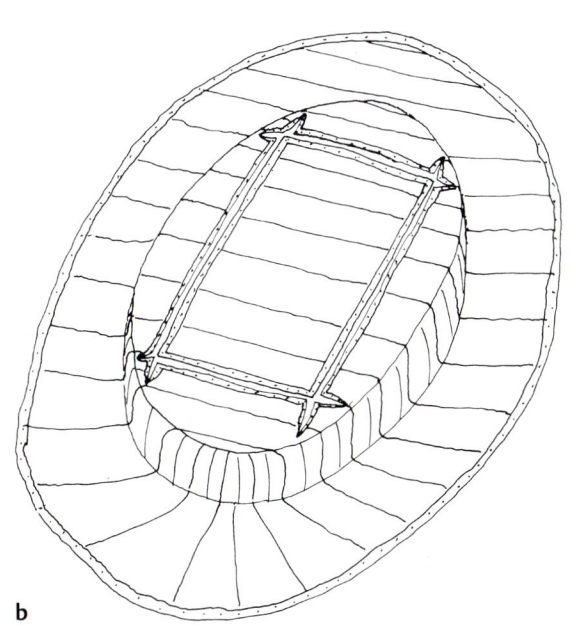

b Cuts are made in the perichondrium to prevent curling.

surgical method may yield good and stable anatomical results in the long term.

Unless and until clinical studies of this method show poorer postoperative hearing results, the on-lay technique is recommended without reservation.

Surgical Techniques of On-lay Tympanoplasty with Island Grafts

None of the on-lay techniques with composite cartilage–perichondrium island grafts have been described previously. Here, proposals for surgery in some typical situations in various types of perforation will be illustrated.

Anterior Perforation

Anterior perforation is the most suitable for the transcanal on-lay tympanoplasty. The perforation can be closed using various incisions and various extents of removal or elevation of the surrounding epithelium, such as total or partial removal of the epithelium, or total (see **Fig. 5.5b, c**; **Fig. 5.7a, b**) or partial elevation of the epithelium flaps (see **Fig. 5.6a, b**) and preservation of as much epithelium as possible.

Two different principles of placement of the island graft in small or middle-sized perforations will be illustrated here: (1) placement of the cartilage disk onto the edge of the eardrum; and (2) placement of the perichondrium flap onto the perforation and lamina propria.

The Cartilage–Perichondrium On-lay Method

Using a small anterior swing-door incision, both skin flaps can be elevated, together with the epithelium flap surrounding the perforation (**Fig. 23.4a**). A half-thickness composite graft is placed onto the denuded lamina propria and the perichondrium flap covers the edge of the cartilage disk and the denuded lamina propria (**Fig. 23.4b**). After replacement of the epithelial flaps, the perichondrium of the graft will readily be epithelialized (**Fig. 23.4c**). The side view in **Fig. 23.4d** shows a very firm and minimally invasive closure of the perforation.

The Perichondrium-Cartilage On-lay Method

After elevation of the anterior skin flaps, together with the epithelium surrounding the perforation (**Fig. 23.5a**), the

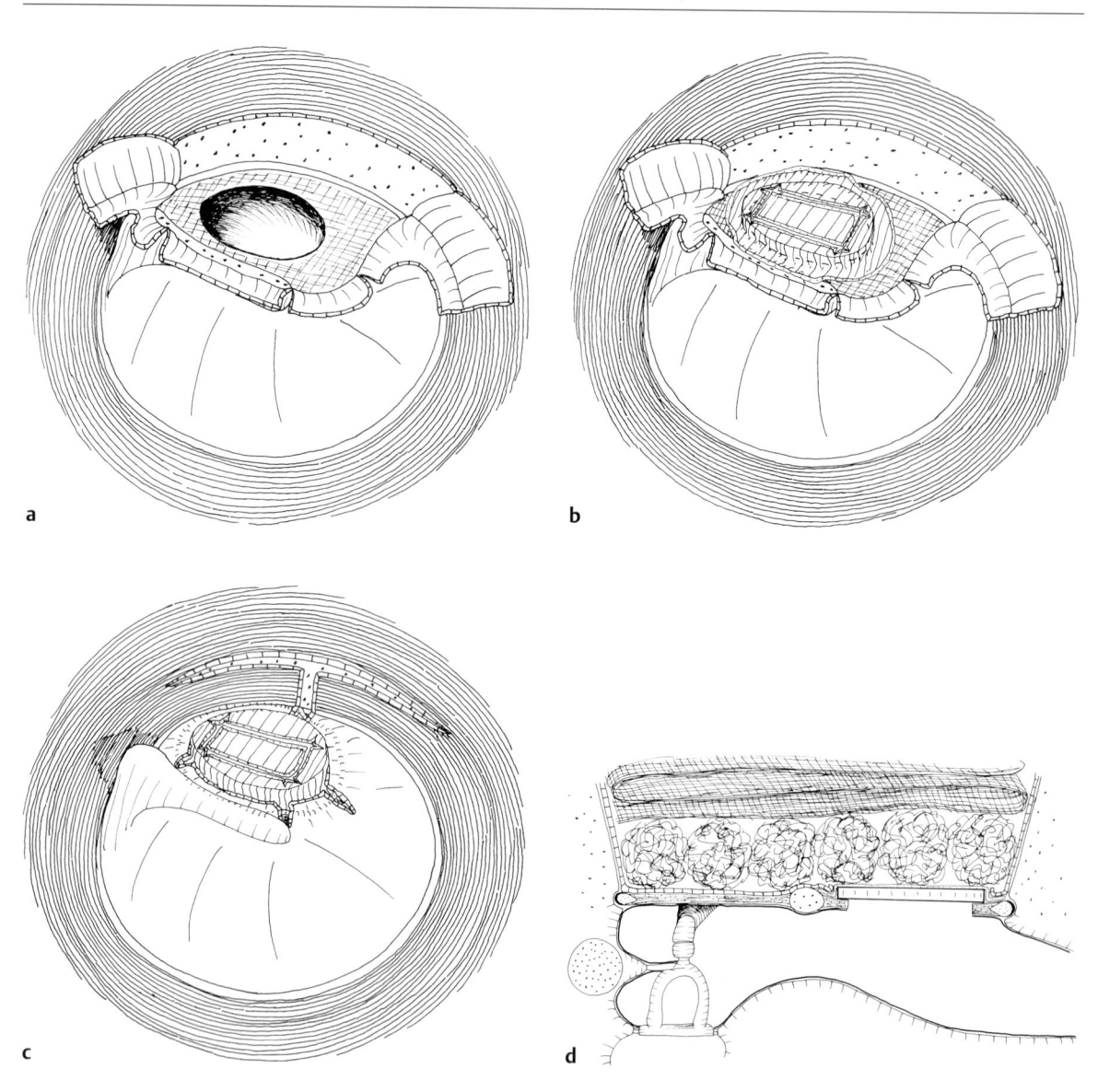

Fig. 23.4a–d Closure of an anterior perforation with an on-lay cartilage–perichondrium composite island graft.

a After an anterior swing-door incision is made, superior and inferior skin flaps are elevated, together with the epithelium surrounding the perforation. The lamina propria and the edge of the perforation are cleaned of the epithelium.

b The half-thickness composite graft, covered with perichondrium on the ear canal side, is placed onto the edges of the perforation. Four incisions are made in the perichondrium to prevent curling. The perichondrium flap is placed onto the denuded lamina propria.

c The epithelial flaps and the two skin flaps are replaced, covering the perichondrium. The perichondrium covering the cartilage disk is scarified to prevent curling.

d Side view of the closure of the anterior perforation with a half-thickness on-lay composite cartilage–perichondrium graft. The perichondrium covers the edges of the cartilage disk and the denuded lamina propria. The replaced epithelial flaps cover the perichondrium. The medial end of the ear canal is covered with Gelfoam, the lateral part is covered with gauze moistened with hydrocortisone–tetracycline ointment.

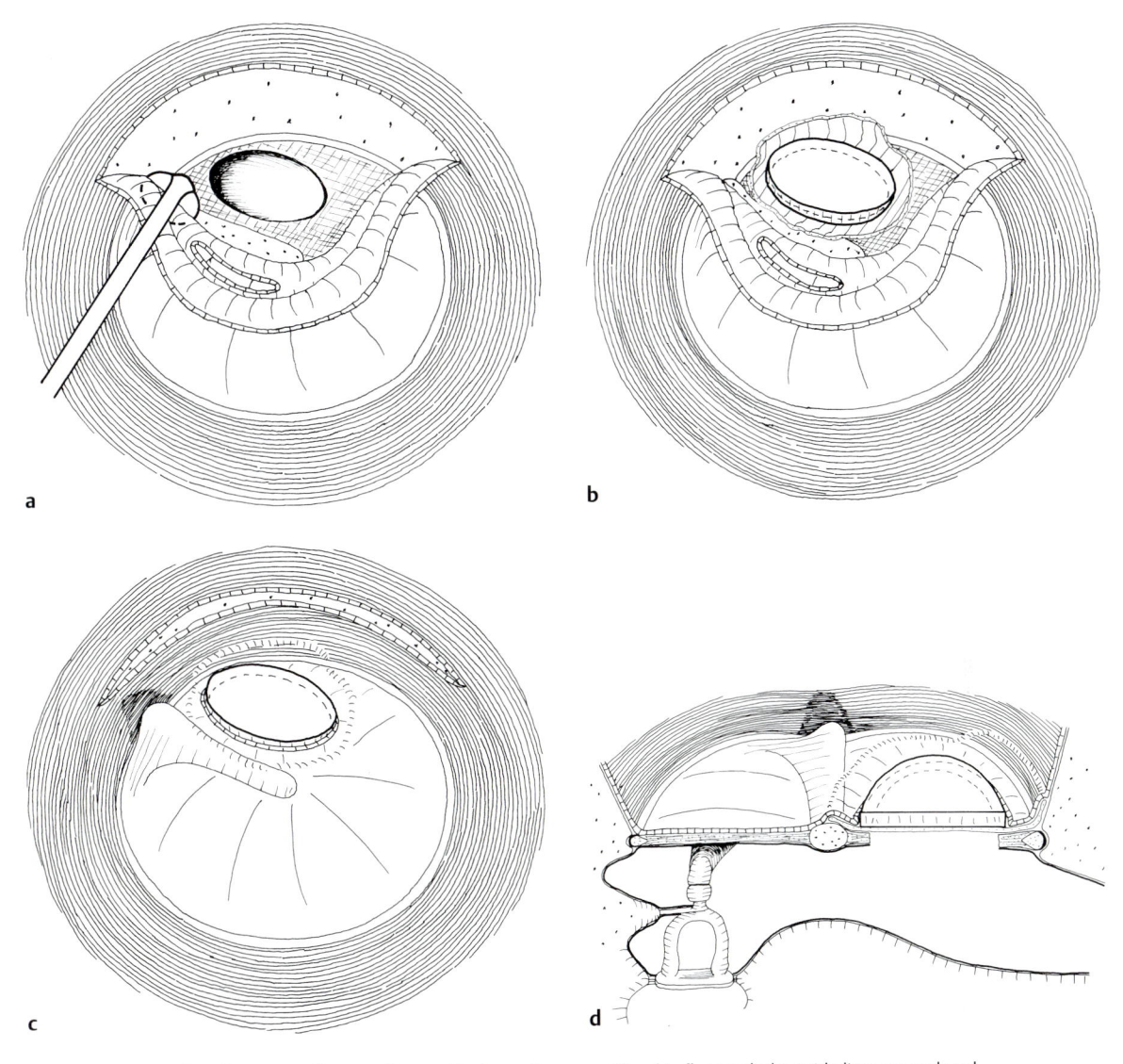

Fig. 23.5a–d Perichondrium–cartilage on-lay method in closure of an anterior perforation.
a A large anterior skin flap is elevated together with the epithelium surrounding the perforation, exposing the lamina propria.
b The perichondrium flap with the adjacent cartilage disk is placed onto the denuded lamina propria around the perforation. The disk is positioned onto the edges of the perforation.
c The skin flaps with the epithelium are replaced.
d Side view with some perspective after closure of the anterior perforation with perichondrium-cartilage on-lay method. The perichondrium flap with the adjacent cartilage disk is placed onto the denuded lamina propria. The cartilage disk is not covered by the perichondrium.

perichondrium with the cartilage disk is placed onto the denuded lamina propria (**Fig. 23.5b**). After replacement of the elevated skin flaps and epithelial flaps (**Fig. 23.5c, d**), the naked cartilage disk will gradually be epithelialized.

Inferior Perforation

Inferior perforation is very suitable for on-lay technique and several types of incisions and means of handling the epithelium surrounding the perforation are used. A few will be illustrated here.

Outward Elevation of the Epithelial Flaps

After the edges of the perforation are cleaned of epithelium, five small vertical incisions along the inferior annulus are made and the epithelial flaps are elevated. Epithelial flaps are also elevated along the superior edge of the perforation (**Fig. 23.6a**). The half thickness cartilage–perichondrium graft is placed onto the edge of the perforation and the perichondrium flap covers the edges of the cartilage disk and the lamina propria (**Fig. 23.6b**). The preserved epithelial flaps are replaced (**Fig. 23.6c**).

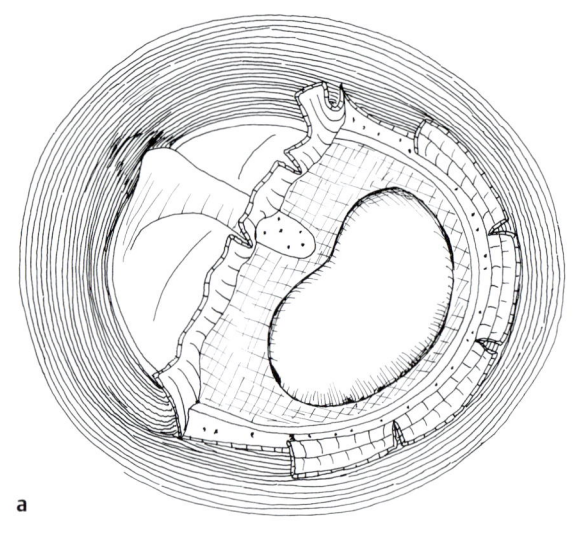

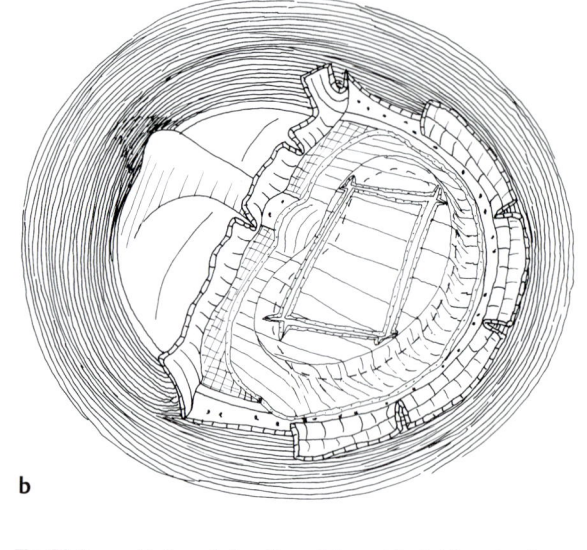

Fig. 23.6a–c Outward elevation of the epithelial flaps in a large inferior perforation.
a   Several small radial incisions are made and the epithelium is elevated as several small flaps.
b   The half-thickness cartilage–perichondrium graft is placed onto the denuded edge of the perforation and the perichondrium flap is folded out.
c   The epithelial flaps are replaced, covering the entire perichondrium flap.

Elevation of a Large Tympanomeatal Flap with the Surrounding Epithelial Flaps in Cartilage–Perichondrium On-lay Method

After elevation of the epithelium (**Fig. 23.7a**), the cartilage–perichondrium on-lay method is used, placing the cartilage disk onto the edge of the perforation. The perichondrium with four incisions covers the cartilage disk and the edges as well as the lamina propria (**Fig. 23.7b**). After replacement of the tympanomeatal and the epithelial flaps (see **Fig. 21.7c**), the chances for rapid epithelialization of the cartilage disk are good.

The Perichondrium-Cartilage On-lay Method; the Alternative Placement of the Island Graft

After elevation of the epithelium as shown in **Fig. 23.7a**, the perichondrium flap with the adjacent cartilage disk is placed onto the denuded lamina propria, covering the perforation. The cartilage disk is positioned onto the perichondrium and onto the edges of the perforation. The ear canal side of the cartilage disk is not covered with perichondrium (**Fig. 23.8a**). After replacement of the tympanomeatal flap and the epithelial flap (**Fig. 23.8b**), the naked cartilage disk will gradually be epithelialized.

Total and Subtotal Perforations

The total perforation can be closed in retroauricular, endaural, and transcanal approach with the fixed ear speculum. This last method represents the most minimally invasive surgery. Several incisions and methods of elevation of the epithelial flaps are used, some of which are illustrated here.

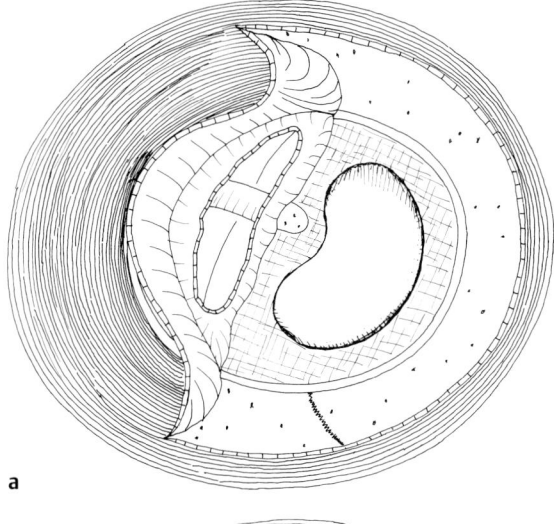

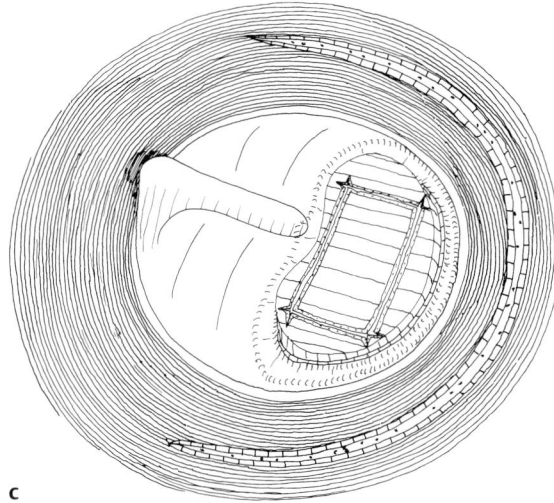

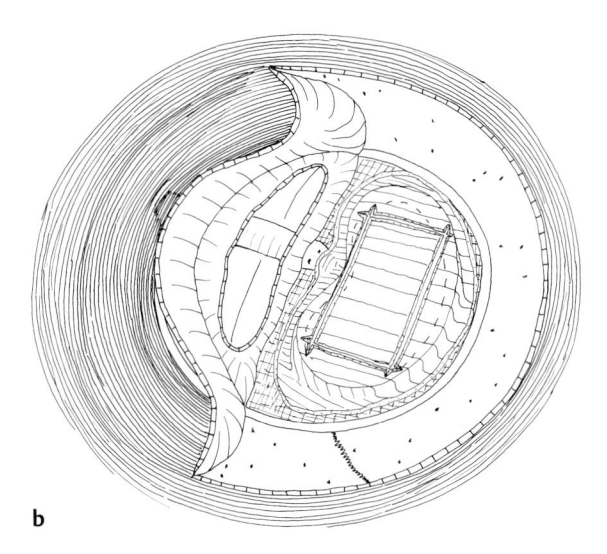

Fig. 23.7a–c Closing of a large inferior perforation with a cartilage–perichondrium on-lay method by elevation of a large tympanomeatal flap with the epithelium surrounding the perforation.

a A circumferential incision is made between the 9-o'clock and 3-o'clock positions and the lamina propria is carefully cleaned of epithelium.

b The half-thickness cartilage–perichondrium graft with the four anti-curling incisions of the perichondrium is placed onto the edges of the perforation. The perichondrium flap covering the edges of the graft is folded out, covering the denuded lamina propria.

c The tympanomeatal flaps and the epithelial flaps are replaced.

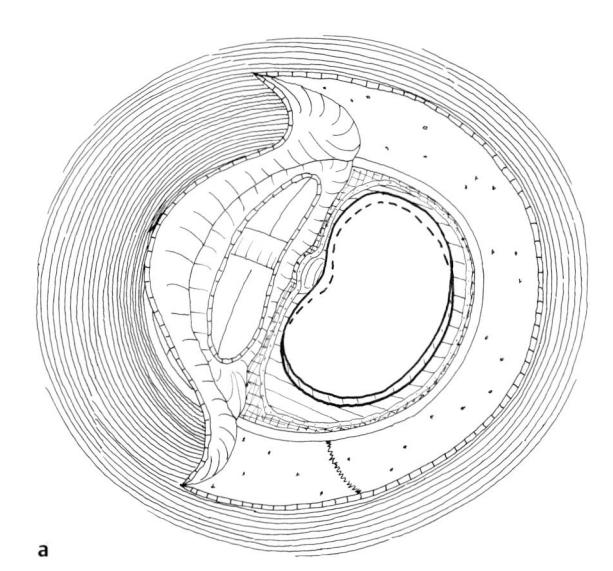

Fig. 23.8a, b The perichondrium-cartilage on-lay method for closure of a large inferior perforation.

a The skin incision and elevation of the epithelial flaps are the same as shown in **Fig. 23.7a**. The perichondrium flap with the cartilage disk is placed onto the denuded lamina propria. The half-thickness cartilage disk is positioned along the edge of the perforation.

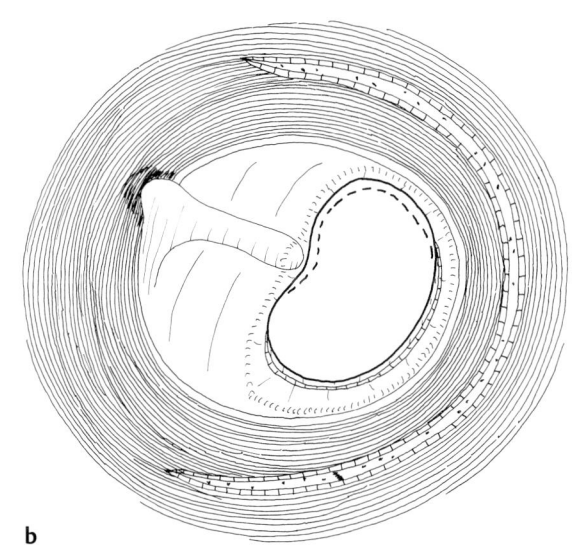

b The tympanomeatal flap with the epithelium is replaced. The edges of the epithelium are positioned close to the cartilage disk.

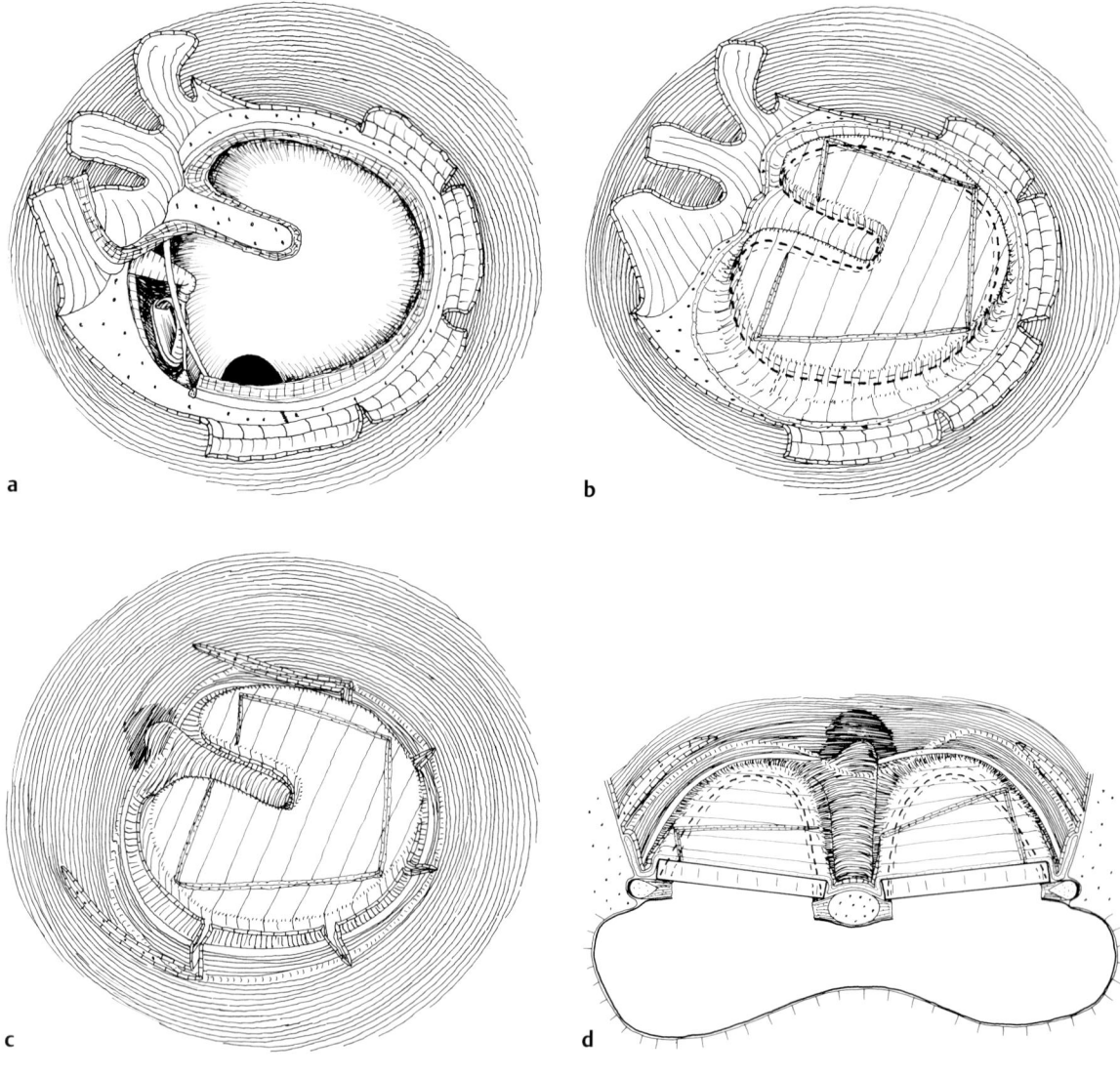

Fig. 23.9a–d On-lay closure of the total perforation with a composite cartilage–perichondrium island graft.
a The three superior skin flaps are elevated. Four epithelial flaps are elevated along the inferior annulus.
b A half-thickness cartilage–perichondrium graft, with some incisions of the perichondrium and shaped to accommodate the malleus handle, is placed onto the lamina propria along the edge of the perforation. The perichondrium flap is placed onto the lamina propria, the fibrous annulus, and the bone of the ear canal.
c The tympanomeatal flaps and the epithelial flaps are replaced. The graft protrudes slightly into the ear canal.
d Side view with some perspective of the on-lay placement of the total cartilage–perichondrium island graft at the level of the umbo. The perichondrium covers the malleus handle and the surround of the perforation.

Elevation of Superior and Inferior Epithelial Flaps

After elevation of the epithelium around the perforation and cleaning of the edges of the perforation (**Fig. 23.9a**), the fibrous annulus is cut at the 9-o'clock position and temporarily elevated to provide an overview of the lateral sinus. The half-thickness cartilage disk with some incisions of the perichondrium to prevent curling of the graft, and a wedge cut-out to accommodate the malleus handle, is placed onto the edge of the perforation (**Fig. 23.9b**). The surrounding perichondrium covers the edge of the cartilage disk, the lamina propria, the fibrous annulus, and the bone. The malleus handle is also covered with the perichondrium. After replacement of the epithelial flaps (**Fig. 23.9c, d**), the conditions are good for rapid epithelialization.

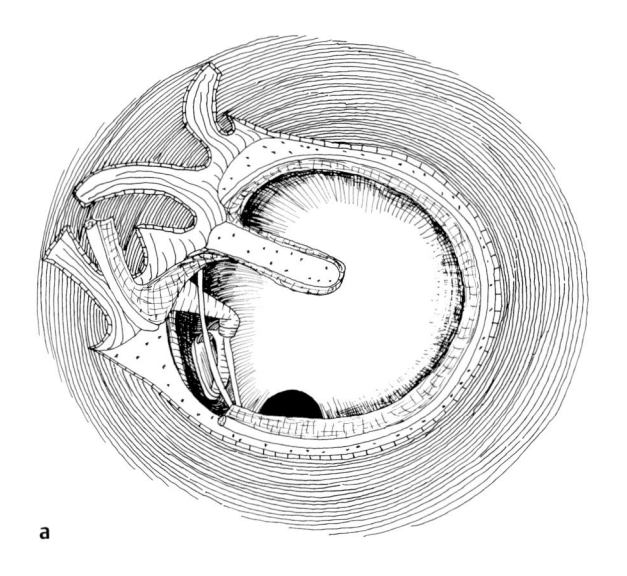

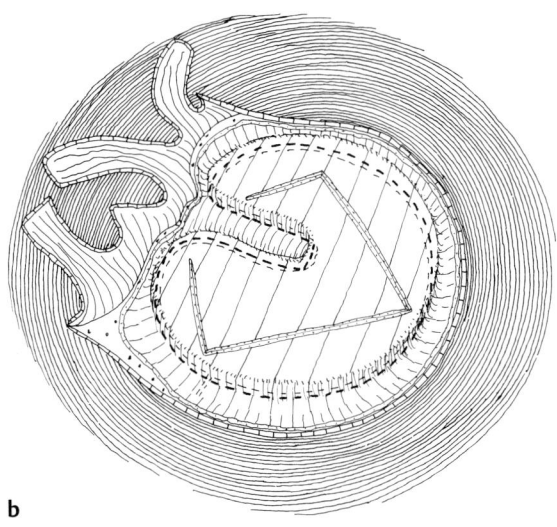

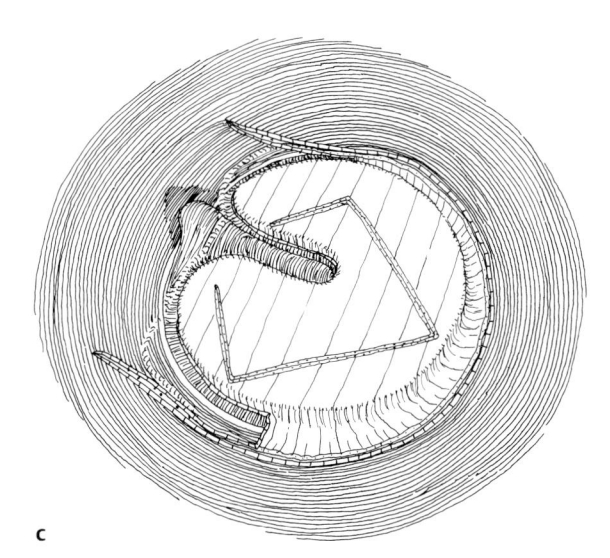

Fig. 23.10a–c Elevation of three superior flaps and removal of inferior epithelium.

a A large medial circumferential incision and two vertical incisions at the 9-o'clock and 3-o'clock positions are made and three flaps are elevated. The inferior skin is removed, cleaning the eardrum of all epithelium.

b The half-thickness cartilage–perichondrium graft with a wedge cut-out for the malleus handle and incisions in the perichondrium is placed onto the edges of the perforation and the perichondrium flap is folded out.

c The tympanomeatal flaps are replaced and Gelfoam balls will cover the eardrum.

Elevation of Superior Flaps Only and Removal of the Inferior Epithelium

This method, which I introduced (Tos 1980), has been widely used in fascia and perichondrium grafting. After a large circumferential incision, the three superior flaps are elevated. The skin and the epithelium along the inferior border of the perforation are elevated (**Fig. 23.10a**). A cartilage–perichondrium graft with a wedge cut-out for the malleus handle is placed onto the edges of the lamina propria and the perichondrium flap is folded out, covering all denuded bone and the lamina propria (**Fig. 23.10b**). After replacement of the epithelial flaps, the epithelialization of the inferior part of the graft will be slow, but the fixation of the perichondrium flap with Gelfoam balls is firm (**Fig. 23.10c**).

Elevation of a Large Tympanomeatal Flap with the Surrounding Epithelium, and Tympanoplasty Type 2 with Incus Interposition

Epithelium surrounding the perforation is elevated together with the tympanomeatal flap. The posterosuperior fibrous annulus is elevated to allow visualization of the footplate. The shaped autogenous incus is placed onto the stapes head, with the short process under the malleus handle (**Fig. 23.11a**). The island graft is placed onto the edge of the lamina propria, the perichondrium flap is folded out (**Fig. 23.11b**), and the tympanomeatal flap with the eardrum epithelium is replaced (**Fig. 23.11c**). The cartilage will subsequently be epithelialized.

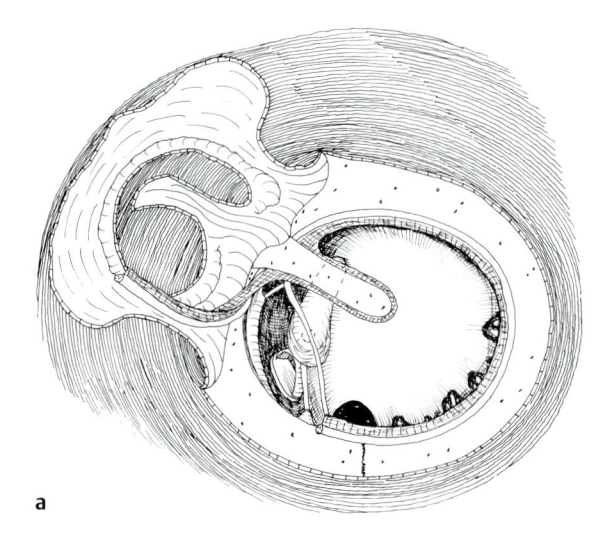

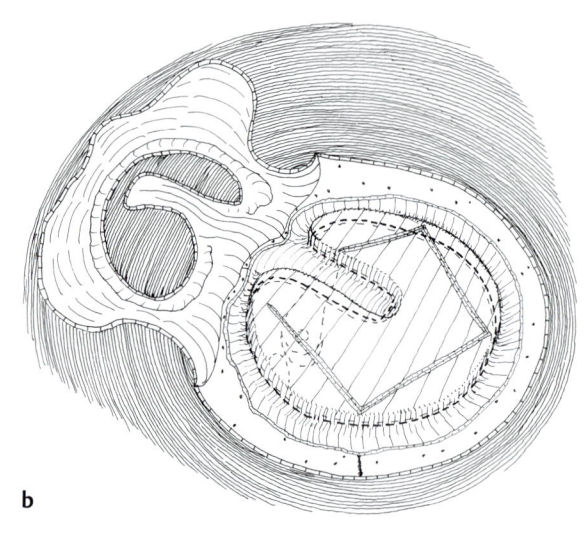

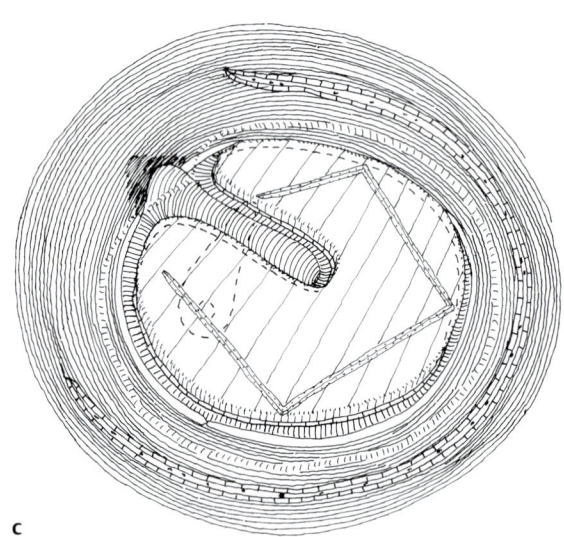

Fig. 23.11a–c Elevation of a large tympanomeatal flap in on-lay tympanoplasty type 2 with incus interposition and closure of a total perforation with a cartilage–perichondrium composite island graft.
a The incus is removed, shaped, and interposed between the head of the stapes and the malleus handle.
b The cartilage–perichondrium island graft, with four incisions of the perichondrium and a wedge cut-out to accommodate the malleus handle, is placed onto the edge of the denuded lamina. The perichondrium flap covers the edge of the cartilage disk, the fibrous annulus, and the ear canal bone.
c The tympanomeatal flap is replaced. The edge of the cartilage graft is covered by the epithelium.

Elevation of a Large Tympanomeatal Flap with the Surrounding Epithelium and Tympanoplasty Type 3 with Placement of a Kurz Titanium Columella

After elevation of the tympanomeatal flap, the epithelium around the perforation is carefully elevated along with the tympanomeatal flap. The incus remnant is removed and the footplate is cleaned. A Hüttenbrink cartilage guide (Hüttenbrink 1984) is shaped from a 4 mm × 4 mm piece of cartilage (**Fig. 3.37**; see also **Fig. 3.38**) and placed onto the footplate. The foot of the titanium columella is placed, through a 0.8 mm hole of the guide, onto the footplate (**Fig. 23.12a**). Because the composite graft is placed onto the lamina propria (instead of under it), the shaft of the columella should be longer, as in underlay grafting (**Fig. 23.12b–d**). Here a full-thickness cartilage graft is used and brought into contact with the head of the columella. The edge of the cartilage disk is covered with the perichondrium flap. After replacement of the tympanomeatal flap (**Fig. 23.12c**) the edge of the cartilage disk is partly covered by the epithelial flaps. The titanium prosthesis will vibrate together with the malleus handle (**Fig. 23.12 d**).

Results of Surgery with On-lay Techniques

Desarda and Bhisegaonkar (2005) found a re-perforation in 4% of 172 cases with on-lay and in 4% of 128 cases with underlay technique. The authors were extremely satisfied with the cartilage–perichondrium composite graft. The success rate was 96%. No details were reported on the size of the perforations.

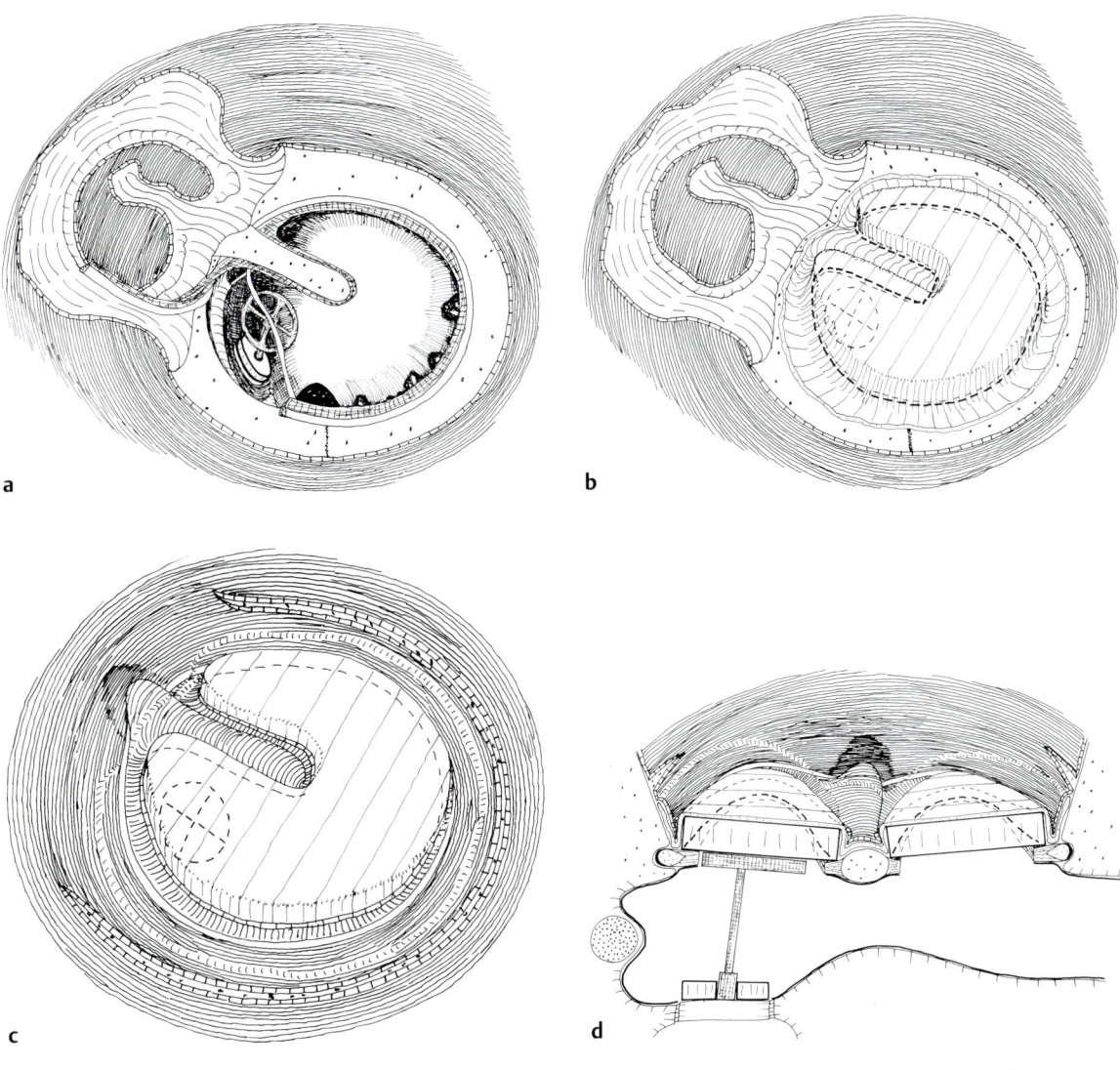

Fig. 23.12a–d On-lay tympanoplasty type 3 with a Kurz titanium TORP and a full-thickness cartilage-perichondrium composite graft in total perforation and missing stapes.

a A large tympanomeatal flap is elevated together with the epithelium. A cartilage guide and a titanium TORP are placed onto the footplate (Hüttenbrink et al. 2004). The perichondrium covers the edges of the full-thickness cartilage graft and the ear canal bone.

b A full-thickness cartilage–perichondrium composite graft, with a wedge cut-out to accommodate the malleus handle, is placed onto the edges of the denuded lamina propria. The perichondrium flap covers the edge of the cartilage disk, the denuded lamina propria, and the ear canal bone. The cartilage graft protrudes slightly into the ear canal.

c The tympanomeatal flap with the surrounding epithelium is replaced.

d Side view with some perspective of tympanoplasty type 3 and on-lay closure of a total perforation with full-thickness cartilage-perichondrium composite graft. The cartilage disk is placed onto the denuded lamina propria and onto the head of the titanium TORP. The foot of the prosthesis first is placed onto the footplate through the hole of the cartilage guide (Hüttenbrink et al. 2004). The perichondrium covers the edges of the full-thickness cartilage graft and the ear canal bone.

Author's Comments and Recommendations

I am still a great fan of on-lay tympanoplasty, and use it whenever possible. In case of a posterior perforation I prefer underlay technique, but in anterior and inferior perforation I prefer the on-lay technique. In total and subtotal perforations I use both the underlay and the on-lay techniques. In on-lay tympanoplasty a transcanal approach with a fixed ear speculum is recommended (see **Figs. 3.1–3.4**). This allows surgery with both hands, and the surgery is minimally invasive. There are no incisions in the lateral part of the ear canal and no risk of a lateral postoperative stenosis, which may occur in endaural or retroauricular approaches.

The transcanal approach, without a lateral incision, is especially recommended in tympanoplasty in children. There is practically no other postoperative intervention than removal of the dressing.

It is my impression that underlay technique dominates completely in otosurgical courses and the practical teaching of on-lay technique is therefore impossible. For this reason, in this book on-lay cartilage tympanoplasty methods are described and illustrated in six chapters (Chapters 5, 8, 11, 12, 23, 24).

In half-thickness composite grafts I recommend four incisions of the perichondrium to prevent possible curling of the thin cartilage–perichondrium graft, though this is not based on documentation or knowledge of the cause and the mechanism of curling.

Research on Epithelialization of the Cartilage Grafts is Needed

If the on-lay cartilage–perichondrium cartilage composite island graft is placed with the cartilage side onto the denuded lamina propria, the ear canal side will be covered by the perichondrium (**Fig. 23.1**). The epithelialization will begin from the border of the epithelium, and continue onto and along the perichondrium.

If the island graft is placed with the perichondrium side turned toward the middle ear (**Fig. 23.2**), the epithelialization will take place along the "naked" cartilage disk, both along the edge and along the platform of the graft.

It is possible that epithelialization of the "naked" graft is delayed or incomplete compared with the graft covered with perichondrium. Simple inspection of the epithelialization at the same postoperative time in "naked" disks and comparison with that in perichondrium disks of the same diameter will provide important otomicroscopic or histopathological information on epithelialization of the grafts. For the butterfly cartilage technique (see **Fig. 25.11c**), poor epithelialization of the cartilage graft has been reported (Chapter 25).

The simplest and the easiest response to the possibility of poor epithelialization of the "naked" cartilage disk might be to cover the composite grafts with perichondrium on both sides, as used by Tolsdorff (1983) in the very first tensa cartilage–perichondrium composite graft (Chapter 17).

References

Desarda KK, Bhisegaonkar SG. Tragal perichondrium and cartilage in reconstructive tympanoplasty. Indian J Otolaryngol Head Neck Surg 2005;57:9–12.

Hüttenbrink K-B. Die operative Therapie der chronischen Otitis media. III. [Surgical treatment of chronic otitis media. III: Middle ear reconstruction] HNO 1994;42:701–708.

Hüttenbrink K-B, Zahnert T, Beutner D, Hofmann G. The cartilage guide: a solution for anchoring a columella prosthesis on the footplate. Laryngorhinootologie 2004;83:450–456.

Tolsdorff P. Tympanoplastik mit Tragusknorpel-Transplantat: "Knorpeldekkel-Plastik. Laryngol Rhinol Otol (Stuttg) 1983;62:97–102.

Tos M. Stability of myringoplasty based on late results. ORL J Otorhinolaryngol Relat Spec 1980;42:171–181.

24 In-lay On-lay Tympanoplasty Techniques with Cartilage–Perichondrium Composite Island Graft

Definition

The in-lay on-lay composite graft consists of a cartilage disk that is placed into the perforation. On the ear canal side the cartilage is covered with perichondrium, which surrounds the cartilage as a 1–2 mm wide flap (**Fig. 24.1**). The cartilage disk is positioned in the perforation, and the perichondrium flap is placed onto the 1–2 mm margin of deepithelialized lamina propria around the perforation.

My co-worker Per Larsen started with the in-lay on-lay technique in 2001, first on small and medium-sized perforations then on subtotal perforations. The name "in-lay on-lay" technique that I apply precisely describes the procedure. No papers on such techniques have been published in the literature. However, the tympanoplasty procedure is an on-lay technique and cannot be performed as an underlay procedure without elevation of a tympanomeatal flap.

The procedures for de-epithelialization of the lamina propria will be illustrated for anterior, posterior, inferior, subtotal, and total perforations.

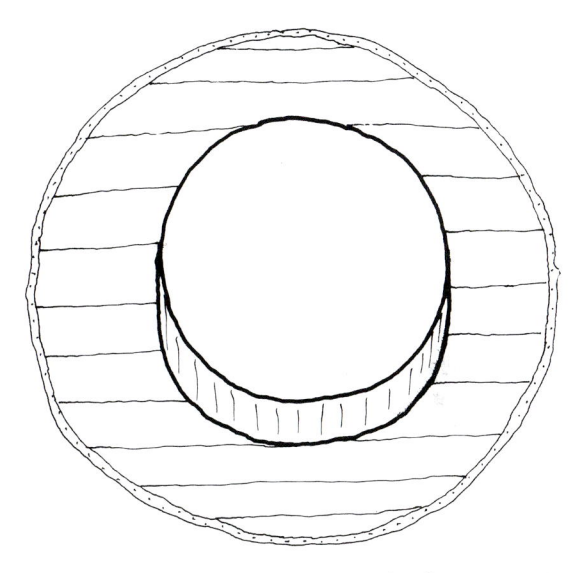

Fig. 24.1 The in-lay on-lay cartilage–perichondrium composite island graft for closure of a small round perforation. The round cartilage disk is covered with perichondrium surrounding the cartilage as a flap. The perichondrium flap will be placed onto the denuded lamina propria.

Harvesting and Elaboration of the Graft

The cartilage is harvested either from the tragus or from the concha. Since the tympanoplasty will most often be a transcanal procedure, the tragal cartilage will often be used.

A horizontal incision 3 mm medial to the tragus dome is made through the skin, the perichondrium and the cartilage in one sweep (see **Fig. 25.1**). A piece of cartilage covered on both sides with perichondrium is removed. Perichondrium is removed from the convex side. The cartilage–perichondrium graft is trimmed and shaped immediately before application when the definitive shape and size of perforation and extent of the deepithelialization of the eardrum are known. With the use of a large hook, the size of the perforation can be determined and marked on the graft as small holes made with a pick. The superfluous cartilage is gradually removed and the graft is shaped to fit exactly into the perforation (**Fig. 24.2**).

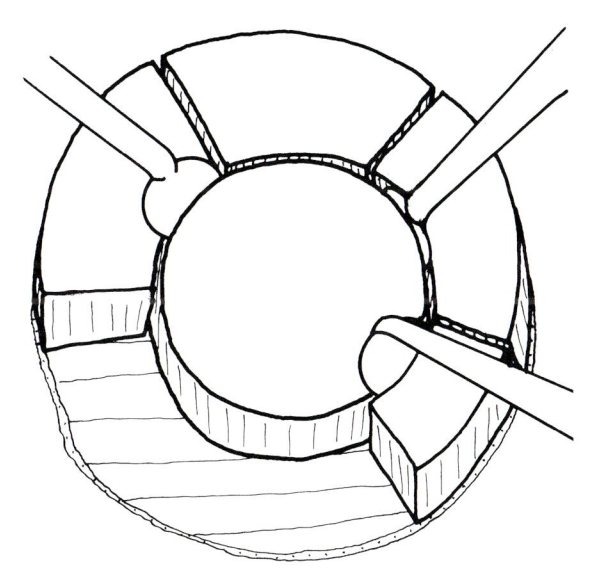

Fig. 24.2 Trimming and shaping the cartilage disk using a round knife. The perichondrium flap remains intact.

a b

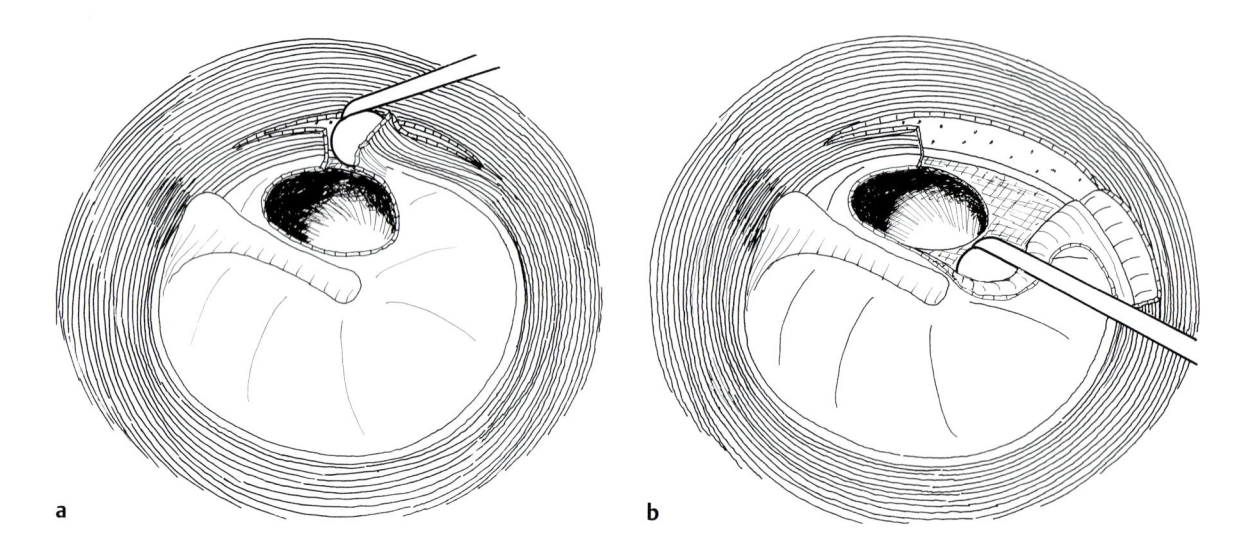

The peripheral perichondrium flap is trimmed in relation to the width of the deepithelialized belt of eardrum remnant around the perforation.

The thickness of the cartilage disk may be reduced to as little as one-third of the full thickness of the tragal or conchal cartilage. Because the perichondrium will grow together with the denuded lamina propria and will subsequently be epithelialized, there is only small risk of curling in the case of a thinned cartilage disk. However, there are no systematic studies on curling in grafts of various thicknesses; such studies are needed to resolve the mystery of curling.

Indications for Application of the In-lay On-lay Graft

Small and middle-sized perforations without suspicion of cholesteatoma can be operated with in-lay on-lay technique, especially anterior and inferior perforations. Posterior perforation with intact ossicular chain and without remnants of an eventual previous retraction can also be operated. In fact, the posterosuperior pars tensa composite underlay island graft (Chapter 15) has the same goal—to prevent postoperative retraction—as the in-lay on-lay graft. Poor preoperative tubal function, expressed as negative preoperative Valsalva or negative deflation test is an obvious indication for cartilage tympanoplasty.

Patients with subtotal perforation were operated on with this technique in 2004 and 2005. Total perforation can easily be treated with in-lay on-lay technique.

The In-lay On-lay Technique

The principle of the method is to suspend the cartilage disk onto the denuded eardrum by the perichondrium flap. The extent of elevation or removal of the squamous epithelium may differ in various perforations.

Anterior Perforation

In on-lay technique the epithelium around the anterior perforation may be totally elevated or totally removed or partly removed and partly elevated.

Here a method with total elevation of the epithelium will be illustrated. Using a small anterior circumferential incision between the 1-o'clock and 4-o'clock positions and a radial incision at the 2-o'clock position, two skin flaps are elevated (**Fig. 24.3a**). First the inferior flap with the adjacent inferior epithelium is elevated, (**Fig. 24.3b**), then the superior flap with the superior epithelium. The elevation of the epithelium continues along the malleus handle (**Fig. 24.3c**). The cartilage disk is placed into the perforation and the perichondrium flap is folded out onto the denuded eardrum remnant (**Fig. 24.3d, e**). The epithelial flaps are replaced (**Fig. 24.3f**). In the side view (**Fig. 24.3g**) the myringoplasty looks rather firm, because the cartilage disk is suspended by the perichondrium flap and this flap is covered by all replaced epithelial flaps.

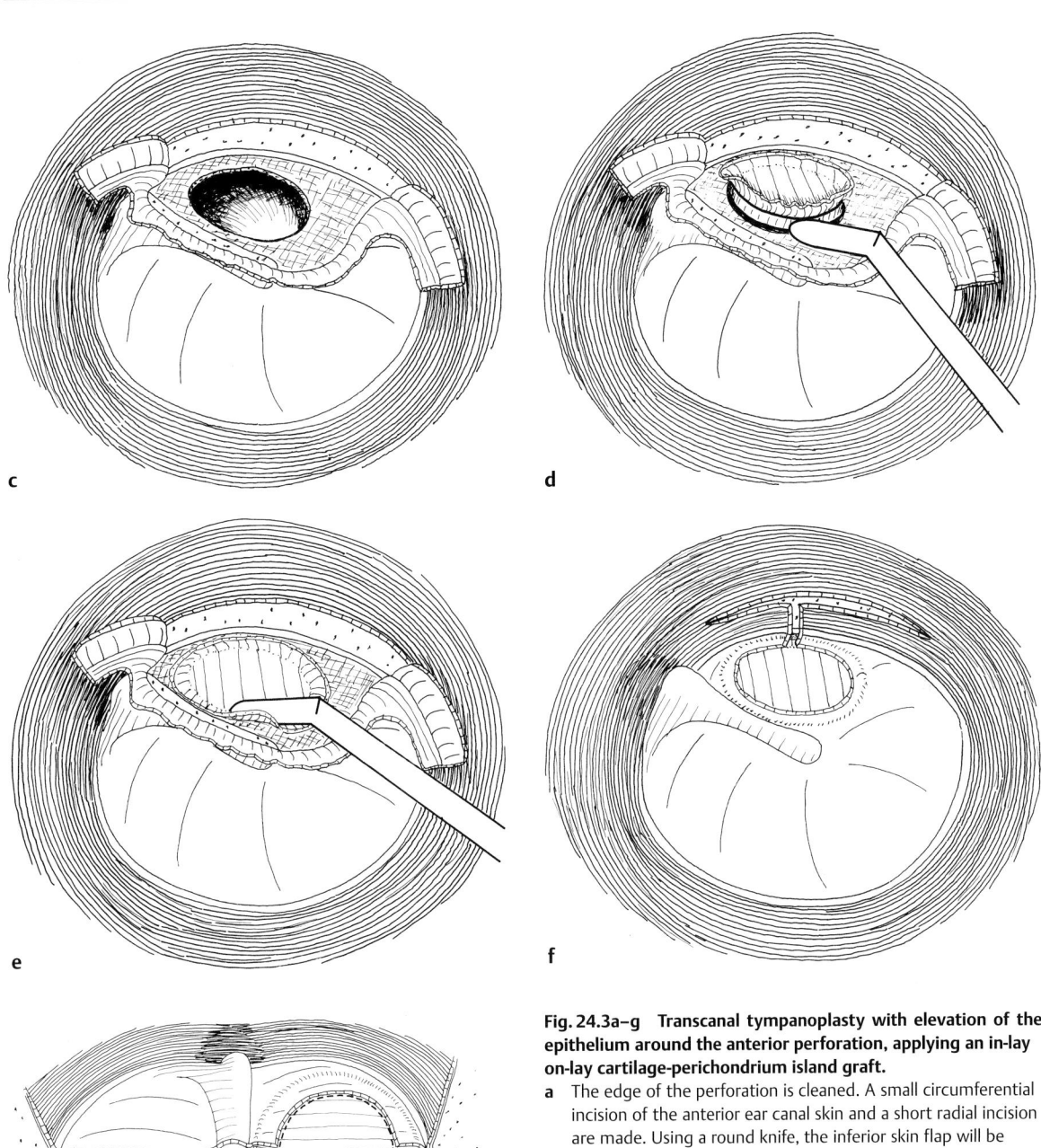

Fig. 24.3a–g Transcanal tympanoplasty with elevation of the epithelium around the anterior perforation, applying an in-lay on-lay cartilage-perichondrium island graft.

a The edge of the perforation is cleaned. A small circumferential incision of the anterior ear canal skin and a short radial incision are made. Using a round knife, the inferior skin flap will be elevated together with the epithelium of the eardrum surrounding the inferior half of the perforation.

b The inferior elevation of the skin and of the eardrum epithelium is completed.

c The superior skin flap is elevated together with the epithelium surrounding the superior and anterior parts of the perforation and the epithelium from the anterior half of the malleus handle.

d The in-lay on-lay graft is first placed into the anterior part of the perforation and the anterior part of the perichondrium is folded out.

e The posterior edge of the cartilage disk is gently pushed into the perforation and the remaining perichondrium is folded out.

f The epithelial flaps are replaced and will be covered with moist Gelfoam balls.

g Side view with some perspective of closure of the anterior perforation with the in-lay on-lay cartilage–perichondrium composite island graft. The cartilage is trimmed to the size and shape of the perforation and is positioned like a plug into the perforation. The cartilage is suspended by the perichondrium flap and by the preserved epithelial flaps.

| a | b |

Posterior Perforation

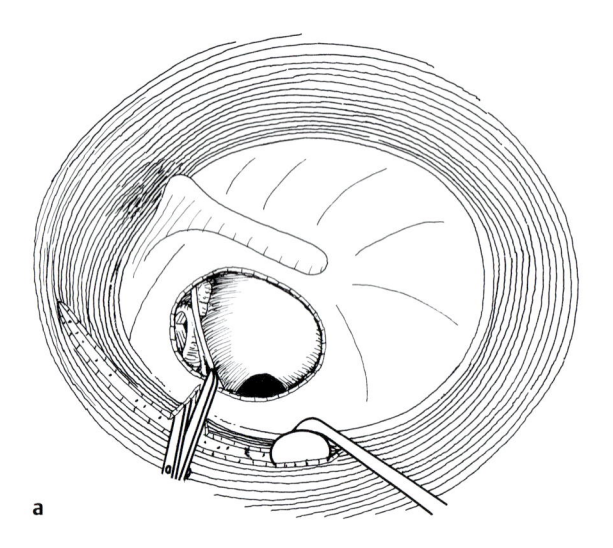

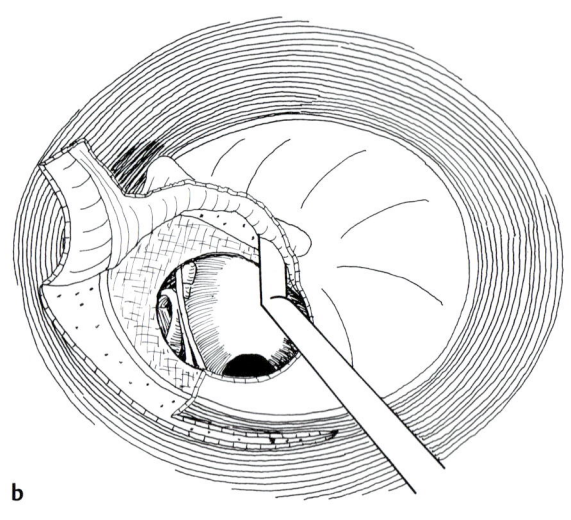

Posterior perforation is usually treated with underlay technique, but it can be treated with in-lay on-lay technique, either with elevation or with removal of the surrounding eardrum epithelium.

After a small circumferential incision between the 11-o'clock and 7-o'clock positions and a small vertical incision are made (**Fig. 24.4a**), the superior skin flap with the superior eardrum epithelium is elevated. The anterior epithelium and the malleus handle epithelium are also elevated (**Fig. 24.4b**). The inferior flap with the inferior epithelium and epithelium from the umbo region is elevated (**Fig. 24.4c**). After further cleaning of the edge of the perforation, the cartilage disk is positioned into the perforation and the perichondrium flap is folded out, then the skin flaps with the epithelial flaps are replaced (**Fig. 24.4d–f**).

Another possibility is to remove a belt of the epithelium around the perforation, clean the edge of the perforation (**Fig. 24.5a**), place the cartilage disk in the perforation, and adapt the perichondrium flap to the denuded area around the perforation (**Fig. 24.5b**).

Between total elevation and total removal of the epithelium surrounding posterior perforation, there may be several combinations of removal or elevation of the epithelium. One such modification is elevation of a posterior and an anterior epithelial flap and removal of the epithelium from the superior and inferior remnants of the perforation (**Fig. 24.6a**). After placement of the cartilage disk into the perforation, the perichondrium flap is folded out and the epithelial flaps are replaced (**Fig. 24.6b**).

Inferior Perforation

Small or medium-sized inferior perforations are easily closed with in-lay on-lay technique with elevation of the epithelium all the way around the perforation (**Fig. 24.7a**). In medium-sized perforations the fibrous annulus is usually exposed. An oval cartilage disk closes the perforation and the perichondrium flap covers the denuded eardrum remnant (**Fig. 24.7b**); the replaced epithelial flaps fixate the perichondrium and provide rapid epithelialization (**Fig. 24.7c**).

Methods involving removal of the epithelium around the inferior perforation may also be applied.

Subtotal Perforation

In subtotal perforation, the edges of the perforation are cleaned and the epithelium from the posterosuperior border, from the umbo, and the anterosuperior border of the perforation is elevated (**Fig. 24.8a–c**). The epithelium around the eardrum remnant is elevated all the way around the perforation, with exposure of the fibrous annulus (**Fig. 24.8d**).

The composite cartilage–perichondrium island graft is trimmed and a rectangular wedge is cut out for the umbo and lower part of the malleus handle (**Fig. 24.8e**). The cartilage–perichondrium graft is placed in the tympanic cavity (**Fig. 24.8f**). The perichondrium of the wedge covers the malleus handle and the umbo. The peripheral perichondrium flap covers the denuded eardrum remnant around the perforation and is itself covered and fixated by the replaced epithelial flaps (**Fig. 24.8 g, h**).

The epithelium around the perforation can either be totally removed or elevated superiorly and removed inferiorly in subtotal perforation, as will be demonstrated in total perforation below.

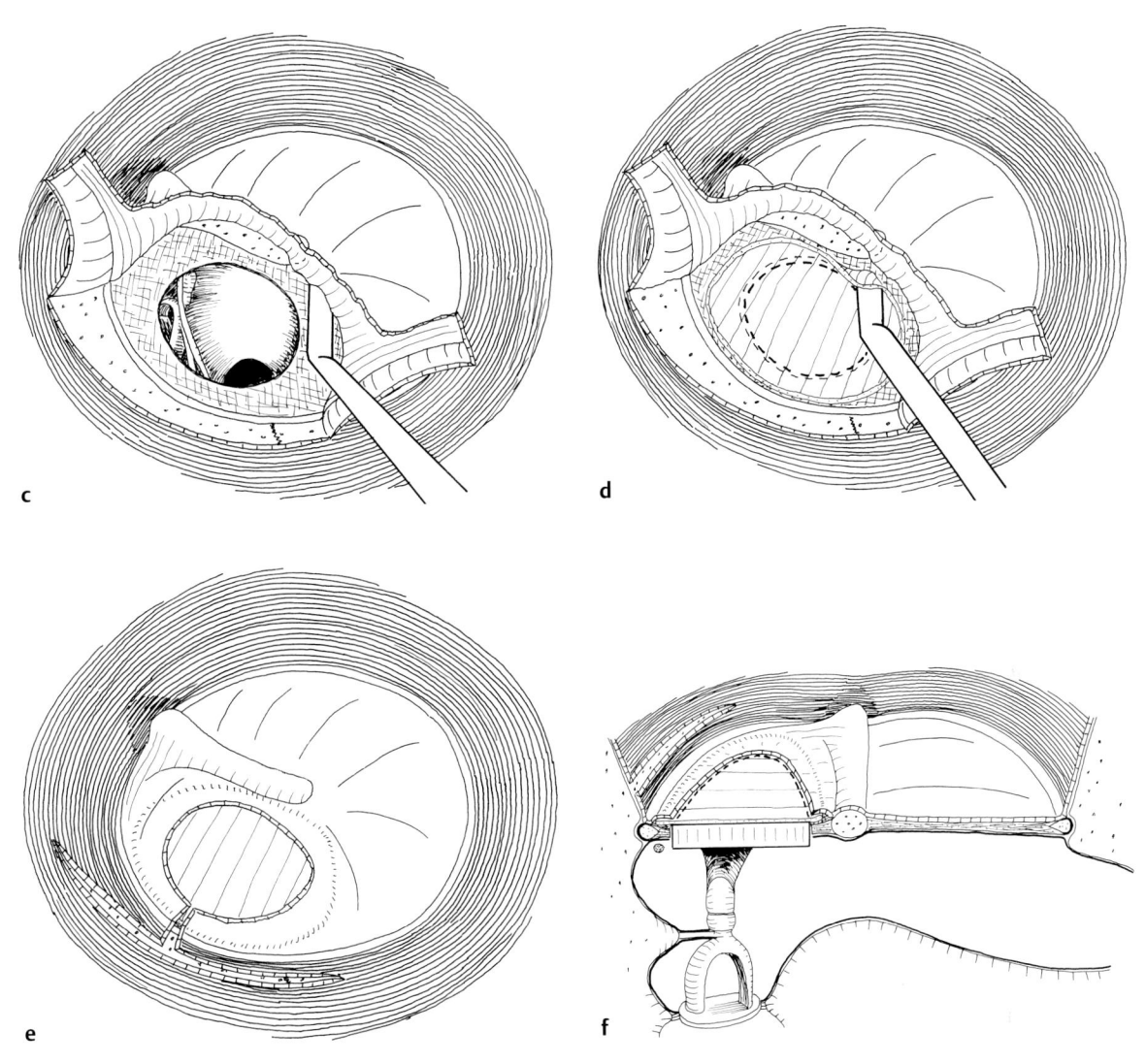

Fig. 24.4a–f Tympanoplasty type 1 applying in-lay on-lay technique in posterior perforation with intact ossicular chain.

a A small circumferential incision is made between the 11-o'clock and 7-o'clock positions and 1 mm lateral to the fibrous annulus. At the 9-o'clock position a small radial incision divides the skin into a superior and an inferior flap.

b The superior skin flap and the superior epithelium are elevated. The epithelium along the anterior edge of the perforation and along the posterior half of the malleus handle is also elevated.

c The inferior skin flap, together with the inferior epithelium up to the umbo region, is elevated.

d The cartilage disk is positioned into the perforation and the perichondrium is folded out.

e All epithelium flaps and the skin flaps are replaced.

f Side view with some perspective of tympanoplasty type 1 of a posterior perforation with intact ossicular chain applying in-lay on-lay graft technique. The cartilage disk does not touch the intact long process of the incus. The perichondrium flap is positioned on the deepithelialized belt around the perforation. The disk is suspended by the perichondrium flap.

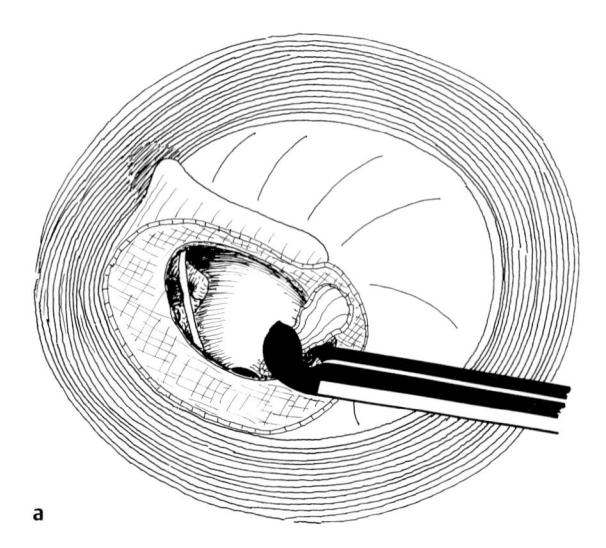

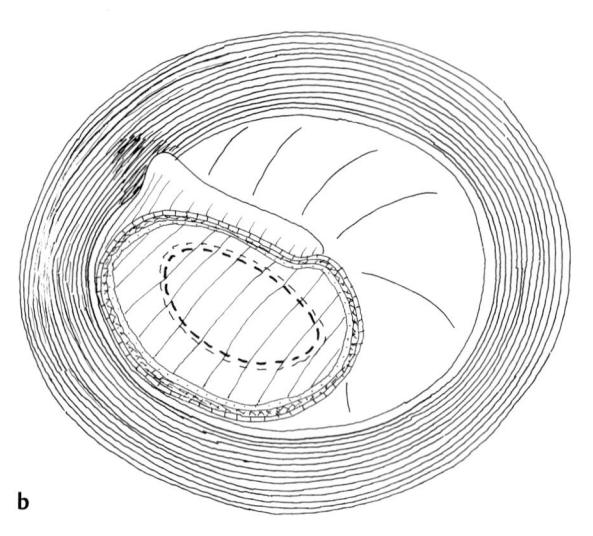

Fig. 24.5a, b Removal of the epithelium around a posterior perforation with intact ossicular chain.
a The deepithelialized margin around the perforation is large enough for the perichondrium flap.
b The cartilage disk is placed into the perforation and the perichondrium is placed on the denuded belt around the perforation.

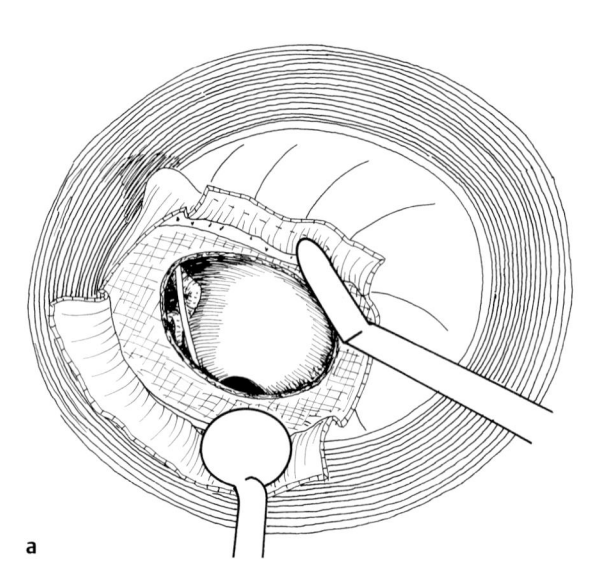

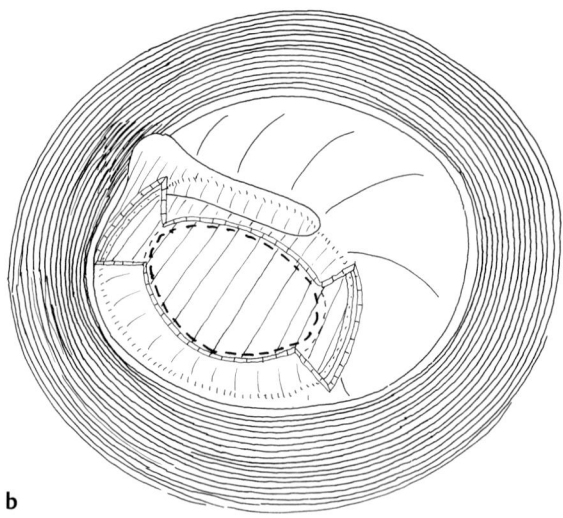

Fig. 24.6a, b Elevation of a posterior and an anterior epithelial flap combined with removal of the epithelium from the superior and inferior borders of the posterior perforation.
a After two small radial incisions have been made, a posterior skin flap is elevated. An anterior epithelial flap is elevated from the malleus handle. The epithelium is removed around the superior and inferior edges of the perforation.
b The cartilage graft is positioned into the perforation; the perichondrium flap is folded out and is covered with two epithelial flaps.

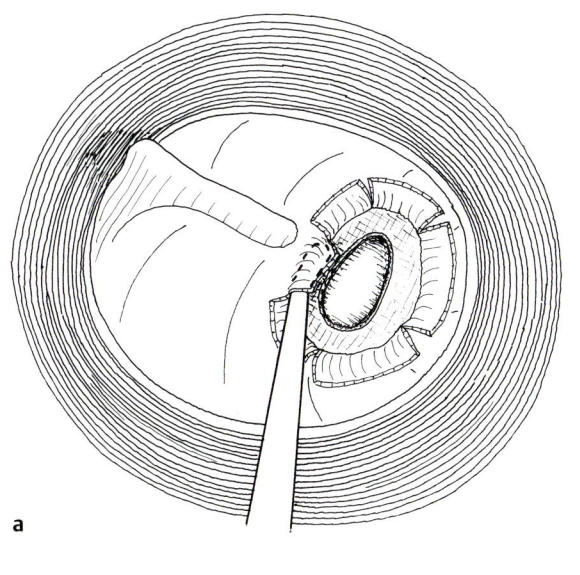

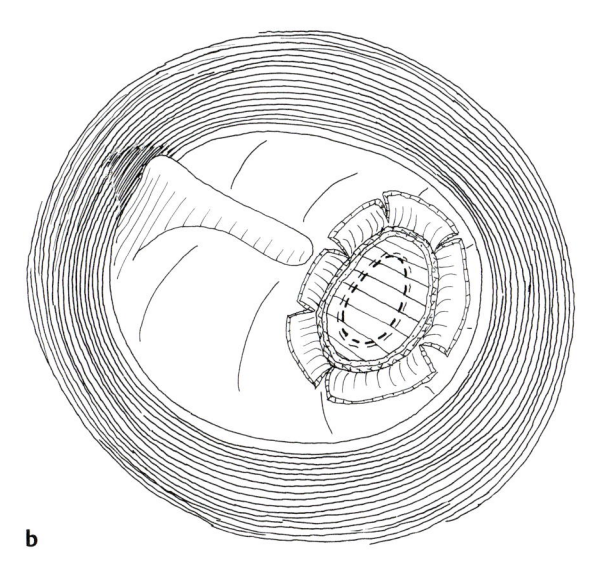

Fig. 24.7a–c Application of an in-lay on-lay graft in an inferior perforation.
a The edges of the oval perforation are cleaned and the epithelium is elevated from a band around the perforation.
b An oval in-lay-on-lay graft is positioned in the perforation. The perichondrium flap is folded out and covers the denuded band of the eardrum.
c The epithelial flaps are replaced.

Total Perforation

The in-lay on-lay graft can be used to close a total perforation. Since the early 1960s, I have performed a myringoplasty with elevation of three superior epithelial flaps (**Fig. 24.9a, b**): the posterior and anterior skin flaps and the malleus flap (Tos 1980). Epithelium is removed along the inferior border of the perforation, but it could also be elevated as shown in **Fig. 24.8d**. A large cartilage–perichondrium flap with a wedge cut-out for the malleus handle is placed in the tympanic cavity at the level of the lamina propria. The perichondrium covers the malleus handle and the cut-out (**Fig. 24.9c**). The peripheral perichondrium covers the denuded eardrum remnant and the fibrous annulus as well as the surrounding ear canal bone (**Fig. 24.9d**). After replacement of the two skin flaps and the malleus flap (**Fig. 24.9e**), the reconstructed eardrum is covered with Gelfoam balls (**Fig. 24.9f**) and gauze moistened with hydrocortisone–tetracycline and polymyxin ointment for a period of 3 weeks.

Pediatric Interleave Tympanoplasty

Gaslin et al. (2007) applied a modification of in-lay on-lay tympanoplasty technique with cartilage–perichondrium island graft in 42 children with a median age of 7.9 years, (range 3–16 years). A portion of tragal cartilage is removed via an incision on the medial aspect of the tragus. Perichondrium is preserved on both sides, but on the anterior side it is elevated and it remains connected via the tragal dome with the posterior perichondrium. The size of the graft is adapted to the size of the perforation. The diameters of the graft must be 2 mm larger than the respective diameters of the perforation. The graft is shaved in a cartilage cutter to a thickness of 0.7 mm. Finally, 1 mm of

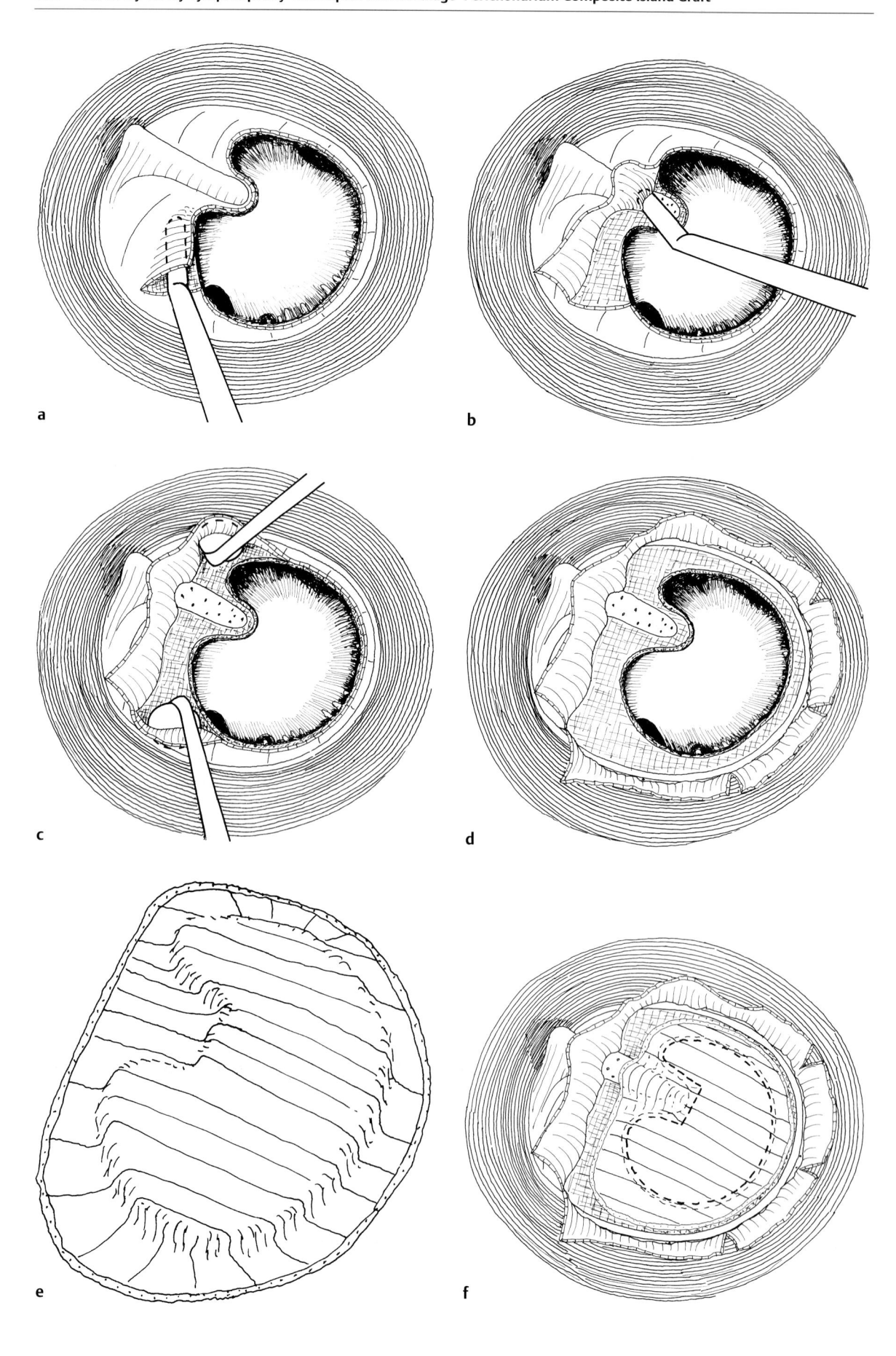

372 24 In-lay On-lay Tympanoplasty Techniques with Cartilage–Perichondrium Composite Island Graft

a

b

c

d

e

f

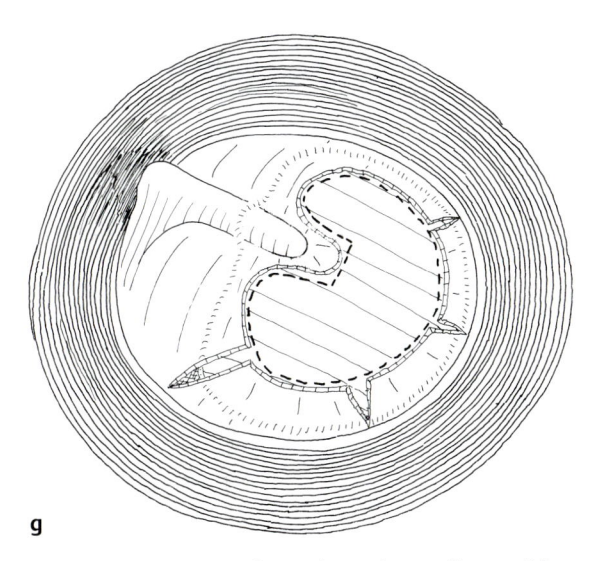

Fig. 24.8a–h Placement of an in-lay on-lay cartilage-perichondrium composite graft in a subtotal perforation.

a The edges of the perforation are cleaned. Elevation of the epithelium is started at the superoposterior border of the perforation and continued toward the umbo.
b The posterosuperior epithelium and the epithelium covering the umbo are elevated.
c Further elevation of the anterosuperior epithelium and the start of elevation of the epithelium along the anterior and posterior fibrous annulus.
d All epithelium of the eardrum remnant is elevated, exposing the fibrous annulus.
e A cartilage–perichondrium composite island graft with a rectangular cut-out for the umbo and a peripheral perichondrium flap is trimmed to fit exactly into the perforation.
f The in-lay on-lay graft with a rectangular cut-out is positioned in the perforation. On the ear canal side the graft is covered with perichondrium, which continues as a flap and is placed onto the denuded eardrum remnant and onto the malleus handle.
g The epithelial flaps are replaced.
h Side view with some perspective of tympanoplasty type 1 closing a subtotal perforation with in-lay on-lay island graft with a cut-out.

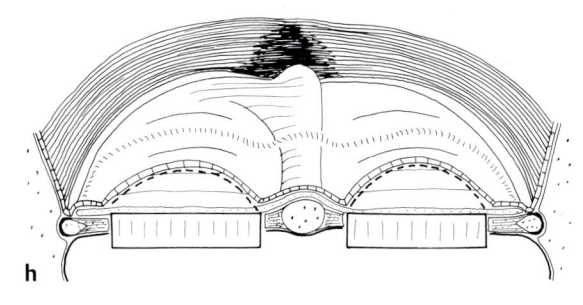

the edge of the cartilage island is removed, leaving the perichondrium intact (see **Figs. 24.1** and **24.2**). The composite cartilage–perichondrium island graft is ready to be placed into the perforation

The tympanoplasty is performed in transmeatal approach, but can be performed in all approaches. The edge of the perforation is scarified. Using the round knife, the epithelium is elevated by pulling it up to 5 mm toward the periphery of the eardrum. An area of the denuded lamina propria is thereby exposed around the perforation. These procedures are illustrated in *Manual of Middle Ear Surgery*, Vol. 1 (Tos 1993), and I have used them widely in on-lay tympanoplasties since the early 1960s; they are shown here for the anterior (**Fig. 24.3a–f**), posterior (**Figs. 24.4a–f, 24.5a, b, 24.6a, b**), inferior (**Fig. 24.7a–c**), subtotal (**Fig. 24.8a–h**), and total perforations (**Fig. 24.9a–f**). If the perforation is total or even marginal, then the squamous epithelium is also elevated from the external ear canal.

The cartilage disk is placed into the perforation and the surrounding perichondrium flap is placed onto the denuded lamina propria; then the elevated epithelial flaps are replaced. They cover the perichondrium and they fixate the graft.

The tympanic membrane and the graft are covered with a thin layer of absorbable packing (FloSeal, Baxter, Germany) or Sepragel (Genzyme, Cambridge, MA, USA). The graft is integrated within 10–14 days after surgery.

Results of Surgery

There are no publications on the in-lay on-lay method or on the surgical results of this method.

During the 4-year period from April 2002 to April 2006, Larsen and Lyneborg performed 46 in-lay on-lay operations (Larsen and Lyneborg, personal communication).

At the last follow up 25 months (range 12–53 months) after surgery, the take rate was 91%. The mean PTA improved 13 dB and the air–bone gap 11 dB (Larsen and Lyneborg, personal communication).

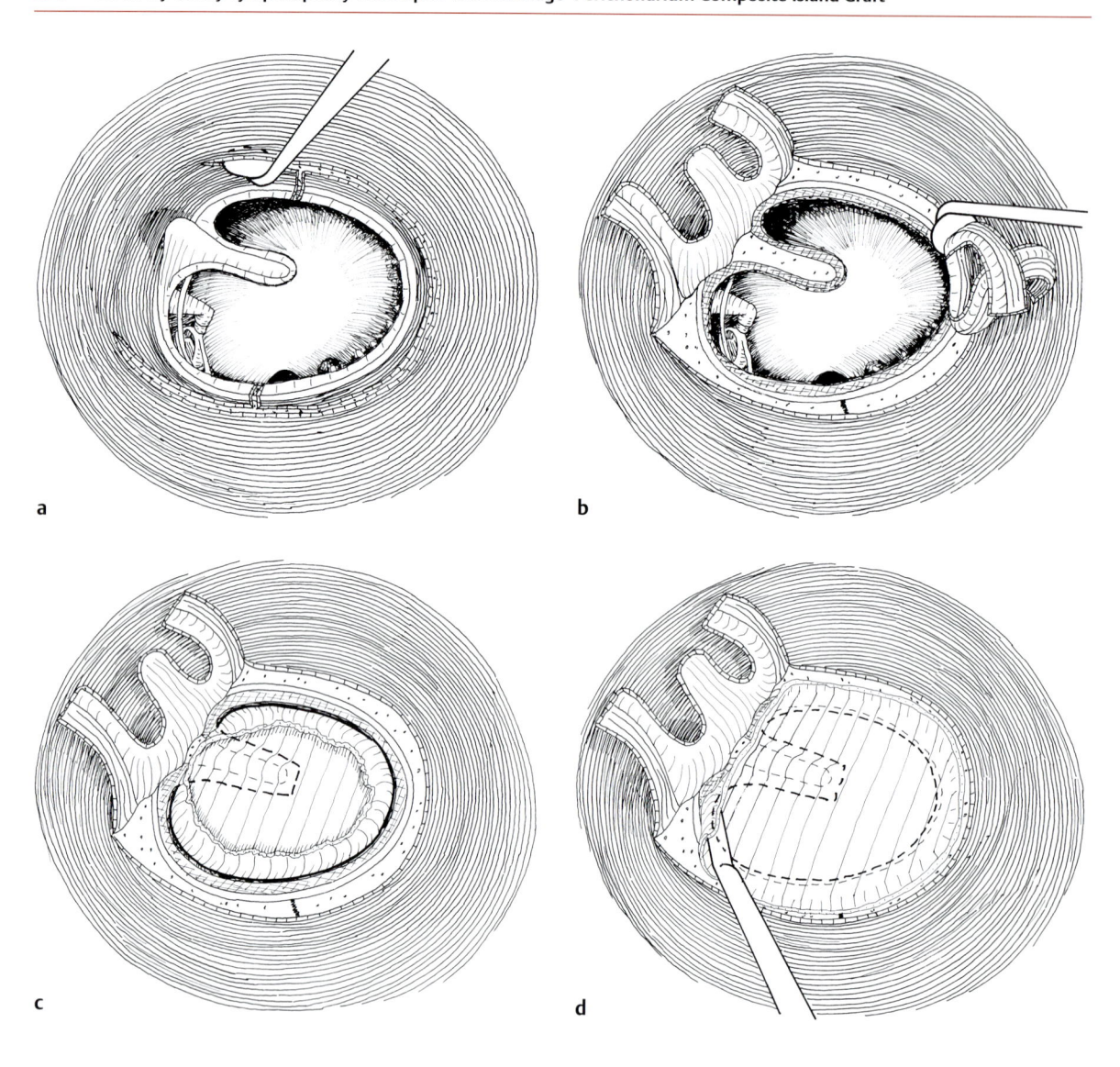

Results of Pediatric Cartilage Interleave Tympanoplasty

During the 3-year period from August 2002 to July 2005, 42 children were operated with a minimum follow-up period of 12 months (mean 30.3 months). Mean size of perforation was 21.3% of the eardrum. The ears were apparently dry at the time of operation. Tympanic membrane was primarily closed in 40 patients (95%); 35 patients (85.7%) maintained an intact, stable tympanic membrane at the follow-up (Gaslin et al. 2007).

In 31 children with audiometric results at follow-up, a mean preoperative average ABG of 10 dB or less was found in 6.4% of the 31 children; the same mean postoperative ABG was found in 80.6%. Mean improvement in PTA was 10.7 dB. Mean improvement in SRT was 9.03 dB. Both the anatomical results and the hearing results were very good.

Pediatric cartilage interleave tympanoplasty represents a very small modification of the in-lay on-lay tympanoplasty technique with cartilage–perichondrium composite island graft as defined, described, and illustrated in this chapter. The small differences are:
1. Elevation of the squamous epithelium around the perforation is in my technique 1–1.5 mm, never 5 mm. Elevation of a large area of the epithelium is not easy and can cause new perforations in addition to the existing perforation, especially in atrophic and thin areas of the eardrum.
2. A large epithelium flap can tear off during the elevation.
3. A large epithelium flap is not necessary for suspension of a small cartilage island graft.

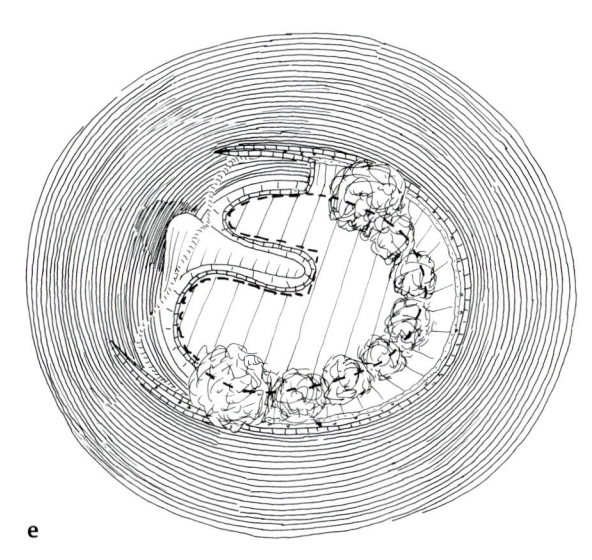

Fig. 24.9a–f In-lay on-lay technique in total perforation with intact ossicular chain applying myringoplasty with elevation of three superior epithelial flaps (Tos 1980).

a A medial circumferential incision between the 11-o'clock and 1-o'clock positions and two radial skin incisions at the 9-o'clock and at 3-o'clock positions are made.

b The three superior epithelial flaps are elevated and the ear canal skin with the epithelium from the eardrum remnant between the 3-o'clock and 9-o'clock positions is removed.

c A large cartilage–perichondrium in-lay on-lay compound graft, with the surrounding perichondrium folded inward, is positioned in the tympanic cavity close to the lamina propria of the eardrum. The wedge cut-out surrounds the malleus handle and is covered with the perichondrium.

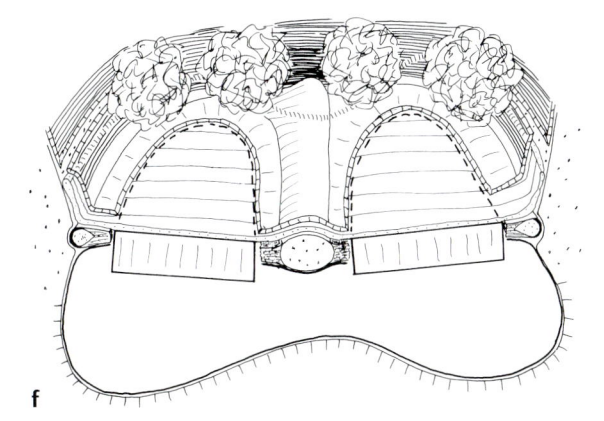

d The perichondrium is folded out to cover the denuded remnant of the eardrum, the fibrous annulus, and the bone of the ear canal.

e The three superior skin flaps are replaced. The perichondrium flap is covered with Gelfoam balls.

f Side view with some perspective at the level of the umbo of tympanoplasty type 1 with in-lay on-lay cartilage-perichondrium graft. The cartilage is covered with perichondrium that also covers the malleus handle. The peripheral perichondrium flap covers the denuded remnant of the eardrum and the ear canal

Author's Comments and Recommendations

Minimally Invasive Surgery

Minimally invasive surgery is popular in all surgical specialities, including otolaryngology and head and neck surgery. As microsurgery, middle ear surgery is often minimally invasive. The transcanal in-lay on-lay technique with minimal incision of the ear canal skin, often without raising a tympanomeatal flap, is a minimally invasive technique, but it involves meticulous separation of the squamous eardrum epithelium from the lamina propria.

Composite Island Grafts for Small and Medium-sized Perforations

In this book, four methods using composite cartilage–perichondrium island grafts are described for closing small and medium-sized perforations, such as anterior, posterior, and inferior perforations. These methods are in-lay on-lay method (this chapter), on-lay method (Chapter 23), in-lay underlay method (Chapter 22), and underlay method (Chapter 21). For scientific rigor it is important to be able to compare the anatomical and audiological results among these four methods and between them and methods using fascia or perichondrium grafting. It is possible that a small cartilage disk included in a part of the tympanic membrane may have excellent vibratility and provide good postoperative hearing. Since the cartilage disk can be of various thicknesses, clinical research is needed into the influence of the thickness of small grafts on postoperative hearing.

References

Gaslin M, O'Reilly RC, Morlet T, McCormick M. Pediatric cartilage interleave tympanoplasty. Otolaryngol Head Neck Surg 2007;137(2):284–288.

Tos M. Stability of myringoplasty based on late results. ORL J Otorhinolaryngol Relat Spec 1980;42:171–181.

Tos M. Manual of Middle Ear Surgery. Vol. 1. Approaches, Myringoplasty, Ossiculoplasty and Typanoplasty. New York, Stuttgart: Thieme; 1993.

25 In-lay Butterfly Cartilage Tympanoplasty

Definition

Eavey (1998) described an original technique that involves placing a specially shaped cartilage–perichondrium composite graft both under and onto the eardrum. Thus, this technique is partly on-lay and partly underlay. However, most of the graft is on the level of the perforation as an in-lay graft, and the technique is therefore called in-lay. The circumferentially incised edges of the cartilage curl apart, like the wings of a butterfly, and hence the name "in-lay butterfly technique."

Indications

Eavey (1998) maintains the following practical advantages for this technique:
- The graft can be inserted onto a hostile eardrum.
- There is no need to remove myringosclerotic plaques; in fact, the stiffness of the plaque enhances the procedure.
- The procedure is minimally invasive, transcanal, without an ear canal skin incision and can, in children, be performed using mask-anesthesia in an outpatient surgery setting.
- No external ear canal packing or support for the graft in the tympanic cavity is needed, because the graft is instantly stable.
- The technique is faster and less expensive than underlay techniques.
- The technique is applied in small or medium-sized dry perforations with an intact ossicular chain, i.e., in easier and smaller pathologies than in those series treated with cartilage palisades or cartilage strips.

On the basis of a recent paper from the Eavey group (Ghanem et al. 2006), the indications for in-lay butterfly grafting can be expanded to large eardrum perforations, annular perforations, and perforations in conjunction with middle ear exploration and mastoidectomy. Such cases were most often operated with a retroauricular approach.

Harvesting and Shaping of the Butterfly Cartilage Graft

A relatively small piece of cartilage, covered on both sides with perichondrium, is needed to shape an Eavey butterfly graft. Using a 15-blade scalpel, an incision is made in one sweep through the skin, perichondrium, and cartilage, about 5 mm medial to the dome of the tragus (**Fig. 25.1a**). The lateral part of the cartilage with the tragal dome is retracted with a hook. Using a pair of small scissors, an extraperichondral plane is created on both sides of the medial part of the cartilage (**Fig. 25.1b**). The medial tragal cartilage is grasped with the flat forceps and small, sharply pointed scissors are used to spread the soft tissues. It is important to include perichondrium on both sides of the cartilage graft. The graft is then excised with scissors (**Fig. 25.1c**). A round graft of the tragal cartilage is cut (**Fig. 25.2**). The size of the graft has to be larger than the perforation and has to have the same shape as the perforation. The diameter should be 2 mm larger than the diameter of the perforation, thus allowing the creation of the butterflies. The round graft, covered on both sides with perichondrium, is grasped and placed under the microscope so that the surgeon can view the edges of the cartilage while holding it in the fingers and cutting it. A thin blade must be used to incise the edge of the cartilage, midway and parallel to the two outlying sheets of perichondrium (**Fig. 25.3a, b**). The attached perichondrium and cartilage on either side will then curl away from the incision line made by the blade. The spreading of the two cartilage surfaces resembles the wings of a butterfly, giving the name to Eavey's technique (**Fig. 25.4a–c**) The depth of the incision should be 1–2 mm to allow the edge of the tympanic membrane to penetrate into the circumferential groove and secure the cartilage graft. In medium-sized and large perforations, the cartilage graft is considerably larger (**Fig. 25.5a–c**).

Harvesting and Shaping of the Butterfly Cartilage Graft 377

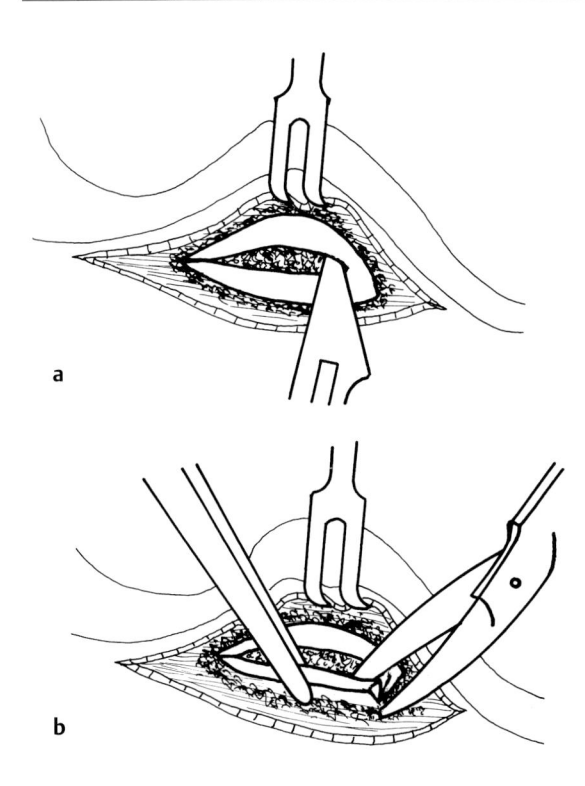

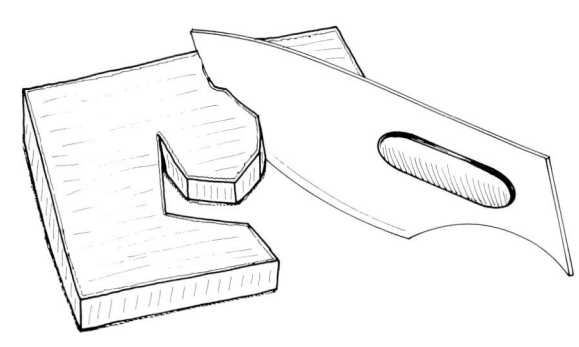

Fig. 25.2 Shaping the butterfly cartilage prosthesis. A round tragal cartilage graft is cut.

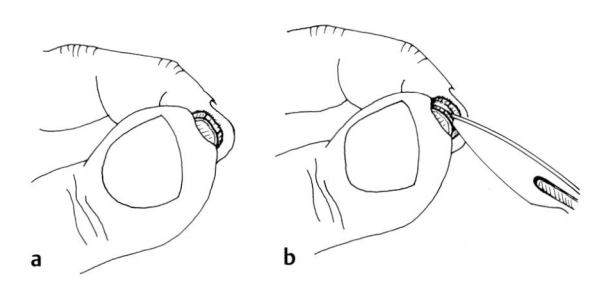

Fig. 25.3a, b The round cartilage graft is held with the fingers (a) and cut in the middle, parallel to the perichondrium on either side (b).

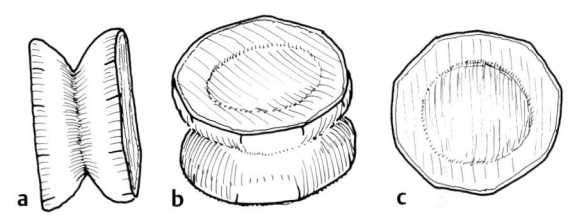

Fig. 25.4a–c The butterfly prosthesis.
a Side view.
b Oblique view.
c View from above.

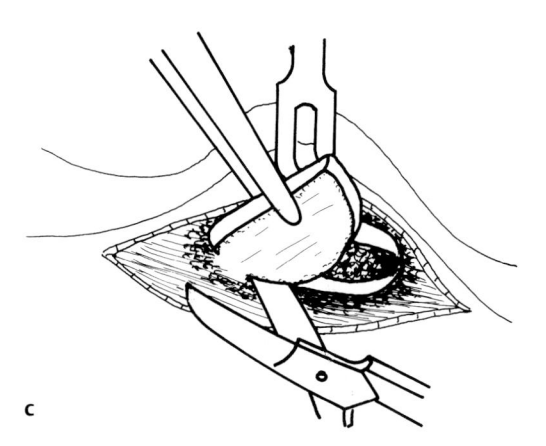

Fig. 25.1a–c Harvesting the butterfly cartilage graft.
a Incision of the skin and tragal cartilage 5 mm medial to the tragal dome.
b An extraperichondral plane is created.
c The cartilage is excised with scissors.

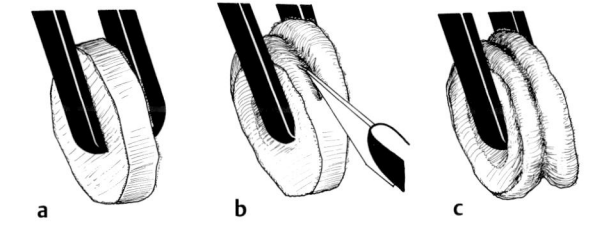

Fig. 25.5a–c Harvesting a Large butterfly cartilage graft.
a A larger piece of a round tragal cartilage is grasped with a non-tooth forceps parallel to the outer perichondrium sheets.
b The cartilage is cut all the way around.
c The result is a larger butterfly cartilage graft.

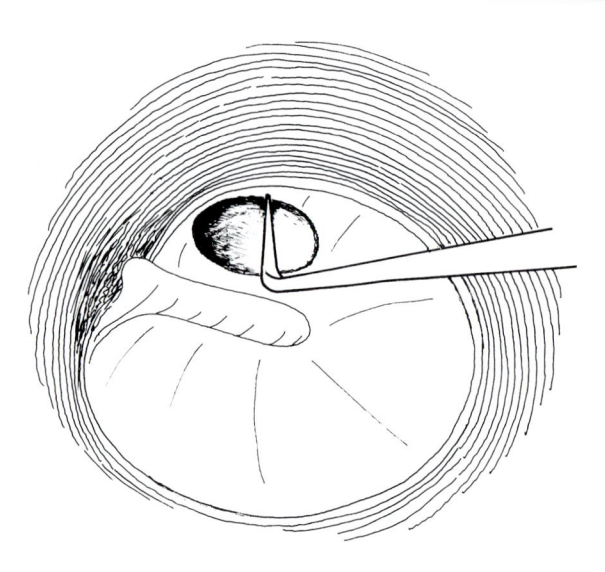

Fig. 25.6 Measurement of the size of the perforation.

The In-lay Butterfly Cartilage Technique

Grafting of a Small Anterior Perforation

The procedure is performed via a transcanal approach, without elevation of a tympanomeatal flap. The size of the perforation is measured using a 4 mm hook (**Fig. 25.6**). The edges of the perforation are removed. The epithelium around the perforation is also removed (**Fig. 25.7a**), using a cup forceps, a sickle knife, or suction.

The Eavey butterfly prosthesis is placed onto the perforation (**Fig. 25.7b**), to be manipulated under the superior and anterior edge of the eardrum initially (**Fig. 10.7c**). Finally, the butterfly prosthesis is pushed under the posterior and inferior edge of the denuded eardrum (**Fig. 25.7d**), similar to placing a grommet. Rotation of the prosthesis indicates its firm position (**Fig. 25.7e**). Displacement of a well-placed prosthesis is difficult.

Finally, the Eavey graft is covered with a split-skin graft (**Fig. 25.7f**) taken from the posterior side of the auricle or elsewhere.

The position of the Eavey graft in the side view illustrated without (**Fig. 25.8a**) and with the split-skin graft (**Fig. 25.8b**).

Whereas Eavey (1998) places a small split-skin graft onto the perichondrium of the butterfly prosthesis, Lubianca-Neto (2000), Mauri et al. (2001), and Couloigner et al. (2005) do not do this.

In the case of a small perforation caused as a complication of grommet insertion, the butterfly graft will have the same shape and size as a grommet. The placement of such a grommet-like graft is similar to grommet insertion.

Grafting a Medium-Sized Inferior Perforation

In an inferior perforation involving the inferior edge of the umbo, the edge of the perforation is removed and the umbo is carefully cleaned of remnants of the epithelium. A band of keratinized epithelium around the perforation is removed (**Fig. 25.9a**). The perforation is prepared for the butterfly graft. A large Eavey butterfly cartilage graft is placed onto the perforation and the in-lay-part of the graft is pushed under the superior border and anterior border of the perforation and under the umbo (**Fig. 25.9b**). The inferior and posterior parts of the graft are then pushed under the edges of the perforation (**Fig. 25.9c**). The grafting is now completed (**Figs. 25.9d, 25.9e**).

Couloigner et al. (2005) indicated that results might be better if cartilage is covered with a split-skin graft as suggested by Eavey (1998). They also suggested that the graft should be at least 2 mm larger than the perforation (**Fig. 25.10**).

Butterfly Technique in Large Perforations

The Eavey group described the butterfly technique for large perforations, performed in a retroauricular approach (Ghanem et al. 2006). After careful measurement of the size and shape of the perforation, a margin of squamous epithelium is removed all the way around the perforation and its edges are cleaned (**Fig. 25.11a**). A butterfly cartilage graft, 2 mm larger than the perforation and covered with perichondrium on both sides, is made as for a small perforation (see **Figs. 25.4, 25.5**). This butterfly graft (**Fig. 25.11b**), of the same shape as the perforation, is placed into the edges of the perforation and the inner wing of the cartilage is gradually pushed under the medial surface of the eardrum remnant (**Fig. 25.11c**). A split-skin graft is placed onto the perichondrium of the lateral side of the graft and the ear canal skin flap is replaced (**Fig. 25.11 d, e**).

Butterfly Prosthesis Placed onto the Bony Annulus

After cleaning the edges of the perforation all the way around and after removal of a margin of the epithelium along the anterior border of the perforation, a tympanomeatal flap is elevated (**Fig. 25.12a, b**). The butterfly prosthesis, previously shaped to fit exactly into the larger defect, made by the elevation of the tympanomeatal flap, is placed into the perforation (**Fig. 25.12c**). The medial wing of the prosthesis is first pushed under the anterior border of the perforation, then under the superior and inferior border and finally under the posterior bony annulus. The lateral perichondrium is covered with a split-skin graft (**Fig. 25.12 d**), and the tympanomeatal flap is replaced. The fibrous annulus is placed under the outer wing of the butterfly prosthesis, the epithelium close to the outer wing (**Fig. 25.12e**).

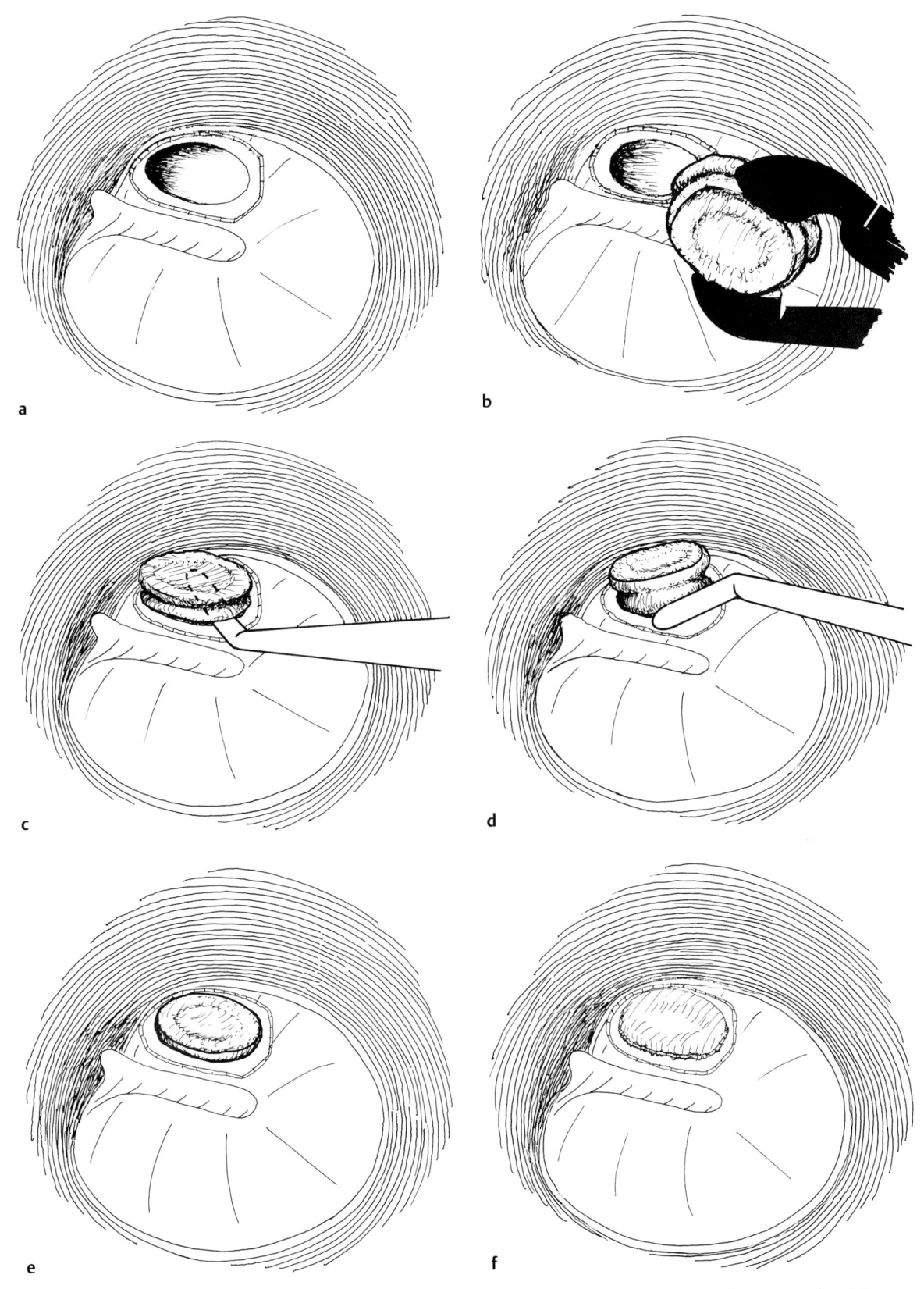

Fig. 25.7a–f Myringoplasty in an anterior perforation applying the in-lay butterfly cartilage technique.

a The edges of the perforation are removed. The epithelium around the perforation is also removed.
b The butterfly prosthesis is placed onto the perforation.
c The graft is pushed inward under the anterior edge of the perforation.
d The graft is pushed under the posterior edge of the perforation.
e The graft is in place.
f The cartilage graft is covered with a split-skin graft.

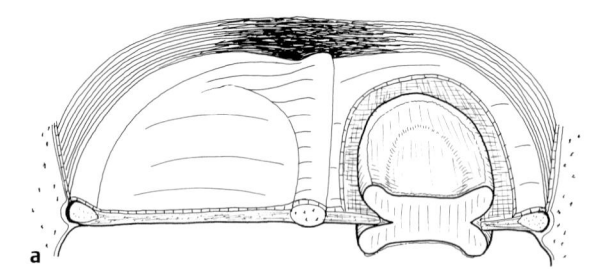

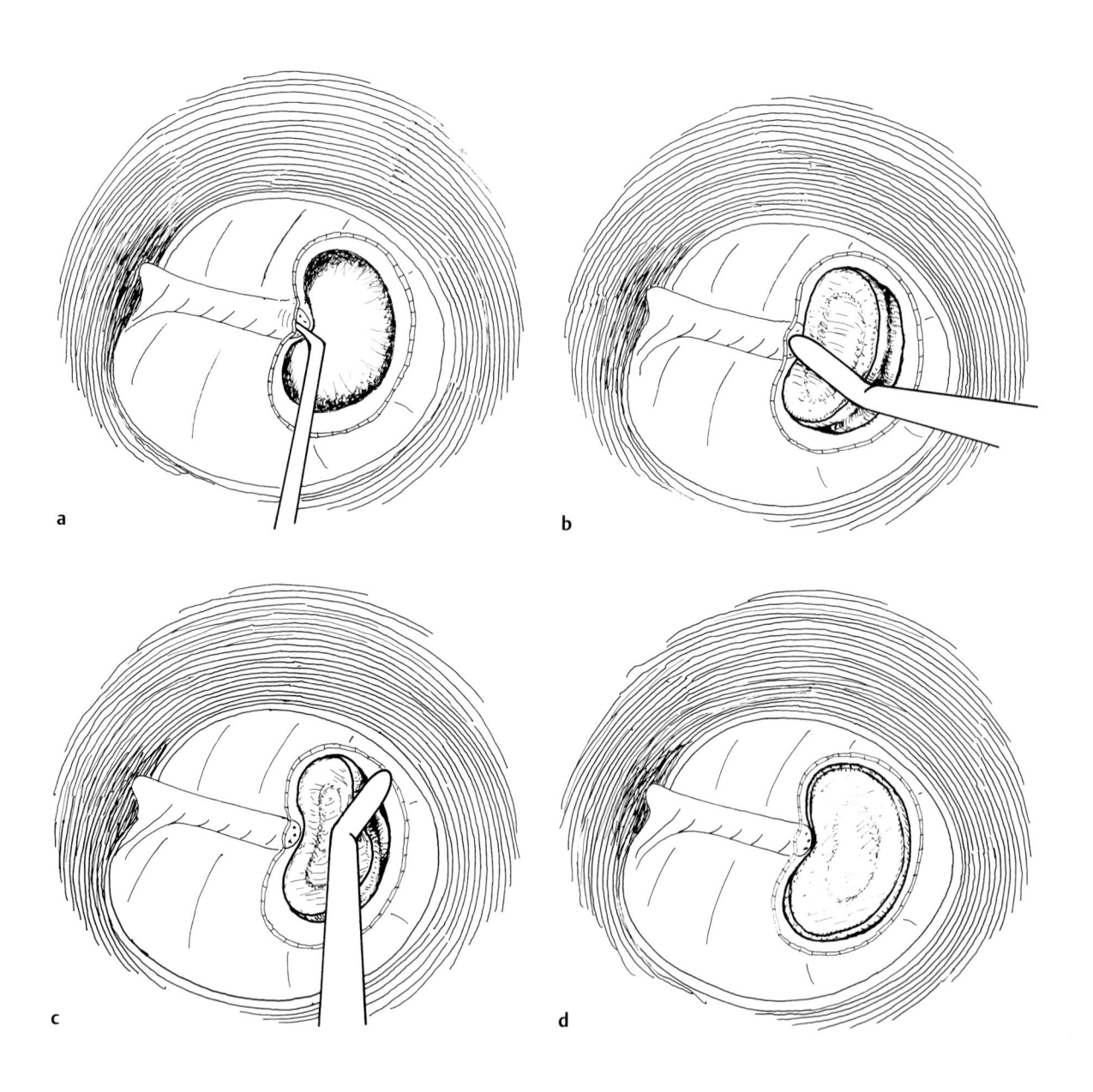

Fig. 25.8a, b Side view of the in-lay butterfly technique in an anterior perforation.

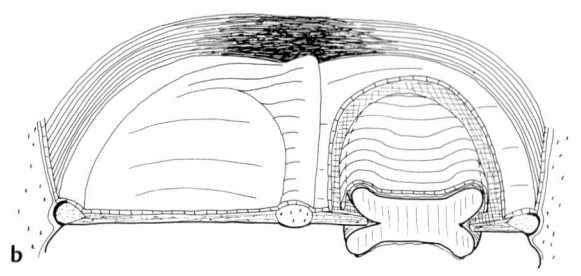

a The cartilage butterfly graft is suspended on the edge of the perforation.
b Side view of the graft covered with split skin graft.

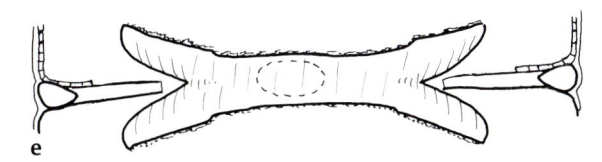

Fig. 25.9a–e The in-lay butterfly technique in an inferior perforation.
a The edges of the perforation are removed and the epithelium around the perforation is removed. The end of the umbo is cleaned of epithelium using a hook.
b The butterfly graft is placed onto the edges of the perforation and its medial wing is pushed under the superior edge of the perforation.
c The medial wing of the butterfly graft is pushed under the inferior edge of the perforation.
d The butterfly prosthesis is positioned into the perforation.
e Side view of the butterfly cartilage graft in an inferior perforation. The graft hangs on the edges of the freshened perforation.

Results of the In-lay Butterfly Technique

Although the method is relatively new, six papers have been published in the world literature on the primary results of the butterfly technique.

The first primary results in 10 children with small anterior and inferior perforations were good, and Eavey (1998) achieved a 100 % "take" rate with good hearing.

In a series of 20 adult patients with small and medium-sized dry central perforations, with diameters of 2–4 mm, a "take" rate of 90 % was achieved after a median follow-up of 7 months. The cartilage graft was healed at the next visit and the hearing was good (Lubianca-Neto 2000).

In a randomized prospective study, Mauri et al. (2001) compared results in 34 adult patients treated with the in-lay technique with 36 patients treated with the underlay fascia technique. The size of the perforation was less than 50 % of the eardrum area. The "take" rate on the 30th postoperative day was 88 % for the in-lay butterfly technique and 86 % for the underlay fascia technique. At the last follow-up, at 7.5 months after the operation, the take rates were 85 % and 83 % respectively. There were no significant differences in the hearing results between the two techniques, but hearing at the first postoperative week was significantly better with the in-lay technique than with the underlay technique. Postoperative pain was less extensive with the in-lay than with the underlay technique.

Couloigner et al. (2005) compared the results of the transcanal in-lay butterfly technique (without any tympanomeatal flap) in 59 children with 29 children treated with an underlay fascia graft. The size of the eardrum perforations was the same in the two groups. The "take" rate was 71 % at 27 months after the in-lay butterfly myringoplasty. In the underlay fascia myringoplasty group the "take" rate was 83 % at 22 months after surgery. The difference in "take" rates is not significant, nor is the difference in hearing between these two series.

Karakullukcu and colleagues presented good results for butterfly technique in 11 adults with perforations of 2–6 mm diameter: 9 months after surgery the take rate was 90 % (Karakullukcu et al. 2006).

In an analysis of 90 patients (99 ears) with a mean age of 10 years (range 2–20 years) and with medium-sized or large perforations closed with butterfly technique, 92 % "take" rate was found 27.6 (range 6–108) months after surgery (Ghanem et al 2006). The mean preoperative to postoperative four-tone air–bone gap improved from 23 to 21 dB, a mean gain of 2 dB, which was not statistically significant.

Author's Comments and Recommendations

It is encouraging that a completely new transcanal, minimally invasive myringoplasty method has been presented, but I do not share the enthusiasm of the surgeons mentioned above for the following reasons:

- The perforations were small and medium-sized, with no ossicular pathology, or infection.
- In the transcanal on-lay technique with fascia or perichondrium, without elevation of a tympanomeatal flap, a higher "take" rate than 71 % should be and could be achieved (Smyth and Hassard 1980; Raine and Singh 1983; Lau and Tos 1986; Tos and Lau 1988, 1989; Ørntoft et al. 1999).

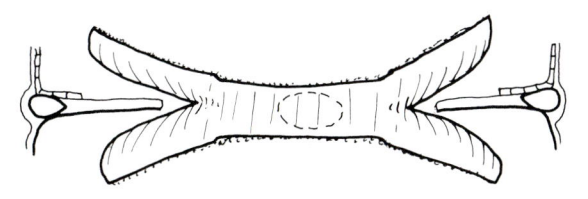

Fig. 25.10 Side view of a butterfly cartilage graft at least 2 mm larger than the perforation, as suggested by Couloigner et al. The wings curl both on the inner and on the outer side of the perforation and thus the epithelialization of the graft may be hampered.

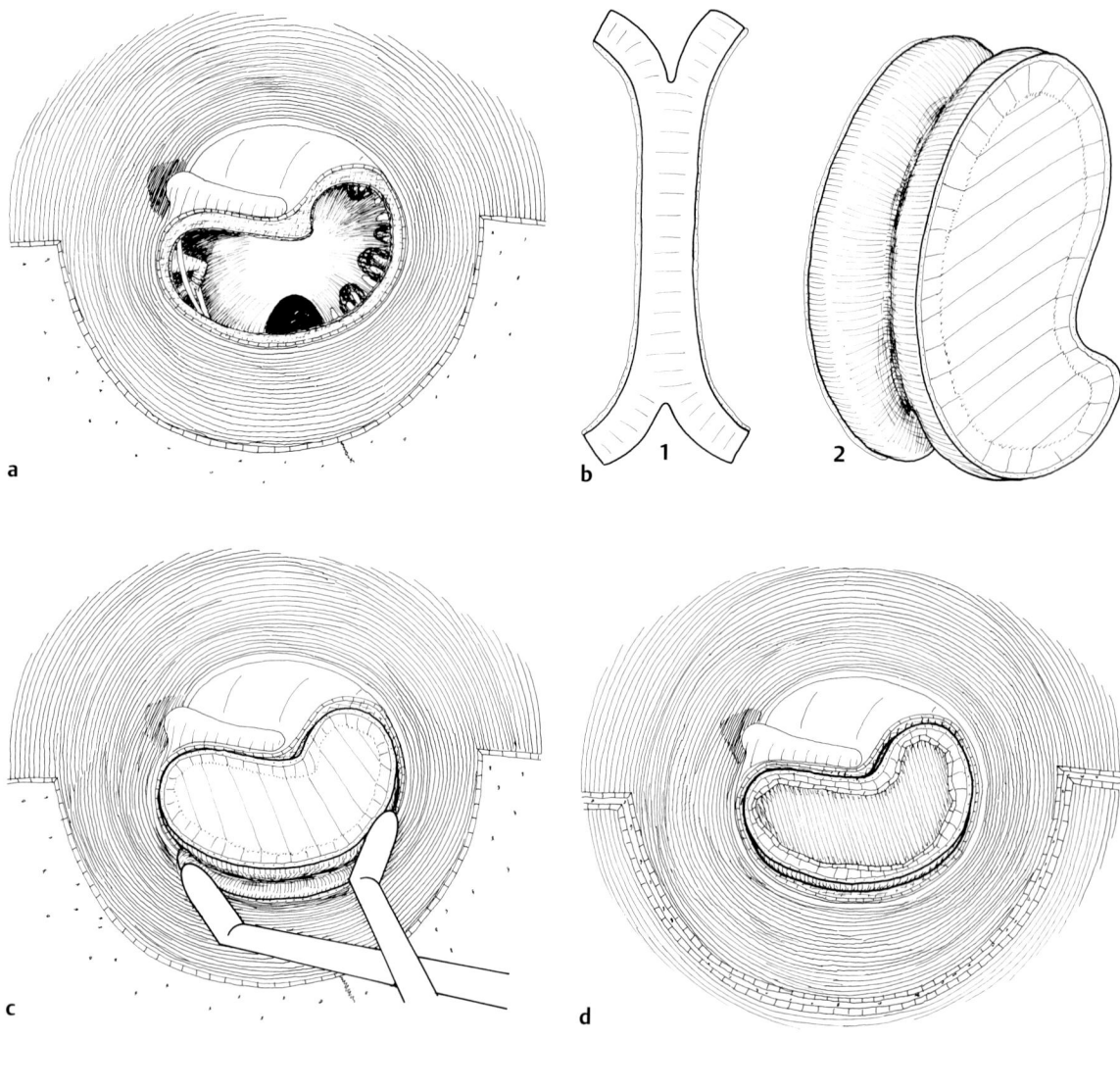

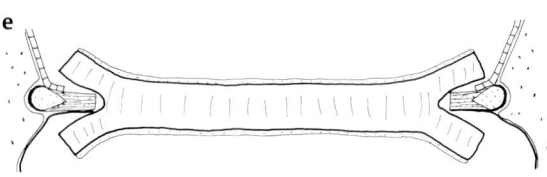

Fig. 25.11a–e The in-lay butterfly technique in a large perforation and intact ossicular chain.

a The edges of the perforation are cleaned. A 0.5–1 mm broad belt of epithelium around the perforation is removed.

b A large butterfly in-lay prosthesis: (**1**) Side view: the graft is covered on both sides with the perichondrium, including the medial and the lateral wing. (**2**) Oblique view.

c Along the anterior edge of the perforation the medial wing of the prosthesis is already positioned under the lamina propria. Along the posterior edge the medial wing is being pushed under the lamina propria.

d The butterfly prosthesis is positioned in the edges of the perforation; its lateral surface and the lateral wing are covered by a split-skin graft. The posterior ear canal skin graft is replaced.

e Side view of the in-lay butterfly technique in a large perforation at the edge of the umbo. The graft is suspended on the edge of the eardrum and is covered with a splint skin graft.

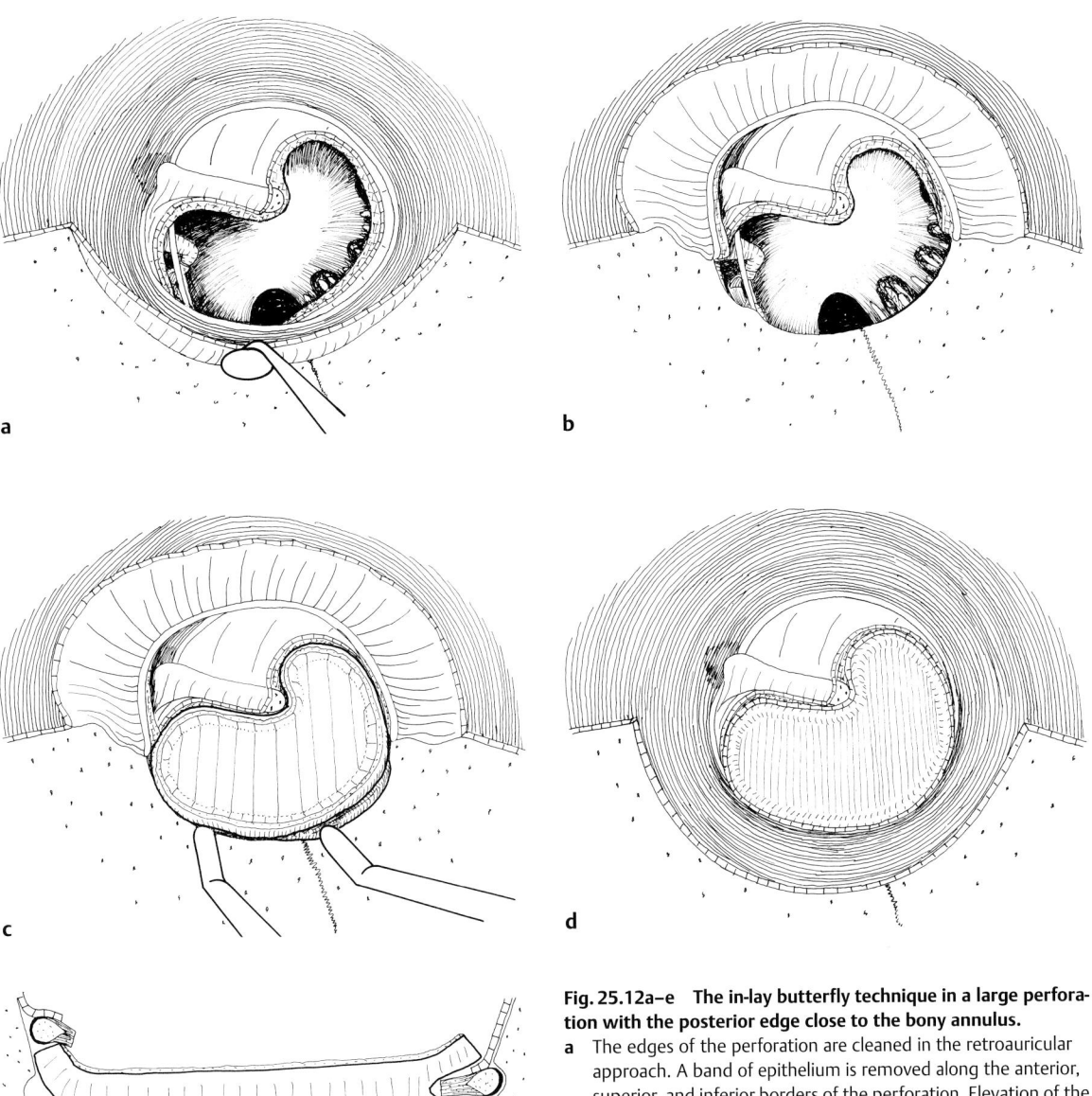

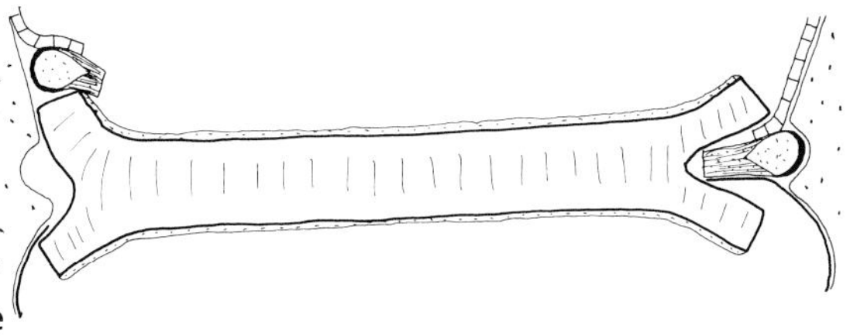

Fig. 25.12a–e The in-lay butterfly technique in a large perforation with the posterior edge close to the bony annulus.

a The edges of the perforation are cleaned in the retroauricular approach. A band of epithelium is removed along the anterior, superior, and inferior borders of the perforation. Elevation of the tympanomeatal flap is started.
b The tympanomeatal flap is elevated, exposing the posterior bony annulus.
c The medial wing of the graft is placed under the anterior, inferior, and superior edges of the lamina propria and is pushed under the posterior bony annulus. The lateral wing is positioned on the outer side of the bony annulus.
d The tympanomeatal flap is replaced and the posterior border of the eardrum is placed under the outer wing of the graft. A split skin graft covers the outer side of the butterfly graft.
e Side view of the butterfly technique closing a large perforation with the posterior edge placed onto the bony annulus. Along the anterior edge of the perforation the wings are placed onto and under the eardrum remnant. Along the posterior edge of the perforation the wings are placed under and over the bony annulus. The butterfly graft is covered on both sides with perichondrium. The lateral perichondrium is further covered with a split skin graft.

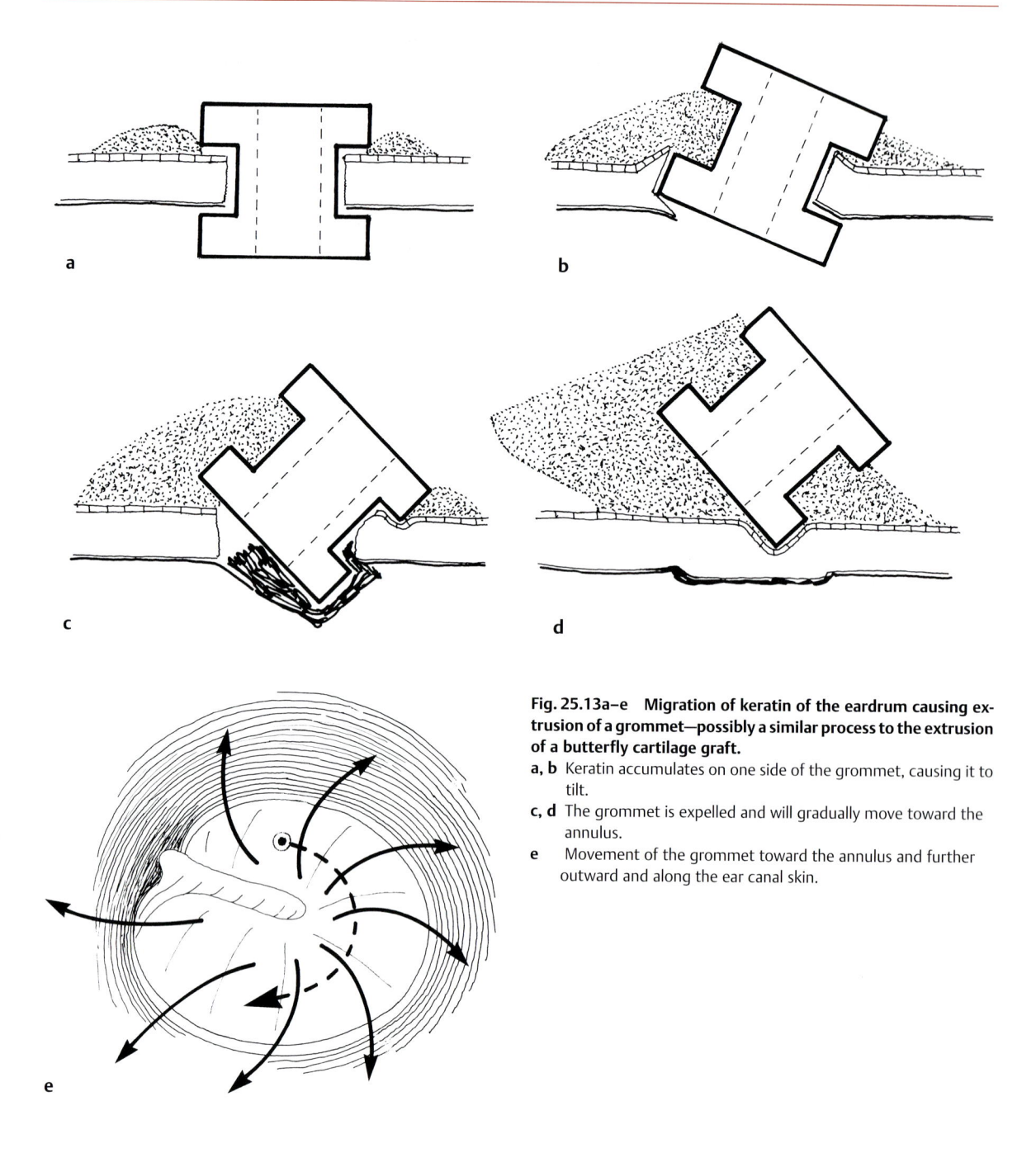

Fig. 25.13a–e Migration of keratin of the eardrum causing extrusion of a grommet—possibly a similar process to the extrusion of a butterfly cartilage graft.
- **a, b** Keratin accumulates on one side of the grommet, causing it to tilt.
- **c, d** The grommet is expelled and will gradually move toward the annulus.
- **e** Movement of the grommet toward the annulus and further outward and along the ear canal skin.

Problems with Epithelialization of the Graft

As indicated by Couloigner et al. (2005), there is a problem with epithelialization of the graft and the possible accumulation of keratin around the graft, similar to what we often observe in the extrusion process and the outward migration of a grommet (**Fig. 25.13a–e**). Such migration or self-cleaning of the eardrum and the ear canal is a fascinating active process at the cellular level in the deeper nucleated cell layers of the epidermis (Alberti 1964; Johnson and Hawke 1985a, b; Jonson 1989). Epithelialization of the cartilage graft, starting from the denuded area of the eardrum, continuing to the edge of the perforation and then outward along the outer wing of the butterfly prosthesis, and finally to the surface of the graft (**Fig. 25.14**) may take longer or may even be impossible if the space between the wing and the graft is occupied by keratin.

My skepticism was confirmed by Effat (2005), who reported poor results 23 months (range 8–38 months) after in-lay butterfly tympanoplasty performed during a period from 2001 to 2004 on 21 patients (28 ears) with simple and dry, small and middle-sized perforations. At the follow-up only 43% of ears showed closure of the perforation. Furthermore, 6 of the 12 closed perforations were not epithelialized. The same author found a "take" rate of 83% in underlay grafting with fascia.

Elevation of the Epithelium Instead of Removal

I am an enthusiast for on-lay myringoplasty techniques and try to elevate the epithelium around the perforation and replace it onto the graft, either fascia or perichondrium. The epithelialization of such a graft is faster and myringoplasty is safer. Instead of removal of the large band of epithelium around the perforation, I propose elevation of the epithelium as small flaps (**Fig. 25.15**), which can be replaced after placement of the butterfly graft. Epithelialization may be faster and there is not the risk of ingrowths of the epithelium into the tympanic cavity.

I applaud Eavey (1998) and Lubianca-Neto (2000) for presenting comprehensive reports on their primary results of surgery, and especially Mauri et al. (2001) and Couloigner et al. (2005) for comparing the results of the Eavey butterfly method with fascia. These two papers and two other papers from our group (Uzun et al. 2003; Andersen et al. 2004), comparing the late results of cartilage palisades and results with fascia in children with sinus and tensa retraction cholesteatoma, are the only publications of such type in the field of cartilage tympanoplasty (see Chapter 4). Also, Kazikdas et al. (2007) has recently compared results of the underlay cartilage strip method with fascia grafting (see Chapter 7).

Closure of Large Perforations and Postoperative Hearing

It is surprising that the mean hearing gain in large perforations is not larger than 2 dB (Ghanem et al. 2006). Successful closure of a large perforation should provide a large hearing gain, especially in cases with intact ossicular chain. The explanation could be that the in-lay butterfly graft in large perforations is firmly fixed to the bony annulus and fibrous annulus, with diminished vibration. Most cartilage perichondrium composite grafts are suspended by the perichondrium flaps and are intended to vibrate. In small and medium-sized perforations the butterfly graft vibrates together with the mobile and intact eardrum, with the result of good hearing gain.

Future Research Needed

Clinical research on the long-term hearing results of such surgery is desired, especially for large perforations.

One can expect that, after the graft in small perforations is completely integrated into the remnant eardrum, there should be no problems with migration of keratin such as we see in the case of grommets. If there are some obstruc-

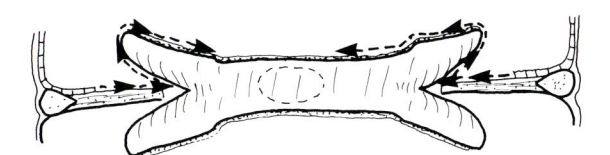

Fig. 25.14 Possible development of epithelialization of the butterfly graft. The epithelialization starts from the border of the eardrum epithelium, first covering the denuded area, continuing on the medial aspect of the lateral wing of the graft (arrows), and then continuing on the lateral aspect of the graft.

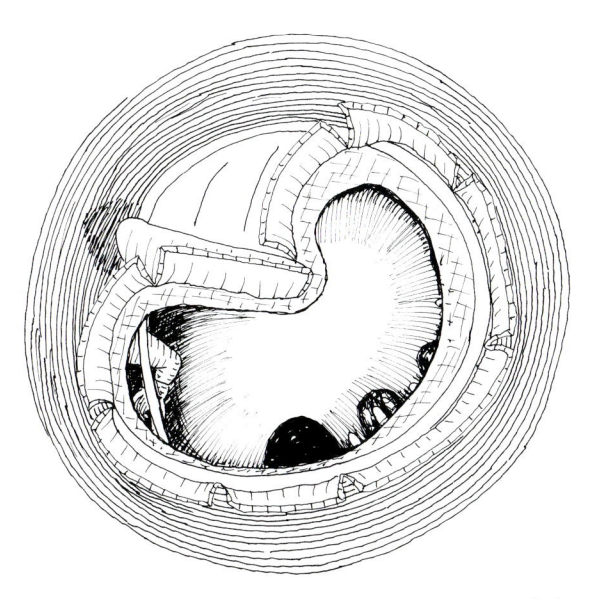

Fig. 25.15 Proposed elevation of epithelial flaps around the perforation instead of removal of the epithelium. After placement of the butterfly graft, the epithelial flaps are replaced.

tions from the wing of the graft, keratin accumulation might occur.

The mechanism of extrusion of the graft has to be investigated otomicroscopically and histopathologically.

The mechanism of epithelialization of the graft should be investigated otomicroscopically and histopathologically on extruded grafts and also experimentally in animals. It can be hoped that this very interesting graft will initiate new research on epithelialization.

The recently published results on medium and large perforations (Ghanem et al. 2006) with a mean observation time of 27.6 (range 6–108) months indicated no migration problems around the graft.

References

Alberti PW. Epithelial migration on the tympanic membrane. J Laryngol Otol 1964;78:808–830.

Andersen J, Cayé-Thomasen P, Tos M. A comparison of cartilage palisades and fascia in tympanoplasty after surgery for sinus or tensa retraction cholesteatoma in children. Otol Neurotol 2004;25:856–863.

Couloigner V, Baculard F, Bakkouri WE, . Inlay butterfly cartilage tympanoplasty in children. Otol Neurotol 2005;26:247–251.

Eavey RD. Inlay tympanoplasty: cartilage butterfly technique. Laryngoscope 1998;108:657–661.

Effat KG. Results of inlay cartilage myringoplasty in terms of closure of tympanic membrane perforations. J Laryngol Otol 2005;119:611–613.

Ghanem MA, Monroy A, Farmaz SA, Nicolau Y, Eavey RD. Butterfly cartilage graft inlay tympanoplasty for large perforations. Laryngoscope 2006;116:1813–1816.

Johnson A, Hawke M. Cell shape in the migratory epidermis of the external ear canal. J Otolaryngol 1985a;14:273–281.

Johnson A, Hawke M. An ultrastructural study of the skin of the tympanic membrane and external ear canal in guinea pig. J Otolaryngol 1985b;14:357–364.

Jonson AP. The Mechanism of migration in the external ear canal: a critical appraisal. In: Tos M, Thomsen J, Peitersen E, eds. Cholesteatoma and Mastoid Surgery. Amsterdam: Kugler & Ghedini; 1989.

Karakullukcu B, Acioglu E, Pamukcu M. Transcanal butterfly cartilage tympanoplasty. Kulak Burun Bogaz Ihtis Derg 2006;16:160–164.

Kazikdas KC, Onal K, Boyraz I, Karabulut E. Palisade cartilage tympanoplasty for management of subtotal perforations: a comparison with the temporalis fascia technique. Eur Arch Otorhinolaryngol 2007;264:985–989.

Lau T, Tos M. Tympanoplasty in children. An analysis of late results. Am J Otol 1986;7:55–59.

Lubianca-Neto JF. Inlay butterfly cartilage tympanoplasty (Eavey technique) modified for adults. Otolaryngol Head Neck Surg 2000;123:492–494.

Mauri M, Lubianca-Neto JF, Fuchs SC. Evaluation of inlay butterfly cartilage tympanoplasty: A randomized clinical trial. Laryngoscope 2001;111:1479–1484.

Ørntoft S, Tos M, Stangerup S-E. Results 20 years after tympanoplasty in children. In: Tos M, Thomsen J, Balle V, eds. Proceedings of the Third Extraordinary Symposium on Recent Advances in Otitis Media. Den Haag: KBugler Publications; 1999:581–586.

Raine CH, Singh SD. Tympanoplasty in children. A review of 114 cases. J Laryngol Otol 1983;97:217–221.

Smyth GD, Hassard TH. Tympanoplasty in children. Am J Otol 1980;1:199–205.

Tos M, Lau T. When to do tympanoplasty in children? Adv Otorhinolaryngol 1988;40:156–161.

Tos M, Lau T. Stability of tympanoplasty in children. Otolaryngol Clin North Am 1989;22:15–28.

Uzun C, Cayé-Thomasen P, Andersen J, Tos M. A tympanometric comparison of tympanoplasty with cartilage palisades or fascia after surgery for tensa cholesteatoma in children. Laryngoscope 2003;113:1751–1757.

26 Composite Chondroperichondrial Clip Tympanoplasty: The Triple "C" Technique

Definition

In 2003, Fernandes from Newcastle, Australia, published a new, interesting, and easy technique, applying a composite graft with perichondrium on the lateral side of the cartilage. The graft is both an on-lay and an underlay graft. The diameter of the cartilage graft should be 2 mm larger than the size of the perforation, allowing elevation of a 1 mm belt of the perichondrium along the periphery of the graft. After removal of the epithelium surrounding the perforation, the graft is placed at the edge of the perforation and the cartilage disk is carefully rotated under the eardrum. The perichondrium is placed onto the denuded ring of the eardrum and the cartilage hangs from the perichondrium.

The perforations are usually round or slightly oval, and the Fernandes grafts should be of corresponding shape and appropriate size (**Figs. 26.1a–c**). The cartilage disk can be thinned to the half the thickness of the tragal cartilage.

Indications for the Triple "C" Techniques

Fernandes performs the surgery by transcanal approach, without entering the tympanic cavity. In such situations the transcanal approach with fixed ear speculum (MMES_1, Figs. 13–24) is the most appropriate and minimally invasive approach. Endaural and retroauricular approaches can be used as well.

Fernandes recommends the following selection criteria:

1. Small to medium-sized dry perforations. The maximal size of the perforation should not exceed one-half of the tympanic membrane.
2. No marginal perforations, with clear view of all margins. Retractions, and remnants of retractions, with any suspicion of squamous keratinizing epithelium should not be operated by this method.
3. Dry ears and no granular myringitis.
4. Conductive hearing loss no greater than 35 dB at any frequency.
5. At least 12 months of clinical observation for nonhealing of the perforation.

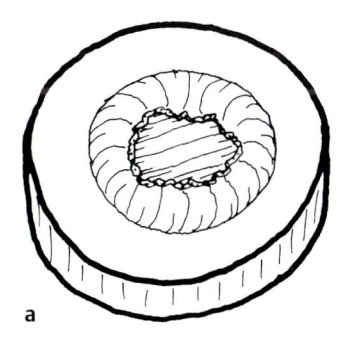

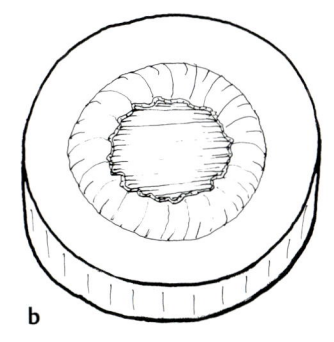

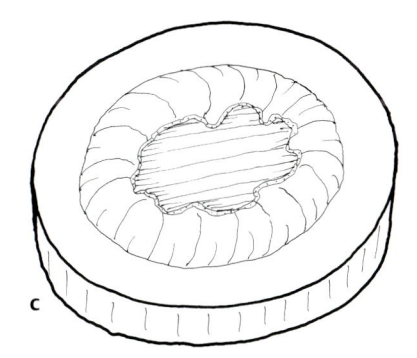

Fig. 26.1a–c Fernandes composite chondroperichondrial grafts for transcanal triple "C" technique.
a A small round graft for a 2 mm perforation. The round cartilage disk has a diameter of 4 mm and the perichondrium is elevated from the periphery of the disk. The cartilage disk is thinned somewhat from the original thickness of the tragal cartilage.
b, c Medium-sized round (**b**) and oval (**c**) Fernandes grafts.

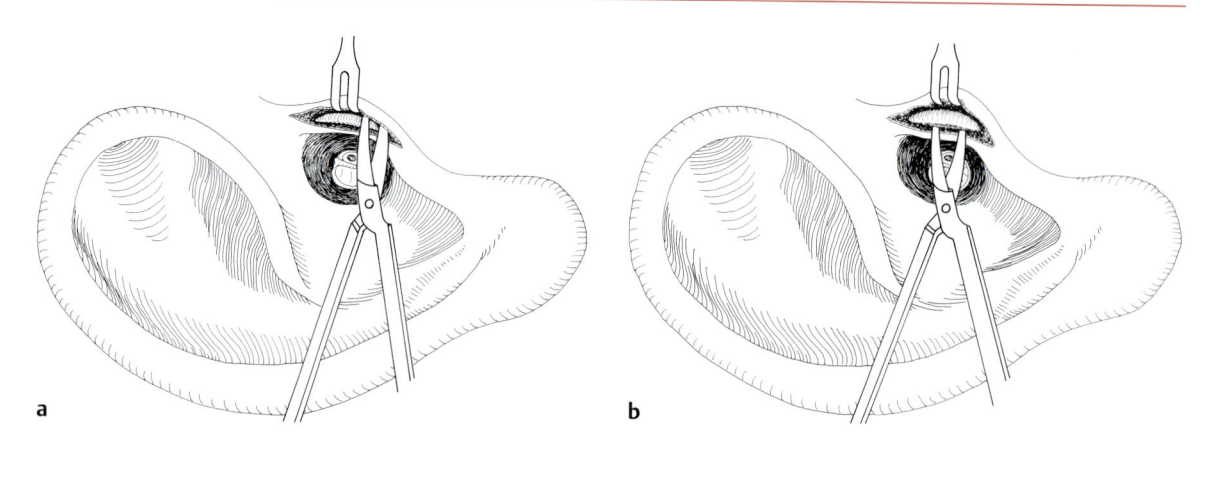

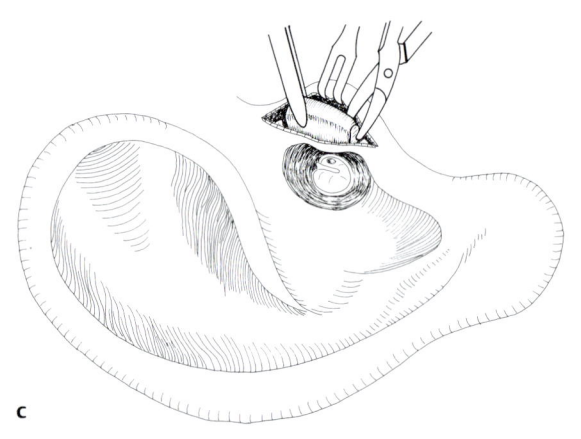

Fig. 26.2a–e Harvesting the Fernandes graft.
a A skin incision is made 2 mm medial to the dome. After pulling the skin with a double skin hook in the anterior direction, the tragal dome is exposed. Using iris scissors, the anterior extraperichondrial space is established and the anterior surface of the tragus visualized.
b With the scissors placed into the extraperichondrial space between the cartilage and the posterior ear canal skin the posterior aspect of tragal cartilage is visualized.
c With a nontoothed forceps the tragal cartilage is pulled slightly out, allowing cutting of a substantial part of the dome and the tragus cartilage, covered on both sides with perichondrium.
d A removed piece of tragal cartilage with the dome (arrow), covered on both sides with perichondrium.
e For a small or medium-sized perforation the perichondrium on one side is elevated and removed along the dotted line.

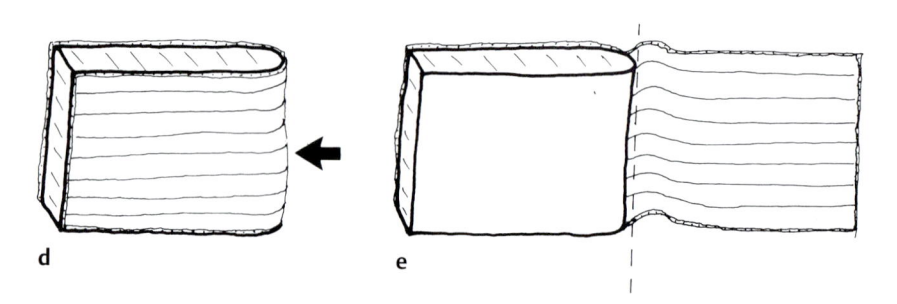

Harvesting and Preparation of the Graft

The tragus skin is incised 2 mm medially to the tragal dome. With a pair of iris scissors and skin hooks, a plane is created at the extraperichondrial level on the anterior side of the dome region (**Fig. 26.2a**) and then on the posterior side (**Fig. 26.2b**). Using a nontoothed forceps to grasp the cartilage to be removed and pulling it outward, a substantial part of the tragus with the dome can be removed (**Fig. 26.2c**). The harvested cartilage is covered with perichondrium on both sides and on the dome region (**Fig. 26.2d**). If the perforation is small or medium-sized, the perichondrium has to be elevated and cut off from the inner (tympanal) side (**Fig. 26.2e**). If the perforation is large or surrounded by atrophic and thin eardrum remnant, the attached perichondrium is applied either as onlay graft or underlay graft.

In the great majority of the cases the cartilage is large enough; in such cases the tragal dome can be left intact for cosmetic reasons. The incision of the skin and the tragal cartilage is made 2 mm medial to the dome. Using a double skin hook, the dome cartilage is pulled laterally (**Fig. 26.3a**) and the medial part of the cartilage is extraperichondrially separated from the subcutaneous tissue and excised with a pair of scissors (**Fig. 26.3b**).

After measurement of the diameters of the perforation (**Fig. 26.4**), the cartilage–perichondrium graft is trimmed and converted to a Fernandes graft by elevating the perichondrium from a 1 mm broad belt of the peripheral area of the cartilage (**Fig. 26.5a–d**).

Before starting the removal of the epithelium around the perforation, the trimmed graft may be placed onto the perforation to determine the necessary extent of removal of the epithelium in relation to the posterior border of malleus handle graft and the anterior fibrous annulus (**Fig. 26.6**).

Surgical Techniques

I will describe the surgical techniques separately for the anterior, the inferior, and the posterior perforations on the basis of the only paper that has been published on the triple "C" technique (Fernandes 2003).

Anterior Perforation

Anterior perforations are often oval with the longest diameter superoinferior. The perforation is usually caused by atrophy of the lamina propria due to long-term tubal dysfunction and secretory otitis during childhood. In our epidemiological studies of otherwise healthy children we found very high incidence of secretory otitis: 90% of Danish children have had at least one episode of secretory otitis and 10% of these children have had atrophy of the ear drum, and in 3% the atrophy was localized to the anterosuperior part of the eardrum (Tos 1981). For various reasons, such as acute otitis or barotrauma, such asymptomatic atrophy may perforate and become a permanent perforation.

There are two different principles of management of the epithelium surrounding the perforation: removal or elevation of the epithelium. Sometimes removal of the epithelium is easier, sometimes elevation is easier; sometimes both methods are necessary at the same time.

Removal of the Epithelium around the Perforation

Usually removal of the epithelium starts peripherally with an incision of the epithelium, pulling it toward the edge of the perforation (**Fig. 26.7a**). Removal of the epithelium continues along the anterior (**Fig. 26.7b**) and the posterior edge (**Fig. 26.7c**). Finally a belt of 1 mm and the edge of the perforation itself are cleaned of epithelium.

Placement of the Fernandes Graft

The principle of placement of the Fernandes graft through an oval anterior perforation is to insert the graft anteriorly along the longest diameter (**Fig. 26.8a**), then to push and manipulate its anterior end toward the tubal orifice

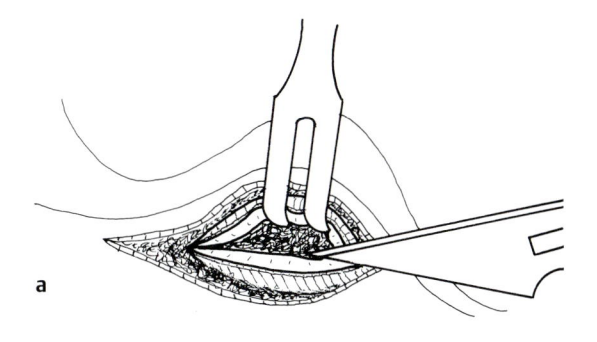

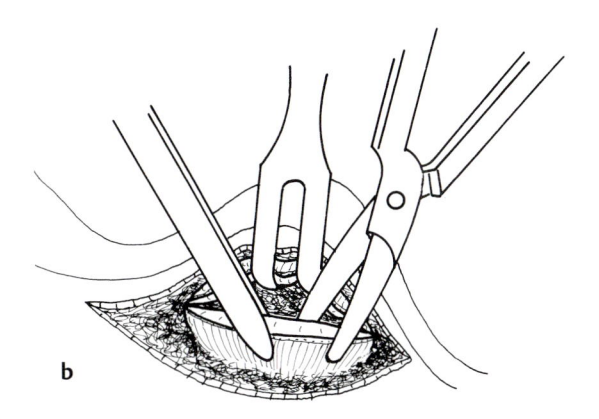

Fig. 26.3a, b Harvesting of a small piece of tragal cartilage without removal of the dome.
a An incision is made 2 mm medial to the dome through the skin and the cartilage at the same time. The anterior and posterior sides of tragal cartilage are exposed and the extraperichondrial space is created on both sides.
b A piece of cartilage with perichondrium is removed with scissors.

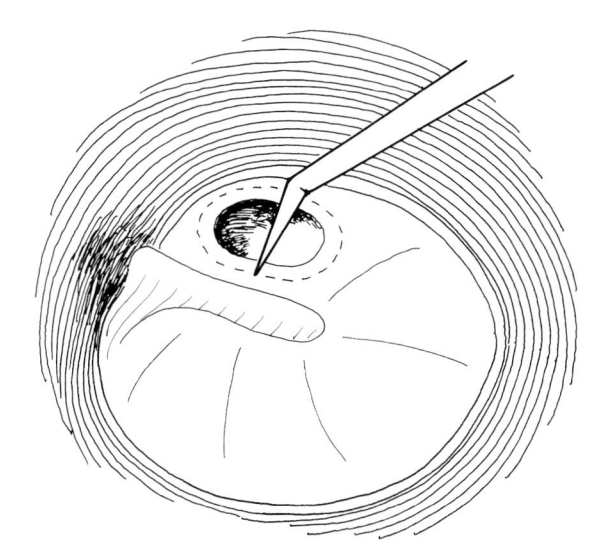

Fig. 26.4 Measurement of the diameters of the oval anterior perforation. Using a large hook, the anteroposterior and the superoinferior diameters of the perforation are measured. One millimeter is added to the sizes of both diameters to provide the sizes of the cartilage disk.

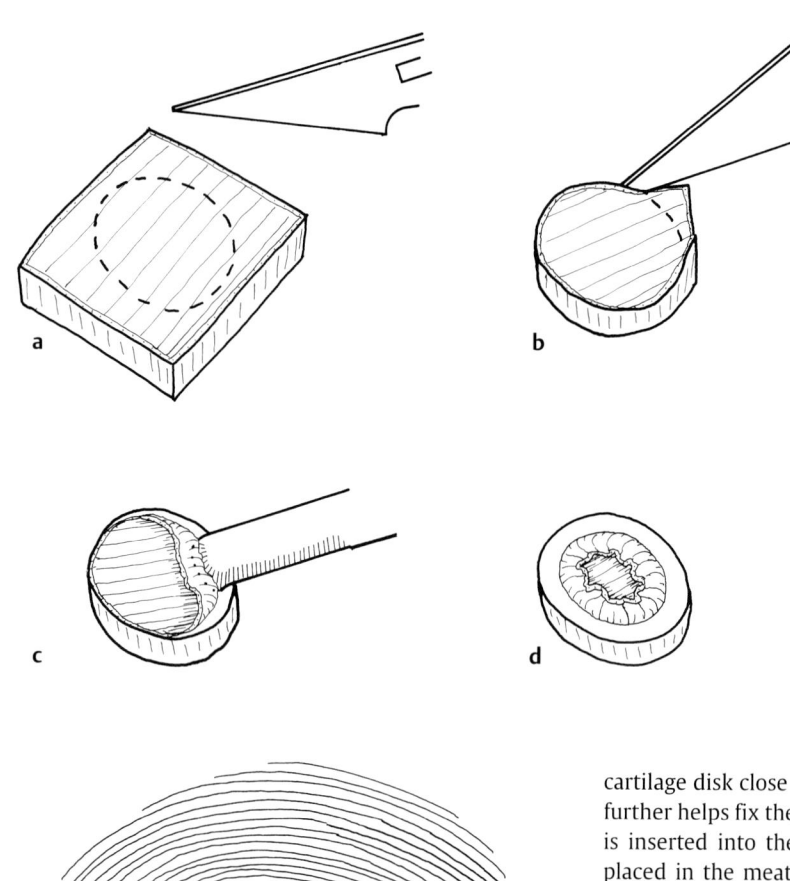

Fig. 26.5a–d Trimming of the cartilage-perichondrium composite graft to the correct size and shape and converting it to a Fernandes graft.

- **a** Superfluous cartilage with perichondrium (outside the broken-line circle) is gradually removed by piecemeal cutting with a scalpel.
- **b** The appropriate size and shape of the cartilage disk is achieved after removal of the last small piece of excess cartilage. The cartilage is covered with perichondrium on one side.
- **c** Most of the perichondrium belt is elevated using a small round knife.
- **d** All the perichondrium from a 1 mm margin of the cartilage is elevated and the Fernandes graft can be placed onto the perforation.

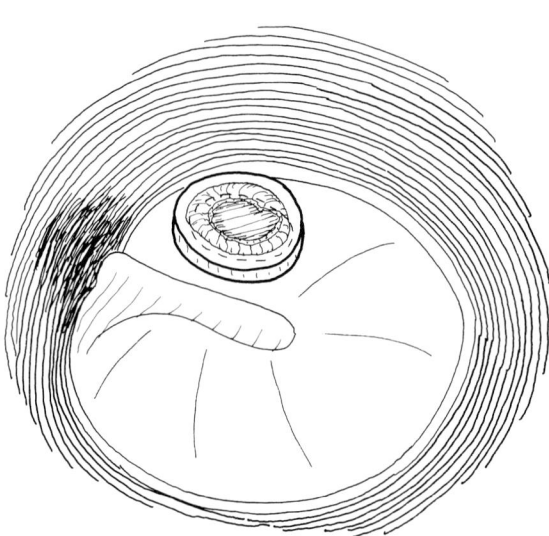

Fig. 26.6 Final measurement of the trimmed graft in relation to the removal of the epithelium surrounding the perforation. The graft is placed onto the perforation, indicating exactly where to start removal of the epithelium.

(**Fig. 26.8b**) until the posterior end of the graft can be pushed under the posterior edge of the perforation (**Fig. 26.8c**). The posterior end is pulled further backward (**Fig. 26.8d**), establishing a balance between the anterior and the posterior position of the cartilage disk, allowing rotation of the graft in a superior direction (**Fig. 26.8e**).

Finally, the perichondrium is folded out and pulled onto the denuded belt of the eardrum (**Fig. 26.8f**), fixing the cartilage disk close under the mucosa. A plate of Gelfoam further helps fix the graft (**Fig. 26.8g**). Antibiotic ointment is inserted into the ear canal and a cotton-wool ball is placed in the meatus. A careful Valsalva maneuver may press the cartilage disk to the undersurface of the eardrum.

A side view (**Fig. 26.8h**) shows an underlay cartilage disk hanging from the perichondrium flap placed as an on-lay.

Elevation of the Epithelium around the Perforation

Some anterior perforations are relatively large and reach the posterior border of the malleus handle and the anterior fibrous annulus. In such cases elevation and saving of the epithelial flaps is an advantage. A small circumferential skin incision in the anterior ear canal (**Fig. 26.9a**) allows elevation of two small skin flaps (**Fig. 26.9b, c**) as well as other small epithelial flaps.

After placement and adjustment of the Fernandes flap (**Fig. 26.9d**), the perichondrium is folded out over the relatively large denuded area around the perforation (**Fig. 26.9e**) and the skin flaps are replaced. They cover and fix the perichondrium and contribute to rapid epithelialization of the eardrum (**Fig. 26.9f**).

A side view (**Fig. 26.9g**) illustrates the position of the cartilage disk close to the malleus handle and anterior fibrous annulus.

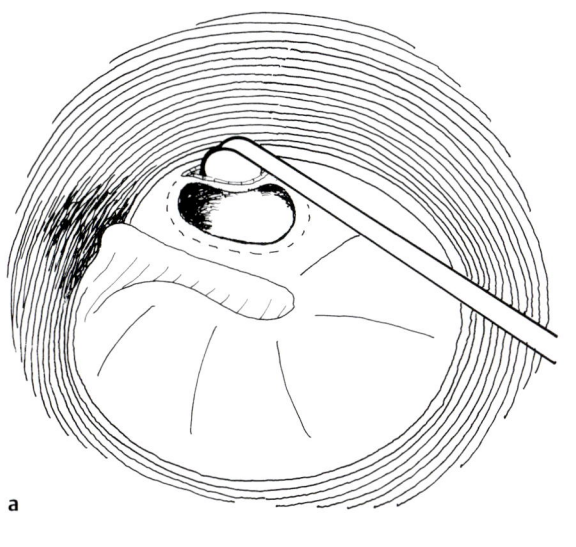

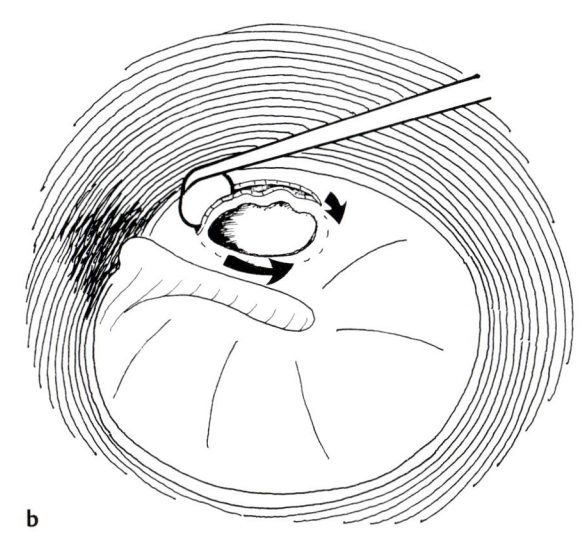

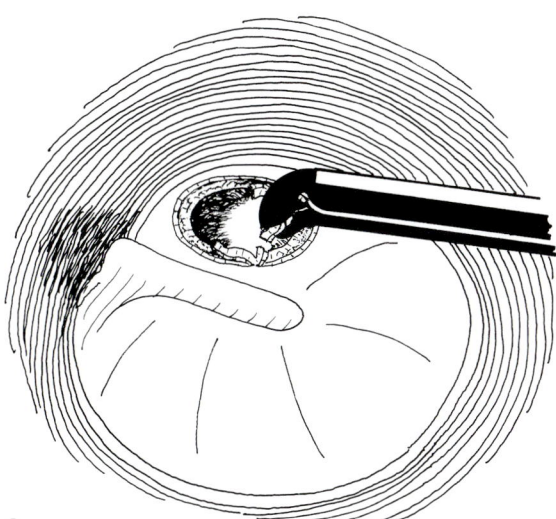

Fig. 26.7a–c Removal of the epithelium from a 1 mm broad belt around the oval anterior perforation.
a Placing a small round knife into the squamous epithelium 1 mm anterior to the anterior edge of the perforation, the epithelium is separated from the lamina propria and can easily be pulled toward the edge and removed.
b After further elevation of the epithelium from the anterior edge of the perforation, further elevation is continued along the malleus handle. The directions of removal of the epithelium are indicated with arrows.
c Removal of the last elevated piece of the squamous epithelium. At the end of the procedure the denuded 1 mm wide margin will be covered with perichondrium of the Fernandes graft.

Inferior Perforation

Many inferior perforations are small, like anterior perforations, and the triple "C" technique is an appropriate method.

In a **small, round perforation**, the Fernandes graft has to be rotated in order to bring it under the eardrum (**Fig. 26.10a–d**). Once the entire graft is under the edges of the perforation, the perichondrium is placed onto the deepithelialized belt of the eardrum, stabilizing and fixing the cartilage disk (**Fig. 26.10e, f**). Further stabilization by packing with a Gelfoam plate is sufficient (**Fig. 26.10g, h**).

Larger inferior perforations require some planning of how to rotate the even larger cartilage disk within the tympanic cavity. Most larger inferior perforations have an oval shape with two markedly different diameters (**Fig. 26.11a**). This is an advantage because the Fernandes graft can first be introduced into the tympanic cavity along its longest diameter (**Fig. 26.11b**). Such an oval cartilage disk can be gently pushed far up under the malleus handle using a hook or a pick. This maneuver allows placement of the inferior edge of the graft under the inferior edge of the perforation (**Fig. 26.11c**), and by further rotation the entire graft is placed under the eardrum (**Fig. 26.11d, e**). Finally, the graft is fixed with the perichondrium flap and a Gelfoam plate (**Fig. 26.11f–h**).

Triple "C" Technique in a Large Inferior Perforation with Involvement of the Malleus Handle

Protrusion of the umbo and inferior part of the malleus handle is common in large inferior perforations and a cutout wedge or rectangular excision of the cartilage graft is necessary for correct placement of the cartilage disk. To achieve removal of the epithelium in a large perforation, it is best to perform a circumferential incision at the level of

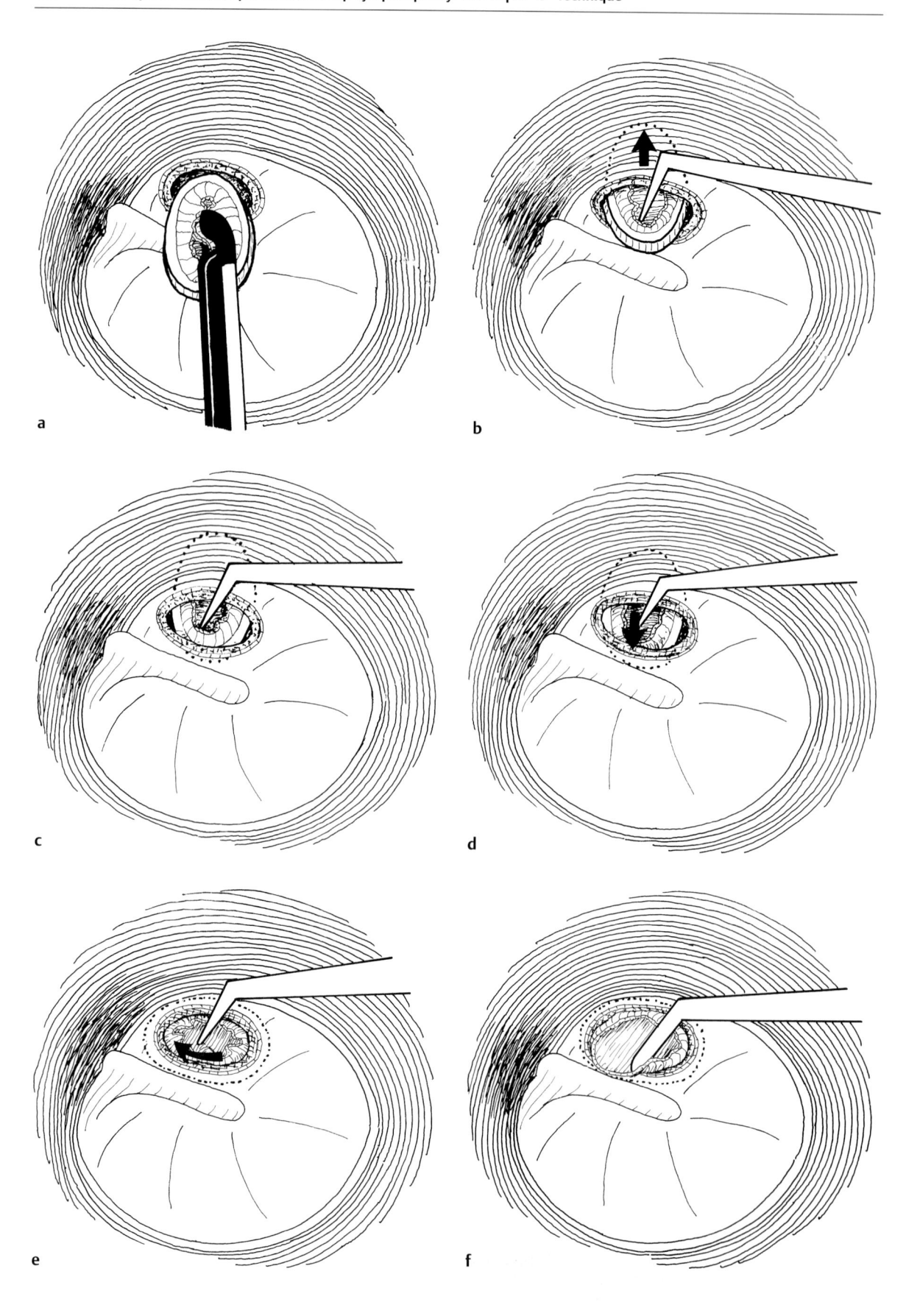

26 Composite Chondroperichondrial Clip Tympanoplasty: The Triple "C" Technique

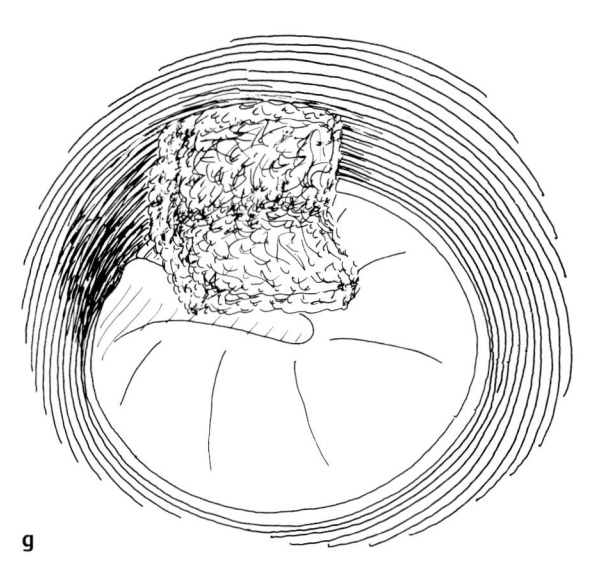

Fig. 26.8a–h Placement of the Fernandes graft under the eardrum.

a Using a forceps, the oval cartilage graft is placed close to the anterior border of the perforation, with the longest diameter of the oval graft in anteroposterior direction.

b With a small hook the anterior part of the graft is pushed under the anterior border of the perforation and then further in the anterior direction toward the tubal orifice (arrow).

c The posterior border of the graft is pushed under the posterior border of the perforation with the small hook. The entire graft is under the eardrum, but it has to be pushed further in the posterior direction.

d The graft is pulled further posteriorly, close to the malleus handle (arrow).

e Rotation of the underlay Fernandes graft. With the hook, the graft is rotated in the superior direction (arrow). The graft is now in the optimal position; its longest diameter is in alignment with the longest diameter of the oval perforation and the cartilage graft lies close to the mucosa of the eardrum.

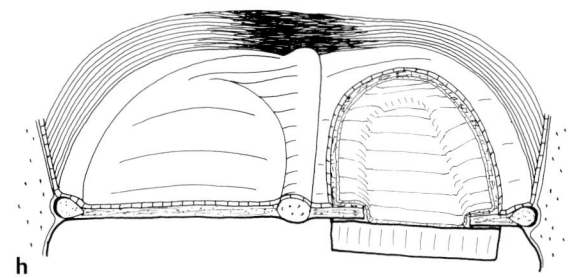

f Fixation of the Fernandes graft with on-lay perichondrium flap. The elevated belt of perichondrium is placed onto the denuded eardrum remnant and carefully adapted to the borders of the keratinized epithelium. The cartilage disk of the Fernandes graft hangs from the central area of the perichondrium.

g The anterosuperior part of the eardrum is covered with moist plate of Gelfoam.

h Side view of triple "C" technique in an oval anterior perforation with removal of the epithelium around the perforation. The perichondrium lies on the denuded remnant of the eardrum, the cartilage disk hangs from the perichondrium and closes the perforation.

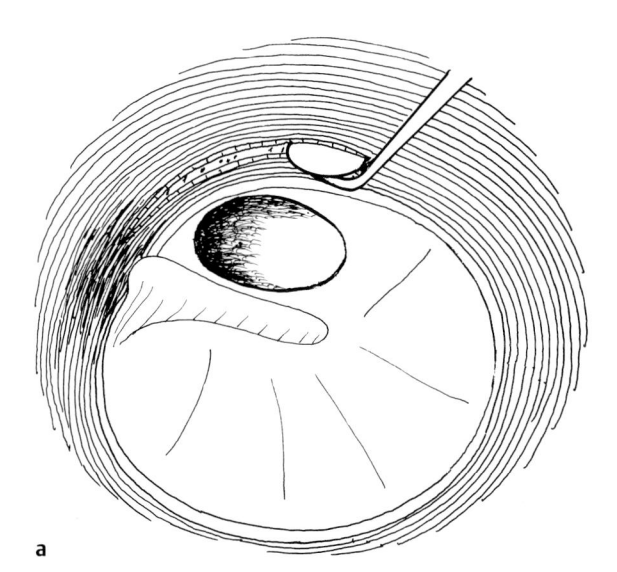

Fig. 26.9a–g Elevation of the epithelial flaps around a larger anterior oval perforation.

a The edge of the perforation reaches the anterior fibrous annulus and posterior border of the malleus handle. An anterior circumferential incision is made 2 mm lateral of the anterior fibrous annulus.

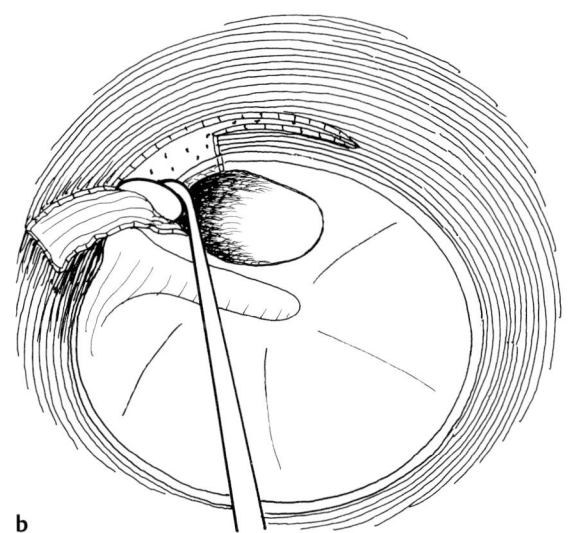

b After a small radial incision at the 3-o'clock position, a small superior skin flap is elevated together with the epithelium surrounding the perforation.

Fig. 26.9c–g ▷

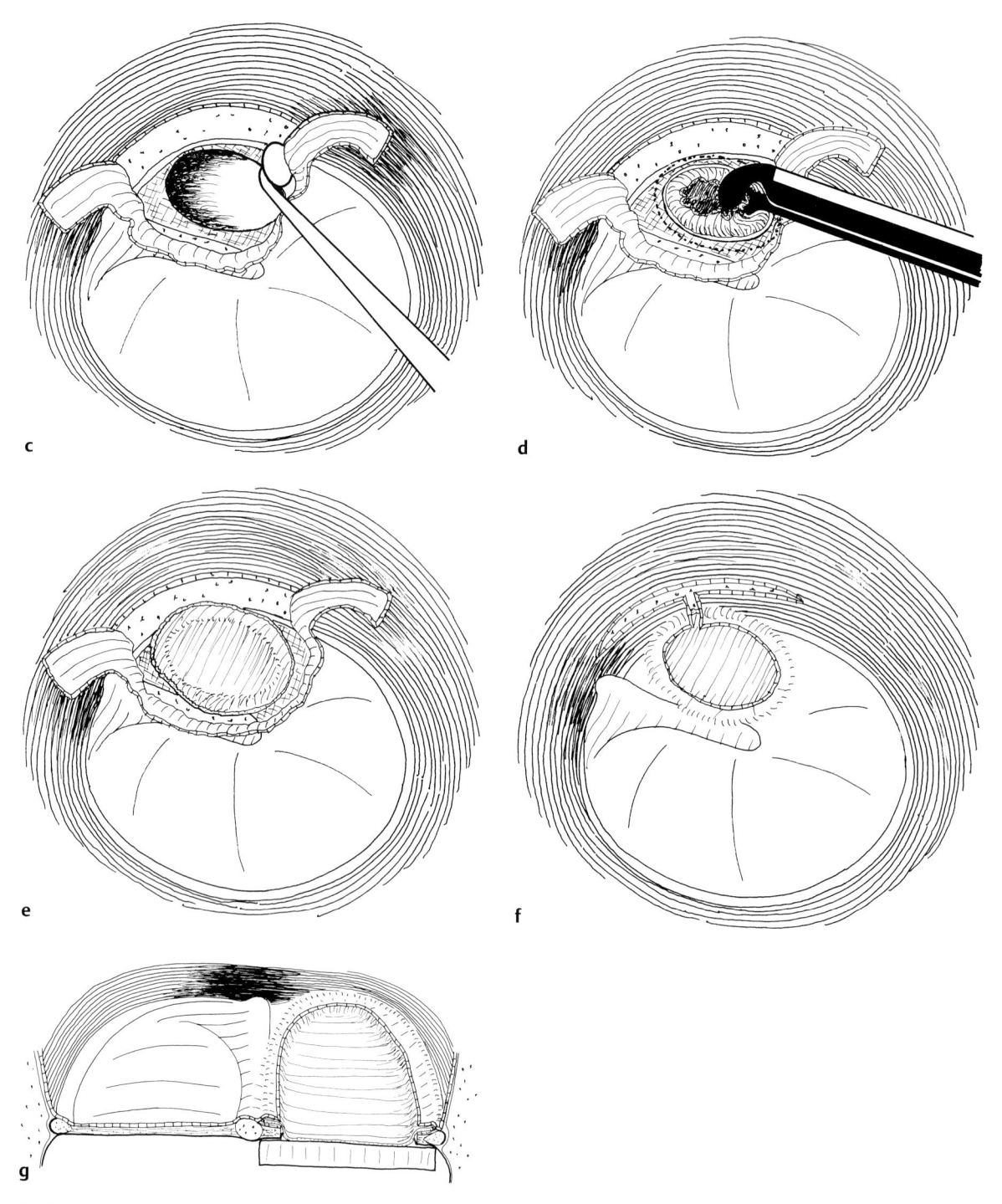

Fig. 26.9c–g

c With further elevation of the epithelium around the perforation and along the malleus handle and of the inferior skin flap, enough denuded area is ready to be covered with the graft perichondrium.

d The oval Fernandes graft is placed, with the cartilage under the eardrum (dotted line). By gentle pulling of the attached perichondrium, the cartilage disk is pulled up to and stabilized closely with the mucosa under the eardrum.

e The perichondrium is placed onto the relatively large denuded area of eardrum, malleus handle, and anterior fibrous annulus.

f The skin flaps and the epithelial flaps are replaced, fixing the perichondrium.

g Side view of triple "C" technique in a relatively large oval anterior perforation with elevation of epithelial flaps. The cartilage is placed under the eardrum, close to the malleus and anterior fibrous annulus. The perichondrium solidly fixes the cartilage and the epithelial flaps stabilize and cover the perichondrium.

Surgical Techniques 395

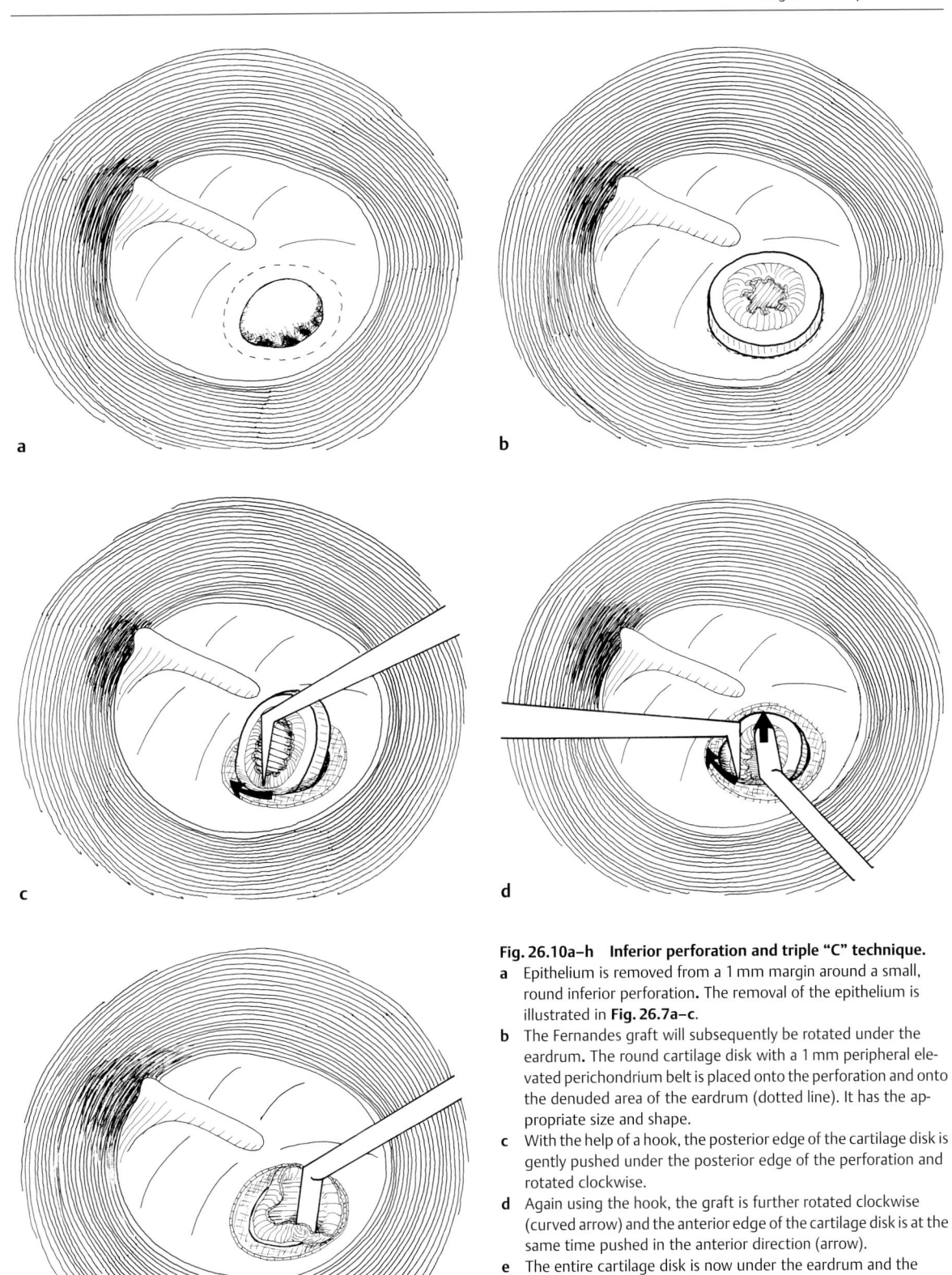

Fig. 26.10a–h Inferior perforation and triple "C" technique.
a Epithelium is removed from a 1 mm margin around a small, round inferior perforation. The removal of the epithelium is illustrated in **Fig. 26.7a–c**.
b The Fernandes graft will subsequently be rotated under the eardrum. The round cartilage disk with a 1 mm peripheral elevated perichondrium belt is placed onto the perforation and onto the denuded area of the eardrum (dotted line). It has the appropriate size and shape.
c With the help of a hook, the posterior edge of the cartilage disk is gently pushed under the posterior edge of the perforation and rotated clockwise.
d Again using the hook, the graft is further rotated clockwise (curved arrow) and the anterior edge of the cartilage disk is at the same time pushed in the anterior direction (arrow).
e The entire cartilage disk is now under the eardrum and the perichondrium can be folded out.

Fig. 26.10f–h ▷

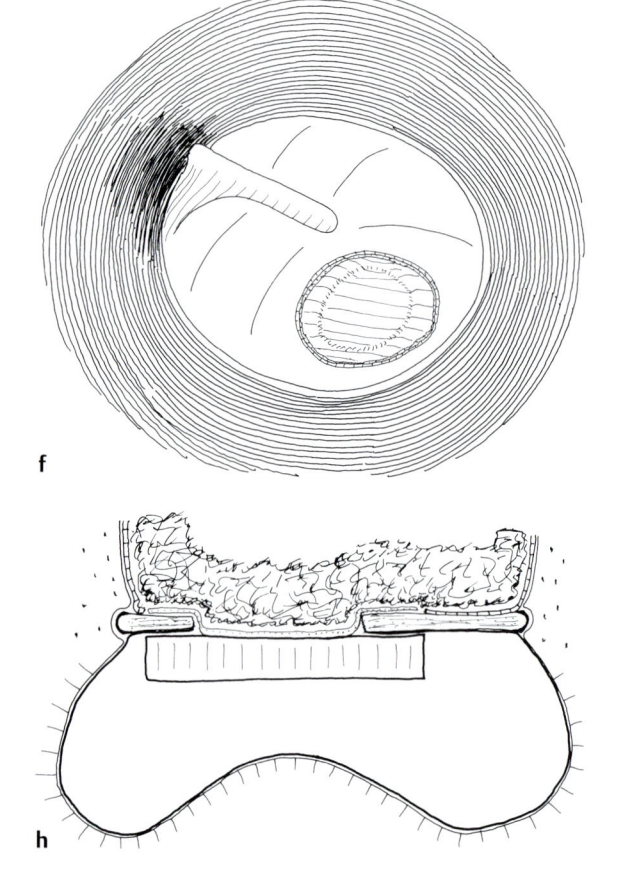

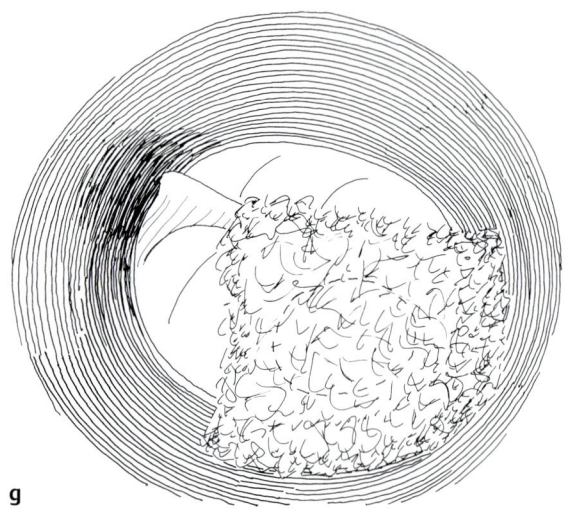

Fig. 26.10f–h

f The entire perichondrium is folded out and the cartilage disk under the eardrum is hanging from the perichondrium.
g A slightly moist Gelfoam plate covers the inferior half of the eardrum, further stabilizing the graft.
h Side view of the inferior half of the tympanic cavity with an inferior perforation closed with the Fernandes graft. The perichondrium elevated from the cartilage disk is placed onto the denuded eardrum.

the fibrous annulus (**Fig. 26.12a, b**). Superiorly the epithelium can easily be elevated (**Fig. 26.12c–e**). After adaptation of the Fernandes graft (**Fig. 26.12f**), the graft is placed with its longest diameter under the umbo (**Fig. 26.12g**) and then pushed upward under the malleus handle (**Fig. 26.12h, i**) and rotated into the proper position in relation to the umbo (**Fig. 26.12j**). The perichondrium is laid onto the deepithelialized margin of the eardrum and the superior epithelial flaps are replaced (**Fig. 26.12k**). The eardrum is covered with a slightly pressed and slightly wet Gelfoam plate (**Fig. 26.12l**).

Posterior Perforation

Because of presence of the incudostapedial joint, posterior malleus ligament, chorda tympani, and bony prominence surrounding the exit of the chorda tympani, there is limited space for rotation of a major cartilage disk in the posterosuperior region. Furthermore, there will be a considerable possibility of adhesions between the eardrum remnant and the incudostapedial joint and remnants of previous retractions.

As stressed previously in describing the pathogenesis of the anterior perforation, the common secretory otitis and chronic tubal dysfunction causes retraction and atrophy of the eardrum (Tos 1981). Atrophy is irreversible and will always remain atrophy, but it may become retracted or perforated. Anterior atrophy will hardly ever end as retraction with adhesion, simply because the medial wall is far too deep. Posterior atrophy is common and will very often retract and adhere to the incudostapedial joint. Such retraction can perforate, or it can progress and end as a sinus cholesteatoma or adhesive otitis.

In a relatively small round posterior perforation, the removal of the epithelium from a 1 mm belt around the perforation extends anteriorly to the malleus handle and posteriorly to the fibrous annulus (**Fig. 26.13a**). The Fernandes graft is placed under the anterior edge of the perforation and rotated clockwise (**Fig. 26.13b, c**). The entire cartilage graft will gradually become an underlay graft and can be stabilized by placement of the perichondrium onto the deepithelialized belt of the eardrum (**Fig. 26.13d**) and further supported with a Gelfoam plate (**Fig. 26.13e**).

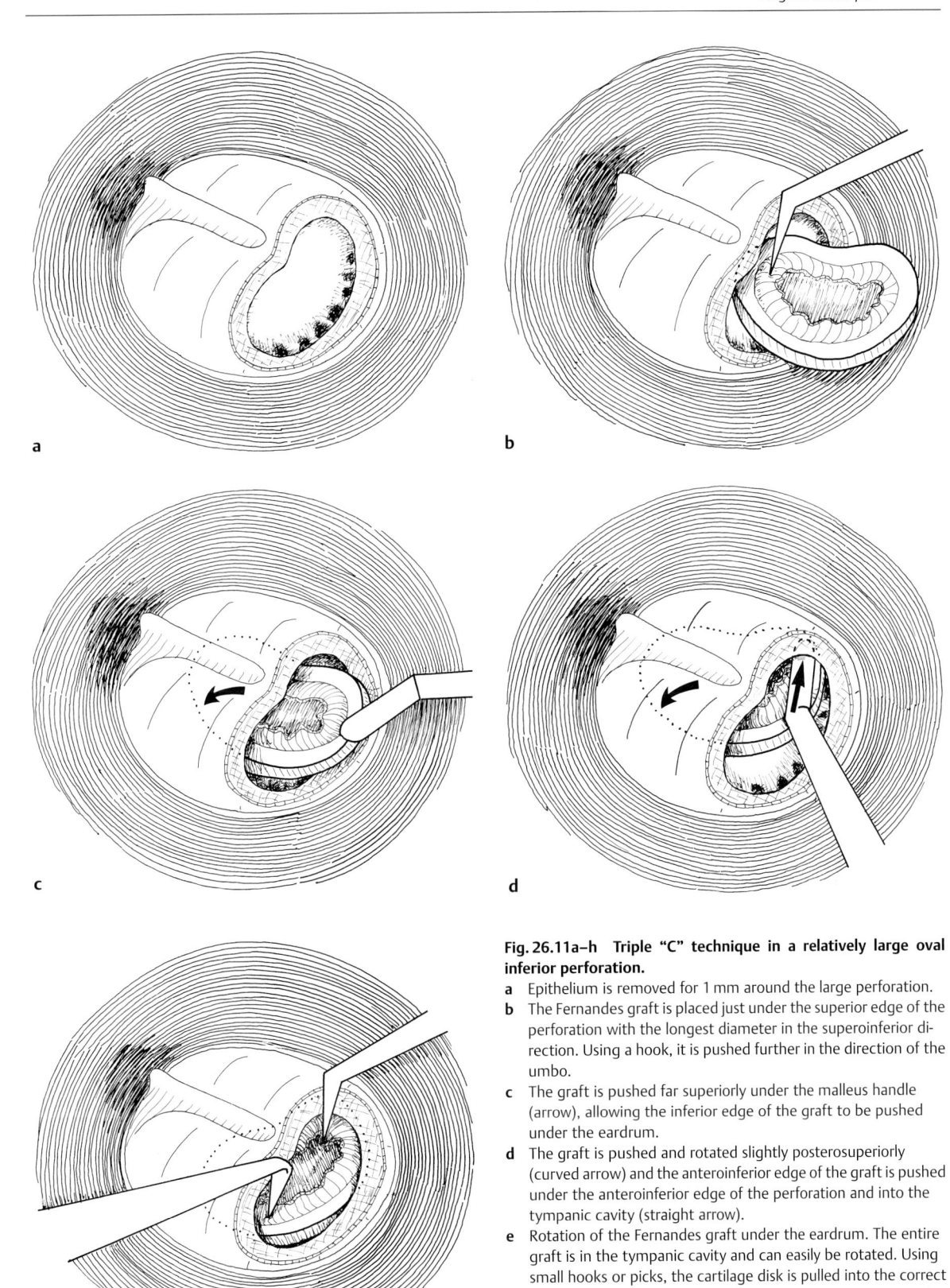

Fig. 26.11a–h Triple "C" technique in a relatively large oval inferior perforation.
a Epithelium is removed for 1 mm around the large perforation.
b The Fernandes graft is placed just under the superior edge of the perforation with the longest diameter in the superoinferior direction. Using a hook, it is pushed further in the direction of the umbo.
c The graft is pushed far superiorly under the malleus handle (arrow), allowing the inferior edge of the graft to be pushed under the eardrum.
d The graft is pushed and rotated slightly posterosuperiorly (curved arrow) and the anteroinferior edge of the graft is pushed under the anteroinferior edge of the perforation and into the tympanic cavity (straight arrow).
e Rotation of the Fernandes graft under the eardrum. The entire graft is in the tympanic cavity and can easily be rotated. Using small hooks or picks, the cartilage disk is pulled into the correct position with the perichondrium protruding through the perforation.

Fig. 26.11f–h ▷

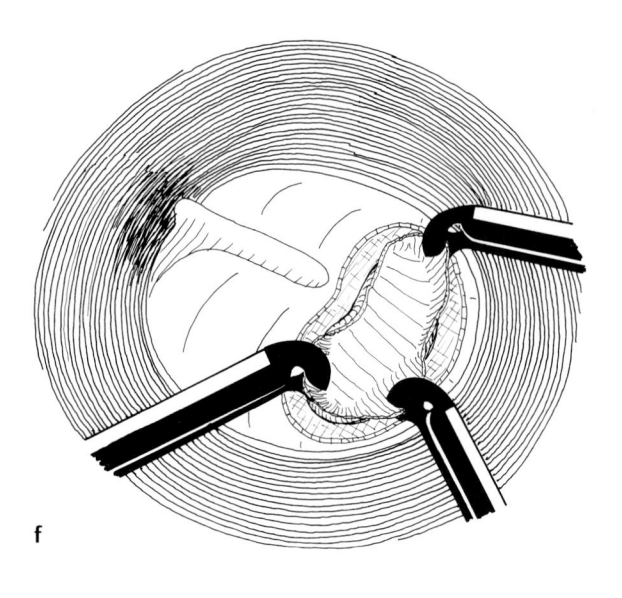

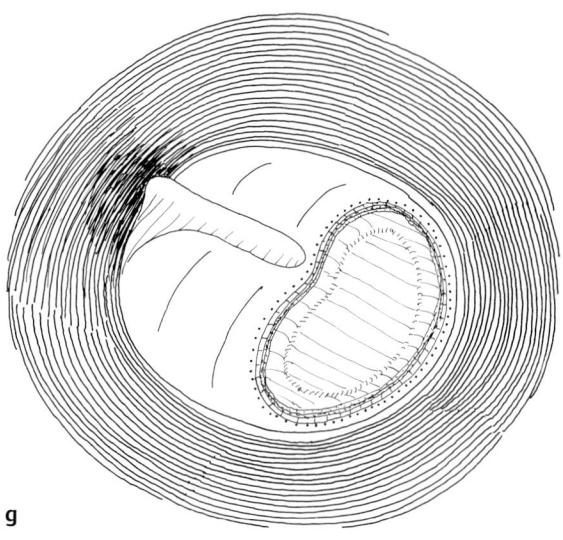

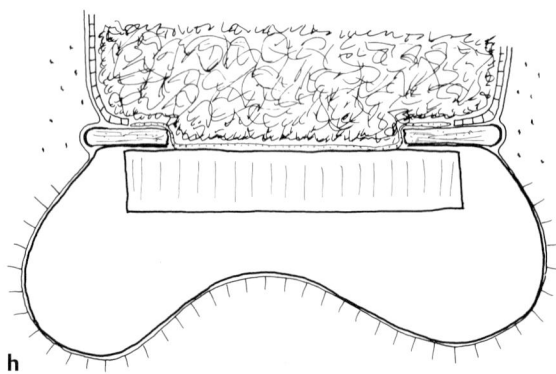

Fig. 26.11f–h

f Using cup forceps, the perichondrium is pulled onto the deepithelialized ring of the eardrum.

g The final situation with the perichondrium adapted to the epithelium. The position of the cartilage disk under the eardrum is indicated by dotted lines.

h Side view of the inferior part of the tympanic cavity with a large inferior perforation grafted with triple "C" technique. A large cartilage composite graft is hanging from a belt of perichondrium lying as an on-lay graft on the deepithelialized belt of ear drum. The graft is covered with a lightly pressed and slightly wet Gelfoam plate, fixing the perichondrium to the eardrum.

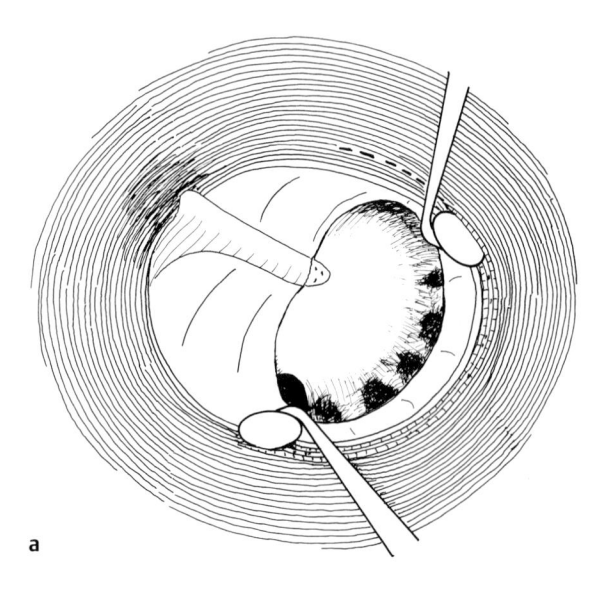

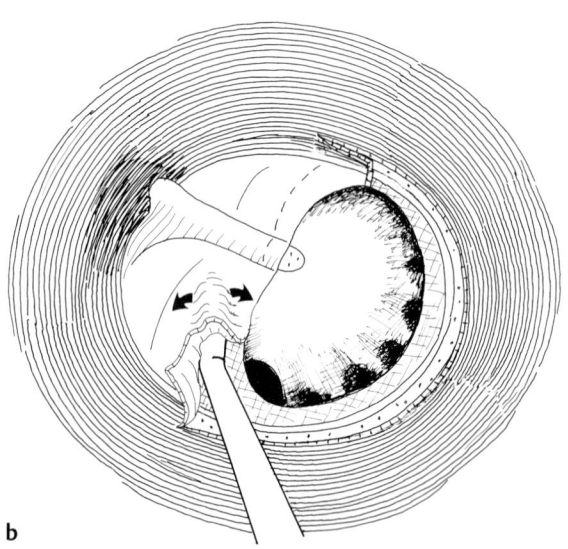

Surgical Techniques 399

Fig. 26.12a–l Triple "C" technique in a large inferior perforation with involvement of the malleus handle.

a Using a round knife, a circumferential incision is made at the level of the fibrous annulus, between the 9-o'clock and 3-o'clock positions.
b Epithelium is removed from a margin of 1 mm around the inferior half of the perforation. Superiorly, the epithelium is elevated by placing an incudostapedial knife between the lamina propria and the epithelium. The epithelium will gradually be elevated as the knife is moved.
c Further elevation of the epithelium from the malleus handle and cleaning of the umbo.
d Elevation of the epithelium in the anterosuperior part of the perforation is continued.
e Elevation of the epithelium is completed.
f The Fernandes graft is adapted to the protrusion of the umbo with a part of the malleus handle into the perforation. A rectangular piece of the cartilage is cut out, but the belt of perichondrium is preserved.
g The graft is placed under the umbo.

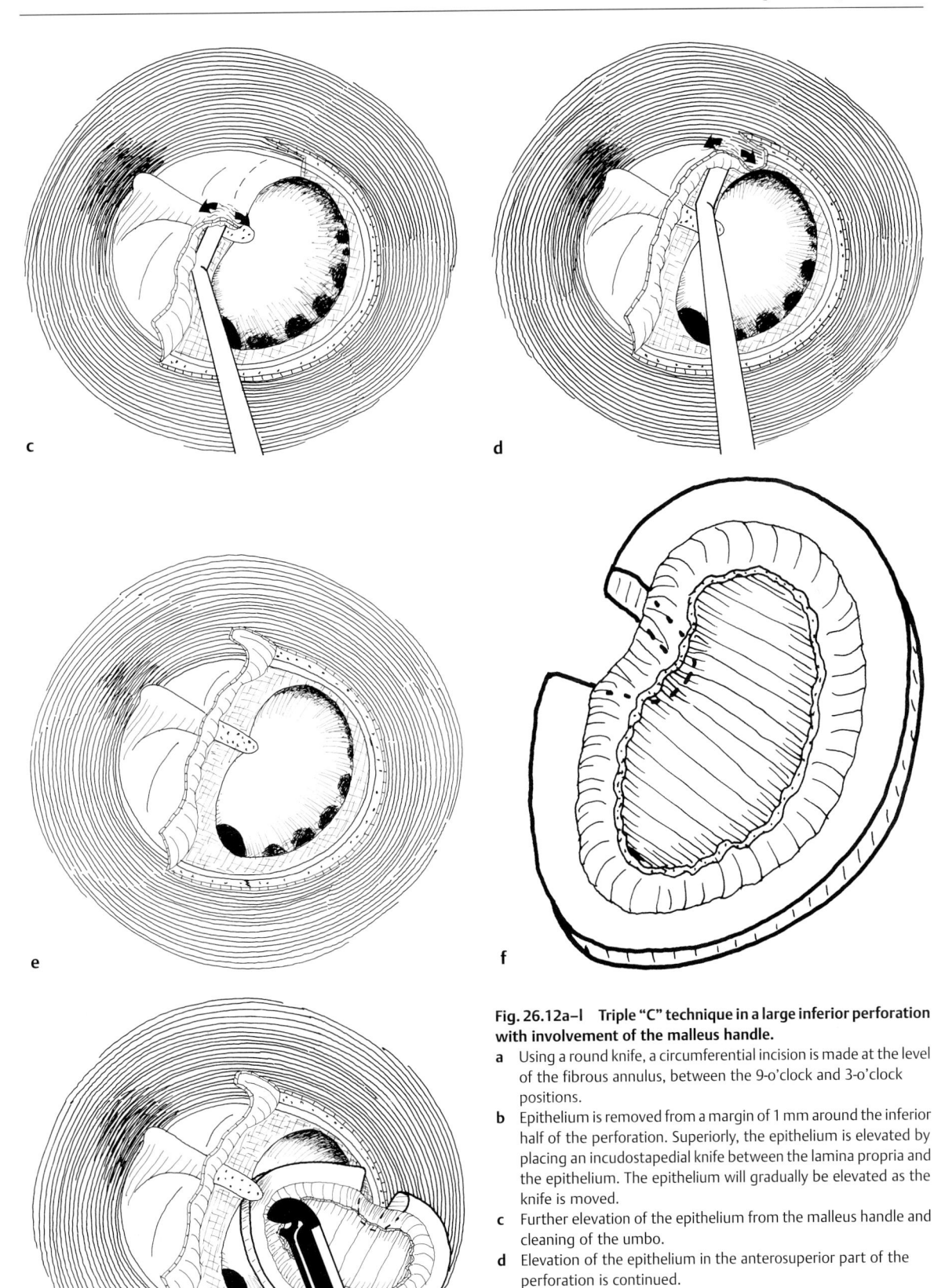

Fig. 26.12h–l ▷

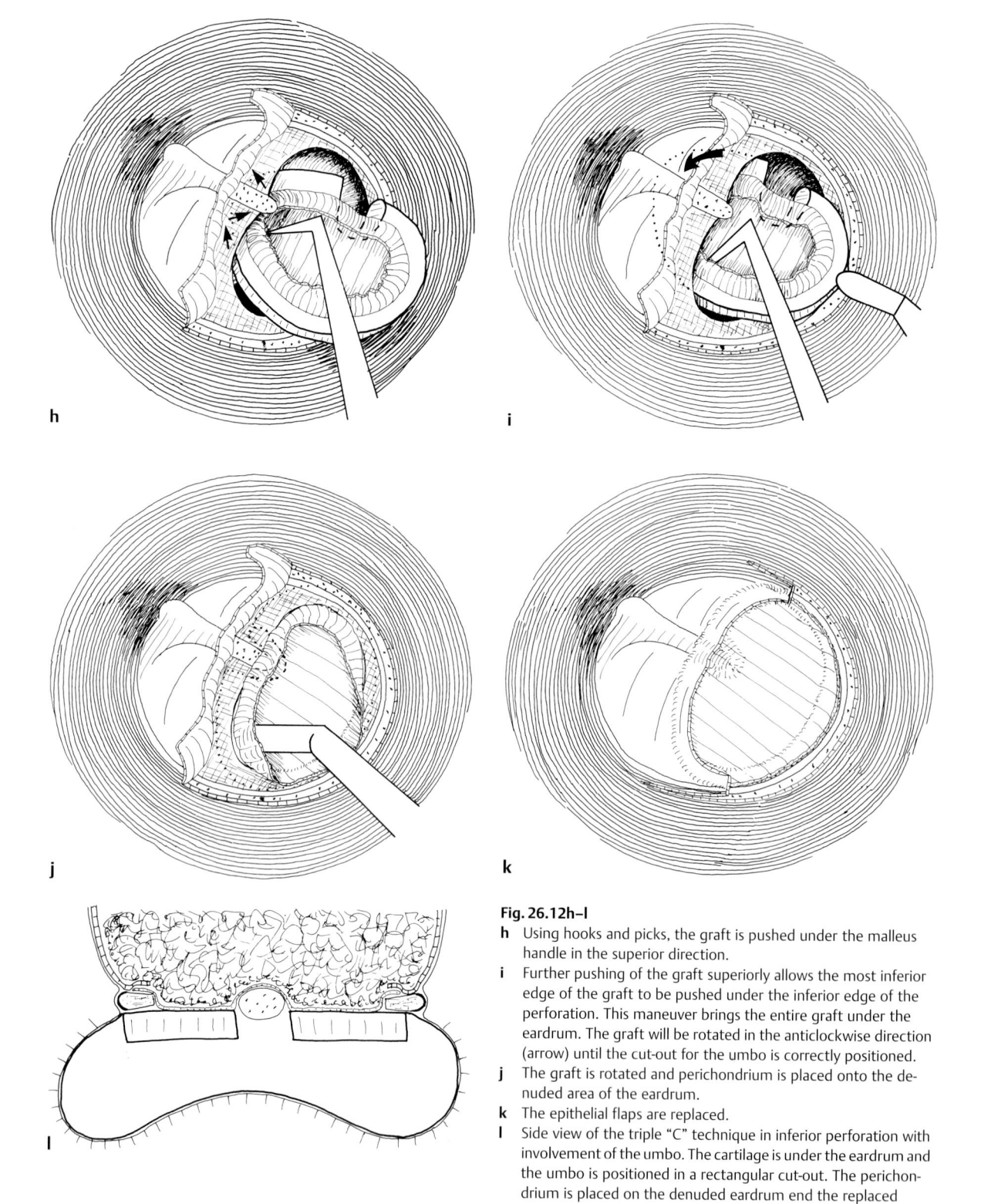

26 Composite Chondroperichondrial Clip Tympanoplasty: The Triple "C" Technique

Fig. 26.12h–l

h Using hooks and picks, the graft is pushed under the malleus handle in the superior direction.

i Further pushing of the graft superiorly allows the most inferior edge of the graft to be pushed under the inferior edge of the perforation. This maneuver brings the entire graft under the eardrum. The graft will be rotated in the anticlockwise direction (arrow) until the cut-out for the umbo is correctly positioned.

j The graft is rotated and perichondrium is placed onto the denuded area of the eardrum.

k The epithelial flaps are replaced.

l Side view of the triple "C" technique in inferior perforation with involvement of the umbo. The cartilage is under the eardrum and the umbo is positioned in a rectangular cut-out. The perichondrium is placed on the denuded eardrum end the replaced epithelial flaps provide additional stability to the tympanoplasty. A Gelfoam plate covers the eardrum.

Surgical Techniques 401

Fig. 26.13a–e Triple "C" technique in a small posterior perforation.
a The epithelium is removed from a 1 mm margin around the perforation ready for a round Fernandes graft to be placed under the anterior edge of the perforation.
b Using a hook, the graft is rotated clockwise to gradually bring it under the eardrum.
c The posterior edge of the cartilage disk is pushed under the posterior edge of the perforation and adapted to the perforation.
d The perichondrium is placed onto the denuded area of the eardrum around the defect.
e Side view of the triple "C" technique in a small posterior perforation. The cartilage disk is hanging from the perichondrium. The eardrum is covered with a Gelfoam plate.

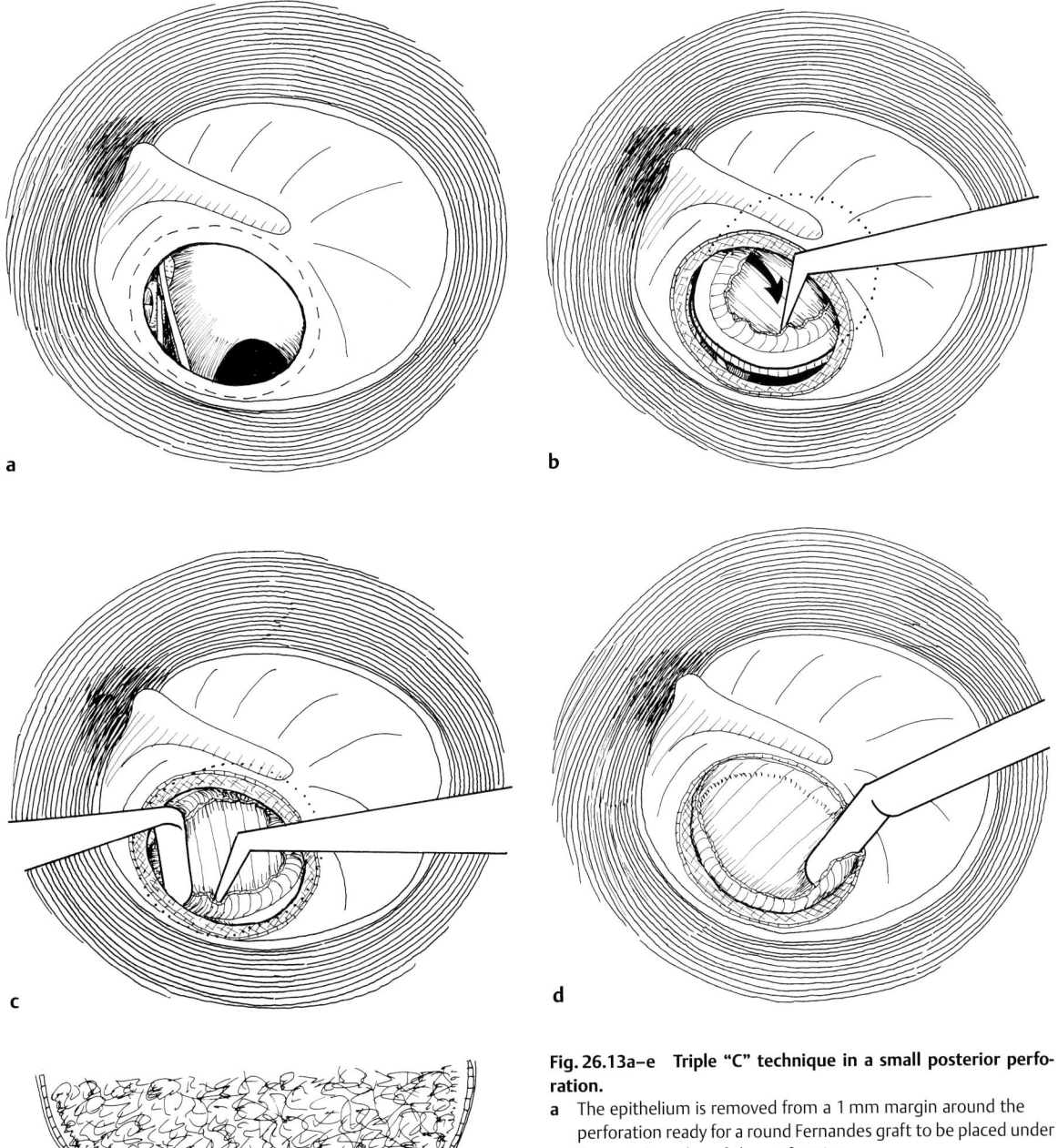

Results of Triple "C" Technique

Only one published paper exists on the triple "C" technique (Fernandes 2003). Fernandes reports on his first 15 patients, operated under general anesthesia, at a median age of 33 years (range 8–58 years). All perforations were anterior, posterior, or inferior.

A transcanal approach was applied in all patients and in no patient was a tympanotomy performed.

One patient had previously undergone a myringoplasty on the same ear, six patients had previously had a grommet inserted. Tubal patency is not mentioned.

Results were excellent, with 100 % take rate at the median follow-up of 15 months (range 8–29 months). Postoperative air–bone gap was reduced to within 10 dB at all frequencies. Postoperative absolute hearing was better than preoperative hearing in all patients.

Some patients with the longest observation times had slightly thinner cartilage than before (Fernandes, personal communication, 2006).

Author's Comments and Proposals

It is a splendid idea to hang and fixate a cartilage plate under the eardrum by an on-lay procedure. I am convinced that triple "C" technique will be widely accepted and used. For this reason, the method is extensively illustrated for the most common and typical anterior and inferior perforations.

There are many excellent otosurgeons with "on-lay phobia" who operate on any small and harmless perforation of the eardrum by retroauricular approach, with elevation of the ear canal skin and eardrum to place a large fascia graft under the eardrum. The underlay and on-lay triple "C" technique could in such cases be the most appropriate and minimally invasive solution.

The triple "C" technique is limited to dry ears and perforations not larger than half of the eardrum with intact ossicular chain and small preoperative hearing loss caused by the perforation (Fernandes 2003). Accordingly, future comparison of the hearing results achieved in triple "C" technique with the results of myringoplasty with fascia or with perichondrium, or with inlay butterfly cartilage technique (Chapter 25), should be between more or less identical series.

In particular, the two cartilage techniques—the inlay butterfly cartilage technique and the triple "C" technique—with similar indications should be compared in prospective studies on identical series.

I propose that the Fernandes cartilage–perichondrium island graft can be applied in total perforations and other more severe middle ear pathologies in the following way:

a) Removal or elevation of the epithelium around a 1–2 mm margin around the perforation.
b) Elevation of a posterior tympanomeatal flap with the eardrum.
c) Removal of the pathology or/and reconstruction of the ossicular chain.
d) Placement of the Fernandes graft of the appropriate size and shape through the posterior tympanotomy under the perforation.
e) Closure of the posterior tympanotomy by pulling the elevated tympanomeatal flap with the fibrous annulus back into the proper position.
f) Pulling the elevated perichondrium of the Fernandes graft onto the denuded belt on the lateral side of the eardrum.
g) Adaptation of the perichondrium to the borders of the eardrum and replacement of any elevated epithelial flaps.

References

Fernandes SV. Composite chondroepithelial clip tympanoplasty: The triple "C" technique. Otolaryngol Head Neck Surg 2003;128: 267–272.

Tos M. Relationship between secretory otitis in childhood and chronic otitis and its sequelae in adults. J Laryngol Otol 1981;95:1011–1022.

27 The Fate of Implanted Cartilage Grafts

The Nourishment of the Cartilage

The nourishment of cartilage is achieved by diffusion, with the help of the perichondrium. For this reason the nourishment of the graft will be optimal if the cartilage graft is covered on both sides with perichondrium. This is very seldom the case in cartilage tympanoplasty of today: Tolsdorff (1983) was the only surgeon to use the total pars tensa composite graft covered on both sides with perichondrium (Chapter 17). In fact, several grafts that are employed are not covered with perichondrium at all, such as thin cartilage foils (Chapters 10 and 11) and thick cartilage plates (Chapters 12 and 13). Cartilage strips, as described in Chapters 7 and 8, have very small perichondrium covering.

Poor nourishment as result of poor covering of perichondrium in the methods mentioned may cause late changes in the graft, such as necrosis and perforations of the reconstructed eardrum. At the time of writing, there are no reports on late anatomical failures after cartilage tympanoplasty except on late deterioration of hearing after insertion of cartilage columellae and cartilage struts (Steinbach and Pusalkar 1981, Steinbach et al. 1992).

The viability of cartilage depends on direct diffusion of tissue fluids into the fibrous matrix, thus nourishing the chondroblasts and chondrocytes (Adams 1993). Cartilage that has been morphologically modified by physical force, such as crushing (Park 1995) or pressure (Kleinfeldt et al. 1975) (Chapter 12), can survive and function as a total pars tensa graft.

Experiments on the Fate of Transplanted Cartilage

The very extensive literature during the period 1865–1939 was summarized by Peer (1939). He categorized the experiments into four groups and pointed to very different findings concerning the fate of the grafts in the different groups: (1) living cartilage transplanted into animals; (2) living cartilage transplanted into humans; (3) dead cartilage transplanted into animals; (4) dead cartilage transplanted into humans. Only experiments with living cartilage will be summarized here.

Living Cartilage Implanted into Animals

Bert (1865) concluded that a cartilage graft retained its viability and led to the formation of bone. Both Ollier (1867) and Zahn (1884) contested the previous view and both found degenerative changes in the grafts that led ultimately to their resorption.

The theory that the survival of the cartilage graft is dependent on the presence of the perichondrium originates from Fischer in 1882. In his experiments, the costal cartilage degenerated after about 8 weeks when transplanted as a homograft without its perichondrium. Cartilage transplanted with its perichondrium showed little alteration in structure over the same period.

By transplanting cartilage from one part of an animal to another part of the same animal (autograft), Mannheim and Zypkin (1926) found that cartilage transplanted **without** its perichondrium was better preserved than cartilage transplanted with its perichondrium.

Loeb (1926) transplanted (autogenous) cartilage in the same guinea pig, and (homogenous) cartilage in other pigs. Such tissue reaction as did occur was extremely mild. After transplantation of the homograft, the reaction began early, reached maximum at 3 weeks, and then disappeared. Both grafts remained in place for up to 5 months.

Mannheim and Zypkin (1926) transplanted cartilage from the same guinea pig to another site in the same animal (autologous grafting), with the following results: (1) Up to one year the cartilage retained its specific structure in all cases. (2). Both degenerative and regenerative processes took place. (3) Cartilage implanted into soft tissue was better preserved than that transplanted in the skull base. (4) As mentioned previously, in this case cartilage implanted without perichondrium was better preserved than that with perichondrium. (5) Free cartilage autografts formed good material for reconstruction.

Living Cartilage Implanted into Humans

The first use of cartilage transplants in humans is credited to Konig (1896), who used them to repair tracheal defects with successful results.

Nelaton and Ombredanne (1904) placed costal cartilage in forehead flaps, which were later swung down to the nose.

After an extensive survey of the literature, Neuhof and Hirschfeld (1923) concluded that simple cartilage grafts remain unaltered in appearance and in staining reactions for many weeks after implantation. Only in grafts that are several months old does fibrosis of the cartilage begin. There is a gradual death of the chondrocytes and they ultimately disappear. The outstanding feature in the histological fate of cartilage transplants is the long period of quiescence that precedes the final phase of degeneration and substitution. The cartilage is absorbed slowly, allowing adequate time for replacement by dense fibrous tissue that maintains the architecture of the graft.

Contrary to the view of Neuhof and Hirschfeld, as early as 1917 Davis gave clinical evidence of the permanence of rib cartilage transplanted into the nose.

Peer (1938, 1939) buried living autogenous rib cartilage beneath the chest skin in two patients operated for deformity of the nose. Histological investigation 4.5 years and 6 years later revealed living cartilage.

Otological Research on Cartilage Grafts

Research on the fate of implanted cartilage in the century from 1850 to 1950 was concentrated on rhinology and plastic surgery to implant the cartilage in congenital and traumatic nasal deformities. After the introduction of modern tympanoplasty by Wullstein (1952) and Zollner (1954), the conditions for cartilage tympanoplasty were first established.

The first otosurgeon to use autologous conchal cartilage in ossiculoplasty was Utech (1959, 1960, 1961). Utech elaborated small cartilage struts, termed cartilage "plastic prosthesis" or "mobile cartilage." The struts were covered with perichondrium and were used to replace a partly or a totally missing crus of the stapes, or to replace the entire stapes with a cartilage strut between the footplate and the long process of the incus. In the case of missing stapes and incus, Utech used a columella between the footplate and the eardrum or the malleus handle. The columella was covered with perichondrium.

Davidson (1959) reviewed the extensive literature up to 1959 and investigated the fate of autogenous cartilaginous transplants in the external ear of rabbits and determined whether the union that takes place between a carefully approximated autogenous graft and its host cartilage is fibrous or whether new cartilage is formed. Using a 7 mm cork-borer, a round piece of cartilage, with the perichondrium, was removed in five rabbits and implanted in a similar defect of the cartilage on the opposite side. The rabbits were sacrificed at intervals of 30 days and the cartilage was removed.

The conclusions of this fascinating and unique study were that:

1. Cartilage union occurred between host and graft.
2. At the point of union, bone formation occurred in 2 cases (at 60 and 120 days).
3. The perichondrium of the host cartilage proliferates and produces new cartilage, which is under way in 30 days.
4. The perichondrium of the graft is also active, but less so, at the point of union with the host cartilage.
5. The older cartilage cells at the border of the graft appear to undergo degenerative changes with encroachment of the newly formed cartilage.
6. The remainder of the cells of the graft retain viability, and at 150 days there was no evidence of replacement over a 90-day specimen.
7. It is possible that the cell degeneration at the periphery of the graft may be due to tissue injury, while the cells more centrally located maintain their integrity.
8. Vascularity was moderate in the areas from which the cartilage grafts were taken and also in those to which they were transplanted. Initially there was some proliferation of fibrous tissue and small blood vessels in the region of contact with the host area. Following this, perichondrial cells proliferated and new cartilage formation occurred with bi-nucleated chondrocytes.

These findings indicate that cartilage grafts evoke very little cellular response and demonstrate that the presence of an intact and established blood supply of the host area contributes to and hastens the union (Davidson 1959).

Guilford et al. (1966) showed that implanted bone and autogenous hyaline (costal) cartilage or elastic (auricular) cartilage retained their viability 3–8 months after implantation into the bulla of a dog. The structural patterns of the implanted cartilage were similar to those of undisturbed cartilage at the original site.

The Fate of Cartilage Columellae and Struts

Cartilage struts used as columellae in tympanoplasty type 3 often became too soft for satisfactory sound transmission and several patients had to be re-operated.

Kerr et al. (1973) found evident fibrous tissue replacement in 2 out of 10 removed homologous septum struts. This occurred mainly from the lacunae within the strut. The same two struts also had erosion. In addition, two other struts had erosion of the cartilage. In all these four cases the time of reoperation was 2¼–4¼ years after the first operation. In four other cases with primary operation less than 2 years previously, no major fibrosis of the strut was found. Because the fibrosis and erosion of cartilage struts may progress with time, Kerr reinforced the strut with a metal wire, but not long after Smyth et al. (1975) from the same clinic started to raise doubts about the use of cartilage as a columella.

Six autograft tragal cartilage struts and two preserved homograft nasal cartilage struts were histologically examined 6–18 months after the primary ossiculoplasty in the House Clinic, Los Angeles (Don and Linthicum 1975). The cause of failure in five patients was displacement of the cartilage struts. Two of these struts were too short. The macroscopic shape was preserved with no gross evidence of resorption. No inflammatory reaction and no resorption of cartilage were found. Chondrocytes were present within the lacunae and there was active cell division in autografts, indicated by double chondrocytes within the lacunae. Histochemical study with staining for polysaccharides with PAS-alcian blue revealed mucopolysaccharides in the matrix in the same amount as in normal cartilage. The appearance of the elastic fibers was the same in the autograft as in the normal cartilage.

The conclusion of this work was that the autograft remained viable in the middle ear, while the homograft remained in a nonvital state. There were two important differences from the Kerr series that may explain the differences in severity of histopathological findings: four cases had luxated or too short columellae, without any vibration of the columella. Furthermore, the interval between the first and second operations was much shorter than in the series of Kerr et al. (1973).

An electron-microscopic study of two cartilage columellae, inserted 3 and 8 years earlier, revealed progressive deposition of the calcium salt in the matrix of the cartilage and degenerative changes in the nuclei, cytoplasm, and walls of the chondrocytes. The authors do not believe that autograft cartilage will be resorbed with time (Belal et al. 1981).

In the Plester Clinic in Tübingen, cartilage was used for ossicular reconstruction from 1963 until 1970; since that time it has been used only infrequently because of very disappointing results (Steinbach and Pusalkar 1981). The authors performed histological studies on 52 cartilage struts, removed in recurrent surgery at various periods after primary surgery: one strut less than one year after surgery, 31 struts 1–7 years after, and 19 struts 8–15 years after primary surgery. Thirty-nine cartilages were autologous tragal cartilage, 13 were septum cartilage. Forty-six struts had gross macroscopic defects, from complete disappearance to irregular shape.

Microscopic appearance: The grafts were covered with normal mucosa, and there were no inflammatory reactions. The number of chondrocytes diminished and the cartilage become grossly hypocellular. The nucleus was pyknotic in some and absent in others. The paired character, with two nuclei, became single, indicating fewer cell divisions of chondrocytes. The borders of chondrocytes were poorly defined. The rows of chondrocytes had become irregular and they occupied only parts of the cartilage. In many specimens the cartilage became replaced by fibrous tissue. There were lacunae in some specimens, indicating resorptive processes. The reason for degenerative changes is the poor nourishment of the strut, simply because the two points—the footplate and the eardrum—are not sufficient to provide the nourishment. This conclusion is logical and seems the only one possible, but none of the studies showed that the strut with attached perichondrium has less degeneration than the strut without such covering. In a later study (Steinbach et al. 1992), of 30 autogenous and homogenous cartilage struts with median implantation time of 8 years (maximum 25 years), 47% of the struts had vital and 63% nonvital chondrocytes. Severe resorption of the matrix was found in 3%, moderate resorption in 50%, and none in 20%. Necroses in the matrix were found in 50% of the vital and in 31% of the nonvital struts.

By implanting autogenous cartilage columellae in the middle ears of 32 cats and measuring their vital and metabolic activity of the chondrocytes by the activity of the enzyme lactic dehydrogenase, Elwany (1985) showed that presence of the perichondrium on both sides of the columella increases the chance of survival of chondrocytes. On the other hand, middle ear infection has a very bad influence on the viability of chondrocytes. In the same paper, Elwany (1985) also reported on 59 cartilage struts removed at reoperation 6 months after the primary operation. Among the 27 dry ears, 18 struts were of normal shape, and 9 had necrosis at the medial end. Among 32 wet ears, only two struts had normal shape, 17 were totally necrotic, and 11 had medial and 2 had lateral necrosis of the strut.

The Fate of Cartilage Grafts after Myringoplasty

Yamamoto et al. (1988) investigated the fate of microsliced homograft cartilage implants 6 months after primary tympanoplasty (Yamamoto et al. 1984). There was no sign of any foreign body reaction and there were no marked histological changes of the matrix, although chondrocytes showed degenerative changes. There was partial resorption of the cartilage and replacement by fibrous connective tissue. Implanted homologous grafts maintained their stiffness for 6 months.

In three autologous cartilage grafts, Yamamoto et al. (1988) found only slight changes of chondrocytes 2 and 8 years after the primary surgery in comparison with homografts and there were no marked changes in the matrix.

Using light and electron microscopy, Hamed et al. (1999) investigated six pieces of cartilage graft, removed at recurrent surgery, 10–15 months after (and one graft 3.5 years after) primary myringoplasty. Additionally, pieces of autogenous or homogenous costal cartilage were implanted in the middle ears of 20 guinea pigs for 1, 3, and 6 months.

Animals: In light microscopy neither autografts or homografts showed signs of inflammatory reaction, but there was degeneration of chondrocytes, while the matrix with its fibrils was preserved in all specimens. On electron-microscopic examination the chondrocytes showed variable degrees of degeneration. The cytoplasm was homogeneous and nuclei were absent or crenated. The matrix was in good condition and its fine structure was preserved.

Humans: In gross the seven human autograft samples collected were of normal healthy cartilage. On light-microscopic examination the specimens removed after 10–15 months showed that the chondrocytes were degenerated with vacuolated cytoplasm and absent nuclei, while the matrix was preserved. Electron-microscopic examination confirmed these findings.

The specimen removed after 3.5 years showed viable chondrocytes and healthy matrix on light and electron microscopy.

The recent thesis of F. Hitari from the University of Olomouc, Czech Republic, had the title [in translation] "Posttransplant histomorphological changes of elastic cartilage after myringoplasty." In Olomouc, Klacansky has used various cartilage tympanoplasty methods since the early 1990s. Annular cartilage–perichondrium composite grafts (Chapter 18) and total pars tensa composite grafts (Chapter 17) were used routinely, but cartilage palisades were also used (Chapters 4 and 5) (Klacansky 1995; Klacansky et al. 1998; Hitari et al. 2004).

During a 4-year period Hitari collected the implanted **autologous cartilage at revision surgery** of 26 patients aged 13–71 years at revision. The primary surgery was performed 10–84 months before the revision surgery. In 13 patients a pair of grafts consisting of a fresh and a previously implanted cartilage graft were investigated. In 10 patients only transplanted grafts were investigated. In addition, four fresh cartilage grafts from the remaining patients were investigated. Two cartilage transplants were taken from one patient who underwent two revision operations.

A **quantitative study on chondrocytes** revealed statistically significant loss of chondrocytes. The loss of chondrocytes was not significantly correlated with the age of the grafts. The same results were obtained with normal and giant lipid vacuoles in transplanted cartilage. In the acellular components of the cartilage, a statistically non-significant difference in the decomposition of the elastic fibers was found between the two types of specimens. The dead chondrocytes were replaced by the fibrous tissue or by the amorphous material of the cartilage.

The study confirms the degenerative and atrophic changes in cellular and acellular components of the transplanted cartilage, caused by a long-term ischemic disorder of graft trophy. The study also confirms the loss of chondrocytes and subsequent replacement with the fibrous tissue and amorphous material.

It remains unclear whether these changes are related to mass reduction of the cartilage. Hitari suggests that a cartilage imaging analysis study will lead to a better explanation.

Based on the good functional clinical results of cartilage tympanoplasty with solid closure of the perforation and stable hearing, it can be speculated that wide replacement of chondrocytes by the fibrous tissue and the loss of lipid vacuoles makes the cartilage a more homogeneous tissue, which transfers acoustic energy better than normal cartilage (Hitari 2006).

Author's Comments and Recommendations

Davidson's (1959) work is a good experimental study, sending several signals to surgeons. I here summarize some aspects of epithelialization of the grafts on the basis of those signals.

1. Work as atraumatically as possible both with the graft and at the donor place.
2. Use grafts with perichondrium covering, which may be on both sides. Arguments against having perichondrium on the tympanic side involve the potential for formation of adhesions between the possibly retracted new eardrum and the middle ear mucosa. However, the retraction of an eardrum reconstructed with cartilage is extremely rare. In contact with the middle ear mucosa an adhesion of the cartilage to the promontory will very seldom occur.
3. Provide good conditions for the epithelialization of both sides of the cartilage graft.
4. Save the keratinized squamous epithelium of the eardrum remnant for outer covering of the cartilage with the epithelium.
5. In on-lay techniques, which are very suitable for cartilage tympanoplasty, the elevation of the squamous epithelium around the perforation can usually be done carefully. The cartilage graft is placed on the denuded edge of the lamina propria and the epithelium is replaced onto the perichondrium or close to it. The mucosa will easily grow along the undersurface of the graft, whether covered with perichondrium or not.
6. In underlay techniques, epithelialization of the outer side of the cartilage is easy if the graft is in close contact with the undersurface of the eardrum remnant. If there is a gap, the squamous epithelium may grow around the edge of the eardrum under the lamina propria, either delaying the epithelialization or causing a perforation at the border of the cartilage graft.

The covering of the undersurface of the cartilage graft should be promoted by scarification or removal of the mucosa around the edge of the undersurface of the perforation. It has to be admitted that we do not know how efficient such scarification is in fact; but on the other hand we do most often observe a solid closure of the perforation. We must also admit that we do not know whether the inner side of the cartilage always is covered by mucosa.

Another interesting situation is an underlay placement of a cartilage graft that is too large in relation to the perforation. The intact mucosa cannot grow around the edge of the graft to epithelialize the undersurface of the graft; it may be that the underside will never be covered completely with the mucosa or that the covering will continue from the other areas of the grafts.

The Fate of the Implanted Cartilage and Clinical Consequences

Some publications indicate that the changes of the implanted cartilage grafts have various clinical consequences. Accordingly, after cartilage tympanoplasty, the fates of implanted cartilage grafts should be evaluated separately in various groups and subgroups as detailed below.

- **Group 1:** Cartilage **columellae**, or struts, used in ossiculoplasty, form a well-defined and already well-documented group in clinical and histological terms (Kerr et al. 1973; Don and Linthicum 1975; Smyth et al. 1975; Steinbach and Pusalkar 1981; Hildmann et al. 1992; Steinbach et al. 1992). It is clearly demonstrated that, because of fibrosis of the cartilage, the columellae become soft, which changes the shape and the function. The transmission of vibrations is inadequate, resulting in hearing loss. The cartilage columellae between the footplate and the eardrum or malleus handle used in tympanoplasty type 3 have been or should be abandoned.

  Full-thickness cartilage plates of 2 mm × 2 mm or 1.5 × 1.5 mm with perichondrium interposed between the stapes head and the eardrum function well and do not suffer change of shape.

  Full- or half-thickness cartilage plates placed onto the head of a TORP or PORP prosthesis may be changed by fibrosis, but extrusion of the prosthesis is very rare.

- **Group 2:** The cartilage grafts and various methods used in **reconstruction of the eardrum** are classified in several subgroups:

  - **Cartilage palisades**, with full-thickness cartilage covered with perichondrium on one side (Chapters 4, 5, 6, and 9).
    There are no studies on the fate of cartilage palisades and no long-term studies (10 years) on the resultant hearing.
  - **Cartilage strips**, cut in an oblique manner, are thinner than palisades. They are covered with a small belt of perichondrium (Chapters 7 and 8).
    Tympanoplasty with cartilage strips is a relatively new method, and there is no publication of long-term hearing results or studies on the fate of these thin cartilages. Because the strips are thinner than palisades, and because of the small belt of perichondrium, the strips may became fibrotic: the late hearing results will be of great interest.
  - **Cartilage foils and thin plates** without perichondrium (Chapters 10 and 11).
    Tympanoplasty with autogenous cartilage foils is a new method without any published description of the results or any publication on the fate of the foils. Six months after tympanoplasty with micro-sliced homologous foils, Yamamoto et al. (1988) found degenerative changes of the cartilage, with partial resorption and fibrosis.
  - **Thick cartilage plates** without perichondrium. The plates can be half- or full-thickness cartilage grafts (Chapters 12 and 13). No histological study on the fate of the cartilage plates has been published, and there is no description of late (10 years) hearing results.
  - **Cartilage–perichondrium composite island grafts**, covered with perichondrium on one side only, and with **full-thickness** cartilage (Chapters 14–17, 21–23). Hitari (2006), in histopathological studies of full-thickness composite island grafts, found degenerative changes of the cartilage and replacement of the cartilage with fibrous tissue, which may make the total cartilage a more homogeneous tissue. Change in the cartilage with increasing fibrosis does not necessarily lead to hearing loss; it can even cause improvement of hearing.

    The cause of the revision operations was either a hearing loss for various reasons or an anatomical failure causing a perforation due to infection. The fibrosis of the cartilage was not the reason for re-operation.

    Even Hitari (2006) found good hearing results in the majority of patients with healed and intact grafts. A long-term follow-up of the entire series with composite grafts and with annular grafts is needed to confirm this report.

    If the fibrosis of the total island graft continues, the hearing is maintained or even improves. The same may be the case after grafting of small and medium-sized posterior, anterior, and inferior perforations treated with various composite island grafts (Chapters 14–16, 21–23).
  - **Cartilage–perichondrium composite island grafts** as in subgroup (e), but with **thinner cartilage disk (one-third, one-half, two-thirds thickness)** (Chapters 14–16, 21–23).
    The fate of the cartilage has not yet been investigated, but the outcome and the late hearing results may be the same as in full-thickness island graft.
  - **Special island grafts** such as in-lay butterfly, full-thickness grafts covered with the perichondrium on both sides (Chapter 25), and the graft for the triple "C" method (Chapter 26) with perichondrium partly covering one side only.
    The butterfly graft may be extruded initially, but later, after the graft is fully epithelialized, there will be hardly any hearing problems even with slight fibrosis of the graft. The graft for the triple "C" technique will retain its position and produce stable hearing. Descriptions of any late hearing results will be appreciated!

- **Group 3A:** Cartilage plates or composite grafts to **reconstruct the bony defects of the posterosuperior scutum region or the attic region**.
  Full-thickness cartilage–perichondrium composite grafts positioned onto the remaining ear canal bone will not change their positions in case of fibrosis of

the cartilage (Chapters 14 and 16). If the autogenous graft is still positioned over the bone in the way it was placed at the primary surgery a year before, then under pressure in the attic it will hardly move inside the scutum because of the eventual fibrosis of the cartilage. Various animal experiments on the fate of the cartilage have shown that the process of increasing fibrosis within the cartilage graft takes many years.

- **Group 3B:** Cartilage–perichondrium composite grafts to **reconstruct the entire ear canal wall**.
  Reconstruction of the entire ear canal wall, after a canal wall down mastoidectomy, together with the total or partial obliteration is a common procedure. A large tragus cartilage graft, with two large perichondrium flaps is usually the main graft, often supported by a large temporalis fascia and temporalis muscle. Many methods of ear canal wall reconstruction are described in MMES_2, Chapters 14–22, and illustrated by 30 drawings. The two large perichondrium flaps are attached to the cartilage and the total graft is placed onto the medial wall of the attic. The two perichondrium flaps are placed on the superior and inferior wall of the cavity. A large fascia graft covers the ear canal and the tympanic cavity. The cavity behind the cartilage graft is obliterated with the pedicle muscle grafts (MMES_2, Figs. 729, 730, 825–835).

  The conditions for nourishment of the cartilage graft are good, with fascia covering the cartilage graft on the ear canal side and the pedicle and vascular muscle graft on the mastoid side. The fate of the autogenous cartilage graft is presumably good and its function should remain satisfactory. Even in extensive replacement of the cartilage several years after primary surgery, the graft will not change its position.

- **Group 4:** Cartilage in **obliteration of the cavity** will presumable not change shape after any fibrosis. Previously, a small cavity with intact bony ear canal wall was easy to obliterate with homogenous cartilage. The amount of autogenous cartilage, harvested around the ear, is not sufficient for a total obliteration of a cavity after intact canal wall mastoidectomy, but it can play a major role in separating the tympanic cavity from the attic and antrum. Several larger pieces of cartilage, covered with perichondrium, are placed onto the medial attic wall vertically and parallel to the thinned ear canal bone. The attic and the antrum can be solidly obliterated with the cartilage plates. The remaining cavity is obliterated by the pedicled muscle grafts (MMES_2, Figs. 971–980). Over a period of some years, fibrous tissue may replace some cartilage without any consequence for the obliteration.

References

Adams JS. Grafts in the head and neck. In: Bailey BJ, ed. Head and Neck Surgery – Otolaryngology. Philadelphia: Lippincott; 1993: 1895–1912.

Belal A Jr, Linthicum FH Jr, Odnert S. Fate of cartilage autografts for ossiculoplasty: an electron microscopic study. Clin Otolaryngol 1981;6:231–236.

Bert P. Sur la greffe animal. C R Acad Sci Paris 1865;61:587–589.

Don A, Linthicum FH. The fate of cartilage grafts for ossicular reconstruction in tympanoplasty. Ann Otol Rhinol Laryngol 1975; 84(2 Pt 1):187–191.

Davidson M. A study of the fate of autogenous cartilage grafts. Laryngoscope 1959;69:1259–1277.

Elwany S. Histochemical study of cartilage autografts in tympanoplasty. J Laryngol Otol 1985;99:637–642.

Guilford FR, Shortreed R, Halpert B. Implantation of autogenous bone and cartilage into the bullae of dogs. Arch Otolaryngol 1966; 84:144–147.

Hamed M, Samir M, El Bigermy M. Fate of cartilage material used in middle ear surgery. Light and electron microscopy study. Auris Nasus Larynx 1999;26:257–262.

Hildmann H, Karger B, Steinbach E. Ossikeltransplantate zur Rekonstruktion der Schallübertragung im Mittelohr. Eine histologische Langzeituntersuchung. Laryngorhinootologie 1992;71:5–10.

Hitari F. Posttransplantacni histomorfologicke elasticke chrupavky po myringoplastice. [Posttransplant histomorphological changes of elastic cartilage after myringoplasty]. Thesis. Medical School Olomouc; 2006.

Hitari F, Klacansky J, Novotny J, Proskova M, Chrapkova P. Posttransplantacne zmeny elastickej chrupky. Choroby hlavy a krku (Head and Neck Diseases) 2004; 3/4: 39–43.

Kerr AG, Byrne JE, Smyth GD. Cartilage homografts in the middle ear: a long-term histological study. J Laryngol Otol 1973;87: 1193–1199.

Klacansky J. Kirurgia uha. In: Chern J, ed. Specialna chirurgija; Part 4. Chirurgia hlavy a krku. Osveta; 1995: 281–327.

Klacansky J, Kucera J, Starek I. Rekonstrukcia blanky bubienka chrupkovymi transplantati. [Reconstruction of the eardrum with cartilage transplants] Otorinolaryngolologie a Foniatrie 1998;47: 59–63.

Kleinfeldt D, Vick U, Lübcke P-F. Zur Verwendung von autologem Ohrmuschelknorpel zur Doppeltransplantatplastik des Trommelfelles. HNO 1975;23:13–15.

Konig F. Zur Deckung von Defekten in der vorderen Trachealwand. Berlin Klin. Wochenschr 1896;33:1129–1139.

Loeb L. Autotransplantation und homotransplantations of cartilage in guinea-pig. Am J Pathol 1926;2:111–122.

Mannheim A, Zypkin B. Free autoplastic cartilage transplantation. Arch Klin Chir 1926;141:668–672.

Nelaton C, Ombredanne L. La rhinoplastie. Paris: G. Steinheil; 1904.

Neuhof H, Hirschfeld S. The Transplantation of Tissues. New York: D Appleton & Comp.; 1923:205–215.

Ollier L. Traite experimental et clinice de la regeneration des os et de la production artificielle du tissue osseoux. Paris: V. Masson & Fils 1867;1:162–185.

Park MS. Tympanoplasty using autologous crushed cartilage. Rev Laryngol Otol Rhinol (Bord) 1995;116:365–368.

Peer LA. Cartilage transplanted beneath the skin of the chest in man. Arch Otolaryngol 1938;27:42–58.

Peer LA. Fate of living and dead cartilage transplants in humans. Surg Gynecol Obstet 1939;68:603–610.

Smyth GDL, Pahor A, Law KE. Ossiculotympanic transplantation. Laryngoscope 1975;85:540–550.

Steinbach E, Pusalkar A. Long-term histological fate of cartilage in ossicular reconstruction. J Laryngol Otol 1981;95:1031–1039.

Steinbach E, Karger B, Hildmann H. Zur Verwendung von Knorpeltransplantaten in der Mittelohrchirurgie. Eine histologische Langzeituntersuchung von Knorpelinterponanten. Laryngorhinootologie 1992;71:11–14.

Tolsdorff P. Tympanoplastik mit Tragusknorpel-Transplantat: "Knorpeldeckel-Plastik. [Tympanoplasty with tragus cartilage transplant: "cartilage cover plasty"] Laryngol Rhinol Otol (Stuttg) 1983;62:97–102.

Utech H. Über diagnostische und therapeutische Möglichkeiten der Tympanotomie bei Schalleitungsstörungen. Z Laryngol Rhinol Otol 1959;38:212–221.

Utech H. Endhörergebnisse bei der Tympanoplastik durch Veränderungen bei der Operationstechnik. Z Laryngol Rhinol Otol 1960; 39:367–371.

Utech H. Über die Verwendung von Knorpelgewebe bei der Tympanoplastik und Stapeschirurgie. HNO 1961;9:232–233.

Wullstein HL. Operationen am Mittelohr mit Hilfe des freien Spaltlappentransplantates. Arch Ohren Nasen Kehlkopfheilkd 1952; 161:422–435.

Yamamoto E, Iwanaga M, Morinaka S. Use of micro-sliced homograft cartilage plates in tympanoplasty. Acta Otolaryngol Suppl 1984;419:123–129.

Yamamoto E, Iwanaga M, Fukumoto N. Histologic study of homograft cartilages implanted in the middle ear. Otolaryngol Head Neck Surg 1988;98:546–551.

Zahn FW. Ueber das Schicksal der in den Organismus implantierten Gewebe. Wirchows Arch Pathol Anat 1884;95:369.

Zollner F. Die Schalleitungsplastiken 1. [Plastic surgery for sound conduction I.] Acta Otolaryngol 1954;44:370–384.

28 Clinical Research in Cartilage Tympanoplasties

The application of various cartilage tympanoplasty methods in middle ear surgery has been increasing rapidly in the first decade of this century (Neumann et al. 2002, 2003; Bernal-Sprekelsen et al. 2003; Dornhoffer 2003, 2006; Ferekidis et al. 2003; Uzun et al. 2003, 2004; Andersen et al. 2004; Tos et al. 2005; Kirazli et al 2005; Kazikdas et al. 2007). At the 8th Cholesteatoma Conference in Antalya, Turkey, in June 2008, 25 papers on cartilage tympanoplasty were presented. The technique was rarely mentioned at previous Cholesteatoma Conferences.

In this chapter selected clinical research papers on cartilage tympanoplasty methods will be described. Looking forward, several clinical research projects will be elaborated and proposed for six cartilage tympanoplasty methods with palisades and strips of group A (see Chapter 2). There are three levels of reporting of the results after cartilage tympanoplasty:

1. Reporting the results without comparing them with other series. The comparison is focused on the preoperative and postoperative data. Such results have been discussed in the respective chapters.
2. Reporting the results of a cartilage tympanoplasty and comparing them with a similar series treated with tympanoplasty with fascia or with perichondrium.
3. Reporting the results of a cartilage tympanoplasty and comparing them with similar series treated with another cartilage tympanoplasty.

Postoperative Results without Comparison with Other Series

Early anatomical and functional results (1–3 months after surgery) and **late** results (more than 2 years) are reported. The preoperative absolute hearing and/or preoperative air–bone gap are compared with the postoperative data; the hearing gain may be separately reported (Amedee et al. 1989). Such reports are described for most methods in the respective chapters. However, the primary results are not yet published for several new methods: cartilage palisades in on-lay tympanoplasty technique (Chapter 5); cartilage strips in on-lay technique (Chapter 8); underlay and on-lay tympanoplasty with foils and thin plates (Chapters 10 and 11); underlay tympanoplasty and in-lay underlay tympanoplasty with cartilage–perichondrium composite island graft (Chapters 21 and 22); on-lay tympanoplasty and in-lay on-lay tympanoplasty with cartilage–perichondrium island graft (Chapters 23 and 24).

Comparison of Functional Results within the Same Cartilage Tympanoplasty in Relation to the Preoperative Tubal Function

Testing is important and any recognized test can be used, such as simple preoperative positive or negative Valsalva. The main reason for the use of cartilage tympanoplasty is to prevent postoperative retraction of the graft caused by poor tubal function. Therefore, the testing of the tubal patency or tubal function is mandatory before and after surgery. I am aware that Valsalva testing of the eustachian tube is rather simple, but the test can divide patients into two groups: one with positive Valsalva and better hearing, and one with negative Valsalva and poorer hearing (Tos 1970, 1974).

Deflation test or aspiration test can grade the tubal function into four grades:

- *Grade 1:* Completely positive aspiration and deflation tests.
- *Grade 2:* Partly positive aspiration test and positive deflation test.
- *Grade 3:* Negative aspiration test and partly positive deflation test.
- *Grade 4:* Negative aspiration test and negative deflation test.

Comparison of Functional Results within the Same Cartilage Tympanoplasty in Relation to the Postoperative Tubal Function

Here the postoperative tubal function is measured by tympanometry. In our studies (Uzun et al. 2003, 2004; Tos et al. 2005) after surgery of tensa cholesteatoma in children, we found significantly ($p < 0.01$, chi-squared test) more retractions (36%) in reconstruction with fascia than in the group reconstructed with underlay cartilage tympanoplasty. In the palisade group with poor tubal function, the anatomical results were as good as in ears with good tubal function.

Comparison of the Results in Cartilage Tympanoplasty Methods with the Results in Tympanoplasty Methods Using Fascia or Perichondrium Graft

Four such studies have been published.

Tympanoplasty with Total Pars Tensa Cartilage–Perichondrium Composite Island Graft Compared with Tympanoplasty with Perichondrium Graft

Dornhoffer (1997) was the first to compare the results of tympanoplasty with total cartilage–perichondrium composite island graft and the results of tympanoplasty with fascia graft. In 22 patients with total perforation and intact ossicular chain treated with total pars tensa cartilage–perichondrium island graft, he found better, but not significantly better, hearing than in 20 similar cases treated with perichondrium (Chapter 17).

Underlay Tympanoplasty with Cartilage Palisades Compared with Underlay Tympanoplasty with Fascia Graft

In our series at Gentofte Hospital of 32 children with tensa cholesteatoma reconstructed with underlay cartilage palisade tympanoplasty, the results 37 months after surgery were better than in 32 ears with similar pathology reconstructed with fascia (Chapter 4) (Andersen et al. 2002, 2004). The mean hearing gain in the cartilage group was 11.5 dB, and in the fascia group was 4.9 dB. Ten-year results of these series are shown on p. 84.

Tympanoplasty with Total Pars Tensa Cartilage-Perichondrium Composite Island Graft Compared with Tympanoplasty with Fascia Graft

In 15 patients with subtotal perforation and intact ossicular chain, treated with total pars tensa cartilage–perichondrium composite island graft, Kirazli et al. (2005) found a postoperative hearing gain of 11.9 dB, compared with 11.5 db in 10 similar patients treated with underlay tympanoplasty with fascia graft (Chapter 17).

Underlay Tympanoplasty with Cartilage Strips Compared with Underlay Tympanoplasty with Fascia

In 23 patients with subtotal perforation and intact ossicular chain treated with underlay cartilage tympanoplasty with strips (Chapter 7), Kazikdas et al. (2007) found better hearing, but not significantly better, than in 28 patients with similar pathology treated by underlay tympanoplasty with fascia graft.

Thus three studies showed slightly better postoperative hearing in the cartilage groups, and one (Andersen et al. 2002, 2004) showed significantly better hearing 37 months after tympanoplasty with cartilage palisades than that achieved in tympanoplasty with fascia.

It is evident that many more such comparisons are needed, both of primary results and of long-term results.

Comparison of Results between Various Cartilage Tympanoplasty Methods

It is hoped that the classification presented in Chapter 2 will inspire clinical research comparing the results achieved between the many cartilage tympanoplasty methods for similar pathology. There are as yet no descriptions of results achieved with any one cartilage tympanoplasty method in comparison with some other cartilage method.

It will be of great interest to compare a series of total perforation treated by cartilage palisade methods with a similar series treated with cartilage foil methods or with total pars tensa cartilage–perichondrium composite island graft.

Proposals for the Methods of Clinical Research in Cartilage Tympanoplasty

In Chapter 2, the 23 cartilage tympanoplasty methods were classified into six groups, each with some specific characteristics (Tos 2008). **Proposals for clinical research are here elaborated for group A only.**

Comparison of Results within Group A

Group A consists of six cartilage tympanoplasty methods (Tos 2008), which include the underlay and the on-lay palisade methods (Chapters 4 and 5), tympanoplasty with broad palisades (Chapter 6), the underlay and on-lay cartilage strip methods (Chapters 7 and 8), and the underlay cartilage slice mosaic tympanoplasty (Chapter

9). Group A is the oldest and the largest group and is therefore the most appropriate for cross comparisons between methods.

Although all of the few known clinical studies on cartilage tympanoplasty with palisades, strips, and slices showed good anatomical results, with few reperforations, few retractions, and few reoperations, we do not know enough about the postoperative hearing after cartilage tympanoplasty. If the postoperative hearing is as good in cartilage tympanoplasty as in tympanoplasty with fascia or perichondrium, then the indications for cartilage tympanoplasty should be widened to include ears with normal tubal function.

The proposed comparisons on clinical studies (Tos 2007) can be spread over several other subgroups (a) to (d).

Group (a): Comparison of Series within the Same Cartilage Method

1. Studies within the same underlay palisade method with the ends of the palisades placed onto the bony annulus (see **Fig. 4.7e**) compared with placement of the palisade ends at the level of the bony annulus (see **Fig. 4.7h**). The size of the perforation, tubal function, and middle ear mucosa should be the same. The ossicular chain is normal.
2. Comparison within the same underlay cartilage palisade method between using full-thickness palisades and using half-thickness palisades.
3. Comparison within the same on-lay cartilage palisade method between using full-thickness palisades and using half-thickness palisades.

The inferior ends of the palisades can be placed (a) onto the bony annulus, or (b) at the level of the bony annulus (see **Fig. 4.7h**), or (c) under the bony annulus (see **Fig. 4.18 f, g**), as shown by Ferekidis et al. (2003). One can imagine that the vibration of the palisades will be smaller in the modification (a), where the palisade ends become much more firmly fixed to the ear canal wall, than in the modifications (b) and (c), where the ends of the palisades may become loosely fixed to the denuded eardrum remnant. A clinical study with comparison of postoperative hearing results of identical series with total perforation and intact ossicular chain would be welcomed.

Group (b): Comparison of the Six Methods of Group A with Each Other

4. Comparison between cartilage palisades in the underlay tympanoplasty technique of Heermann (**Fig. 4.7e**) or in my own technique (**Fig. 4.7h**) and palisades in on-lay tympanoplasty (**Figs. 5.14, 5.15, 5.16**). The size of the perforation, normal ossicular chain, and tubal function should be the same in both series.
5. Comparison between tympanoplasty with broad cartilage palisades (**Fig. 6.2e**) and the small palisades in underlay tympanoplasty (**Fig. 4.7e, h**). The perforation, tubal function, and normal ossicular chain should be the same in both series.
6. Comparison between cartilage palisades (**Fig. 4.7f**) in underlay tympanoplasty and cartilage strips in underlay tympanoplasty (**Fig. 7.14c**).
7. Comparison between cartilage underlay strips (**Fig. 7.15b**) and the on-lay strips (**Fig. 8.7b**). The perforation, tubal function, middle ear mucosa, and normal ossicular chain should be the same in both series.
8. Comparison between the Dornhoffer underlay cartilage mosaic slice tympanoplasty (**Figs. 9.1 and 9.8a**) and the underlay palisade methods (**Figs. 4.7e, h**).
9. Comparison between the Dornhoffer underlay cartilage mosaic slice tympanoplasty (**Figs. 9.1 and 9.8a**) and cartilage palisades in on-lay tympanoplasty (**Figs. 5.14, 5.15, 5.16**).
10. Comparison between the Dornhoffer underlay cartilage mosaic slice tympanoplasty and the method of broad palisades of Bernal-Sprekelsen (**Fig. 6.2e**).
11. Comparison between the Dornhoffer underlay cartilage mosaic slice tympanoplasty and the method of underlay cartilage strip tympanoplasty (**Fig. 8.9**).
12. Comparison between the Dornhoffer underlay cartilage mosaic slice tympanoplasty and the method of on-lay cartilage strip tympanoplasty (**Fig. 8.10b**).
13. Comparison between cartilage strips in underlay tympanoplasty and cartilage palisades in on-lay tympanoplasty.
14. Comparison between cartilage strips in on-lay tympanoplasty and cartilage palisades in underlay tympanoplasty.
15. Comparison between tympanoplasty with broad palisades and cartilage palisades in on-lay tympanoplasty.
16. Comparison between tympanoplasty with broad cartilage palisades and cartilage strips in underlay tympanoplasty.
17. Comparison between tympanoplasty with broad palisades and cartilage slices in on-lay tympanoplasty.
18. Comparison between cartilage strips in on-lay tympanoplasty and cartilage palisades in underlay tympanoplasty.
19. Comparison between cartilage strips in on-lay tympanoplasty and cartilage palisades in on-lay tympanoplasty.

Group (c): Comparison of the Six Cartilage Tympanoplasty Methods of Group A with the Fascia or Perichondrium Tympanoplasty Methods

The size of the perforations, middle ear mucosa, tubal function, and intact ossicular should be identical in the series being compared.

1. Cartilage palisades in underlay tympanoplasty compared with tympanoplasty with fascia or perichondrium. Our group has performed such studies on cholesteatoma surgery in children (Andersen et al. 2002, 2004).

2. Cartilage palisades in on-lay tympanoplasty compared with tympanoplasty with fascia or perichondrium.
3. Tympanoplasty with broad palisades compared with tympanoplasty with fascia or perichondrium.
4. Cartilage strips in underlay in underlay tympanoplasty compared with tympanoplasty with fascia or perichondrium. One such study has been performed by Kazikdas et al. (2007).
5. Cartilage strips in on-lay tympanoplasty compared with fascia or perichondrium.
6. Dornhoffer mosaic cartilage tympanoplasty compared with fascia or perichondrium.

Group (d): Comparison of the Six Cartilage Tympanoplasty Methods of Group A with Series of Normal Preoperative Tubal Function and Series with Abnormal Tubal Function

1. Cartilage palisades in underlay tympanoplasty and normal tubal function compared with series with the same surgery but with abnormal tubal function. Our group has performed such studies on cholesteatoma surgery in children reconstructed with cartilage palisades underlay tympanoplasty (Andersen et al. 2002, 2004).
2. Cartilage palisades in on-lay tympanoplasty and normal tubal function compared with the same tympanoplasty but with abnormal tubal function.
3. Tympanoplasty with broad palisades and normal tubal function compared with the same tympanoplasty but with abnormal tubal function.
4. Cartilage strips in underlay tympanoplasty and normal tubal function compared with the same tympanoplasties but with abnormal tubal function.
5. Cartilage strips in on-lay tympanoplasty and normal tubal function compared with the same tympanoplasty but with abnormal tubal function.
6. Dornhoffer underlay cartilage slice mosaic tympanoplasty with normal tubal function compared with the same tympanoplasty but with abnormal tubal function.

There is no limit to further clinical research, such as cartilage tympanoplasty in cholesteatoma surgery; in various ossicular defects in tympanoplasty type 2, type 3, or type 4; in canal wall up or canal wall dawn mastoidectomy and in other mastoidectomy methods.

Similar proposals for clinical research could be elaborated for Groups B to E. Such research can be undertaken after more reports on results of the new methods are published.

References

Amedee RG, Mann WJ, Riechelmann H. Cartilage palisade tympanoplasty. Am J Otol 1989;10:447–450.

Andersen J, Cayé-Thomasen P, Tos M. Cartilage palisade tympanoplasty in sinus and tensa retraction cholesteatoma. Otol Neurotol 2002;23:825–831.

Anderson J, Cayé-Thomasen P, Tos M. A comparison of cartilage palisades and fascia in tympanoplasty after surgery for sinus or tensa retraction cholesteatoma in children. Otol Neurotol 2004;25:856–863.

Bernal-Sprekelsen M, Lliso MDR, Gonzalo JJSG. Cartilage palisades in type 3 tympanoplasty: anatomic and functional long-term results. Otol Neurotol 2003;24:38–42.

Dornhoffer JL. Hearing results with cartilage tympanoplasty. Laryngoscope 1997;107:1094–1099.

Dornhoffer J. Cartilage tympanoplasty: indications, techniques, and outcomes in a 1000 patient series. Laryngoscope 2003;113: 1844–1856.

Dornhoffer JL. Cartilage tympanoplasty. Otolaryngol Clin North Am 2006;39:1161–1176.

Ferekidis EA, Nikolopoulos TP, Kandiloros DC, . Chondrotympanoplasty: a modified technique of cartilage graft tympanoplasty. Med Sci Monit 2003;9:73–78.

Kazikdas KC, Onal K, Boyraz I, Karabulut E. Palisade cartilage tympanoplasty for management of subtotal perforations: a comparison with the temporalis fascia technique. Eur Arch Otorhinolaryngol 2007;264:985–989.

Kirazli T, Bilgen C, Midilli R, Ogüt F. Hearing results after primary cartilage tympanoplasty with island technique. Otolaryngol Head Neck Surg 2005;132:933–937.

Neumann A, Hennig A, Schultz-Coulon H-J. Morphologische und funktionelle Ergebnisse der Knorpelpalisadentympanoplastik. HNO 2002;50:935–939.

Neumann A, Schultz-Coulon H-J, Jahnke K. Type 3 Tympanoplasty applying the palisade cartilage technique: A study of 61 cases. Otol Neurotol 2003;24:33–37.

Tos M. Tubal function and tympanoplasty. J Laryngol Otol 1974; 88:1113–24.

Tos M. Need for clinical research in cartilage tympanoplasty. Trakya Univ Tip Fak Derg 2007;24:179–189.

Tos M. Cartilage tympanoplasty methods. Proposal of a classification. Otolaryngol Head Neck Surg 2008;139(6):747–758.

Tos M, Uzun C, Cayé-Thomasen P, Andersen J. Tympanometry after tympanoplasty with cartilage palisades or fascia after surgery for tensa cholesteatoma in children. In: Lim DJ, Bluestone CD, Casselbrant M, eds. Recent Advances in Otitis Media. New York: Decker; 2005:321–322.

Uzun C, Cayé-Thomasen P, Andersen J, Tos M. A tympanometric comparison of tympanoplasty with cartilage palisades or fascia after surgery for tensa cholesteatoma in children. Laryngoscope 2003;113:1751–1757.

Uzun C, Cayé-Thomasen P, Andersen J, Tos M. Eustachian tube function in tympanoplasty with cartilage palisades or fascia after cholesteatoma surgery. Otol Neurotol 2004;25:864–872.

Index

Page numbers in *italics* refer to illustrations or tables

A

Adkins superior cartilage–perichondrium composite island graft 180, *181–182*
annular composite graft tympanoplasty 16, 17, *17*, 243–279, *243*
   Borkowski underlay annular graft technique 258–263, *264, 266–267*
   definition 243
   Goodhill's on-lay annular graft technique 247, *248–249*
   harvesting and shaping of graft *243*, 244–246, *245–246*
   indications 246–247
   Klacansky annular graft technique 258, *260–262*
   malleus absence and 265, *272–273*
   malleus handle abnormalities and 263–265
     missing malleus handle 263–265, *269–271*
     retracted malleus handle 263, *268–269*
   need for research 278–279
   previous applications 244
   results 277–278
   tympanic cavity reconstruction after mastoidectomy 272–277, *274–277*
   type 2 tympanoplasty 247–253, *249–256*
   type 3 tympanoplasty 253–258, *257, 259*
   U-shaped annular graft *243*, 246
     large inferior perforation 265, *274*
annulus, drilling a hole or groove in 341, *341*
anterior perforation *see* perforation
approaches *see* surgical approaches
atelectasis
   total pars tensa composite graft results 240
   tympanoplasty with U-graft 316–320
     grade 2 atelectasis 316–318, *316–317*
     grade 3 atelectasis 318–320, *318–321*
atresia
   congenital 285, *286*
     crown cork tympanoplasty 286–288, *287, 288, 289–290*
     type 2 a 286–288, *286, 287*
     type 2 b 288, *288, 289–290*
   postinflammatory acquired solid atresia 285
   postoperative 285
attic approaches 187
attic cartilage–perichondrium composite island graft *see* cartilage–perichondrium composite island grafts

attic cholesteatoma 179, 187
   pathogenesis 224
attic precholesteatoma 177–179, 224
attic retractions 177, *179*
   classification and grading 222–223
   epidemiology 223–224, *223*
   incidence 190
   preventive surgery 186–187
     indications 189
attic wall reconstruction 120, *123*
atticotomy
   closure with broad cartilage palisades 108, *110*
   transmeatal 187
auricle, harvesting cartilage from 42–44, *43*
   conchal cartilage 42–43, *43*
   cymba cartilage 43, *44*
   fossa triangularis cartilage 43–44, *44*
   scapha cartilage 44, *44*

B

Bernal-Sprekelson broad palisade techniques *see* broad cartilage palisades
biocompatible materials
   columella 258
   prostheses 253
Black superior cartilage–perichondrium composite island graft 180–182, *184*
blunting 285
   fibrous tissue removal and crown cork tympanoplasty 288, *291–292*
bony tissues 27
Borkowski underlay annular graft technique 258–263, *264, 266–267*
broad cartilage palisades 101–110, *102*
   Bernal-Sprekelson broad palisade techniques 102–106
     total perforation with intact ossicular chain 102, *104–104*
     total perforation with missing long process of the incus 102–104, *107*
     total perforation with missing ossicles 102, *106*
     total perforation with retracted and adherent malleus handle 104–106, *108*
   definition 101
   harvesting and shaping of palisades 101–102, *102*
   indications 102
   research needed 110

   results 108–110
     anatomical results 108
     complications 110
     functional results 108–110
butterfly cartilage graft *14*, 19–20, *20*
   epithelialization problems 382–383, *383*
   harvesting and shaping the graft 374, *375*
   see also in-lay butterfly cartilage tympanoplasty

C

canal wall *see* ear canal
cartilage
   harvesting 38–50
     from the auricle 42–44, *43–45*
     Groningen Cartilage Cutting Device 49–50, *50*
     Hüttenbrink Cartilage Guide 47–49, *49*
     in endaural approaches 44–45, *45–46*
     thinning the cartilage 45–47, *46–48*, 87
     tragal cartilage 38–42, *41–42*, 87
     see also cartilage grafts; *specific techniques*
   hidden 26
   homogenous 160
   nourishment of 401
   see also fate of implanted cartilage grafts
cartilage boards on-lay technique 161, *164*
cartilage foils and thin plates 13, *24*, 145, *146*
   fate of 405
   on-lay technique 14, *14*, 153–159
     anterior perforation 154, *155*
     definition 153
     harvesting and elaboration 153
     indications 153
     inferior perforation 154–155, *156*
     results 157
     total perforation 155–156, *157–159*
   underlay technique 13–14, *14*, 145–152
     definition 145
     harvesting and elaboration 146, *147*
     indications 147
     inferior perforation 147, *149*
     posterior perforation 147, *149*
     results 150–151
     total perforation 147–149, *150–150*
cartilage grafts 10–11, *23*
   see also cartilage palisades; cartilage strips; cartilage–perichondrium composite island grafts; *specific techniques*

cartilage mosaic tympanoplasty *see* Dornhoffer cartilage mosaic tympanoplasty
cartilage palisades 11–12, *23*, *45*, *113*
    fate of 405
    history 6–7, *8*
    see also broad cartilage palisades; cartilage grafts; on-lay palisade grafting; underlay palisade grafting
cartilage shield T-tube tympanoplasty 171, 294–327
    cartilage shield T-tube graft 16, 17–18, *18*, 175
    classification 175–176
    complications 320–322
        granulation tissue formation 321
        infection and otorrhea 322
        medialization of the cartilage graft 322
        removal of tube 320–321, *322*
        tube malfunction 321
    definition 294–295
    Dornhoffer technique 296, *297*, 314, *314–315*
    Duckert technique 295–296, *296*, *297*, 300–311, *300–313*
    Elsheikh U-shaped T-tube graft 296, *298*, 316–320, *317–321*
    Hall technique 295, *295*, 298–300, *299*
    harvesting and construction of grafts 295–296, *295–298*
    indications 297–298
    inferior cartilage shield graft proposal 324, *324*, *325*
    postoperative care 320
    results 322–323, *324*
    tubal function 324–327
        long-term research on 326–327
        need for testing 326
        tubal mucosa influence 326–327
cartilage strips 12–13, *12*, *24*, *113*
    fate of 405
    on-lay cartilage strip method 13, *13*, 125–135
        anterior perforation 126, *128–128*
        definition 125
        harvesting and shaping of strips 125–126, *126*
        indications 126
        inferior perforation 126, *130–130*
        need for research 135
        results 132
        total perforation 126–131, *132–135*
    underlay cartilage strip method 13, *13*, 112–123, *114*
        covering strips with perichondrium 120–121
        definition 112
        eardrum and attic wall reconstruction 120, *123*
        harvesting and shaping of strips 112–113, *115–115*
        indications 113
        inferior perforation 115, *118–118*
        posterior perforation 115, *117–117*
        results 121–123
        total perforation 116–119, *119–120*
        tunnelplasty 119, *122*
        versus fascia 409

    see also Dornhoffer cartilage mosaic tympanoplasty
    see also cartilage grafts
cartilage tympanoplasty
    classification 10, 20–22
    clinical research 408–411
        proposals for research methods 409–411
        research needed 84–85
    type 1 20, *21*, 59
        Dornhoffer cartilage mosaic method 137, *138*, 141, *142*
        in-lay on-lay composite island graft *366–367*
        modification without perichondrium flaps 336–339
        underlay cartilage strip technique 115, 116, *117*, *119*
    type 2 20–21, *21*, 59, 194
        annular graft in 247–253, *249–256*
        cartilage palisades and incus interposition 60–67, *66–72*
        cartilage shield T-tube tympanoplasty with PORP 308–311, *312*
        Dornhoffer cartilage mosaic method 138, *139*, 141, *143*
        malleus handle abnormalities and 263, 265, *269*, *270*
        on-lay cartilage strip technique 131, *136*
        on-lay composite island graft 359, *360*
        on-lay method with foils 155–156, *158*
        thick cartilage plates and 161, *163*
        underlay cartilage strip technique 116–119, *120*
        underlay method with foils and thin plates 147, *150*
        with intact stapes 1, *2–4*, *6*
    type 3 21–22, *21*, 59
        annular graft in 253–258, *257*, *259*, 276–277, *276–277*
        cartilage palisades and columella 67–70, *73–74*
        cartilage shield T-tube tympanoplasty 311, *313*
        Dornhoffer cartilage mosaic method 138, *140*, 141–142, *144*
        in-lay underlay composite island graft *349*
        missing malleus handle and 265, *271*
        on-lay cartilage strip technique 130, *135*
        on-lay composite island graft 360, *361*
        on-lay method with foils 156, *159*
        thick cartilage plates and 161, *163*
        underlay cartilage strip technique 115, *118*, 119, *121*
        underlay method with foils and thin plates 149, *151*
        with missing stapedial arch 1, *5*
    type 4 *21*, 22, 59, *250*
        without ossicles 22
    type 5A 22, 59
    type 5B 22
    see also cartilage grafts; cartilage palisades; Dornhoffer cartilage mosaic tympanoplasty; Ferekidis chondrotympanoplasty

cartilage–perichondrium composite island grafts 15–20, *25*, *329*
    annular graft *see* annular composite graft tympanoplasty
    butterfly technique *see* in-lay butterfly cartilage tympanoplasty
    cartilage shield T-tube graft *see* cartilage shield T-tube tympanoplasty
    crown cork graft *see* crown cork cartilage-perichondrium composite graft
    fate of 405
    in-lay on-lay technique *see* in-lay on-lay composite island graft
    in-lay underlay technique *see* in-lay underlay composite island graft
    missing malleus handle and 265
    on-lay technique *see* on-lay composite island graft
    posterior composite island graft 15, *16*, 192–211, *192*
        cartilage ossiculoplasty and myringoplasty by lever method 201–203
        cartilage titanium mesh graft 199–201
        definition 192
        harvesting and shaping the graft 193, *195*
        indications 193–194
        results 203–206
        sinus cholesteatoma removal 195–199, *196–205*
    superior and posterior composite island graft 16, 213–225, *213*, *214*
        definition 213
        harvesting and shaping of the graft 213, *214*
        indications 213–215
        Levinson technique 215–217, *216–219*
        Poe and Gadre technique 217–218, *220–221*
        results 218–222
        two separate grafts of Couloigner 218, 222
        vibratile and non-vibratile island grafts 222
    superior or attic composite island graft 15, *16*, 177–190, *178*
        closure of scutum defects 179–183, *179–186*
        definition 177
        difficulties in comparison of series 187–190
        indications 177–179
        results 183–186
        see also scutum surgical defects
    underlay technique *see* underlay composite island graft
    see also total pars tensa composite island graft; triple "C" technique
cholesteatoma 187–190
    attic cholesteatoma 179, 187
        pathogenesis 224
    broad cartilage palisade techniques 108
    CT-scanning 188
    entire tensa retraction cholesteatoma 188
    in postinflammatory acquired atresia 285
    incidence 189–190, 224–225
    removal techniques 187
    sinus cholesteatoma 188, 194

pathogenesis 210–211
removal 195–199, *200–205*
total pars tensa composite graft results 240
tubal function testing and 188
tympanic membrane reinforcement with plates after removal 174
underlay palisade tympanoplasty results in children 80–82, *81*, 84
cartilage palisades versus fascia 81–84, 409
chondrotympanoplasty *see* Ferekidis chondrotympanoplasty
chronic hyperplasia of the eustachian tube mucosa 327
circular annular graft 243, *244–246*
columella 21–22
autogenous incus columella 253, *257*
biocompatible materials 258
cartilage columellae 257–258
cartilage stapes columella 1, *5*
fate of cartilage columellae 402–403, 405
metal 258
titanium columella 161, *163*, 258, *259*
tympanoplasty type 3 67–70, 73–74, 79, 250
annular graft technique 253–258, *257, 259*
columella stabilization 161, *164, 165*
missing malleus handle and 265, *271*
on-lay cartilage strip technique 130, *135*
on-lay method with foils 156, *159*
thick cartilage plates and 161, *163, 164, 165*
underlay cartilage strip technique 115, *118, 119, 121*
underlay method with foils and thin plates 149, *151*
composite cartilage titanium mesh graft 199–201
composite chondroperichondrial clip tympanoplasty *see* triple "C" technique
composite island grafts *see* cartilage-perichondrium composite island grafts
conchal cartilage harvesting
endaural approach 45–46, *46*
for crown cork graft 280, *284*
retroauricular approach 42–43, *43*, 87
congenital malformations 285
crown cork cartilage-perichondrium composite graft 16, *17, 18*, 280–293, *281*
congenital type 2 a atresia 286–288, *287*
congenital type 2 b atresia 288, *288, 289–290*
definition 280
fibrous tissue removal in blunting 288, *291–292*
harvesting and construction of graft 280, *281–284*
conchal cartilage grafting 280, *284*
tragal cartilage harvesting 280, *281–283*
indications 285
results 288–293
curling of the cartilage grafts 88, 167–168
cymba cartilage harvesting 43, *44*

D

Dornhoffer cartilage mosaic tympanoplasty 13, 136–144, *137*
definition 136
harvesting and trimming the cartilage 136, *138*
indications 137
inferior perforation 139, *141*
posterior perforation 137–138, *138–139*
results 142
subtotal perforation 139, *141*
total perforation 141–142, *142–143*
Dornhoffer cartilage shield T-tube graft 296, *297*, 314, *314–315*
results 323
Dornhoffer cartilage-perichondrium composite island graft 226, *227*, 234, *238*
results 239–240
shaping of *227–228, 231*
Duckert compound cartilage-perichondrium graft with T-tube 294, *294*, 300–311, *300–313*
anterior perichondrium flap fixation *307, 308, 309*
anterior perichondrium flap placement 306, *308–309*
cartilage shield T-tube tympanoplasty type 2 with PORP 308–311, *312*
cartilage shield T-tube tympanoplasty type 3 with TORP 311, *313*
construction 295–296, *296, 297*
contouring of the anterior sulcus 300, *308*
notched cartilage disk 308, *310–311*
results 322–323
widening of the anterior annular sulcus 300–306, *308*
with anterior radial skin incisions 306, *306–307*
without anterior radial skin incisions 300, *305*

E

ear canal
incision 33, *33*
wall reconstruction 199–203
Eavey butterfly graft 14
see also butterfly cartilage graft
Elsheikh U-shaped T-tube graft 296, *298*, 316–320
grade 2 atelectasis 316–318, *316–317*
grade 3 atelectasis 318–320, *318–321*
results 323
endaural approach with intercartilaginous incision 33–35
cartilage harvesting 44–45, *45–46*
Farrior incision 34, *35*
Heerman intercartilaginous incisions 33, *33, 34*
Lempert incision 34, *34*
mastoidectomy and 34–35
Shambaugh incision 34, *34*
epithelia 26
epithelialization of graft
butterfly graft 382–383, *383*
on-lay composite island graft 362
eustachian tube mucosa, chronic hyperplasia 327

F

Farrior endaural approach 34, *35*
cartilage harvesting 45, *46*
Farrior retroauricular approach 35, *39*
fascia
cartilage palisades and 75–77, *82–83*, 409
cartilage plate covered with 170–171, *171, 172*
versus perichondrium graft 81–84, 241, 340, 409
fate of implanted cartilage grafts 401–406
after myringoplasty 403–404
cartilage columellae and struts 402–403
clinical consequences 405–406
living cartilage implanted into animals 401
living cartilage implanted into humans 401–402
nourishment of the cartilage 401
otological research 402
Ferekidis chondrotympanoplasty 71–75
chondrotympanoplasty type 1 71–74, *76–77*
ossiculoplasty and 74
chondrotympanoplasty type 2 74–75, *78*
chondrotympanoplasty type 3 75, *79*
intratympanal tubal chondroplasty 75, *79*
Fernandes graft 385
harvesting and preparation of 386–387, *386–388*
see also triple "C" technique
Fisch technique 35
Fleury superior composite cartilage island graft 179, *181*
foils *see* cartilage foils and thin plates

G

Gelfoam 85
Gerlach suspension of underlay cartilage island graft 335, *338*
Glasscock tragal cartilage prosthesis 1, *4, 5*
Glasscock posterior cartilage-perichondrium composite island graft 192, *194*
results 203–205
Goodhill annular graft technique 6, *8–9*, 247, *248–249*
Goodhill tragal cartilage strut as columella 1, *5*
granulation tissue formation, tube–perichondrium interface 321
grommet extrusion 382, *382*
Groningen Cartilage Cutting Device 49–50, *50*

H

Hall cartilage shield T-tube graft 294, *294*, 298–300, *299*
construction 295, *295*
results 322
Heerman approach
cartilage harvesting 44, *45*
Heerman A intercartilaginous incision 33, *33*
Heerman B intercartilaginous incision 33, *33, 34*
Heerman C intercartilaginous incision 33, *33*

Heerman cartilage tympanoplasty 22
  late results 84
Heermann stapes–annulus cartilage bridge 3–4, *6*
  broad stapes–annulus cartilage bridge 4–6, *7*
helix spine interposition 247–253, *255*
Hildmann cartilage clamp 47, *47*
homogenous cartilage 160
homogenous eardrum implantation 160
Honda scutumplasty 182, *185*
Hüttenbrink Cartilage Guide 47–49, *49*
hyperplasia, eustachian tube mucosa 327

I

in-lay butterfly cartilage tympanoplasty 14, 19–20, *20*, 374–384
  anterior perforation 376, *377–378*
  definition 374
  epithelialization problems 382–383, *383*
  epithelium elevation instead of removal 383, *383*
  future research needed 383–384
  graft placed onto the bony annulus 376–379, *381*
  harvesting and shaping the graft 374, *375*
  indications 374
  inferior perforation 376, *378–379*
  large perforations 376, *380*
    postoperative hearing 383
  results 379
in-lay on-lay composite island graft *18*, 19, *20*, 363–373, *363*
  anterior perforation 364, *364–365*
  applications 364
  definition 363
  harvesting and elaboration of graft 363–364, *363*
  inferior perforation 366, *369*
  pediatric interleave tympanoplasty 369–371, *372*
  posterior perforation 364–366, *366–368*
  results 371–372
  subtotal perforation 366, *370–371*
  total perforation 366–369, *370–373*
in-lay underlay composite island graft 18–19, *19*, *20*, 343–350, *343*
  anterior perforation 344, *345–346*
  definition 343
  harvesting and shaping the graft 343
  indications 344
  inferior perforation 344–347, *347–348*
  posterior perforation 349, *349*
  subtotal perforation 349–350, *350*
incisions, ear canal 33, *33*
  Farrior incision 34, *35*
  Heerman incisions 33, *33*, *34*
  Lempert incision 34, *34*
  medial circumferential 36–37
  retroauricular flap incisions 35, *36*
  retroauricular fold incision 35, *36*
  Shambaugh incision 34, *34*
  see also surgical approaches
incus interposition 102–104, *107*, *108*
  annular graft technique 247, *249–250*
    missing malleus handle and 265, *270*

cartilage palisade technique and 60–67, *66–72*
on-lay cartilage strip technique and 131, *136*
on-lay tympanoplasty with foils 155–156, *158*
underlay cartilage strip technique and 116–119, *120*
underlay tympanoplasty with foils and thin plates 147, *150*
infection, T-tube and 322
inferior perforation *see* perforation
interposition
  helix spine 247–253, *255*
  incus *see* incus interposition
  prostheses made of biocompatible materials 253
  prostheses made of metals 253
  with cartilage 247, *254*
intratympanal tubal chondroplasty 75, *79*

J

Jahnke total tensa cartilage–perichondrium composite graft 226, *227*
Jansen cartilage plate on-lay tympanoplasty 160–161, *162*
Jansen septal cartilage prosthesis 1, *3*, *5*

K

Klacansky annular graft technique 157, *260–262*
Klacansky chondrotome 244, *245–246*
Klacansky small total pars tens composite island graft 228–230
Kurz PORP prosthesis 66, *71*
Kurz Precise Cartilage Knife 47, *48*

L

lateral attic reconstruction (LAR) technique 186–187
Lempert approach 34, *34*
  cartilage harvesting 44
lever method 201–203
  results 206
Levinson cartilage–perichondrium composite graft 213, *213*, 215–217, *216–219*, 222
  results 218–219, *219*
Linde posterior cartilage–perichondrium composite island graft 192, *192*, *193*
  results 203

M

McCleve attic island graft 179, *179–180*
malleus handle abnormalities
  floppy malleus handle with remnant stapes 272–276, *275*
  missing malleus handle 263–265, *269–271*
    incidence 263–265
  retracted and adherent malleus handle 104, 263
    annular graft 263, *268–269*
    Bernal-Sprekelson broad palisade technique 104–106, *108*

malleus, missing 265, *272–273*
mastoidectomy
  annular graft in tympanic cavity reconstruction 244–277, *272–277*
  endaural approach and 34–35
  intact canal wall up 187
  modified combined approach 187
  retrograde mastoidectomy on demand 187
  transmeatal retrograde canal down 187
'Mercedes-Benz' graft 230, *232*
metal columella 258
metal prostheses 253
  titanium PORP prostheses 66, *71*, 253, *256*
minimally invasive surgery 372
mosaic tympanoplasty *see* Dornhoffer cartilage mosaic tympanoplasty; Portmann mosaic underlay cartilage tympanoplasty
myringocruropexy 207, *209–210*
myringoincudopexy 207, *207*
myringoplasty 58, *274*
  fate of cartilage grafts 403–404
  history 2, *6*
  in-lay butterfly cartilage technique 377
  lever method 201–203
myringoplatinopexy 207, *211*
myringostapediopexy 207, *208–209*

N

Nitsche total pars tensa cartilage–perichondrium composite graft 226, *228*, 230, *232–234*
notched cartilage disk 308, *310–311*

O

on-lay cartilage strip method *see* cartilage strips
on-lay composite island graft 19, *20*, 351–362, *351*, *352*
  anterior perforation 353–355
    cartilage–perichondrium on-lay method 353, *354*
    perichondrium–cartilage on-lay method 353–355, *355*
  definition 351–352
  epithelialization of the cartilage graft 362
  harvesting and elaboration of graft 352, *353*
  indications 352–353
  inferior perforation 355–356, *356–357*
  results 360
  total/subtotal perforations 356–360, *358–361*
on-lay palisade grafting 12, *12*, 87–100
  curling of the cartilage grafts 88
  definitions 87
  full-thickness palisades 87, *88*
  half-thickness palisades 87, *88*
  harvesting of the palisades 87–87
  incus interposition and 247, *251*
  indications 88
  perichondrium flaps 87, *88*
  research needed 100
  results 99
  shaping of the palisades 87–88, *88*, *89*
  surgical techniques 88–99

anterior perforation 89, *91–94*
inferior perforation 89–94, *96–97*
total perforation 94–99, *99–100*
see also cartilage palisades
ossiculoplasty
history 1–6, *2–7*
lever method 201–203
underlay cartilage palisade technique and 58–70
chondrotympanoplasty 74
columella in tympanoplasty type 3 67–70, *73–74*
incus interposition in tympanoplasty type 2 60–67, *66–72*
preservation of intact ossicular chain 59–60
see also interposition
otorrhea, T-tube and 322

P

'Pac Man' graft 222
partial ossicular replacement prostheses (PORPs) 1
titanium 66, 71, 253, *256*
pediatric interleave tympanoplasty 369–371
results 372
perforation
anterior 89
in-lay butterfly cartilage technique 376, *377–378*
in-lay on-lay composite island graft 364, *364–365*
in-lay underlay composite island graft 344, *345–346*
on-lay cartilage strip technique 126, *128–128*
on-lay composite island graft 353–355, *354–355*
on-lay palisade grafting 89
on-lay tympanoplasty with foils and thin plates 154, *155*
swing-door technique 126, *129*
technique with elevation of a large anterior skin flap 89, *93*
technique with partial removal of epithelium 89, *92*
technique with small epithelial flaps 89, *91*, 126, *128*
triple "C" technique 387–388, *389–392*
underlay composite island graft 329–335, *330–334*, *336–337*
with bulged ear canal 89, *94–94*
inferior 53–55, 89–94
Dornhoffer cartilage mosaic tympanoplasty 139, *141*
elevation of superior epithelial flaps 126, *130*
in-lay butterfly cartilage technique 376, *378–379*
in-lay on-lay composite island graft 366, *369*
in-lay underlay composite island graft 344–347, *347–348*
large tympanomeatal flap technique 54–55, *60–61*, 92, 97, 115, *119*, 126, *131*, 335, *338*
on-lay cartilage strip technique 126, *130–130*
on-lay composite island graft 355–356, *356–357*
on-lay palisade grafting 89–94
on-lay tympanoplasty with foils and thin plates 154–155, *156*
outward elevation of epithelium and skin 92–94, *98*
palisades with perichondrium flaps on both ends 94, *98*
partial elevation of superior epithelial flaps 91–92, *96*
swing-door technique 54, *58–59*, 335, *338*, 347, *348*
technique without tympanomeatal flap 53–54, *57*, 115, *118*
triple "C" technique 389–394, *393–398*
U-shaped annular graft 265, *274*
underlay cartilage strip technique 115, *118–118*
underlay composite island graft 335, *337–339*
underlay palisade grafting 53–55
underlay tympanoplasty with foils and thin plates 147, *149*
posterior 53, 194
Dornhoffer cartilage mosaic tympanoplasty 137–138, *138–139*
in-lay on-lay composite island graft 364–366, *366–368*
in-lay underlay composite island graft 349, *349*
large tympanomeatal flap technique 53, *56*
swing-door technique 53, *54–55*
triple "C" technique 394, *399*
underlay cartilage strip technique 115, *117–117*
underlay tympanoplasty with foils and thin plates 147, *149*
subtotal
Dornhoffer cartilage mosaic tympanoplasty 139, *141*
in-lay on-lay composite island graft 366, *370–371*
in-lay underlay composite island graft 349–350, *350*
on-lay composite island graft 356–360, *358–360*
underlay cartilage island graft 335–336*340*
total 55–58, 94–99, 102–106
annular graft 272–276, *275*, 276–277, *276–277*
broad palisade techniques 102–106, *104–107*
Dornhoffer cartilage mosaic tympanoplasty 141–142, *142–143*
elevation of three superior epithelial flaps 94, *99*, 128, *133*
in-lay on-lay composite island graft 366–369, *370–373*
large tympanomeatal flap technique 57–58, *64–65*, 96, *100*, 116, *119*, 130, *134*
on-lay cartilage strip technique 126–131, *132–135*
on-lay composite island graft 356–360, *358–360*
on-lay palisade grafting 94–99
on-lay tympanoplasty with foils and thin plants 155–156, *157–159*
outward elevation of eardrum epithelium and skin flaps 127–128, *132*
palisades with perichondrium flaps 96–99, *101*
swing-door technique 57, *62–63*
underlay cartilage strip technique 116–119, *119–120*
underlay palisade grafting 55–58
underlay tympanoplasty with foils and thin plates 147–149, *150–150*
with granulations 285
total pars tensa composite graft results 240
perichondrium flaps
anterior flap fixation *307*, 308, *309*, 330, *332*
anterior flap placement 306, *308–309*
anterior perforation 330, *332*
inferior perforation 94, *98*
on-lay palisade grafting 87, *88*
posterior flap, attached to malleus handle 332, *333–334*
total perforation 96–99, *101*
trimming 88, *89*
plates see cartilage foils and thin plates; thick cartilage plates
Plester technique 35, *37*
Poe and Gadre double-island composite graft 213, *214–215*, 217–218, *220–221*
results 219, *219*
Portmann mosaic underlay cartilage tympanoplasty 150, *152*
Portmann's posterosuperior incision 146, *147*, 150, *152*
posterior composite island graft see cartilage–perichondrium composite island grafts
posterior perforation see perforation
posterior retraction 194
classification and management 206–210, *207–211*
posterosuperior retraction *316–317*
transmeatal removal 195, *198–199*
when to operate 211
postinflammatory acquired solid atresia 285
precholesteatoma
attic 177–179, 224
sinus 194

Q

Quinn scutumplasty 183, *186*

R

reinforcement 192
tympanic membrane, after cholesteatoma removal 174
retractions see attic retractions; posterior retraction
retroauricular approach 35–38, *36*
Farrior technique 35, *39*
Fisch technique 35

retroauricular approach
 medial circumferential incision 36–37
 medial tympanomeatal flap management 37–38, *37–39*, *40*
 Plester technique 35, *37*
 posterosuperior retraction *316–317*
 removal of ear canal skin 36
  in cartilage tympanoplasty 36, *38*, *39*
 swing-door technique 35, *38*
 Wullstein–Kley technique 37, *40*
retrograde atticoantrotomy 197–199, *204–205*
rib cartilage plates 173, *174*
Richards speculum holder 30–31, *31*, *32*

S

Salen cartilage tympanoplasty 2, *6*
scapha cartilage harvesting 44, *44*, 87
scutum surgical defects 179, 192
 closure methods 179–183, 192, *193*
  Adkins technique 180, *181–183*
  Black technique 180–182, *184*
  Fleury technique 179, *181*
  Honda scutumplasty 182, *185*
  McCleve technique 179, *179–180*
  proposals 187, *189*
  Quinn technique 183, *186*
Shambaugh approach 34, *34*
 cartilage harvesting 44, *46*
simmering 7, *8*, 52
 placement 85
sinus cholesteatoma 188, 194
 pathogenesis 210–211
 removal 196–197, *202–203*
  retrograde atticoantrotomy 197–199, *204–205*
  transmeatal removal 195–196, *200–201*
sinus precholesteatoma 194
soft tissues 26–27
strips *see* cartilage strips
subtotal perforation *see* perforation
superior cartilage–perichondrium composite island graft *see* cartilage–perichondrium composite island grafts
surgical approaches 30–38
 endaural, with intercartilaginous incision 33–35, *33–35*
 retroauricular 35–38, *36–40*
 transmeatal, through fixed ear speculum 30–33, *30–33*
swing-door technique 35, *38*
 anterior perforation 126, *129*
 inferior perforation 54, *58–59*, 335, *338*, 347, *347–348*
 posterior perforation 53, *54–55*
 total perforation 57, *62–63*

T

T-tube *see* cartilage shield T-tube tympanoplasty
Texido Cartilage Cutter 47
thick cartilage plates 13, *24*, 145
 fate of 405
 on-lay technique 14, *14*, 160–168
  cartilage boards on-lay technique 161, *164*
 clinical research on thickness 167–168
 columella stabilization 161, *164*, *165*
 definitions 160
 full-thickness cartilage plate 161, *165*
 harvesting and elaboration of plates 160
 Jansen cartilage plate on-lay tympanoplasty 160–161, *162*
 optimal thickness 168
 problems with curling 167–168
 results 163–165
 thickness effect on hearing 165
 titanium columella and 161, *163*
 tympanoplasty type 2/3 and 161, *163*
 underlay technique 15, *15*, 170–176
  cartilage plate covered with fascia 170–171, *171*, *172*
  cartilage shield tympanoplasty of Moore 171
  definitions 170
  harvesting and elaboration of plates 170
  results 174–175
  tympanic membrane reinforcement after cholesteatoma removal 174
  tympanoplasty with cartilage plates only 171, *173*
  tympanoplasty with crushed autogenous cartilage plate 171–173, *174*
  tympanoplasty with irradiated homogenous rib cartilage plates 173, *174*
thin plates *see* cartilage foils and thin plates
titanium columella 161, *163*, 258, *259*
titanium mesh 199–201
titanium PORP prostheses 66, *71*, 253, *256*
Tolsdorff total pars tensa cartilage–perichondrium composite island graft 226, *228*, 231, *234–235*
 shaping of 226–227, *228*, *230*
total pars tensa composite island graft 16, *16*, *17*, 226–241, *227*
 definitions 226
 Dornhoffer technique 234, *238*
 indications 230
 Nitsch graft 226, *228*, 230, *232–234*
 results 235–241
  outcome by surgical indication 240
  pediatric series 240–241
  series with posterior and total pars tensa grafts 241
  versus fascia graft 241, 409
 shaping of the graft 226–230, *232–238*
 Tolsdorff graft 226, *228*, *230*, 231, *234–235*
 Würzburg clinic techniques 233–234, *236–237*
total perforation *see* perforation
tragal cartilage harvesting 38–42, *41–42*, 87
 for crown cork graft 280, *281–283*
 through an intercartilaginous incision 41–42, *41*, *42*
 tragus dome cartilage and perichondrium 39–41, *41*
transmeatal approach through fixed ear speculum 30–33
 as minimally invasive surgery 31–33
 Richards speculum holder 30–31, *31*, *32*
 tilting of the ear speculum 31, *31*, *32*
 Treace speculum holder 31
triple "C" technique *15*, 20, *20*, 385–400, *385*
 anterior perforation 387–388, *389–392*
 definition 385
 harvesting and preparation of the graft 386–387, *386–388*
 indications 385
 inferior perforation 389–394, *393–398*
 posterior perforation 394, *399*
 results 394–400
tunnelplasty 6, *8*, 119, *122*
tympanic membrane reconstruction evaluation 166–170
 methods 166, *166*
 sound pressure response 166–167
  cartilage composite island grafts 167, *167*
  cartilage palisades *166*, 167
  cartilage plates 166–167, *166*
  perichondrium 166, *166*
 see also cartilage tympanoplasty
tympanomeatal flap
 anterior perforation 330, *332–333*, 344, *346*
 inferior perforation 54–55, *60–61*, 92, 97, 115, *119*, 126, *131*, 335, *338*
 medial flap management 37–38, *37–39*, *40*
 posterior perforation 53, *56*
 total perforation 57–58, *64–65*, 96, *100*, 116, *119*, 130, *134*, 359–360, *360–361*
tympanoplasty *see* cartilage tympanoplasty

U

U-graft *see* Elsheikh U-shaped T-tube graft; U-shaped annular graft
U-shaped annular graft 243, 246
 large inferior perforation 265, *274*
underlay cartilage strip method *see* cartilage strips
underlay composite island graft 18, *19*, *20*, 329–342
 anterior perforation 329–335, *330–334*, *336–337*
 definition 329
 harvesting and shaping of the graft 329, *330*
 indication 329
 inferior perforation 335, *337–339*
 modifications of techniques 342
 recommendations 341–342
 results 339–340
 versus fascia 340
 subtotal perforation 335–336, *340*
 see also cartilage–perichondrium composite island grafts
underlay palisade grafting 11–12, *11*, 52–85
 definition 52
 harvesting and shaping of palisades 52–53
 indications for surgery 52
 inferior perforation 53–55, *57–61*
 modifications 71–77
  cartilage palisades and fascia 75–77, *82–83*, 409
  covering palisades with perichondrium 75, *76–79*, *80–81*

Ferekidis chondrotympanoplasty 71–75, 76–79
ossiculoplasty and 58–70
  columella in tympanoplasty type 3 67–70, 73–74
  incus interposition in tympanoplasty type 2 60–67, 66–72
  preservation of intact ossicular chain 59–60
placement of the palisades 85
posterior perforation 53, 54–56
research needed 84–85
results 77–84
  cartilage palisades versus fascia 81–84
  cholesteatoma in children 80–82, 81, 84
  late results 84
  total perforation 55–58, 62–65
  see also cartilage grafts; cartilage palisades
Utech cartilage prostheses 1, 2–3, 5

V

ventilation tubes *see* cartilage shield T-tube tympanoplasty

W

Waltner method of cartilage thinning 46, 46
Waltner type 2 ossiculoplasty 1, 4
'wheel' graft 230, 232
Wiegand palisade technique covered with fascia 75–77, 82–83
Wullstein-Kley technique 37, 40
Würzburg clinic techniques 233–234, 236–237
  results 239